SHELF-LIFE
DATING OF FOODS

F
N
P

JOURNALS AND BOOKS IN FOOD SCIENCE AND NUTRITION

Journals

JOURNAL OF FOOD SERVICE SYSTEMS, G.E. Livingston and C.M. Chang

JOURNAL OF FOOD BIOCHEMISTRY, H.O. Hultin, N.F. Haard and J.R. Whitaker

JOURNAL OF FOOD PROCESS ENGINEERING, D.R. Heldman

JOURNAL OF FOOD PROCESSING AND PRESERVATION, T.P. Labuza

JOURNAL OF FOOD QUALITY, M.P. DeFigueiredo

JOURNAL OF FOOD SAFETY, M. Solberg and J.D. Rosen

JOURNAL OF TEXTURE STUDIES, P. Sherman and M.C. Bourne

Books

RECENT ADVANCES IN OBESITY RESEARCH, VOL. III, P. Bjorntorp, M. Ciavella and A.N. Howard

RECENT ADVANCES IN OBESITY RESEARCH, VOL. II, G.A. Bray

RECENT ADVANCES IN OBESITY RESEARCH, VOL. I, A.N. Howard

ANTINUTRIENTS AND NATURAL TOXICANTS IN FOOD, R.L. Ory

UTILIZATION OF PROTEIN RESOURCES, D.W. Stanley, E.D. Murray and D.H. Lees

FOOD INDUSTRY ENERGY ALTERNATIVES, R.P. Ouellette, N.W. Lord and P.E. Cheremisinoff

VITAMIN B_6: METABOLISM AND ROLE IN GROWTH, G.P. Tryfiates

HUMAN NUTRITION: 3RD ED., R.F. Mottram

DIETARY FIBER: CURRENT DEVELOPMENTS OF IMPORTANCE TO HEALTH, K.W. Heaton

FOOD POISONING AND FOOD HYGIENE, 4TH ED., B.C. Hobbs and R.J. Gilbert

FOOD SCIENCE AND TECHNOLOGY, 3RD ED., M. Pyke

POSTHARVEST BIOLOGY AND BIOTECHNOLOGY, H.O. Hultin and M. Milner

THE SCIENCE OF MEAT AND MEAT PRODUCTS, 2ND ED., J.F. Price and B.S. Schweigert

SHELF-LIFE DATING OF FOODS

by

Theodore P. Labuza, Ph.D.
DEPARTMENT OF FOOD SCIENCE AND NUTRITION
UNIVERSITY OF MINNESOTA
ST. PAUL, MINNESOTA 55108

FOOD & NUTRITION PRESS, INC.
WESTPORT, CONNECTICUT 06880 USA

FOOD & NUTRITION PRESS, INC.
Westport, Connecticut 06880 USA

Library of Congress Catalog Card Number: 81-71 470
ISBN: 0-917-678-14-1

Printed in the United States of America

PREFACE

The objective of this book was to review the basic technology and scientific capability that would be applicable for setting open dating regulations for processed foods.

In the first chapter, a review of conferences and opinions on open dating prior to the OTA meetings is categorized and summarized. Basically, consumer groups are strongly in favor of some type of disclosure of a quality-related date on foods. Manufacturers presently use a process/pack date in code which could be converted to a readable date, but most groups served, including regulatory agencies, felt that this system serves no useful purpose except to help promote stock rotation. Industry was most concerned with the excess losses that could occur with the requirement of a "sell by" or "use by" date, when the food might still be edible. The government was concerned with how to determine whether a food went out of compliance before the listed expiration date. Consumers felt that "sell by", "best if used by" and "use by" dates were beneficial, but a major concern was whether the distribution system was adequate to prevent loss of shelf-life prior to the date listed.

In Chapter 2, the major food processing principles are catalogued and the modes of deterioration are listed. These include biological and microbial decay, senescence, and chemical and physical decay. The relationship of these reactions to loss of shelf-life and how they are affected by the environment are examined for each major food process.

Chapter 3 examines the scientific principles involved in predicting shelf-life of foods as a function of the environment and the package system. It is stressed that the reaction order must be known in order to predict shelf-life. The effect of temperature in terms of the rate of loss of shelf-life as defined by Q_{10} is detailed to explain why different foods deteriorate at different rates. The TTT method used to predict shelf-life of frozen foods is given as an example and some commercial shelf-life indicator devices are examined. Equations for shelf-life loss for both zero and first order reactions are derived. In addition, equations for loss of shelf-life as a function of moisture gain/loss are explained with some examples given. Lastly, the effect of oxygen on rate of loss of shelf-life is illustrated.

The subsequent chapters discuss 18 food categories, outlining the typical process/packaging/distribution system for each. Data on shelf-life, mainly as available in the scientific literature since 1960, are presented. Where applicable, the data are analyzed on the basis of the scientific methods explained in Chapter 3. For each food, an analysis of the pros and cons of open dating in relation to pack date, sell date or use by date is made with recommendations based on the scientific shelf-life data. In many cases, a "sell by date" or a "best if used by" date with home storage information seems to be the preferred open date system.

The last chapter contains the results of a survey of about 50 companies giving their current food research and marketing practices with respect to shelf-life and open dating. Little use is currently made of the basic scientific principles involved in shelf-life testing. In many cases the companies felt that most of the food was sold before a reasonable end of shelf-life. The biggest problem was control of the distribution conditions. The chapter ends with general recommendations on open dating from a regulatory standpoint and points out the real problems in monitoring and establishing compliance.

The major recommendation of this study is that open dating be kept voluntary, but that if used, a "sell by" or "best if used by" date with some storage information be required on the package.

THEODORE P. LABUZA

OTHER CONTRIBUTORS TO THIS PROJECT

Scientific Investigators

Katherine Benkler
Dave Bresnahan
Curt Busk
Scott Donnelly
Seth Goldsmith
Jaya Joglekar
Joyce Johnson
Jimbay Loh
Linda N. Kreisman
Robert McIver
Palma Peterson
Wayne Peterson
Craig Rethwill
Miriam Shapero
Mary Tufte
Julianne Wood

Staff Contributors

Alla Petrenko
Jan Swanson
Diane Ford

CONTENTS

CHAPTER 1

INTRODUCTION TO OPEN DATING

GENERAL TYPES OF OPEN DATING SYSTEMS

Over the last 15 years, and especially since the advent of the consumer movement, many different types of open dating systems have been proposed as part of the consumer's "right to know". An open date on a food product is a legible, easily read date which is displayed on the package. Its purpose is to inform the consumer about the shelf-life of the product. The date used can be the manufacturing date ("pack date"); the date the product was placed on the food store shelf ("display date"); the last date on which the product should be sold in order to allow the consumer a reasonable length of time in which to use it ("pull date" or "sell by date"); the last date of maximum high quality ("best if used by date"); or the date after which the food is no longer at an acceptable level of quality (the "use by date" or "expiration date").

Today there is still no uniform or universally accepted open dating system used for food in the United States. There are parts of the country where much of the food supply has some type of open date on it and parts where almost none of the food has any type of open date. Where it is used the dates are found primarily on perishable or semi-perishable items such as dairy products and meats. The open dating systems used now are voluntary in some areas, or mandatory by state, county or municipal statutes or administrative regulations. Some manufacturers voluntarily open date their products and some food stores voluntarily put open dates of display on perishable items. Where voluntary open dating is used by manufacturers and/or retailers, some local governments ignore it, while others enforce the dates.

As can be inferred from the variety of approaches to open dating, a great diversity of opinion exists regarding the benefits and problems involved in the open dating concept.

This chapter will summarize some of the positions taken on the open dating issue by consumers, manufacturers, retailers and government agencies in the United States. It should be noted that presently many manufacturers voluntarily put a closed "code" on their products which indicates to some degree the day it was processed and placed into the final consumer container.

CONSUMERS' POSITION ON OPEN DATING

Consumer groups are the major force behind the push for open dating of foods. Today's consumers, buying in huge impersonal supermarkets, feel they have little control over their food supply. They exhibit a need to know as much as possible about the food they purchase, as a means of combating a feeling of vulnerability. The majority of the consuming public are not willing to expend much energy in educating themselves about modern food processing, but when asked for a preference will overwhelmingly vote in favor of more information being presented to them. They may then not actually take advantage of this information themselves, but will feel better knowing that the information is available to others who will act as the enforcers of the information.

The New York State Consumer Protection Board has recently (1977) published a book translating food manufacturers' codes. Marilyn Maxwell of their staff said that they expected about 10,000 requests for the book. So far they have received over 100,000 requests and more are coming in every day. She feels there should be a law mandating open dating on nonperishable food items as well as on perishable ones. Testimony given by the Minnesota Office of Consumer Services at the Minnesota State Senate hearings on open dating legislation in February/March 1973, shows some further insight into this "need to know."

Keith Ford of the Minnesota Office of Consumer Services feels that overage food is being sold. In a study that his group did of baby formula sold in 1972, 44% being sold was overage and 64% of the store managers were unable to read the date code so they could not rotate the stock. He felt that overage food is not usually unsafe, but that it has little or no nutritive quality, or is unpalatable or nonfunctional. He felt that he did not know how much loss occurs, but surveys have shown lack of freshness to be a substantial problem.

The Minnesota Public Interest Research Group (MPIRG) also reported at these hearings. In a survey of 25 Minnesota stores, they found that 100% had some outdated food products; 100% had outdated cake mix; 50%, cold cereal; 100%, toastettes; and 16%, whipping cream. Date codes were broken using the Consumer's Union Codebook and shelf-lives were taken from the 1973 USDA Food Stability Survey. Their conclusion was that, if the products had open dating on them, then the consumer could determine how old the product was on the shelf and then could decide how long it could be held at home before using it.

It should be noted that MPIRG's use of shelf-lives in the survey is questionable. For example, the Food Stability Survey lists the shelf-life of cake mix as 6 to 18 months and MPIRG used 7 months. Very few of the cake mixes found were older than 18 months.

This use of the shorter shelf-life is understandable in light of the consumer's distrust of shelf-life dates set by manufacturers. This distrust is spelled out in detail in the January/February 1976 publication of the Arizona Consumers' Council, *Freshness dating of perishable food: The consumer issues.*

Not too many years ago a consumer could go to a local bakery to purchase a loaf of fresh baked bread. The baker was probably up early the same day to bake the bread. The same was true with milk. Milk was processed daily by a local dairy and delivered fresh to the consumer. The situation was similar with fresh meat. The butcher at a local market cut the meat to order. Eggs, butter, and other perishable food products were processed and sold locally — fresh daily.

A reputable bakery or dairy would not try to sell day-old products for fresh product prices. But that practice for chain supermarkets has become a way of life. Bread is baked and milk is processed, not locally, but at central locations, and in huge volume, then transported for distribution over a large geographic area to many stores, by a network delivery system. But not fresh daily.

As this chain market distribution system developed, for perishable as well as other products, processors adopted the practice of "code dating" products. Information about the date a product was processed was indicated on the package in a code consumers could not comprehend. Presumably distributors and retailers could.

With code dating food industry representatives talked about the "shelf-life" of bread, milk, and other perishable food products, not about the "freshness". And food processors added chemicals to perishable food products to extend the shelf life. The shelf-life of a product is the length of time it can remain on a store shelf without adverse consumer reaction. This is estimated by the processor. The last day a product should, in the judgment of the processor, be offered for sale is the "pull date". Perishable food products should be pulled from a store shelf on that date. The product is no longer "fresh".

The consumer concern about perishable foods is the freshness of the product offered for sale. In response to demands from consumer organizations some years ago for freshness dating of perishable foods, the industry "voluntarily" went to a system of "open" pull dates. Rather than in codes consumers could not understand, perishable food products were dated openly in a way consumers could understand.

A pull date is put on a perishable food product by the processor, not the retailer. An exception is fresh meat packaged at the store; then the retailer dates the package, if it is dated. However, retailers, not processors, are responsible for monitoring pull dates on packages and removing them from sales when the pull date is reached. Processors, who are frequently distributors as well, assume no responsibility for perishable foods after the pull date expires. No provision is made by processors for return or disposal of outdated food. The retailer is expected to pull the outdated packages, take them off sale, and absorb the loss.

The consumer issue with pull dates is whether or not consumers should pay fresh product prices for perishable foods which are no longer fresh. The pull date system has not worked for the benefit of consumers. But it has been a bonanza for the chain supermarket industry. The pull date system is a deceptive industry practice which allows supermarkets to sell stale products at fresh product prices.

Consumer organizations are renewing their demand that perishable food products be openly dated on the package, and that the date be the first day the product is offered for sale — a freshness date. Consumers have a right to that information. It is not enough for the producer, and perhaps the retailer, to know how long a perishable food product has been on the shelf. The consumer must have that information inorder to make an intelligent marketplace choice to buy or not to buy a product at a price asked by the seller. In the case of perishable products, "freshness" is essential information for a consumer.

The pull date system violates the principle that a consumer has a right to information about a product offered for sale. Producers and processors put pull dates on packages at their discretion. There are no standards. For a half-gallon of milk the pull date can be 5 days or 15 days after the product was first offered for sale; that is entirely up to the processor. In view of the host of marketplace abuses inflicted by the food industry on consumers, there is no reason to believe that producers date perishable products for the benefits of consumers.

The quality of perishable foods offered depends on handling and storing conditions during the distribution process and in the market. Producers of perishable foods may or may not have control over standards for handling and storing products during the distribution process. They have no control over the produce once it enters the retail store. Milk, for example, deteriorates in quality rapidly when not kept properly refrigerated; so do eggs, meat, and delicatessen items. A pull date does not provide information a consumer needs. Pull dates assume standards for handling and storing which may not be observed in fact. Unless the consumer knows the freshness date he has no way of knowing about the quality of the product.

As the term implies, perishable foods in time perish. Even under the best handling and storing conditions, perishable food products lose nutritional value as well as esthetic appeal as time passes. An egg is not the same product twelve months later as it was the day it was laid. Freshness dating is essential for a consumer to make an informed decision in purchasing a perishable food.

Industry interest in removing perishable food products from sale when pull dates are reached is seriously questioned by consumers. The pull date system is enforced, not by producers who date the packages, but by retailers. Retailers have no incentive to pull packages from shelves when the pull date is reached. Perishable food packages remain on store shelves for weeks, even months, after pull dates. They are offered for sale until sold, regardless of pull dates.

It is difficult to obtain from industry spokesmen information about procedures for removing perishable products from sale when the pull date is reached. It is even more difficult to get information about procedures used to dispose of such products removed from shelves because they were unsold when the pull date was reached. It is more profitable to sell stale products at fresh product prices than it is to dispose of garbage.

The decision to purchase perishable food which is fresh or stale is a decision which consumers should make, not producers or retailers. The pull date system does not allow consumers to make that decision. The only way consumers can make that decision is by freshness dating — by openly dating the package the date the product is first offered for sale.

A 1973 survey by the A.C. Nielsen Company pointed out that almost half of the people surveyed had complaints about product freshness.

A.C. Nielsen Company 1973 Study of Consumer Attitudes Toward Product Quality

Types of Product Complaints (each as a percent of total respondents)	
broken or crumbled product	51%
product freshness	47%
contamination	28%
excessive or insufficient carbonation	23%
bulged can	16%
other	9%

A 1973 survey by the ERS and CRI for the USDA also indicated that people felt there was a problem with the freshness of foods (USDA 1973), despite the fact that 93% of them said they had rarely or never brought stale or spoiled food during the past year.

This report also reported shoppers' attitudes and experiences obtained through a telephone survey in June 1971:

Food Dating: Shoppers' Reactions and the Impact on Retail Food Stores (Summer and Fall 1971)

(1) During the last two weeks have you purchased food which spoiled or staled sooner than expected?
18% said yes.

(2) What food categories?

fresh dairy	5.6%	processed meat	2.1%
vegetables	5.1%	baked	2.1%
meat/poultry/fish	4.2%	all other	1.8%
fruit	3.5%		

(3) One-half noticed spoilage on day of sale. More threw it out than returned it; many used it.

(4) 62% knew of store money-back guarantees.

(5) 43% knew of manufacturers' money-back guarantees.

This survey also found that young, affluent, educated suburban shoppers found more stale and spoiled foods and felt it to be more of a problem than did older, poorer, undereducated inner-city or rural shoppers. This is interesting since the first kind of shopper is considered to shop in more efficient, better run stores.

In 1977 the Consumer's Council of Massachusetts (Leverett Saltonstall Building, Government Center, 100 Cambridge Street, Boston, MA 02202) studied the open dating question. The following is a summary of their report to the Department of Health.

Summary of Report on Open Dating for Non-perishable Food Items

A careful analysis of all the materials submitted to the Department of Public Health on the subject of open dating yields the following conclusions:

(1) There is a compelling need for regulations requiring shelf life and storage information on "non-perishable" foods because:
  - (a) both the food itself and its container (can or carton) have limited shelf lives;
  - (b) there is a strong possibility that non-perishables will be stored for periods of time greater than their shelf lives;
  - (c) resulting deterioration causes loss of nutritional value (generally undetectable by consumers), spoilage, change in appearance, and loss of functional properties.

(2) There is broad public support for the concept of open dating for all foods, perishable and nonperishable;

(3) The concept of open dating nonperishables is feasible because:
  - (a) food manufacturers routinely calculate meaningful and accurate shelf-lives for nonperishables, and in a large number of cases already put this information on containers in code for their own use;
  - (b) storage conditions, a most important determinant of shelf-life, can be controlled by the food industry.

(4) Enactment of State open dating regulations will not result in any significant adverse economic impact on the food industry or the Commonwealth of Massachusetts in terms of increased costs or higher food prices.

In a speech at a conference of Food Stability and Open Dating at Rutgers University (October 1971), Cynthia Metzler of the Center for Study of Responsive Law summarized the problem:

> Intricate codes on the vast majority of food products serve to raise consumers' suspicions about what is being held back. consumers unwittingly buying stale, moldy or unfresh food is a common phenomenon. Although deterioration of these products may be visually obvious, consumers can't see through the packages.

Although consumers seem to agree that they should be informed of the freshness of their food, they seem to differ on which type of date should be used.

A 1975 nationwide study by *Response Analysis* for the FDA found that:

> The date stamped on milk is the date by which it *should be sold* (pull date) but 43% of all consumers don't know this and 62% think it should be the date by which milk *should be used* (use date).

Industry and government tend to question whether consumers actually read the labels of food products. A March 1977 survey of Better Homes and Gardens subscribers (Better Homes and Gardens Consumer Report 5, Meredith Corp., 1977) found that 88% always or frequently look for the last sale date of a perishable food product. It should be noted that, although the sample panel profile agrees very well with that of Better Homes and Gardens Subscribers, the subscriber tends to have a higher income than average, be older than the average consumer, and is likely to be married.

James Turner, a consumer advocate, in a speech at a one-day conference "Food: Getting the Picture into Focus" held at the University of Minnesota on October 26, 1977, stated that:

> Industry has used the argument against open dating that it would increase costs and give little or no benefit to consumers. But no one who ever used open dating has found that it raised costs by wasting earlier dated food. The supermarkets using it found that the most tangible result was less loss due to better stock rotation. Also they found that consumers liked it — got positive feedback and decided it wasn't such a bad idea after all.
>
> Consumers do read labels. 30% read nutritional labels and 80% rely on their presence whether they read it or not.

Even though strongly in favor of open dating, today's consumer movement is not always in favor of laws and regulations mandating open dates. In a conversation held at the same conference, Mr. Turner said that:

> A voluntary open dating program on the part of industry would be more effective than governmental regulations. Direct communication and interaction between consumers and industry will allow more flexibility and generate more problem-solving capability than would government regulations which may turn out to be non-enforceable. Consumer/industry task forces can work to encourage technological developments, such as time-temperature integrating devices that would reduce the problems involved in determining the end of shelf life and in implementing open dating systems.

Jay Adelman, New Jersey Food Council, in a telephone conversation on October 28, 1977, in conjunction with information gathering for the U.S. Office of Technology Assessment summarized their position as follows:

> The New Jersey Food Council is strongly in favor of open dating but only on a voluntary basis. The New Jersey Food Council would not formally endorse any law on open dating. If there has to be a law, a Federal law is preferable. Every major food store chain in New Jersey is now using open dating, especially on perishable items. The stores set shelf-life on products where they have direct control (i.e., ground beef = 24 h) and in conjunction with manufacturers on their items. The pull date with some amount of total product life left for consumer storage is the best type of system. Open dating on semi-perishable food would be good if reasonable standards could be set. Standards should be set by manufacturers in conjunction with supermarkets because all are part of the total distribution system.

INDUSTRY POSITION ON OPEN DATING

Manufacturers and retailers face different problems with open dating and therefore have differing positions that must be examined separately. A distinction must also be made between manufacturers of perishable items (namely, less than 3 months shelf-life) and manufacturers of semi-perishables (shelf-life of 3 months to more than 2 years). The retail industry has historically been in favor of open dating and has addressed itself primarily to the open dating of perishable items. Their support has firm grounding in the benefits to them proven by trial runs of open dating in retail stores in 1971. The January 1973 USDA Marketing Research Report reported the following:

In-store Open Dating Experiment: Consumer Reactions

	Percent of consumers with complaints in stores:			
	using pull date	**using pack date**	**using no date but improved handling**	**using no date**
Before study:				
foods to be open dated	19.4	20.1	20.6	24.6
all other foods	3.1	3.7	3.4	4.8
During study:				
open dated foods	9.9	11.0	27.7	21.6
all other foods	1.8	2.0	7.3	4.4
10 months later with open dating at all stores:				
open dated foods	13.4	13.6	16.4	11.4
all other foods	1.5	1.8	1.7	1.0

(1) Both using pull dates and pack dates decreased the percent of food freshness complaints by one-half (pull date 19% to 10% and pack date 20% to 11%). The store which used no open date but tried to improve handling control actually showed an increase in complaints (21% to 28%).

(2) The 50% decrease in the number of complaints about "all other foods" was shown to be statistically significant at the 0.05 probability level.

(3) One year after the 8-week promotional period (with all stores using pull dates for 10 months) complaints had increased again slightly but had not reached the initial level.

"These results indicate that the improved consumer attitude and trust generated by advertising open dating may be more important than gains in actual product freshness."

Economic Impact of Open Dating on Food Store Operations

Dairy foods were the only section in which costs due to overage foods increased.

Bakery goods were handled more but losses were lower due to less being thrown away (sold at lower price when barely overage).

All other sections of foods showed less costs due to wastes — better stock rotation.

It was found that people did not buy freshest and leave older but good food on the shelf.

At the October 1971 Conference on Food Stability and Open Dating at Rutgers University, Clarence Adamy of the National Association of Food Chains (today called the Food Marketing Institute) made a statement about open dating. The following is a summary:

The NAFC are much in favor of open dating — the question is not if, but when, where and how — but doubts the viability of legislative activity.

(1) Local legislation would be terrible because so much food is produced for nationwide distribution (i.e., 70% of the nation's vegetables are grown in California).

(2) Federal legislation is too inflexible — we don't yet know what is the best way to open date — more experimentation needs to be done and that is what supermarkets are doing.

The NAFC favors pull dates over pack or expiration dates. The pack date is the most objective (no judgment necessary and not open to question), but the consumer has the least ability to use this date.

The expiration date would be of the greatest use to the consumer if it could be reliably determined — but there is so much subjectivity and so many unknowns after it leaves the supermarket (consumer abuse) that the NAFC has grave fears of it.

The pull date (with a reasonable amount of time left for the consumer to store before using) is the best compromise.

The conflict between retailers and manufacturers over the open dating issue is illustrated by the following summaries of speeches given by Donald W. Stowbridge of the Stop and Shop Co. and by Harold J. Rafson of Topco Associates, at the October 1971 Rutgers University Conference.

Donald W. Stowbridge, Stop and Shop Co. "Practices and Experiences" Conference Proceedings October 21-22, 1971, Rutgers University.

Stop and Shop puts open pull dates on all its private brand perishable merchandise. Trying to get all suppliers to do the same but problems are involved:

(1) The manufacturers don't want to because they can't control the temperatures and conditions after the food leaves the plant.

(2) The supermarkets are worried about the reliability of the manufacturers' dates because of different grades of ingredients used by different firms in the same product, the quality and integrity of the packaging and the bacterial load. Supermarkets have no control over this.

Harold J. Rafson, Topco Associates. "Practices and Experiences" Conference Proceedings October 21-22, 1971, Rutgers University.

Topco uses the following system of open dating on its products. First, semi-perishables are divided into three classes: (1) 1 mo. to 6 mo.; (2) 6 mo. to 1 yr; and (3) over 1 yr.

Class (1) has first priority in open dating. 80 to 90% now are open dated with a "freshness date". The freshness date indicates the day the *total distribution time* for the product has expired. The maximum supply date is the last date the retailer should accept delivery of the product.

Suppliers have 20% of the total distribution time.
Retailers have 60% of the total distribution time.
Consumers have 20% of the total distribution time.

Thus, Topco is for an open sell date which disagrees with the Rutgers Report. Mr. Rafson asked why is there this difference of opinion between retailers and manufacturers? He stated that part could be due to the fact that the Rutgers Report references 107 manufacturers but only 7 retailers. The prevading viewpoint in the Rutgers report is that temperature and environmental conditions are more important than time. This is true, but it is also true from knowledge of the distribution system that conscientious efforts are made to store products under proper conditions. It is not true that manufacturers have no control over the food after it leaves the processing plant. Retailers have good handling and storage practices just as manufacturers have GMPs. The manufacturer has as much reason to expect this as the retailer does to expect product quality when it leaves the plant. All are parts of the total picture — not separate. There is a *normal* distribution and handling condition that should be used in determining shelf lives.

There are two basic objections to the Rutger's recommendation of date of shelf display:

(1) Ineffective: it doesn't tell stockboy when to remove the product from the shelf.

(2) Inefficient: it adds another handling step that already increases cost to consumer.

Also, it does not account for differences in distribution time to the supermarket. If a shipment got delayed it would be given apparent new life by an unknowing stockboy putting a current stock rotation date on it.

Open dating provides a guideline to freshness, not a gurarantee. Most of the hang-ups about open dating are caused by missing this fact. More research is needed in the area of expected product lives under normal handling conditions and of ways food distribution can be improved (i.e., better refrigerated display cases).

Problem of financial responsibility:

If floating (i.e., abuser pays): companies with financial clout get unfair advantage.

If manufacturer: distributor and retailer will not be careful enough.

If retailer: it ignores fact that the manufacturer has a large part in determining distribution route (type of selling).

The current stand of other retailers on the open dating question is illustrated by the following summaries of telephone conversations with Bob Wunderle of Pathmark, and Jay Rosengarten of Shopwell, representatives of two large coast-to-coast retail food store chains.

Bob Wunderle, Vice President for Public Affairs of Pathmark Food Stores:

Pathmark is in favor of open dating, as demonstrated by their current practice of open dating all perishable (and a number of non-perishable) items in their stores. In development of a law concerning open dating they have questions about what, if any, distinctions would be made concerning products that are unusable when out of code versus those that may simply have passed the peak of quality when out of code.

One major problem they find even with their present open dating system is the confusion it sometimes generates on the part of the consumer. Many people feel that an open date represents a self-destruct date (i.e., ground beef has a one-day life and consumers ask if it will still be good tomorrow night). Educating the consumer is a problem. It takes an 18 in. × 24 in. sign by the delicatessen to explain that the date indicates peak of freshness and to itemize how long 15 of the items will last if kept wrapped and refrigerated. How can you explain this for 9000 items?

Jay Rosengarten, Shopwell (New York) (He has helped draft a proposed state bill on open dating of perishable foods which has passed in the assembly and on which Senate hearings will be held.) comments as follows:

"There has been a problem in New York with local jurisdictions passing laws on open dating that are different from each other. The proposed law is very similar to the New York City law passed in 1971 with a few revisions that are the result of 7 years' experience. For example, the New York City law provides for open dating, but does not provide for disposal of out-of-date food. The new law provides for sale of out-of-date food if it is clearly marked and separated.

The pull date is the best date to use. It is more meaningful to consumers about freshness. A use date cannot take into account the handling conditions after the product leaves the store. Experience has shown that consumers are not as careful about handling as are manufacturers and retailers. The proposed law has the manufacturers set the pull date because they are most familiar with their product and also because it is easier and cheapest for them to print the date on the package. If individual stores put the date on, it would cost more and more mistakes would be made. There is a possibility of giving the New York Department of Agriculture power to step in if they think manufacturers are abusing the pull date.

Experience has been that there is very little wastage due to overage food because managers tend to order more carefully and rotate stock better. Practice has been that the store chain takes the financial responsiblity for overage products that come through the warehouse and vendors take responsibility for overage products that they deliver directly to the stores. Legislation should not have to deal with the question of financial responsibility because the food industry has developed so many different types of practices within itself that legislation would confuse more than it would help.

The time for open dating of nonperishables is getting closer. It can probably be dealt with on a voluntary basis (as the National Canners Association is trying to work out) but if there is legislation it should be on a Federal level. The canning companies are so large that if an individual state sets legislation, either the cost of the nonperishables will go up greatly in that state or the product will not be sold there.

Most of the food industry is in favor to some degree of open dating on perishable items. A pull date is one of the most valuable tools they can provide to their customers."

Most states today have regulations concerning the open dating of some perishable food products, usually dairy and/or bakery goods.

In 1971, when the Rutgers University Food Stability Survey was compiled, most manufacturers of perishable food products seemed to be uniformly against open dating. One manufacturer of baked goods is quoted as stating (page 61, Rutger's Food Stability Survey):

The stamping of the date of a shelf display (DSD) by retail stores is in most of our opinions, more likely to be a disservice to the consumer than a service to him. Such dating could give the consumer a false sense of security that as of the date stamped on the container, the product was of the highest possible quality, when, in effect, much of the damage due to mishandling may have occurred after the product has left the manufacturer's plant and immediately before the date proposed by your team has been placed.

We do not believe that it would help rotation more than the date of manufacture (DOM), but it would really incur wastes because no consumer would pick up an older date the moment a newer date is placed beside it on the shelf.

Another manufacturer of baked goods is quoted as follows on the same page:

. . .However, we do not agree with the adoption of open dating of manufacture, etc. Unless there was universal adoption and consumer education, it could create prejudices vs. a manufacturer with shelf stable products, i.e., refusing to purchase an excellent 3-month old product in favor of a two-week old product, inferior in quality at the time of manufacture.

There is some question, however, whether this would still be the prevailing attitude today after more companies have actually experienced open dating laws. In a telephone conversation on November 1, 1977, Mr. Gordon Skinner of Continental Baking Co., Minneapolis, MN, made the following statement:

Bakeries in Minnesota have been required to open date all products since January 1, 1977. Continental Baking has experienced no problem with the open dating. We do not feel that it has hurt or helped. We do feel, however, that it helps the consumer because now they can see which is the freshest. Consumers do tend to pick the freshest bakery products on the shelf but this is no problem since deliveries are made daily.

Previous to January 1, 1977, the products were color date-coded. Now we use a "fresh through" date. The shelf-life from the day of production is 48 h for breads and 7 days for cakes., Some markets request a 48 h rotation for cakes as well as breads and Continental complies with this. Out-of-code products are collected by drivers and sold at Continental's thrift store.

The dairy industry also was strongly against open dating in 1971. A 1969 nationwide study of milk dating by the Committee for Study of Milk Availability of the Milk Industry Foundation is quoted as follows (page 77, Rutgers University Food Stability Survey):

> The practice of milk dating cannot be justified from public health, quality, or economic considerations.
>
> With respect to quality, research findings have demonstrated conclusively that age of milk is not a reliable index of quality. Furthermore, studies have indicated that the age of milk offered for sale in stores does not differ significantly between dating and non-dating markets. Thus, processor coding is as effective as milk dating as a method of inventory control to assure proper rotation of milk in stores.
>
> Neither does milk dating serve the economic interest of consumers. Dating deters the adoption of more efficient delivery practices and thus directly increases industry costs of delivering milk to stores. In the long run, these increased costs are borne by consumers.

There is the question however, of whether this would still be the prevailing attitude in the milk industry in 1977. In a telephone conversation of November 1, 1977, Jim Hokanson of the Clover Leaf Creamery Company in Minneapolis, made the following observations:

> Clover Leaf Products have always been date-coded. The color of the caps on the old glass bottles were changed daily.
>
> Minnesota has an open dating law that went into effect January 1, 1975. The date used is a pull date and is set 14 days from processing. This leaves about one week for consumer use if milk is stored properly.
>
> The drivers drop-deliver to the stores. It is the drivers' responsibility to maintain an adequate stock in the store cooler. They pull anything out-of-code, pull the old stock forward, and make sure the store personnel are rotating the stock properly.
>
> Clover Leaf has not experienced any problems with the open dating. They have noticed no change in consumer buying habits. Most returns are still due to faulty containers and only rarely is an out-of-date package returned. They do not find that consumers will buy only the freshest packages.
>
> Clover Leaf Creamery will continue to open date their products whether there is a law or not.

Mrs. Arlene Stansfield, Director of Consumer Affairs for Land O' Lakes in Minneapolis, in a telephone conversation on November 2, 1977 said that:

> Open dating has worked well in the dairy industry. They do a better job of stock rotation and their product freshness is more credible to the consumer. She feels open dating would be of benefit to consumers on all food products, not just dairy products. They found that consumers were initially shocked at the length of the shelf-lives of products but once the shock had worn off, they were delighted that products would last that long. Consumers often do not rotate the stock in their home pantries as well as they should. Dates on cans and cake mixes, for example, would help them know when to use or discard products at home.

Even in 1971 when the Rutgers' University Food Stability Survey was compiled, the meat industry seemed to be divided on the merits of open dating. An executive of the American Meat Institute stated (page 26, Rutgers' Food Stability Survey):

My opinion is that the meat packing industry would be opposed to open dating. I think this is true because of the fact that the date is not the most significant piece of information a person can have about a product, and can actually be misleading because it says nothing about handling. In addition, because of the manner in which consumers select products in self-service counters, some products inevitably will be wasted.

In the same report a major meat processing company which was already using a quality assurance date made the following statement (page 27, Rutgers' Food Stability Survey):

The growing popularity of large supermarkets in recent years has placed increasing demands on meat processors to improve the keeping time of their products. As a result, product technology and packaging methods have improved rapidly, and we have been able to meet this challenge through means of improved sanitation, better product refrigeration and advanced packaging materials and methods. It is necessary to achieve satisfactory and dependable product life.

In placing a control date or quality assurance date on our products, we are passing a large share of the benefits of improved technology along to our retailers and customers. All such dates are set so as to assure a reasonable length of time for the sale of the item plus adequate time for the consumer to store and use the product after the expiration of the control date.

It has been our experience that the rotation and movement of our products in stores can be much more easily administered by this system than by working with the date of packaging. The date of pack provides no information regarding the length of time that the manufacturer expects his product to keep. It places the good operator and the careless producer on the same basis and removes much of the reward for maintaining sanitary operating conditions, improving handling methods, developing new packages, and the like.

The trend in at least these three perishable food industries (bakeries, dairies and meats) seems to be one of extreme doubt before actually instituting open dating, then changing to acceptance after using some system of open dating.

At a March 1973 hearing on proposed open dating legislation, Chuck Myberg of the George A. Hormel Co. of Austin, Minnesota gave testimony to the Minnesota State Senate Committee on Health, Welfare and Corrections to the following effect:

He was concerned with the tendency of states to enact legislation which varies from state to state and which impedes interstate commerce. Congress has established a meat code in the 1967 Wholesome Meats Act which in section 678 forbids states from requiring marking or labeling ingredient contents in addition to or different than those required in the Act. In Michigan and New York lawsuits against the state laws have won. Congress has unmistakably ordained that the Federal act fixes the sole standards and completely preempts state laws.

Manufacturers of non-perishables seem to tend to be generally against proposed state legislation.

In 1971 in the Rutgers' University Food Stability Survey (pages 198-199) two manufacturers of dry breakfast foods made the following comments:

We wish to emphasize that our products move very rapidly from manufacturer to consumer and that under present methods we believe our products customarily are purchased on a first-in, first-out basis. If such food products were to bear readable code-dates denoting either the date of manufacture or the date beyond which the product could not be consumed or sold, we fear the natural tendency of consumers would be to purchase most recently manufactured prdoucts. Thus, products would be purchased on a last-in, first-out basis, and greater quantities of our product would unnecessarily fail to meet our own standards. This very real possibility would be undesirable and not in the best interest of consumers. We believe that our present coding and surveillance methods insure that our products meet our high standards upon reaching the consumer.

Quality changes are often so slight and subtle that they are virtually undetected over short periods of time such as the duration of time from purchase to consumer use. Specific dates infer significant quality change taking place at a specific time. Such an assumption would lead to consumer rejection of slightly older packages with good quality merchandise left to be eventually destroyed. The selection process would also lead to increased handling damage of individual packages.

Many food packages are small and irregular in shape with labels currently crowded with mandatory and instructional information. Meaningful code dating would require special coding areas frequently requiring larger labels.

Your statement that "as health hazard problems are low, there is no need to openly date individual packages with date of manufacturing or date of expiry," is quite correct. We believe the same holds true for Date of Shelf Display (DSD). Consumer protection benefits would not justify the added accumulated expenses for implementation. These increased costs would undoubtedly result in higher costs for the consumer.

The following position was given by the National Association of Frozen Food Packers, now known as the American Frozen Food Institute (page 198, Rutgers' Food Stability Survey):

Proposed Resolution of the Board of Directors (Association Policy on Frozen Food Date Labeling)

The National Association of Frozen Food Packers has carefully considered the matter of labeling of frozen food packages with the date of packing in light of the interest of high standards of quality for which the industry strives.

The Commissioner of Food and Drugs and the Administrator of Consumer and Marketing Service, USDA, have not considered it desirable, in the interest of consumers, to include the date of packing on the labels of frozen food packages.

The NAFFP encourages *code* dating of frozen food packages.

The NAFFP has consistently and vigorously opposed all legislative proposals which would require the date of packing to appear on labels of frozen food packages.

In order to establish guidelines for committees and staff of the Association on the matter of requiring the date of pack on the labels of frozen food packages, the Board of Directors adopts the following:

Resolution.

(1) It is a well established scientific fact that the quality of frozen products is dependent upon several factors, among which the most important are the initial quality of the raw material and the integrated effect of the length of time of storage and the storage temperature. Reference is made to "Quality and Stability in Frozen Food" edited by Michael J. Copley, W.B. Van Arsdel and Robert L. Olson, all of the Western Utilization Research and Development Laboratory, ARS of USDA.

(2) It is also well known that quality changes during storage differ widely for different products, depending upon their basic characteristics. Some vegetable products have high quality lives at 0 °F for up to three years, whereas other products, such as fatty fish species, have a high quality life of only a few months at the same temperature.

(3) Historically, a common concept of food date labeling has been related to the term "fresh", as in the case of bread, eggs or milk. However, the term "fresh" relative to its application to frozen food has been considered ambiguous and, therefore, undesirable by the Food and Drug Administration and the United States Department of Agriculture.

(4) Since dating would be considered by consumers to be a means of selecting high quality, but in fact is an unreliable index, it would cause confusion and economic waste.

(5) Under usual conditions of handling frozen food, an "older" product which has been well handled will be superior in quality to a recently frozen product which has been badly handled.

(6) Furthermore, the use of various forms of indicators has been suggested to insure an objective "measurement" of storage temperatures of time/temperature effects. So far, all such indicators tested fall far short of their objective because they reflect quality changes which studies show do not occur. Stability tests of frozen food show that, even a few exposures of higher temperatures (e.g., 10 °F to 20 °F) although generally undesirable, cause little or no detectable change in quality. Reference is made to NAFFP's Technical Service Bulletin No. 51, "A White Paper Report on the Minneapolis-Honeywell Device." The use of such devices could not by itself provide any guarantee to the consumer that the product is of a satisfactory quality at the time of final sale. In fact, this practice could be most misleading.

On August 29, 1973, Jerry Jenko of General Mills Corporation gave testimony to the Minnesota State Senate on the benefits and disadvantages of open dating legislation. He felt that open dating is only good for all "really perishable goods" (those with shelf-lives of less than 90 days).

The disadvantages include:

(1) The expense estimated at $3000 per product line for equipment and $3250 per product line per year for maintenance and operation.

(2) The fact that there is no need because General Mills receives only two complaints per million packages in spite of their unconditional guarantee of products.

(3) Conflicting state laws would force manufacturers to segregate inventories.

This widespread opposition to open dating may still be the major position of the non-perishable food industry today. The Grocery Manufacturers Association came out strongly against the open dating legislation proposed in 1977 in Massachusetts. The following is an outlined summary of a statement of their objections sent on February 3, 1977 by the GMA attorneys Bingham, Dana and Gould, 100 Federal St., Boston, MA 02110, to Dr. Stuart H. Shapiro of the Massachusetts Department of Public Health.

Economic Impact of Open Dating of Non-perishables

(1) Immediate inflationary effects
  (a) Research costs:
    Ralston Purina 1—2 yr ($138,000)
    Nabisco 1½ yr ($2,113,000)
    Lipton 5 yr (over 2 million)
  (b) Equipment costs:
    Biscuit & Cracker Mfg. Assoc. (millions of dollars)
    Lipton ($50,000 equip.); ($2 million label redesign)
    French ($258,000)
    Hunt Wesson (over $1 million)
  (c) Maintenance Costs.

(2) Increased distribution costs
  (a) Cost of segregating Massachusetts produce
    1. could not fill Massachusetts demand from undated inventory
    2. could not take advantage of peak production years
    3. prohibit free movement of produce from state to state
  (b) Possibility of other states enacting different open dating regulations
  (c) Reduction of food products shipped for sale in Massachusetts
    1. small companies that could not afford change-over
    2. large companies for which Massachusetts is small percent of total market would not change over.

(3) Increased food waste
  (a) Because use date must be earliest date, any of the 6 loss criteria occur to any extent and because possible adverse storage conditions cannot be predicted, use date would be very conservative to avoid possible criminal penalties
  (b) Consumers would select freshest dates and acceptable, but later, dates would not be purchased

(c) Increased costs passed on to consumers due to increased waste might be as high as 3 to 5% of retail price.

Application of Proposed "Loss Criteria"

(1) Predictable and significant decline of nutrients, flavor, color, etc. simply does not occur in nonperishables
(2) Quantitative methodologies are not sensitive enough (or simply do not exist) to measure that decline which does occur
(3) Proposed regulation wording of any loss means that the endpoint would be at the time of processing since the criteria are lost in processing
(4) Criteria are more likely to be lost due to temperature, humidity and light in storage than due to time of storage.

Some segments of the nonperishable food industry however, seem to be willing to at least try for voluntary open dating programs to avoid the passing of legislation mandating it.

The National Food Processors Association is studying the possibility of implementing a voluntary program of open dating on canned products. In telephone conversations on October 20, 1977, Dr. Allan Matthys and Roger Coleman said that one committee is working on the problem of setting shelf-lives and another one is working on the problem of where, how, and in what form to print dates on labels. An in-house report was presented to the Board of Directors in November 1978, with further recommendations on how to proceed. In that report a voluntary "best if used by date" was recommended.

The 84 companies that were asked for translations of their date-coding systems by the New York Consumer Protection Board generally showed two basic responses. Some manufacturers did not give any useful information on translating their codes. The companies that translated their date codes almost always indicated the shelf-lives of their products in general terms ("good for at least one year after the date"). These shelf-life guidelines were printed in the book along with the code translations.

STATE GOVERNMENT OPINIONS AND RESPONSES TO OPEN DATING

The diverse, and often conflicting, demands by consumers for open dating and the complexity of the problems faced by industry are reflected in the various approaches to the problem by state governments.

Billy Riddle, Assistant Director of Consumer Protection Division, the Georgia Department of Agriculture, explained the uncertainties of many state officials about whether to work for open dating legislation (telephone conversation, October 21, 1977):

Only fresh eggs, milk and prepared sandwiches are required to be open dated now. However, they enforce dates that are voluntarily placed on foods, in that they ask that out-of-date food be removed from sale when they find it. State inspectors make at least four visits per year to every grocery store in Georgia. Strictly, according to state law, they would have to prove even out-of-date food to be unwholesome before they could force removal. But only rarely have they had any difficulty in getting overage food removed from sale, although they often have to tell store managers that the food is out-of-date. The only difficulty in compliance has been in cases where the store has purchased the food on a "cash and carry" basis and cannot return it to the wholesaler.

Mr. Riddle has mixed feelings about the problem — he feels open dating has benefits for the consumer, especially for perishables and knows consumers are very aware of dates on food (his department gets many complaints). But he cited the problem of long shelf-life for canned food (2—2½ years, most turn over by then). In fact, just because food is in-date does not assure good quality (distribution and warehouse conditions are more important). He feels there are many laws on the books that are there to aid consumers, but he is not sure all of them really are — just raising prices.

An example is the nutritional labeling law. If the information was really used it would certainly benefit consumers. But he feels most consumers either do not understand the information or do not take the time to compare the nutritional content of different products. So the labels are not being used effectively, but prices are increased anyway.

He feels his department would have no problem getting an open dating law passed in Georgia if they decided to ask for it. May be phasing open dating in slowly would be best, perishables first and canned food last.

In some states that have passed laws on open dating, the government officials charged with implementing the law are not satisfied. Carl Farmer, of the Food and Dairy Division of the Oregon Department of Agriculture is one of these officials. The following is a summary of telephone conversations with him on October 19 and October 21, 1977.

Legislation was passed in Oregon in 1973. Mr. Farmer has been enforcing it since 1974. Regulations from statute have been confusing to everyone: consumers, retailers and manufacturers. Some products are required to have the pack date, some (with shelf-lives less than 30 days) are required to have the pull date. For fresh meat (including poultry) the pack date is the date it is packaged in the supermarket. Oregon had a hearing on October 20, 1977 to see if some way they could standardize (i.e., the pull date). Consumers did not make their position known. Industry showed up in bits and pieces. He feels the issue is confusing and that it is hard to know what is the best way to implement the law — everyone has a different idea.

As a result of this hearing, open date labeling for fresh or raw meats, all forms of fresh poultry, fresh fish, crab and shrimp became effective December 1977 in Oregon.

According to the Oregon Department of Agriculture, poultry must bear a specified pull date on each package under the new regulation. All fresh, raw packaged meats, sausage products, seafood products and fresh fish products will be designated with a package or preparation date, so that the shopper will know the exact date that the item was offered for sale.

The changes will also require retailers to specify by placard or label that the date on the package is either a pull date or a package date.

Meat and poultry products could, under previous regulations, be labeled with slaughter date, pack date or pull date, which was confusing to consumers, the department said.

Many government officials in the states with no open dating legislation are ambivalent about the benefits of such legislation. The following are summaries of telephone conversations with four officials who are not wholeheartedly in favor of open dating legislation in their states for various reasons.

Bill Teer, of the Arkansas Health Department (October 19, 1977):

There is no open dating law or regulations in Arkansas. Inspectors have not found a problem. Sometimes they get complaints from consumers, but usually they find there is no problem with the food (it is still good even though out-of-date). He feels if open dating were mandatory it would take a lot of personnel time policing it when there is no problem with the food. He feels that help on a Federal level from the FDA in preventing mislabeled products from coming across state lines (i.e., sorghum), would be more useful.

Dr. George M. Rose of the Division of Inspection of the Florida Food Grades and Standards Bureau (October 19, 1977):

Florida has open dating on milk and all grade A dairy products (expiration date, after which they are not sold). It is entirely unnecessary and wasteful to have required open dating on processed food. No one can predict shelf-life adequately. The pack date doesn't mean anything to the consumer — they just look for the freshest. We don't have that much of a problem with foods and it is hard to educate the public against open dating, particularly for non-perishables; there is some merit in it for perishable foods.

Mr. Kain of the New York State Food Inspection Services (October 19, 1977):

New York State has no open dating regulations now. It is the opinion in the department that open dating does not mean much to the consumer because temperature and other storage conditions are more important.

Joseph Prince of the New Jersey Department of Health Consumer Services (October 28, 1977):

The only type of open dating required in New Jersey at present is on milk and milk products (i.e., 5 days from the date of packaging for milk). Rutgers ran a shelf-life testing study in 1971, but nothing came of it except that voluntary industry dating became more common. The voluntary dating has caused some problems for the Department of Health because when consumers call to complain, there is nothing in New Jersey law to cover taking it off the shelf (unless the food is proven to be actually unwholesome). They might be able to enforce removal under the law on false labeling. Usually the store will remove the food from the shelf as soon as the date is pointed out by the Health Department. They do get some complaints from consumers, but not enormous. They have to rely on consumer complaints because there is not enough money to do routine inspections of stores. Mr. Prince is a proponent of uniformity. U.S. food is distributed over a very large area, sometimes worldwide. Therefore, a uniform application of laws over as large a geographic area as possible is highly preferable to individual states or counties trying to enforce their own regulations. An example is the FDA-coordinated program of interstate milk shippers which has worked very well in helping the individual state agencies. If the situation indicates an excess of unwholesome food being sold overage, then a Federal open dating law is in order. The U.S. food industry does an excellent job.

In a telephone conversation on October 19, 1977, West Horton of the Arizona Weights and Measures section of the Department of Agriculture and Horticulture said:

> Arizona passed legislation in August, 1974 that became effective on January 1, 1975. Through this legislation the state enforces the voluntary dating of perishable products with a shelf-life of less than 60 days. When the products are overage they must be designated as such and sold at a lowered price. There were a lot of problems with this legislation at first but now consumers are aware of it and markets practice good stock rotation. A mandatory open dating law would work in Arizona.

Dr. George Michael of the Massachusetts Department of Public Health is strongly in favor of open dating, but they have gotten a bad response from industry. He feels that industry wants no part of it, and objections are on a purely business and non-scientific basis. Dr. Michael is disappointed that he has not received more support at least from the scientific branches of industry. He feels that open dating is very desirable on all foods. Open datings, along with prescribed temperatures and method of storage, would result in an optimum distribution system. The consumer would then actually get the high quality and nutritional level of food which was intended.

Open dating should be on canned foods also. The National Canners' Association has been studying the problem and Dr. Michael intends to work with and encourage them.

The DPH had an open dating law in the works in Massachusetts this year but aborted it. They thought that perhaps specific regulations on each food would be more flexible and appropriate than a general statutory law.

SUMMARY OF OPINIONS ON OPEN DATING

There are basically three different types of open dates being considered. The date the food is manufactured or processed is known as the "pack date". The date the food is first put on the shelf in the retail food store is known as the "display date", and is similar in principle to the "pack date" for fresh produce such as hamburger. In general, this display date is not used for products manufactured elsewhere. The date by which the product should be sold or removed from the store shelf is known as the "sell by" or "pull date". The product generally has some length of consumer shelf-life left to it after purchase on this date. The date by which the product should either be consumed by or discarded is the third method, and is respectively known as the "best if used by" and the "use by date". Of these basic types of dating, the display date has the fewest number of backers. Opinions are widely divided on the other types.

Consumers across the country strongly support the concept of putting open dates on food products. They may disagree on which type of date is best, or on whether it should be voluntary or legally mandated, but they all agree that they have a right to know something about the age of the food they buy.

The food industry seems to be deeply divided over the question of open dating. The retailing portion of the food industry, especially the larger food store chains, is generally in favor of open dating. Manufacturers of semi-perishable and non-perishable food items are generally against any kind of open dates on their products. However, they are beginning to work on voluntary systems of open dating in order to avoid a mass of conflicting laws in the states where their foods are sold. Manufacturers of perishable goods were generally against open dating six or seven years ago. But today, after many states have adopted open dating regulations concerning their products, they seem to be much more in favor of some form of open dating.

State government officials across the country have varying opinions on the benefits of open dating laws and regulations. Some of them feel any type of open dating would be more wasteful than beneficial. Others feel it would be beneficial but have mixed feelings about implementing regulations. Others are strongly in favor of it and fuel that the time has come for open dating regulations on almost all foods.

Much of the concern about open dating relates to the enforcement of guidelines and on who will set the guidelines. Probably the best system of open dating would be a voluntary basis with regulations stipulating which system should be used, preferably a sell by or best if used by date. Past experience indicates that open dating would tend to improve the distribution system and would not incur excessive waste.

REFERENCES

A.C. NIELSEN COMPANY. 1973. Study of Consumer Attitudes Towards Product Quality.

ARIZONA CONSUMERS' COUNCIL. 1976. Freshness dating of perishable food: The consumer issues.

BETTER HOMES AND GARDENS CONSUMER REPORT NO. 5. 1977. Meredith Corporation.

COMMONWEALTH OF MASSACHUSETTS CONSUMER COUNCIL. 1977. Summary: Open Dating for nonperishable food items.

DHEW. 1975. FDA consumer nutrition knowledge survey, Rep. II, Publ. 76-2059, DHEW.

RUTGERS UNIVERSITY. 1971a. Food Stability and open dating. Conference Proceedings, Oct. 21-22.

RUTGERS UNIVERSITY. 1971b. Food stability survey. Rutgers University.

STATE OF NEW YORK, CONSUMER PROTECTION BOARD. 1977. Blind dates: How to break the codes on the foods you buy.

U.S. GOVERNMENT PRINTING OFFICE. 1979. Open Shelf-LIfe Dating of Foods, Stock No. 052-003-00694-4. Washington, D.C.

USDA. 1973. Food dating: Shoppers' reactions and the impact on retail food stores. Marketing Research Report 984.

VAN ARSDEL, W.B., COPLEY, M.J. and OLSON, R.L. 1969. Quality and Stability in Frozen Food. Wiley-Interscience, New York.

CHAPTER 2

BASIC FOOD PRESERVATION AND DEGRADATION MODES

INTRODUCTION TO THE PRINCIPLES OF PRESERVATION

Because of the size of the country and the separation of the consumer from the producer of foods, some form of preservation must be used to insure that the food consumed is of good quality, is safe to eat and provides the nutritional needs of the consumer. These factors are the basis for preservation. In addition, preservation methods are used to separate foods into edible components and to produce new, more convenient food items that meet the needs and desires of the consuming public. Finally some preserved foods are produced for purely aesthetic reasons, i.e., they meet the psychological desires of the consumer for specific purposes and nutrition, although supplied, is not of concern. It must be pointed out, however, that underlying all preservation methods is the basic principle of food safety. Preserved food is changed or processed into a form that will insure safety from either toxic substances or harmful microorganisms, as long as the distributors, marketers and consumers themselves practice good sanitary and handling habits.

In order to open date a food, knowledge is needed of the major mode of deterioration that would be expected, based on the method of preservation used. This information is needed, to insure that the consumer is able to purchase foods of high enough quality, safety and nutritional value to meet his or her needs. This chapter will describe the general modes of deterioration and the types of preservation used to slow down degradation. Chapter 3 will review the methods for mathematical prediction of shelf-life, based on the factors influencing the speed of deterioration of some of the various classes of foods.

MAJOR MODES OF FOOD DEGRADATION

Preharvest Biological Decay

Prior to harvest and slaughter, plant and animal foods are subject to a myriad of microbiological diseases including viruses, molds, yeasts and bacteria. In addition, some foods before harvest can be attacked and diseased or eaten by insects, birds and rodents. For plants, competition by weeds can result in poor yield. To prevent or control this, one form of processing is the use of chemical or physical means of control or prevention. The use of pesticides, herbicides and rodenticides are examples of chemical control. Another method of chemical control is the use of drugs such as antibiotics to prevent diseases in animals prior to slaughter. Weeding by machine is a physical means of control. These modes of deterioration are not generally considered in regard to shelf-life or open dating. However, if the food is subjected to damage, its initial quality wil be less. Processing does not make low quality foods better, and overall shelf-life will be less after slaughter or harvest than with undamaged foods.

Senescence

Once a fruit, vegetable, cereal grain or animal product is slaughtered, it is separated from its source of nutrients and water. However, since it is still a viable living system, the enzymes present continue to operate and utilize the available carbohydrate and nutrient stores. For fruits this process can be of benefit because they can repair postharvest damages, and more important, fruits can be picked prior to optimum maturity, transported long distances to the marketplace and home, and then develop into a high quality product. If the fruits were picked at optimum ripeness, they could rot before consumption, during the transport. This biochemical process also operates in the aging of meat to achieve the desired degree of tenderness. In this case the state of the animal before slaughter is very important and affects the final product quality.

For all foods, however, eventually enzymatic biochemical processes occurring postharvest lead to degradation, including loss of color, flavor, nutrients and texture. In addition, the breakdown products produced damage the tissues so that the foods become subject to microbiological attack with subsequent more rapid decay. To prevent this mode of deterioration, three major processing methods can be used: (1) lowering of temperature slows the reaction; (2) raising the temperature denatures the enzymes and makes them inactive; and (3) removal or binding of water reduces water availability (or water activity, a_w), which reduces the ability of the enzymes to operate. The mechanism of this will be discussed in Chapter 3.

Other control methods are addition of acid thereby lowering pH, control of carbon dioxide and oxygen level (CA-storage) which is done for many fresh fruits, vegetables and some meat, and substrate control through genetic manipulation to decrease senscence. With respect to open dating, senescence is an important mode of deterioration of fresh fruits and vegetables, whole grain cereals, meat, poultry, fish, and to some degree, dairy products.

Microbiological Decay

Microorganisms constitute a major mechanism by which many foods, especially fresh ones, lose their quality. This is because microbes are ubiquitous in the environment, and can grow rapidly. After a food is harvested or slaughtered, it loses some degree of its ability to fight off microbial attack. If it is physically damaged, then it becomes more susceptible to attack. Bruising, cutting and trimming constitute such damage. Microbes can grow rapidly on foods (starting with one microbe which divides every 10 min, with sufficient available nutrients, in five hours there would be over one billion microbes present). The basic principle of preservation is to control or destroy them. Much the same controls are employed as those used for enzymes:

(1) Lower temperature to slow growth.
(2) Raise temperature to kill them.
(3) Remove or bind water to slow or prevent their growth.
(4) Lower pH to slow or stop their growth by adding acid or through fermentation.
(5) Control O_2 or CO_2 level to control population.
(6) Manipulate food composition to remove nutrients needed by the microbes.

Because in some cases the above methods change the food into a form not desirable by the consumer, chemical means of preservation can be used. These chemicals are used to slow growth or kill the organisms. At the level of use the chemicals should have no ill effect on the consumer. Examples are the use of calcium propionate in bread and sodium benzoate in some soft drinks.

Knowledge of the rate of growth of microbes as a function of the environmental conditions of the food is very important in the prediction of shelf-life and, thus, the open dating of some foods such as: fresh and ground meats and fresh poultry; fresh fish; dairy products such as milk, cheese and yogurt; cured meats such as hot dogs, bacon and bologna; pasteurized fruit drinks; fruits and vegetables; and whole grains.

A second and more serious problem with microorganisms is the fact that some are pathogenic to humans, i.e., they either cause infection when ingested or result in the production of chemicals in the food which are toxic to humans. Most food processes are designed to guard against contamination with pathogens and the subsequent growth of these pathogens after processing, or as important, to treat the food in such a way as to destroy any potentially harmful microbes that might be inadvertently present in the food. For example, fermentation of foods with useful microbes results in alcohol or acid production. The acid and alcohol prevent the growth of pathogens. The major microorganisms pathogenic to humans that are important in foods are:

Intoxicants
Staphylococcus aureus
Clostridium botulinum
Clostridium perfringens
Aspergillus flavus
Infectious
Salmonellae species
Escherichia coli strains

In most cases temperatures below 45 °F, food with a water availability less than 80% equilibrium humidity (or an a_w or water activity ≤ 0.8) and a pH less than 4.5 are sufficient conditions to prevent the growth and multiplication of the pathogens. Open dating should not be based on the growth of these organisms, but the manufacture of the food and subsequent handling should ensure absolute control of the microbes. Unfortunately, if the latter is not done, consumers have have a false sense of security that a food consumed before its open sell by or use by date is safe when, in fact, it could cause food poisoning. This one fact is a "must" in the education of the consumer as to the value of the open dating.

Chemical Deterioration

During the processing of foods, tissue damage occurs which causes the release of various food chemical constitutents into the cellular fluid environment. These chemicals can then react with each other or with external factors to lead to deterioration of the food and result in a shortening of the shelf-life. Many different reactions can occur which lead to quality and nutrient loss. The major ones are classified below.

Enzymatic. — As mentioned above, the normal postharvest enzymatic reactions can lead to a loss in food quality and shelf-life. In addition, destruction of cell tissues releases enzymes which can lead to further deterioration. For example, lipoxidase enzymes released from cell organelles called mitochondria can attack lipids and cause rancidity. Similarly, the polyphenol oxidase enzyme can react with some cell constitutents and oxygen and lead to the production of brown color, which is typically seen as a deterioration reaction in bruised or cut fruits such as apples or bananas. These reactions are usually very rapid at room temperature, but are controlled in the natural state. Once the food is handled, deterioration starts. Enzymatic decay also occurs in the frozen state unless the enzymes are previously denatured by blanching. Enzymatic reactions also lead to the major mode of deterioration of many refrigerated doughs. Unfortunately, heat treatment to denature the enzymes results in loss of dough functionality. Control of the enzymatic reactions is the same as was discussed for senesence. Knowledge of the rate of these reactions as a function of environmental conditions is very important in prediction of shelf-life for open dating. The major environmental factors are oxygen, water, pH and temperature. Other enzymatic degradations include color losses and vitamin losses such as for vitamin C.

Lipid Oxidation. — Many foods contain unsaturated fats, which are important in the nutrition of humans. Unfortunately, these fats are subject to direct attack by oxygen through an autocatalytic free radical mechanism. This results in the production of rancid off-flavors which make the food undesirable to consume. Very little fat has to oxidize for the consumer to detect rancidity and reject the food. Unfortunately, the food will still be very nutritious. The free radicals and peroxides produced in this process can react and bleach pigments, such as occurs in dried vegetables, can destroy vitamins C, E, and A; can result in protein degradation, making it of poorer quality, as can happen in whole dry milk; can cause darkening of the fat as happens in deep fat frying; and can produce toxic substances which have been implicated in some animal studies as potential carcinogens.

Knowledge of the rate of lipid oxidation is important in foods where it might be the principal mode of deterioration; for example: (1) fried snacks (e.g. chips), (2) nuts, (3) dried meats/vegetables/fish/poultry, (4) cereals, (5) wheat germ, (6) frozen vegetables/meats/fish/poultry, (7) some dairy products, (8) semi-moist meat products, (9) pre-cooked refrigerated meats and fish, (10) cured meat and fish, (11) coffee, (12) cooking and salad oils, (13) margarine, (14) spices, and (15) dried vegetables such as potatoes and carrots.

Rancidity development can be controlled directly by elimination of oxygen (which is very difficult to do) and by addition of antioxidants such as BHA, BHT and EDTA. The rate of reaction is also dependent on temperature to some degree (rate increases from 30% to 300% for 10 °C increase in storage temperature for dry foods) and on water availability or water activity. Very dry foods and semi-moist foods are most subject to rancidity. For example, as potato chips gain or lose moisture they become rancid faster. Light and trace metals (such as are used in fortification) also catalyze the reaction. Rancidity can also occur in the frozen state, where the rate can increase 600 to 1000% for a 10 °C increase in temperature. A knowledge of the rate of these reactions can be used to predict shelf-life and to open date foods. A knowledge of the rate of oxygen permeation into the food package is also necessary in order to predict shelf-life. In addition, the consumer must be instructed as to the extent and control of this reaction so as to better maintain the quality and nutritional value of the food in the home.

Nonenzymatic Browning (NEB). — Nonenzymatic browning (NEB) is another major chemical reaction leading to a loss of quality and nutritional value. This reaction is the result of reactions between reducing compounds (such as glucose, fructose and lactose) and proteins or amino acids. Browning can also occur as the result of heating sugars to very high temperatures (carmelization) or through the oxidation of vitamin C. In certain cases the reaction is desirable, such as in the toasting of the bread, the crust formed in roasting meats, malting of barley for beer and spirits manufacture, and the production of syrups, molasses and caramel candies.

Undesirable aspects of NEB lead to the production of bitter off-flavors, darkening of light-colored dry products such as nonfat dry milk, loss of protein solubility, toughening of protein foods and, most significantly, decrease in protein nutritional quality due to the binding of an essential amino acid, lysine, in the reaction. The NEB reaction leads to the end of shelf-life in processed proteins, dry milk and whey powders, dry whole egg, dehydrated meat and fish, frozen meat, fish, and poultry, breakfast cereals, cake mixes, fortified pasta, intermediate moisture breakfast bars and mixes, and some concentrated juices. In juices, ascorbic acid (vitamin C) acts as the reducing compound and results in loss of nutritional value as well.

The environmental factors which control NEB are temperature, pH and water activity (a_w). The rate of NEB is more sensitive to temperature than rancidity. In dry foods it increases in rate 400 to 800% for a 10° increase in storage temperature. In foods in which both reactions can occur, at high temperature NEB predominates while at low temperature rancidity predominates. Thus, during processing, exposure time at high temperature should be minimized since it leads to excessive browning precursors which can shorten shelf-life during subsequent storage. Lowering of pH slows browning but is not a desirable method of processing because of the flavor problem. The major control of browning is through control of the amount of water available in the food in which the reaction can occur. The lower the water content, the slower the reaction rate for the foods mentioned above. However, very moist foods such as fresh or canned products brown slowly because the reactants are diluted at the higher water content.

With respect to open dating, knowledge of the rate of browning as a function of temperature and water content is very important in order to accurately predict shelf-life. The rate of moisture gain through the package will also significantly affect shelf-life for these types of products.

Other Chemical Reactions. — Other chemical reactions that can lead to food degradation include the thermal destruction of vitamins such as

A, B_1 and C; the effect of light on pigments such as occurs in the browning of meat and bleaching of chlorophyll; the direct oxidation of vitamin C; the effect of light on riboflavin; and the direct oxidation of carotenoid pigments and the loss of flavor through some mechanism. In every case the effect of temperature, oxygen level, moisture content, and light must be known for the rate of the reaction to be predicted and the time to reach end of shelf-life measured. Of importance in all these reactions is a decision as to what extent of degradation is considered to be the end of shelf-life. In many cases the data must be correlated with actual organoleptic and sensory testing of the food so that the correct index of deterioration can be chosen.

Physical Degradation

Physical damage can also lead to loss of shelf-life. The types of physical damage can be classified into the following categories.

Physical Bruising/Crushing. — This mode of deterioration is related to physical abuse of the food in harvest, processing, and distribution. It is particularly important to fruits and vegetables, since physical abuse leads to microbial attack and decay. Packaging to prevent abuse is a key to long shelf-life. With dry materials such as chips, crushing can lead to unacceptability based on consumer desires. This cannot be equated to open dating or loss of shelf-life, but proper packaging and care can eliminate this problem.

Wilting. — Fresh leafy and tuber vegetables can deteriorate if subjected to low relative humidity, losing moisture to their surroundings. This results in loss of crispness and an increased rate of senescence reactions with subsequent quality and nutrient losses. Proper knowledge of the rate of moisture loss for various packaging materials and the maximum allowable moisture loss can be used as one means of setting open dates for fresh produce.

Moisture Loss/Gain. — With some food products such as candy, semi-moist pet foods, cakes and bread, moisture loss leads to an increase in hardening. If a limit of hardness is known to be unacceptable then predictions to reach this level based on equations which describe the moisture change with time, can be used as one method of prediction of end of shelf-life. From this, the open date for best quality can be set. These same equations can be used to predict the moisture loss of flour, pasta, and similar dry products for which a natural loss of moisture occurs and a net weight limit is set for sale. Similarly, some products that gain moisture have a textural limit at which they become too soft, such as potato chips, other dried or fried snacks, and crackers. In addition, some crystalline foods such as salt, brown sugar and convenience dry meal mixes, dry coffee, dry teas and dried drink mixes can gain enough moisture to become sticky and caked. Predictions of the end of shelf-life, based on a gain of a critical amount of moisture, can be made if the temperature/relative humidity conditions are known as a function of time, and the permeability of the package to moisture is known.

Temperature Induced Texture Changes. — Temperature fluctuations per se can affect physical modes of deterioration. For example, the continuous rise and fall of temperature around a phase change point leads to melting of fat and the subsequent degradation of quality of some candies and formulated foods. In frozen foods, repeated thawing and freezing causes loss of tissue moisture and increases chemical reaction rates. If the temperature fluctuation does not exceed the thawing point, package ice, which is a result of evaporation of the water from the food into the package space, with subsequent freezing as ice crystals, can occur. This results in consumer unacceptability. In addition, if the water loss is significant from a particular surface region, then freezer burn, an undesirable discoloration due to enhanced chemical reaction, can occur. This also is unacceptable to the consumer. Lastly, some temperature fluctuations can result in emulsion destabilization of products such as mayonnaise, margarine, salad dressings and dessert toppings. Knowledge of the sensitivity of these reactions to the degree of temperature fluctuation and a knowledge of the possible fluctuations occurring in distribution and in the home is needed in order to predict high quality shelf-life. In most cases manufacturers formulate the product to withstand any abuse that may occur. Heating itself can also cause texture changes. In this case the reaction is usually desirable as in the canning and/or cooking of vegetables, meat, fish and poultry. Canning at high temperature is usually undesirable for fruits as they lose their desirable crisp texture and develop a cooked flavor. These texture changes are usually not of concern in the storage deterioration of foods.

Staling. — Staling is a mode of deterioration important in processed wheat flour products such as bread and cakes. The reaction is basically a crystallization of amylopectin, one of the major starches present in wheat flour. The rate is increased as temperature decreases, which is opposite to the chemical, enzymatic, and microbial reactions discussed earlier. Thus, to prevent staling, the food must not be refrigerated. However, this can result in other reactions causing loss of shelf-life.

Chemically Induced Textural Changes. — As mentioned in the section on chemical degradation modes, both lipid oxidation and nonenzymatic browning can result in degradation of proteins, which leads to toughening and loss of shelf-life. Control and prediction were discussed previously.

BASIC FOOD PROCESSING PRINCIPLES

Introduction

The previous section discussed the modes of food deterioration that lead to loss of shelf-life and gave examples of the prevention of these deteriorative reactions. In this section the basic principles of the major food process methods will be outlined. Particular foods preserved by these methods will be discussed in detail in Chapter 4 with respect to modes of deterioration and open dating.

Use of Temperature

Heat Preservation. — The use of heat to preserve foods is based on the principles of: (1) destruction of pathogens; (2) destruction of spoilage microbes; (3) denaturation of enzymes; and (4) softening of tissues to make more of them digestible.

Blanching is the application of heat under mild conditions, or at high temperature for a short time, to achieve enzyme degradation and soften food tissues. It is used as a preprocess step for canning, freezing and drying to minimize loss of quality and nutrients before the product is preserved.

Pasteurization is a mild heat treatment used to reduce the number of live microorganisms in the food so as to extend its shelf-life and destroy important pathogens. The product is not sterile, so organisms can grow back and will eventually lead to the spoilage of the food. The mild treatment is used so as to not induce a cooked flavor. It can also be accomplished at high temperature for a shorter time period. Since microbes are more sensitive to an increase in temperature, this results in the same reduction of organisms but with less cooked flavor.

During canning, food is heat-treated to destroy all organisms of pathogenic nature and most important spoilage organisms. The process safety is based on the time needed to reduce the population of *Clostridium botulinum* by a factor of about ten billion at the most heat resistant point in the food. This organism is the most heat resistant and most harmful of the pathogens. Not all organisms are killed, however, since some are more heat resistant but do not grow under normal canned food storage conditions. They will grow and spoil the food if subjected to high temperature (40–50 °C). Processing to destroy these organisms will destroy the food quality. If adequate heat treatment is used, canned "commercially sterile" foods lose some color; lose 20–30% of some vitamins; have a cooked flavor; and develop a softer texture. Subsequent deterioration is usually confined to chemical modes of decay which do not require oxygen since the can is hermetically sealed.

Cold Preservation. — The basis of refrigeration and freezing is that the lower the temperature the slower the rate of most deteriorative reactions, such as senescence, enzymatic decay, chemical decay and microbial growth. Microbes usually cannot grow below −5 to −10 °C, so that freezing stops microbial growth. In some cases however, lower temperature increases degradation due to fracture of membranes and the subsequent release of degradative enzymes such as occurs in chill injury and freezing of some fresh fruits and vegetables. It has also been found that freezing some foods to just below the freezing point increases degradation rates by chemical reactions. This is because not all the water is frozen out and the chemicals are concentrated in the remaining water. Finally, some degradation microbes grow better at lower temperature since they have a lower optimum temperature, and thus compete better against other spoilage microorganisms.

Control of Water Content

Concentration and Drying. — As water is removed from a food, less of it is available as a solvent and medium for the degradation reactions. Thus, most chemical reactions decrease in rate as the water content decreases. Unfortunately, during the process of water removal, the reactants first begin to concentrate so that the rate of reaction can initially increase. To prevent this the temperature is kept low during the process or the drying is done rapidly to get through the danger zone. The degree of drying or concentration is best represented by a factor which describes the availability of water in the food: water activity (a_w). This is discussed in more detail in Chapter 3 with respect to the prediction of chemical reactions. The a_w is on a scale of 0 to 1, with 1 being the most available. Basically, as a_w is lowered, microbial decay is inhibited, with bacteria being the most sensitive, and molds the most resistant to lowered a_w. Browning, enzymatic activity, lipid oxidation and nutrient loss also decrease as a_w decreases with NEB showing a maximum in rate at an a_w of 0.6 to 0.8.

Concentration is used for foods such as frozen concentrated juices, concentrated canned soups, condensed sweetened milk, and as a preprocess step in the preparation of a liquid concentrate which is to be spray dried such as for dry milk, dry coffee, dry tea and some dry food supplements such as yeast. In these latter processes pre-concentration is used because it is a cheaper way than drying to remove water. However, not all water can be removed, so further drying is required. During concentration, the temperature of exposure is usually low since vacuum is used. Thus, cooked flavor and nutrient losses are diminished.

In drying, heat is applied to supply the energy to remove the water, and the relative humidity surrounding the food is lowered so that the water will be evaporated from the food. To achieve both, the air passing over the food is warmed, thus supplying energy and lowering the humidity. Solid piece materials like vegetables for soup mixes are dried in an air tunnel at 50 to 65 °C for 4 to 8 h. Slurry material (like potatoes) is dried in thin layers on hot rotating drums (120—140 °C) in 2—3 min. Although this process takes place at a higher temperature, less time is involved, so less quality and nutrient damage occurs. Concentrated liquids can be dried by spraying into a vertical tower through which high velocity air at 200 to 250 °C is passed. In this case drying occurs in 3 to 20 sec, so very little damage takes place. Freeze drying creates the least damage, since it occurs at low temperatures in a vacuum.

In each case the principle is to lower the water content and the a_w to a level such that during storage, reactions proceed at a very slow rate. It is therefore imperative that good packaging be used to prevent the chemical reactions described above, to prevent moisture which would allow microbial growth, and to prevent any physical changes caused by moisture gain. If the product contains unsaturated fat, it must also be vacuum packed or nitrogen flushed to slow the reaction. The rate of oxidation does not drop as much as desired at low oxygen pressure, but the lowering of total oxygen availability limits the overall extent of oxidation. Antioxidants actually have a much better effect on limiting the reaction but cannot be incorporated to all dry foods.

Humectant Use. — Rather than removing water by drying, the ability of the water present in foods to act as a medium and solvent can be reduced by adding water binding agents to the food. All dry food solids have this ability, but the lower the molecular weight, the better the water activity lowering effect. The common agents used are called humectants. Sugars and salts have this preservative ability and in fact, have been used in curing since ancient times. The basis of the process is the lowering of the a_w to a level below which pathogens and/or spoilage microbes cannot grow. Control of pH by adding acid and the addition of antimycotics, are usually done in conjunction with the use of humectants. The result is a shelf-stable food which does not require refrigeration. Common examples are the intermediate moisture pet foods, confectionaries, some bakery goods and breakfast tarts. These foods are subject to chemical deterioration because of the high a_w, and to moisture loss if left in a dry environment.

Extrusion. — Extrusion is a process utilized for many cereal foods, dry snacks, dry animal food and semi-moist pet foods. In this process, a dough is passed at high pressure by screw action through a heated cylinder. The heat causes the components to interact, giving the desired flavor, color, and texture. As the product is released from the screw the internal steam in the paste expands and flashes off. This results in further textural changes and drying of the product. In some cases further air drying may be used. Packaging requirements and modes of deterioration are similar to those described for dry foods. Of significance with extruded foods is moisture gain, which can result in a soft undesirable texture.

Other Methods. — Deep fat frying is a drying process, in that the hot oil evaporates off the water. In this process the oil replaces the water in the pores of the food. In baking, the hot air in the oven serves as the drying medium. The longer the baking time, the lower the final moisture of the product. Freezing also can be considered as a drying process. However, in this case the liquid water is converted into a solid which becomes unavailable. It should be noted that for most foods, about 20—30% of the water is still not frozen at —20 °C. Therefore reactions are not stopped by freezing, only slowed down, both to lower water availability and low temperature.

Chemical Preservation

Fermentation. — Fermentation is one of the oldest of the known food processes. In this method, a desirable organism is allowed to partially convert some of the carbohydrates of the food material into acid, alcohol and flavor compounds. This can be done naturally by changing the environment of the food so that the desired organisms can grow (e.g., addition of salt to cabbage inhibits spoilage bacteria and allows the desirable bacteria to grow). Industrially, a starter culture of the desired organism may be added to insure that the proper fermentation takes place. The basic principle of the process is to allow the formation of desirable chemicals, such as acids or alcohol, which prevent the growth of undesirable spoilage or pathogenic organisms. The shelf-life of fermented foods is limited by the growth of the desired organism. In some cases further processing is done, such as in pasteurization of beer, wine, and vinegar, or the product is kept refrigerated, such as with yogurt and cheeses.

Additives. — Chemical additives can be used to preserve and/or prolong the shelf-life of foods. Each has a specific action by which it operates. The various classes are listed below.

(1) Acids, such as citric and phosphoric. These lower the pH and inhibit undesirable microbes as well as slowing undesirable enzymatic and chemical reactions. Acids also contribute to flavor.

(2) Humectants, such as salt, sugar and glycerol. These bind the water present, lowering its activity and thus reducing the rates of microbial growth, enzymatic activity and chemical reactions.

(3) Smoking of foods, a process which deposits chemicals from the

smoke which inhibits microbial action on the surface of foods. The heat also destroys some of the microbes.

(4) Metabolic inhibitors, such as calcium propionate and sodium benzoate. These chemicals act against specific types of microbes. They are used where further processing of the food results in indesirable quality and nutritional changes. Gases can also be used as chemical sterilants and to deinfestate grain. Ethylene oxide is an example, as is chlorine applied in a solution.

(5) Anti-caking agents, such as the silicates. These are high water binding agents used in dry powdered or crystalline foods to prevent caking by selectively binding water.

(6) Antioxidants, such as BHA. These act in the lipid oxidation reaction to slow the rate and thus extend shelf-life.

(7) Chelating agents, such as EDTA and citric acid. These chemicals tie up trace metals to prevent them from catalyzing undesirable reactions such as rancidity.

(8) Other chemicals such as calcium salts are used to prevent softening of fruits and vegetables during the canning process. Sodium polyphosphates help to hold water in cured and canned meats. Sulfite not only inhibits microbes but slows down enzymatic browning reactions. Some additives are used for mainly aesthetic purposes to enhance or restore those flavors or colors lost during normal preservation, or for manufacture of engineered foods. Finally, nutrients can be added to restore those lost during preservation.

Separation

Separation processes are used either to create new foods or ingredients (making butter out of milk) or to transform a raw food into a more digestible or more stable form (making flour from wheat). There are many different processes which incorporate those methods already discussed above. For example, in the manufacture of instant coffee, after harvest the bean is fermented, ground, roasted, leached to form a liquid (the separation step), concentrated, then spray dried and packaged. The shelf-life of the product would depend on the effects of each step.

Gas Atmosphere Control

The shelf-life of many fruits and vegetables is dependent on the rate of respiration after harvest, which uses up the storage energy. This rate can be reduced by reduction of the availability of oxygen or an increase in CO_2 levels. The methods are generally classified as controlled atmospheric storage (CA) and include: (1) Reduction and control of O_2 by use of nitrogen. (2) Hypobaric storage by pulling a vacuum either in a large truck or in a pouch. (3) Use of both increased nitrogen and increased carbon dioxide in the head space.

Carbon dioxide can also be injected into the headspace of diary and meat packages to reduce microbial growth and increase shelf-life. Vacuum packaging with CO_2 injection is used to enhance shelf-life of poultry products. Overall, shelf-life in these cases depends on the degree of maturity after harvest, temperature, and permeability of the package to oxygen and carbon dioxide.

DISTRIBUTION HAZARDS

Once a food is preserved and packaged it is not stable forever. Each food system slowly decays or deteriorates to the point where it is unacceptable. One goal of open dating should be to give consumers information as to the shelf-life of the product so that it is consumed before it is unacceptable. The loss of acceptability however, does not necessarily mean the product is inedible, only that the established consumer quality standard has been passed. The problem is therefore twofold: (1) setting a standard for unacceptability; and (2) determining or predicting the loss that occurs from point of distribution to point of consumption.

Data on actual shelf-life modes and shelf-lives of various products based on some endpoint standards are presented in Chapter 4. Chapter 3 will discuss the second problem, i.e., based on environmental factors, how one can predict changes in shelf-life. The important environmental influences include:

(1) Temperature
- (a) increasing
- (b) decreasing
- (c) fluctuations

(2) Moisture (relative humidity)
- (a) gain
- (b) loss

(3) Oxygen level

(4) Light.

REFERENCES

ANON. 1977. The role of processing in extending the food supply. Dairy Council Dig. *48* (4), July-Aug.

BORGSTROM, G. 1968. Principles of Food Science, Vol. 1. Food Technology. Macmillan Co., New York.

CLYDESDALE, F.M. and FRANCIS, F.J. 1977. Food, Nutrition and You. Prentice-Hall, Englewood Cliffs, N.J.

DESROSIER, N.W. 1977. Technology of Food Preservation, 4th Edition. AVI Publishing Co., Westport, Conn.

DEUTSCH, R.M. 1976. Realities of Nutrition. Bull Publishing Co., Palo Alto, Calif.

LABUZA, T.P. 1977. Food and Your Well Being. West Publishing, St. Paul, Minn.

NICKERSON, J.T.R. and RONSIVALLI, L. 1977. Elementary Food Science. AVI Publishing Co., Westport, Conn.

POTTER, N.N. 1975. Food Science, 2nd Edition, AVI Publishing Co., Westport, Conn.

U.S. GOVERNMENT PRINTING OFFICE. 1979. Open Shelf Life Dating of Foods. No. 052-003-00694-4.

CHAPTER 3

SCIENTIFIC EVALUATION OF SHELF-LIFE

INTRODUCTION

Chapter 2 covered the principles of processing and major modes of deterioration of foods. It can be concluded that one of the major environmental factors that results in increased loss of quality and nutrition for most foods is exposure to increased temperature. The higher the temperature the greater is the loss of food quality. In order to predict the extent of high quality life, and to be able to put a shelf-life date on a product, a knowledge of the rate of deterioration as a function of environmental conditions is necessary. Coupled with this is the need for gaining knowledge of the actual environmental conditions the various classes of foodstuffs are exposed to during processing, distribution and handling.

The U.S. Army supported some major studies during the late 1940s through 1953 to gain this information for the military food supply. The studies are summarized in *Long Term Storage of Military Rations* (Cecil and Woodroof 1962). Basically, for each food item, each mode of deterioration was studied at several temperatures for up to three years. In addition, information as to temperatures in warehouses, boxcars, etc. was gathered. The results of this study included many reports and tables (such as Table 3.1, from Army Technical Manual TM743-200). However, much of this is inapplicable today because the foods are processed differently, different packaging systems are used, and the distribution system has changed. One interesting outcome of the report was a nomograph as in Fig. 3.1 which gives the prediction of quality for various food classes based on some rate of deterioration and a desired shelf-life. What this graph says is that, given a certain rate of loss, if it is constant, one can predict the amount of change. Unfortunately, this simple method is not correct for many foods and for many modes of deterioration such as nutrient loss, color change, and flavor change. The next section will cover the basic principles of how temperature affects the rate of food deterioration.

TABLE 3.1
STORAGE LIFE OF SEMI-PERISHABLE FOODS

Item	Keeping time in months (approximate)			
	Packaging	40 °F	70 °F	90 °F
Almond paste	can	36	9	3
Apple				
Regular pack	can	72	36	21
Butter	can/jar	48	18	10
Sauce	can	72	36	24
Baby food, drained	jar	36	18	12
Dehydrated (instant)	can	36	24	12
Dietetic pack	can	66	42	15
Junior food	jar	36	18	12
Juice	can	60	63	12
Dehydrated	can	60	36	12
Single strength	can	60	36	12
Apricots				
Regular pack				
Baby food, strained	jar	30	18	9
Dietary pack	can	56	30	12
Dried	carton	24	3	1
Freeze dehydrated	can	24	12	5
Apricot nectar				
Regular pack	can	48	24	10
Freeze dehydrated	can	24	12	5
Asparagus	can	60	36	12
Baby formula preparation	can	24	12	3
Bacon				
Sliced	can	48	18	12
Sliced, irradiated	can	48	38	12
Sliced, prefried		48	38	12
Bakery mixes	can	48	36	9
	bag/carton	12	6	3
Baking powder	can	24	12	6
Baking soda	carton	indef.	indef.	indef.
Barley, pearl	bag/carton	36	24	12
Banana, baby food, strained	jar	24	12	6
Beans				
Dried	bag/carton	24	12	9
Green, baby food, strained	jar	30	18	9
Green, regular	can	60	36	12
Green, junior food	jar	30	18	9

continued . . .

TABLE 3.1 (Continued)

Approximate Storage Life, Months	
Apple	18
Apple juice, concentrated	30
Asparagus	10
Bacon	
Slab, type I	5½
Slab, type II	12
Sliced, type I	1½
Sliced, type I vacuum packed	3
Sliced, type II	2¼
Sliced, type II vacuum packed	4½
Beans	
Green	10
Lima	14
Wax	10
Beef	
Boneless, fabricated (without meat)	10
Boneless, fabricated (with ground meat)	8
Carcass, wholesale cuts	10
Corned	6
Dried, sliced	12
Ground	4
Ground patties	3
Liver, whole or portion cut	4
Tongue, fresh	4
Tongue, cured or smoked,	
Type I	6
Type II	4
Blackberries	18
Blueberries	18
Bologna	
Lebanon	8
50% beef	3-4
60% beef	3-4
75% beef	6
Boysenberries	18
Bread dough	6
Bread yeast raised (and rolls fresh)	6
Broccoli	11
Brussel sprouts	11
Butter prints and patties	12
Carrots	24
Cauliflower	14
Cervelat	
Dry	6
Soft (thuringer)	3-4
Cherries, RSP	24
Chicken	
Parts, cut up, ready-to-cook	8
Whole, ready-to-cook	10
Clams, shucked	9
Corn	24
Corn on the cob	9
Cream	8
Dates	12
Duck	10
Eggs	
Whole (including table grade)	9
Whites	12
Yolks	12
Fish, fillets, portions, steaks (varies with species)	3-9
Frankfurters — 50% beef, 50% pork	
Type I, carton	1½
Type I, flexible package	1
Type II, carton	2½
Type II, flexible package	6
Type III, flexible package	12
Type III, can with thaw indicator	15
Grape juice, concentrated	24
Grapefruit juice, concentrated	24
Grapefruit-orange juice, concentrated	24
Grapefruit sections	12
Greens, leafy	14
Hams	
Boneless	6
Smoked, bone in	6
Ice cream, sherbets or ices	9
Lamb	
Boneless, fabricated	6
Carcass, whole cuts	8
Slices, chops	6
Telescoped	8
Lemon juice, concentrated	18
Lime juice, concentrated	18
Lime juice, single strength	18
Lobster tail	8
Lobster, whole	8
Luncheon loaf	3-4
Margarine, prints and patties	12
Meal, precooked (TV dinners, pot pies, etc.	6
Milk fat, anhydrous	12
Milk, pasteurized, homogenized	1

continued . . .

TABLE 3.1 (Continued)

Milk, pasteurized, homogenized, sterilized	3	Liver	3-4
		New England style	4
Milk, whole, concentrated	9	Pork, bulk style	3
Okra	12	Pork, links	
Orange juice, concentrated	24	Type I, carton	3-4
Oysters	9	Type II, carton	2
Peaches	18	Type III, carton	3
Peas		Type III, can	3-4
Black eyed	12	Pork, precooked	3-4
Dehydrofrozen	14	Pork and beef, precooked	6
Green	14	Scallops	8
Peas and carrots	14	Shrimp	
Peppers	12	Raw, peeled/unpeeled	8
Pies, fruit, baked and unbaked	4	Raw, breaded, molded	8
Pineapple	12	Soups	12
Pineapple juice, concentrated	24	Spinach	14
Pizza shells	6	Squash, summer	24
Pork	4	Strawberries	18
Diced	4	Succotash	12
Loin, boneless, fabricated	4	Sweet goods, yeast raised	2
Slices, chops	4	Topping desert	24
Wholesale, cuts	6	Turkey	
Potatoes white, French fries	12	Boneless, cooked	9
Rabbit		Boneless, raw	8
Ready-to-cook	6	Whole, ready-to-cook	10
Ready-to-cook, cut up	5	Veal	
Berries	24	Diced	6
Rhubarb	24	Boneless, fabricated	6
Salami		Carcass, wholesale cuts	8
Cooked	3-4	Semi-boneless	8
Dry	5	Vegetables, mixed	10
Sausage		Waffles	1

BASIC REACTION KINETICS FOR PREDICTING THE LOSS OF FOOD QUALITY

Basic Equation

The loss of food quality for most foods can be represented by a mathematical equation of the following form:

$$\frac{dA}{d\theta} = kA^n \tag{1}$$

where: A = the quality factor measured

θ = time

k = a constant which depends on temperature and water activity

n = a power factor called the order of the reaction which defines whether the rate is dependent on the amount of A present

$\frac{dA}{d\theta}$ = the rate of change of A with time. A negative sign is used if the deterioration is a loss of A and a positive sign if it is for production of an undesirable end-product.

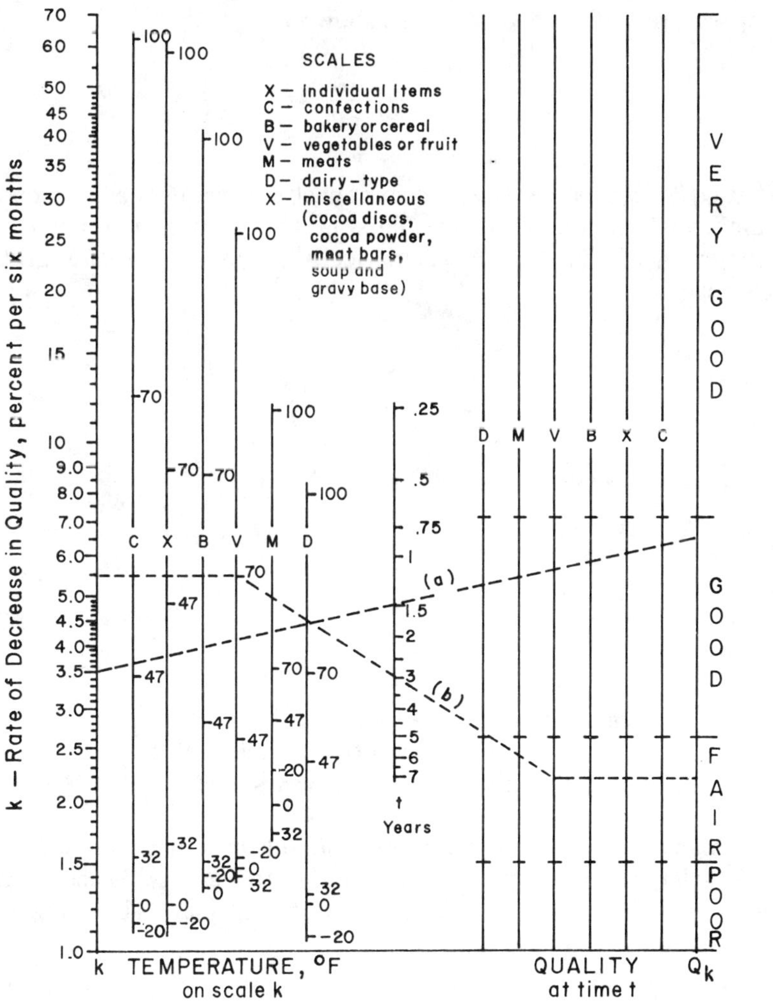

FIGURE 3.1. NOMOGRAM OF TEMPERATURE, TIME, AND QUALITY FOR THE MILITARY RATION ITEMS USED IN THE LONG-TERM STORAGE TESTS.

Usually, results of shelf-life studies are not obtained as a rate but rather as the amount of A as a function to time. Thus, to get the rate of deterioration, one must transform the data into a kinetic plot. Unfortunately, most of the data in the literature for foods have not been analyzed in this way and can lead to erroneous results in prediction of true shelf-life.

Constant Loss of Shelf-Life

Based on eq (1), much of the food literature assumes (without truly measuring it) that the value of $n = 0$. This assumption, called a zero order reaction scheme, then implies that the rate of loss at constant temperature and a_w is constant, as shown in eq (2):

$$-\frac{dA}{d\theta} = k \qquad (2)$$

What eq (2) says is that the percent of shelf-life lost per day is constant at some constant temperature. This is the assumption used in the nomograph of Fig. 3.1. Mathematically, if eq (2) were integrated as follows:

$$-\int_{A_o}^{A_e} dA = \int_0^{\theta_s} k d\theta \qquad (3)$$

then $A = A_o - k\theta$ (4)

or $A_e = A_o - k\theta_s$ (5)

where A_o = initial quality value
A = amount left after time θ
A_e = value of A at end of shelf-life (could be zero or any other defined value)
θ_s = shelf-life in days, months, years, etc.

In many cases A is not a very quantifiable or measurable value and is based solely on human panel evaluation. In this case A_o is assumed to be 100% quality and A_e is just unacceptable quality. Thus, the rate of deterioration or the rate constant is:

$$k = \frac{100\%}{\theta_s} = \text{constant \% per day} \tag{6}$$

This is the assumption of Fig. 3.1. Technically, the major problem in shelf-life testing is to verify that indeed n = 0, so that eqs (4), (5) or (6) can be used. Based on prior work, some modes of deterioration are applicable directly to zero order kinetics. These include: (1) Enzymatic degradation (fresh fruits and vegetables, some frozen foods, some refrigerated doughs); (2) Nonenzymatic browning (e.g. dry cereals, dry dairy products, dry pet foods, loss of protein nutritional value); (3) Lipid oxidation (rancidity development in snacks, dry foods, pet foods, frozen foods).

Based on this knowledge, then, one can predict the shelf-life of a food at a given single temperature if the amount of loss at any time is known. For example, if it is known that a certain food has lost 50% of its quality in 100 days when held at some constant temperature, then:

$$k = \frac{A_o - A}{\theta} = \frac{100-50}{100} = 0.5\% \text{ per day}$$

Based on this we can construct Fig. 3.2, which gives the shelf-life left as a function of time (k is the slope of the line). As seen at 40 days there is 80% shelf-life left, at 160 days there is 20% left, etc.

The problem, of course, in constructing this graph is determining the criteria for establishing what is to be measured (i.e. what is A) or how much of A must be lost to give an end of shelf-life as perceived by the consumer. It must be noted that shelf-life is not a function of time; rather it is a function of the environmental conditions and the amount of quality change that can be allowed. The problem, however, is that food distribution occurs at variable temperature so that the data must be collected at several temperatures to be useful. Methods to apply these equations to variable temperature will be described later.

Variable Shelf-life Loss Function: First Order

As discussed above, the shelf-life in many cases does not follow a simple constant rate of degradation. In fact, the value of n can range for many reactions from zero to any fractional value or whole value up to 2. Many foods that do not deteriorate by zero order follow a pattern where n = 1 which results in an exponential decrease in rate of loss as quality decreases. This does not mean that the shelf-life of foods that follow this scheme is longer than those with a constant rate, since the value of the rate constant k is different. Mathematically for n = 1 or a first order reaction, the rate of loss is:

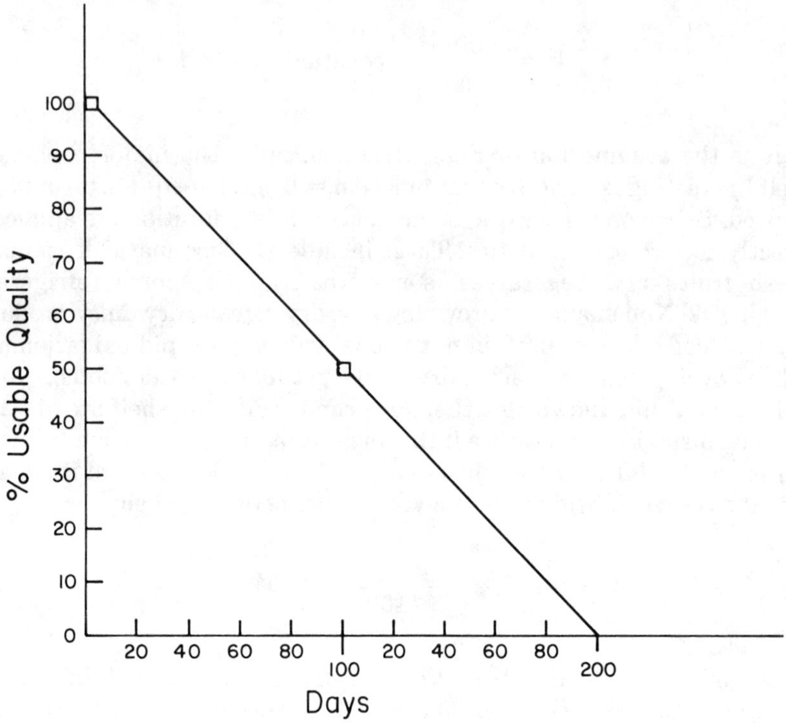

FIG. 3.2. CONSTANT SHELF-LIFE LOST

$$\frac{-dA}{d\theta} = kA^1 \tag{7}$$

Thus, the rate of loss of quality is directly dependent on the amount left. In other words, as quality (A) decreases, the rate of loss of quality slows down. Integration of eq (7) gives:

$$\int_{A_o}^{A} \frac{dA}{A} = -\int_{0}^{\theta} k d\theta \tag{8}$$

$$\ln \frac{A}{A_o} = -k\theta \tag{9}$$

or

$$\ln \frac{A_E}{A_o} = -k\theta_s \tag{10}$$

where A = amount left at time θ
A_E = amount left at end of shelf-life θ_s (not = 0)
k = the rate constant in units of reciprocal time

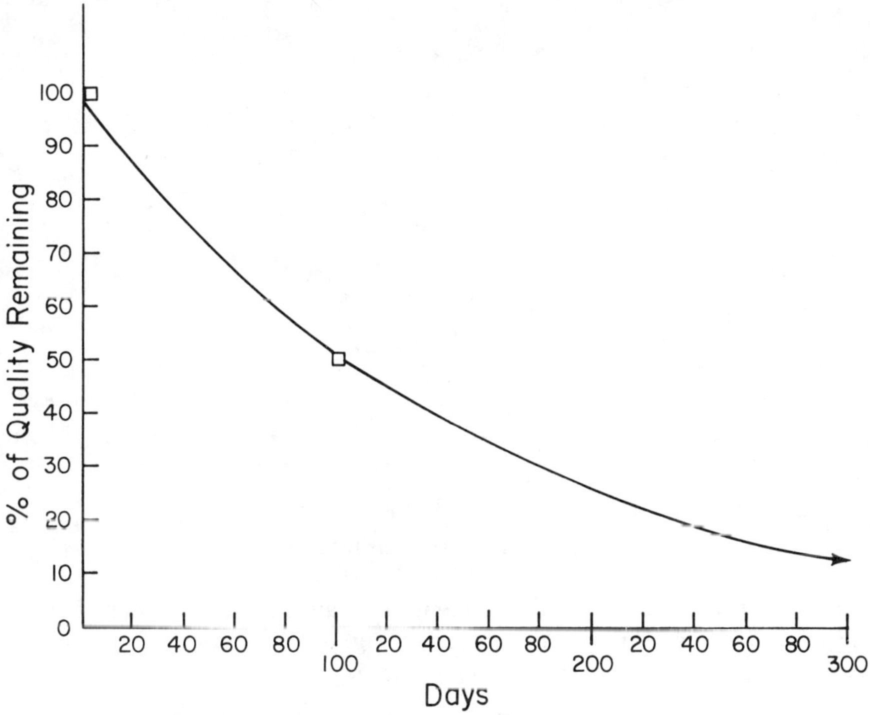

FIG. 3.3. 1ST ORDER DEGRADATION

A plot of amount left vs time is not a straight line, as is illustrated in Fig. 3.3. If 50% of the quality is lost in 100 days as in the previous example, then at 40 days, there is 76% of the quality left, whereas for a constant rate of loss there was 80% left. At 100 days both mechanisms give the same percent left, but after this time the quality loss slows down for the first order mechanism and theoretically never reaches a zero value. For example, at 160 days there is 33% left and at 300 days there is still 12.5% left. This example shows that it is quite important to know the order of the reaction. The types of deterioration that follow n = 1 are:

(1) Rancidity (as in salad oils or dry vegetables).

(2) Microbial growth (fresh meat and fish) and death (heat treatment).

(3) Microbial production of off-flavors and slime, such as in meat, fish and poultry.

(4) Vitamin losses (canned and dry foods).

(5) Loss of protein quality (dry foods).

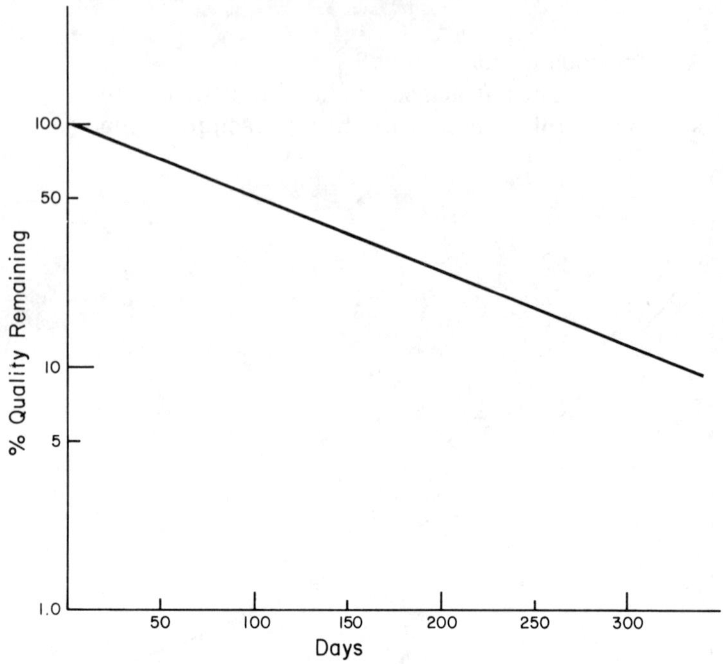

FIG. 3.4. FIRST ORDER LOG PLOT

Another way of representing exponential decay is to plot the loss of quality vs time on semilog paper, as seen in Fig. 3.4. The slope of this line at constant temperature is the value k where:

$$k = \frac{0.693}{\theta_{1/2}}$$

where $\theta_{1/2}$ is the half-life. Mathematically, if one knows the amount of degradation at any time and at some temperature, and that it follows a first order reaction, Fig. 3.4 can be easily constructed. If the end of the shelf-life is defined as being less than 50% of the total change possible, the less the percent change for end of shelf-life the less difference it makes whether the reaction is calculated as zero or first order, as seen in Table 3.2. Obviously, the better the data are at a given temperature, the better is the estimate of the value of n. In essence, the less the change required to reach end of acceptability as compared to the total change that could occur, the less important is the need for knowing exactly what the value of the order of the reaction is.

TABLE 3.2
TIME TO REACH A GIVEN CHANGE IN QUALITY

% Change	Time for Zero Order	Time for First Order	Difference in Days
A. If 20% change in 100 days = end of shelf-life:			
5	25	23	+2
10	50	47	+3
15	75	73	+2
20	100	100	0
B. If 30% change in 100 days = end of shelf-life:			
5	17	14	+3
10	33	30	+3
15	50	46	+4
20	67	63	+4
25	83	81	+2
30	100	100	0
C. If 50% change in 100 days = end of shelf-life:			
10	20	15	+5
20	40	32	+8
30	60	52	+8
40	80	74	+6
50	100	100	0

As stated earlier, first order kinetics can be applied to microbial growth and death. Microbe death is not generally applicable during shelf-life of foods but eq (7) can be rewritten to represent it as:

$$-\frac{dN}{d\theta} = -k_D N \qquad (7A)$$

which in integrated form is:

$$\ln \frac{N}{N_o} = -k_D\theta \qquad (7B)$$

where N_o = initial load
N = load at time θ
k_D = death rate constant in reciprocal time

Most microbiologists deal in a term called D value, where D is the time θ_D to reach a one log cycle destruction in number or:

$$D = \frac{2.3}{k_D} = \theta_D \tag{7C}$$

There is much literature concerning this and it will not be presented here.

Bacterial growth also follows a first order reaction after an initial lag phase. Some data indicating this will be shown in Chapter 4, with regard to fresh foods. The equation representing growth is similar:

$$\frac{dN}{d\theta} = k_G N \tag{7D}$$

where k_G = growth rate constant

also

$$k_G = \frac{\ln 2}{G} = \frac{0.693}{G} = \frac{2.3}{D_G} \tag{7E}$$

G = time for one doubling

D_G = time for 1 log cycle increase in number.

Usually, G is determined from the log phase of growth thus:

$$G = \frac{0.693 D_G}{2.3} \tag{7F}$$

Some values are reported in Table 3.3. As seen, the increase in growth rate for a 10°C increase in temperature (Q_{10}) is around 2—3, but some organisms are more temperature sensitive and could pose problems in food if the generation time was small.

Other Orders

Very few data exist describing food degradation by orders other than zero or first. Lee *et al.* (1977) and Sing *et al.* (1976) have described the degradation of vitamin C in liquid foods such as tomato juice or canned infant formulas by a second order reaction. In this case, the reaction is dependent on both ascorbate and oxygen and thus, as the oxygen is depleted the rate of loss of ascorbate becomes less than that predicted by a first order reaction.

Labuza (1971A) has reviewed the area of lipid oxidation kinetics and has found that oxygen uptake generally follows a half order reaction with respect to oxygen for relatively pure lipids. However, addition of antioxidants changes the order to first order. In complex foods, however, the data best fit zero order kinetics.

TABLE 3.3
MICROBIAL GENERATION TIME IN HOURS[1]

	Generation Time								
	0 °C	2—2.5 °C	4—5 °C	10 °C	14-15 °C	20 °C	30-32 °C	E_a (kcal/mole)	Q_{10}
Clostridium hastiforme	—	—	73.0	25.5	14.5	—	—	25.68	5.05
Clostridium 61	17.0	—	—	9.0	5.0	3.5	—	12.70	2.23
Bacillus W25	23.0	—	8.5	6.0	3.0	2.5	—	17.13	2.94
Bacillus W16B	24.0	—	11.5	7.0	2.8	2.5	—	18.85	3.28
Bacillus coagulans	—	24.0-30.0	—	—	—	—	—	—	—
Bacillus (Group A)	30.0	13.0-19.0	7.5-14.0	4.0-4.5	—	—	—	28.56	6.05
Pseudomonas 92	26.6	—	11.7	5.4	2.3	1.7	0.90	18.87	3.29
Pseudomonas 69	29.1	—	14.7	6.5	2.7	1.9	0.85	20.47	3.63
Pseudomonas fluorescens	—	—	8.2	3.5	2.0	1.5	1.2	12.41	2.19
Pseudomonas fluorescens (P-200)	35.0	13.7	—	4.0	2.0	1.5	0.85	12.41	2.19
Pseudomonas fluorescens	30.2	—	6.7	—	—	1.4	—	22.71	4.18
Pseudomonas fragi	11.3	7.7	5.0	2.6	—	1.1	—	18.17	3.14
Pseudomonas (21-3c)	20.0	9.2	7.3	3.2	2.0	1.3	0.77	16.96	2.91
Pseudomonas (1-3b)	10.3	8.0	7.0	2.7	2.3	1.6	0.93	13.50	2.34
Aerobacter aerogenes (Ps48)	37.7	—	12.2	4.1	2.2	1.3	0.8	21.17	3.80
Gram negative rod									
aerobic	21.2	—	4.3	—	—	1.4	—	19.49	3.42
anaerobic	23.4	—	9.8	—	—	0.6	—	29.27	6.32
Gram negative rod	20.0	—	7.6(6 °C)	1.9(12 °C)	—	—	0.78	16.85	2.89
Achromobacter—7	—	7.1	5.3	2.5	1.8	1.4	1.6	6.73	1.53
Achromobacter 438	—	7.8	6.0	2.5	1.8	1.3	1.5	10.61	1.95
Achromobacter 5	—	—	7.4	3.1	1.8	1.4	—	17.95	3.10
Pseudomonas 451	—	13.8	9.7	4.0	2.0	1.2	0.8	17.75	3.06

[1]Tompkin (1973)

TEMPERATURE DEPENDENCE OF RATE OF DETERIORATION

The above mathematical analyses of loss of quality assumed a constant temperature. The temperature dependent part of either the zero or first order equation is the rate constant k. Theoretically, k obeys the Arrhenius relationship which states that:

$$k = k_o e^{-E_A/RT} \tag{11}$$

where k_o = a pre-exponent constant
E_A = the activation energy in cal/mole
R = the gas constant in cal/mole °K and equals 1.986
T = the temperature in °K (°C + 273)

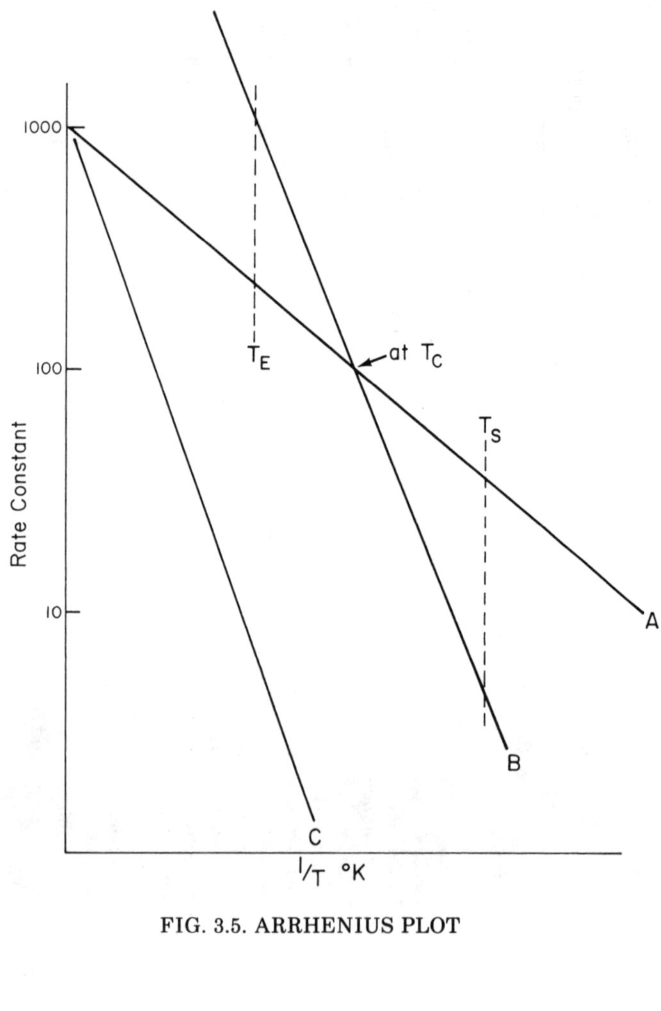

FIG. 3.5. ARRHENIUS PLOT

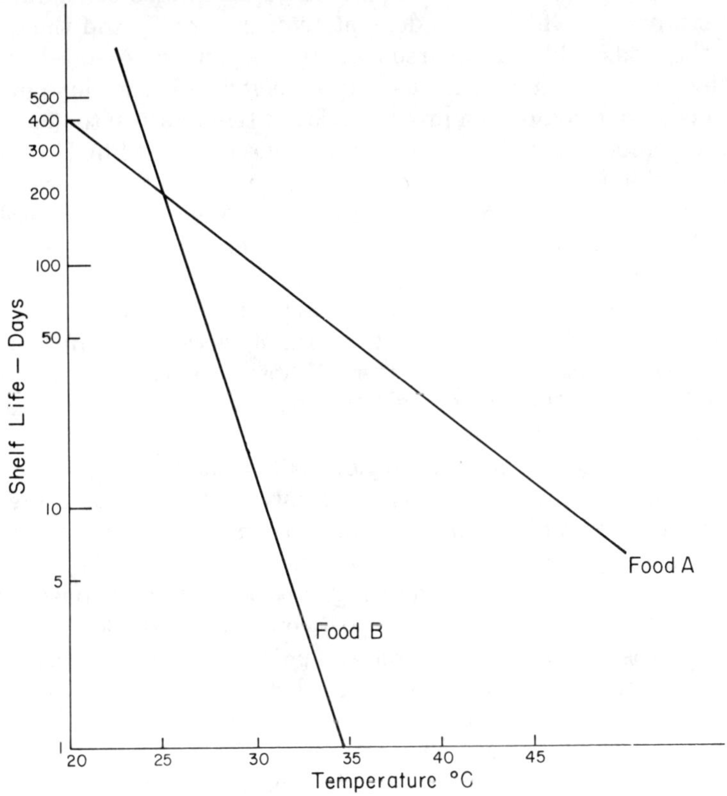

FIG. 3.6. SHELF-LIFE PLOT

Thus, a plot of the rate constant on semi-log paper as a function of reciprocal (absolute) temperature (1/T) gives a straight line. As an example, three systems are theoretically represented in Fig. 3.5. The slope of each line is equal to the activation energy divided by R. A steeper slope means the reaction is more temperature dependent; i.e. as the temperature increases, the reaction increases at a faster rate. Thus, in Fig. 3.5, B and C have the same temperature dependence, and increase in rate more rapidly than A as temperature increases (1/T becomes less).

This graph also illustrates that, for A and B at some possible temperature, the rates are the same; however, above and below this level their relative rates are different. Thus, at temperatures below T_c (i.e. larger 1/T) the rate of loss of A is faster than B; above T_c, B is lost more rapidly than A. What this could mean is that for a food with two modes of deterioration, the mode of deterioration may change with temperature, which could create a problem in predicting shelf-life. For example, if a single study of shelf-life were done at temperature T_E and the quality loss in the food could be measured by both mechanisms A and B, B would be faster and would result in the end of shelf-life. If the slope of line B were known, one could then project to lower temperature to get the rate at T_s (the temperature of storage) and thus get the shelf-life. However, as seen, at T_s the rate of deterioration for mode A is faster than for B, so the true shelf-life could be much less than estimated. Unfortunately not enough data are available on food reactions to determine whether this is a likely occurrence.

Most data for modes of deterioration in the literature do not give rates or rate constants but rather are in the form of overall shelf-life (end-point analysis) as a function of temperature. Villota *et al.* (1980) have recently analyzed the literature for dehydrated foods to try to determine order and shelf-life. Using the above mathematical models the end-point data can be transformed into a shelf-life plot as illustrated by Fig. 3.6, which is usually a straight line. Theoretically, if only a small temperature range from the Arrhenius plot is used (no more than a 20—40 °C change) then the same data will give a fairly straight line on the shelf-life plot.

Two examples are illustrated in Fig. 3.6, both of which pass through 200 days at 25 °C. What is needed to construct this plot is: (1) some measure of loss of quality; (2) some end-point value for unacceptability; (3) the order of the reaction so as to predict the time to reach this end-point; and (4) experiments to measure this loss at least at two temperatures so the line can be constructed.

It is obvious from the graph that the steeper the slope, the more sensitive is the food (or the reaction) to temperature change. A measure of this sensitivity is called the Q_{10} of the reaction, which is defined as:

$$Q_{10} = \frac{\text{rate at temperature } (T + 10\,^\circ\text{C})}{\text{rate at temperature } T\,^\circ\text{C}} \tag{12}$$

The Q_{10} can also be calculated from the shelf-life plot as:

$$Q_{10} = \frac{\text{shelf-life at } T\,^\circ\text{C}}{\text{shelf-life at } (T + 10\,^\circ\text{C})} = \frac{\theta_{s_T}}{\theta_{s_{T+10}}} \tag{13}$$

which assumes that the rate is inversely proportional to the shelf-life. For a zero order reaction this is exactly true since:

$$\text{rate} = k = \frac{\text{amount lost at end-point}}{\theta_s}$$

If the amount lost at θ_s is defined, then the Q_{10} can be calculated as in eq (13). A similar relationship can be derived for first order reactions to also show that Q_{10} can be calculated by eq (13). Thus, the fit of data to Fig. 3.6 gives no clue as to reaction order.

From Fig. 3.6 it can be calculated that for food A the Q_{10} is (for example):

$$Q_{10} = \frac{\theta_s \text{ at } 25\,°C}{\theta_s \text{ at } 35\,°C} = \frac{200}{50} = 4$$

For food B the Q_{10} is:

$$Q_{10} = \frac{800}{3} = 266$$

Thus, food B or reaction B is much more sensitive to temperature change than A is. Theoretically, the Q_{10} and the activation energy can be related by:

$$\log_{10} Q_{10} = \frac{2.19\ E_A}{(T)\ (T + 10)} \tag{14}$$

Figure 3.6 illustrates the usefulness of a shelf-life plot when applied to studying the loss of quality, since it shows that holding a food at a higher temperature causes it to degrade faster. Thus, if studies at two different temperatures are made, the shelf-life at some lower temperature can be predicted if the line is assumed to be straight. One cannot, however, study the deterioration at only one temperature since it is not possible to predict beforehand the slope of the line or the Q_{10} exactly. Table 3.4 illustrates how important the Q_{10} would be for prediction of shelf-life at lower temperature. It should be noted that different reactions may occur at different temperatures to cause end of product acceptability, so the projected line might be incorrect. Therefore, in Fig. 3.6 reaction B would cause end of shelf-life in 12 days at 30 °C, but below 25 °C reaction A is faster and would cause the end of shelf-life.

TABLE 3.4
SHELF-LIFE AT GIVEN TEMPERATURE FOR GIVEN Q_{10}

	Q_{10}				
Shelf-life at	2	2.5	3	4	5
50 °C	2 wk	2 wk	2 wk	2 wk	2 wk
40 °C	4 wk	5 wk	6 wk	8 wk	10 wk
30 °C	8 wk	12.5 wk	18 wk	32 wk	50 wk
20 °C	16 wk	31.3 wk	54 wk	2.5 yr	4.8 yr

SHELF-LIFE PREDICTION FOR VARIABLE TEMPERATURE

Given the data as to the mathematical model of the reaction causing end of shelf-life can be obtained and a shelf-life plot constructed, some simple expressions can be derived to predict the extent of deterioration as a function of a variable time-temperature storage condition.

Zero Order Reaction Prediction

For zero order the expression is as follows:

$$A = A_o - \sum_{i=o}^{i=n} (k_i\theta_i) \qquad (15)$$

where $\sum k_i\theta_i$ = the sum of the product of the rate constant (k_i at each given temperature T_i) × the time interval (θ_i) at the average temperature T_i for the given time period $\Delta\theta$.

The time-temperature history is broken up into suitable time periods as illustrated in Fig. 3.7, and the average temperature in that time period can be found. The rate constant for this period is then calculated from the shelf-life plot using a zero order reaction and this rate constant is multiplied by the time during the period to get $k_i\theta_i$. The increments of $k_i\theta_i$ are added up to get the total amount lost at any time.

If shelf-life is based simply on some time to reach unacceptability, eq (15) can be simplified to give:

$$f_c = \text{fraction shelf-life consumed} = \sum \left(\frac{\theta_i}{\theta_s}\right)_{T_i} \qquad (16)$$

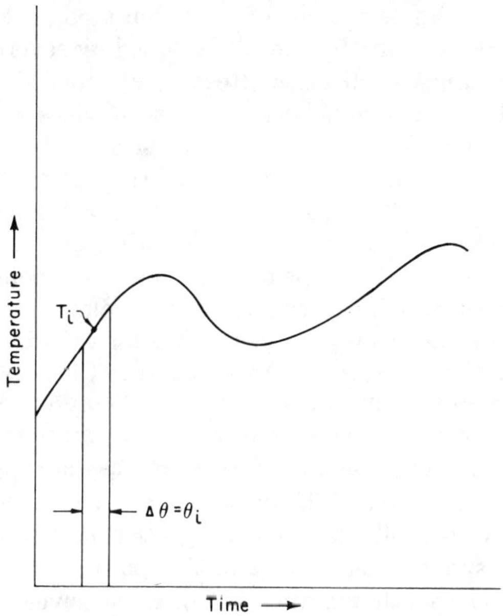

FIG. 3.7. TEMPERATURE-TIME HISTORY

This equation utilizes the same techniques as before. The temperature history is divided into suitable time periods; the average temperature T_i at each time period is evaluated; the time held at that temperature θ_i is then divided by the shelf-life θ_s for that given temperature. The fractional values are then summed up to give the fraction of shelf-life consumed. From this, then:

$$(1 - f_c)\theta_s = \text{days left at temperature } T_s \quad (17)$$

That is, the time left at any temperature is the fraction of life remaining $(1 - f_c)$ times the shelf-life at that temperature from the shelf-life plot. This method was initially developed by the USDA (1960). It is referred to as the TTT method (time-temperature-tolerance). Gutschmidt (1974) applied this to the storage life of frozen chicken with excellent results. It must be remembered, however, that this only applies for reactions with a zero order degradation mechanism.

Zero Order Shelf-Life Devices: Present Technology

A device which can be attached to a frozen food package to integrate time-temperature exposure has been developed by several companies, including the Kockums Chemical Co. (Reston, Virginia). Theirs is called the i-point TTM. Unfortunately, because these devices have only certain Q_{10}s, they can only be used for reactions of the same Q_{10}. One must match the device to the food, if accurate prediction of shelf-life is desired. Recently, Shubert (1977) published an article showing how use of several devices of different Q_{10}s can be used with high accuracy, but the mathematics is beyond the scope of this book. The i-point device uses an enzymatic reaction which causes a change in color.

A different device using the gas diffusion principle which also integrates time and temperature is made by Info Chem (Fairfield, NJ). At 40 °F these devices all have a response life of 750 days, so they probably cannot be used for refrigerated or frozen foods, since they respond very slowly at temperatures below 32 °F. However, they are applicable for semi-perishable foods with a shelf-life of 30 days to 1 yr at 60 °F to 100 °F.

Other devices are available which integrate time-temperature but have much shorter response times. The 3-M Company (Minneapolis, MN) and Tempil Company (South Plainfield, NJ), have developed temperature-time abuse integrators. These devices use the melting point principle, in which a waxy material melts at a given response temperature and is absorbed by a wick and travels along a visible scale as long as the device is held above this critical response temperature. The device does not integrate whole shelf-life as calculated above, it only integrates exposure to some temperature above a set limit. This is useful if the product has a very high Q_{10}, which means it is very sensitive to high temperature.

Several studies have been made on the reliability of these integrators (Hu, 1972; Hayakawa and Wang 1974; Byrne 1976; Kramer and Farquhar 1976; and Farquhar 1977). In essence, many of these indicators became unreliable if they were exposed to high temperature prior to their activation. In addition, the response characteristics in many cases did not match the manufacturers' specifications. Since these studies were published, the indicators have been modified. The performance may be better, but an indicator is still needed that exactly matches the Q_{10} for the food. The Australians have devised an electronic device which has the capability of setting the exact Q_{10} desired (Olley 1976). It is useful as a research tool for monitoring a distribution system, but is not practical for everyday use on packages.

First Order Prediction

As with a zero order prediction, an equation can be developed to predict the amount of shelf-life used up as a function of variable temperature storage for a first order reaction in the form:

$$A = A_o \exp\left[-\sum k_i\theta_i\right] \tag{18}$$

where A is the amount left at the end of the time-temperature distribution, and $\Sigma k_i\theta_i$ is as was shown in Fig. 3.7. Recent work in our laboratory at the University of Minnesota has shown the validity of this equation during storage of whey powder and pasta. However, there are no devices which have a first order response, thus the zero order devices mentioned above should not be used for a food wich decays by first order unless the extent of degradation to end of shelf-life is small.

If the data for the food are based solely on shelf-life, a similar equation to the TTT method can be derived. To do this, however, one cannot define A_E as being zero. Thus:

$$\ln \frac{A}{A_o} = -\sum k_i\theta_i \tag{19}$$

and

$$k_1 = \frac{\ln A_E/A_o}{\theta_s} \tag{20}$$

at time θ fraction of shelf-life consumed = $\ln A/A_o$
at time θ_s fraction of shelf-life consumed = $\ln A_E/A_o$
f_R = fraction of shelf-life remaining is:

$$\therefore f_R = 1 - \frac{\ln A_o/A}{\ln A_o/A_E} = 1 - \sum\left(\frac{\theta_i}{\theta_s}\right)_{T_i}$$

This equation also must be validated for storage of foods, but it has been applied as eq (19) to the calculation of quality losses, nutrient destruction, and microbial death during the thermal processing of canned foods (Lenz and Lund 1977a,b,c). There is no reason to believe that this equation and approach are not applicable to the prediction of storage life of foods.

Sequential Fluctuating Temperatures

In some cases a product may be exposed to a sequential regular

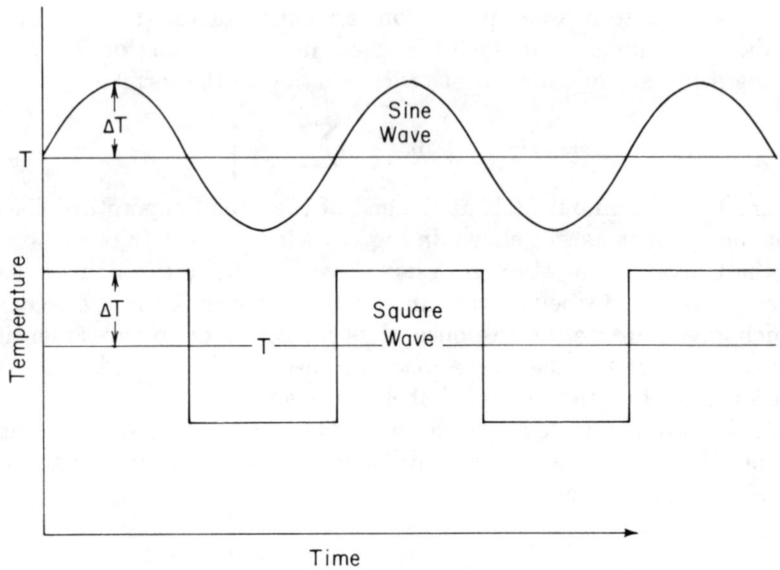

FIG. 3.8. SQUARE WAVE OR SINE WAVE EXEMPLIFYING SEQUENTIAL REGULAR FLUCTUATING TEMPERATURE PROFILE.

fluctuating temperature profile, especially if held in boxcars, trucks, and warehouses because of the daily day-night pattern. Many of these patterns can be assumed to follow either a square wave or sine wave form as is shown in Fig. 3.8. The amount of degradation occurring in these storage sequences can be calculated by the formula previously presented if the proper order of reaction is used.

There have been some papers published that have developed formulas for calculating the amount degraded for either square wave or sine wave functions. The classic papers have been by Hicks (1944), and Powers *et al.* (1965). Although not stated exactly in these papers, the derivations they presented were all for zero order reactions. Unfortunately, subsequent work by the group at Georgia has unknowingly used these equations for predicting changes that occur for first order reactions. Recently Labuza (1979) has derived similar functions for first order reactions and as noted above, they have been tested and found to be reliable.

The equations for a square wave are as follows:

First Order

$$\ln \frac{A}{A_0} = -\tfrac{1}{2}\, k_{T_m} \theta_T \left[Q_{10}{}^{a} + Q_{10}{}^{-a'} \right] = k_{T_m}\, \Gamma_{\text{square}} \cdot \theta_T \qquad (22)$$

Zero Order

$$A = A_o - \tfrac{1}{2}\, k_{T_m}\theta_T \left[Q_{10}^{a} + Q_{10}^{-a} \right] = A_o - k_{T_m}\, \Gamma_{square} \cdot \theta_T \quad (23)$$

where k_{T_m} = rate constant at mean temperature T_m between fluctuations

θ_T = total time of storage

Q_{10} = as before

$a = \left[\dfrac{T+10}{T+\Delta T}\right] \dfrac{\Delta}{10}$ (where T is in °K)

$a' = \left[\dfrac{T+10}{T-\Delta T}\right] \dfrac{\Delta T}{10}$ (where T is in °K)

ΔT = amplitude of the square wave

$\Gamma_{square} = \tfrac{1}{2}\, [Q_{10}^{a} + Q_{10}^{-a'}]$

For the sine wave function the equations are derived as a ratio of the fluctuating condition to the constant condition and take the form:

First Order

$$\frac{(\ln A/A_o)\text{sine}}{(\ln A/A_o)\text{ constant}} = \Gamma_{sine} = 1 + \frac{(\Delta T \cdot b)^2}{2^2} + \frac{(\Delta T \cdot b)^4}{2^2 4^2} + \frac{(\Delta T \cdot b)^6}{2^2 4^2 6^2} \quad (24)$$

Zero Order

$$\frac{(A_o - A)\text{ sine}}{(A_o - A)\text{constant}} = \Gamma_{sine} = 1 + \frac{(\Delta T \cdot b)^2}{2^2} + \frac{(\Delta T \cdot b)^4}{2^2 4^2} + \frac{(\Delta T \cdot b)^6}{2^2 4^2 6^2} \quad (25)$$

where ΔT is the amplitude in Fig. 3.8, and b is the slope of the shelf-life plot (log shelf-life vs temperature) in the same temperature units as is ΔT (i.e., $\theta_s = \theta_o \exp [bT]$ where θ_o = shelf-life at T=0).

The amount of loss is:
for Zero Order

$$A = A_o - k_{T_m}\, \Gamma_{sine}\, \theta_T$$

for First Order

$$A = A_o \exp [-k_{T_m}\, \Gamma_{sine}\, \theta_T]$$

It should be noted that the amount of degradation calculated at the mean temperature (T_m) for the total time of storage is less than that found when the fluctuation is accounted for. This is because the shelf-life (or the reactions causing it) are exponentially related to temperature; and thus the actual amount of degradation is always more. Based on this, the reaction can be assumed to be occurring at some effective temperature that is greater than T mean.

Other Temperature Effects

Two other phenomena which occur in foods as a function of temperature and lead to loss of shelf-life are staling and phase change. Staling is a process which proceeds in bakery items and is related to the crystallization of starch components. A recent review has been published (Knightly 1977). In staling the rate of loss of shelf-life increases as temperature decreases. The kinetics are first order in nature with a Q_{10} of around 2 to 3, but one cannot apply the typical Arrhenius approach. The Avrami equation seems to apply well where:

$$f_R = e^{-k\theta} \tag{26}$$

f_R = fraction uncrystallized

$$= \frac{E_L - E_\theta}{E_L - E_o} \tag{27}$$

where E_o = elasticity at zero time
E_L = elasticity at end of shelf-life
E_θ = elasticity at time θ
and k = rate in reciprocal time units
θ = time

Based on this, it would seem that the equations developed for first order reactions would apply.

A second area is that of phase change, including thawing, freezing and fat melting: solidifying phenomena. No mathematical models can be developed to predict how these would affect loss of shelf-life. It is known, however, that thawed frozen foods are very subject to microbial deterioration and the melted fat can oxidize faster as well as cause loss in desired texture. Commercial devices which indicate whether a frozen product has been exposed to temperatures where it can possibly thaw have been developed by the same companies that have made the time-temperature integrations.

UTILIZATION OF TEMPERATURE DEPENDENCE EQUATIONS

The previous section outlined the mathematical models that could be used to predict shelf-life. Obviously, these equations could be used to set a sell by date in which the fraction of shelf-life used up in the distribution-marketing system could be calculated. From this, information could be included on the package which would indicate the expected shelf-life for given storage conditions in the home. Similarly, the same calculations including specified home storage could be used to set a use by date or best if used by date. Some of the problems that could occur which would make these calculations meaningless are:

(1) The product used to develop any shelf-life data or graph may not be the final product marketed, since the shelf-life studies should start early in the product development.

(2) As in no. 1, the product tested may be produced in the lab or pilot plant and therefore will not be subjected to the same conditions as would the plant product.

(3) The ingredients can vary due to growth conditions, rain, sunshine etc., as well as genetic variety, in addition to their own storage effects.

(4) Labels must usually be made early in the year prior to the growing season so that if effects such as in no. 3 occur, it would be impossible to account for them.

(5) The calculations to set the date must be developed for the average conditions. Some product will thus be out of date before the time on the label due to statistical variation.

(6) Some product will be mishandled by distributors and supermarket personnel and could lose shelf-life before the label date.

(7) Product shelf-life tests can only be done on individual packages. During a large part of the distribution time, these packages are in cartons which are in cases which are in pallets, so that exposure to the external conditions is not as drastic for those cartons in the center. Thus, the product may have shelf-life greater than the label states and good food could be wasted.

Other factors could also be included; therefore, it is obvious that setting a true shelf-life date for an individual package cannot be done. Only averages can be calculated and these only where good kinetic data exist. To collect these data is a very time-consuming and expensive process, especially where expert panel evaluations must be used. Therefore, it is probably best not to require open dating of all food products, but to mandate what can be put on the label if open dating is used. Based solely on kinetic implications with respect to temperature, a best if used by date with home storage information seems most logical. This will be considered in depth for the various classes of food systems.

MOISTURE EFFECTS ON SHELF-LIFE PREDICTIONS

Introduction

Labuza (1971b; 1980) has critically reviewed the effects of water content on storage stability of dry and semi-moist foods. Basically, the rates of degradation are a function of water availability or water activity (a_w) as defined by eq (28):

$$a_w = p/p_o = \frac{\%ERH}{100} \tag{28}$$

where p = vapor pressure of water in the food

p_o = the vapor pressure of pure water at the same temperature of the food

%ERH = the percent relative humidity in equilibrium with the food at which it neither gains nor loses weight

Figure 3.9 depicts a typical moisture sorption isotherm which gives the relationship between moisture content (on a dry basis) and water activity. On a general basis, a considerable amount of water must be removed to lower the a_w significantly below 1 (e.g. at 1 g H_2O/g solids or 50% water, the a_w is still very close to 1.0).

Of consequence is the fact that for most foods in their natural state, the a_w is high and so rates of many reactions including microbial growth are also high. In order to preserve the food, the a_w can be lowered by drying or by adding water binding agents such as sugars and salt. The point on the isotherm of maximum stability is the BET monolayer value (m_o in Fig. 3.9) which is at a low a_w in the range of 0.2 to 0.3. In general, the rates of most chemical reactions follow the pattern shown in Fig. 3.10; i.e., the rate of reaction increases above the monolayer value, reaches a maximum, then decreases again. Rancidity is unusual in that the rate increases again below the monolayer, as seen in Fig. 3.10.

Moisture Gain or Loss Equation to Reach Critical Value

Gain of moisture by dry or semi-dry foods can lead to several modes of deterioration, including microbial growth, loss of crispness, loss of

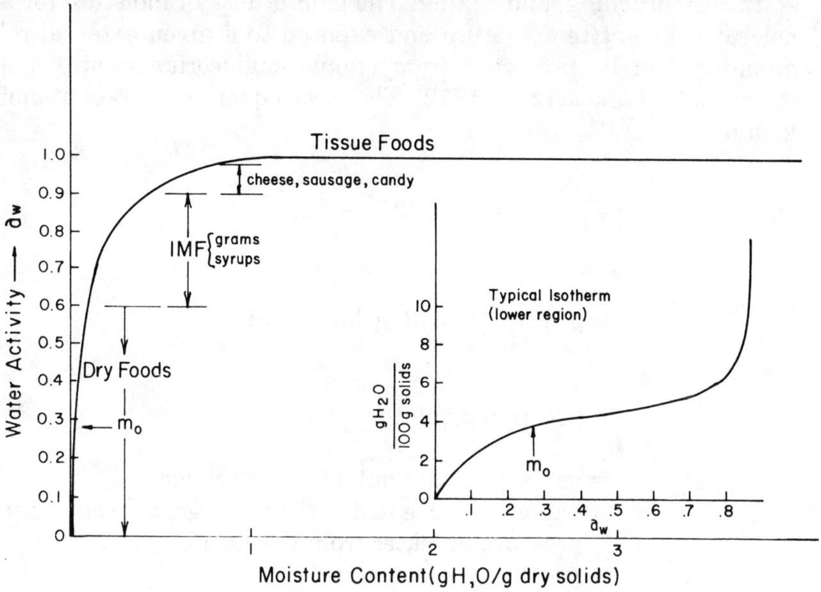

FIG. 3.9. MOISTURE CONTENT VS. WATER ACTIVITY

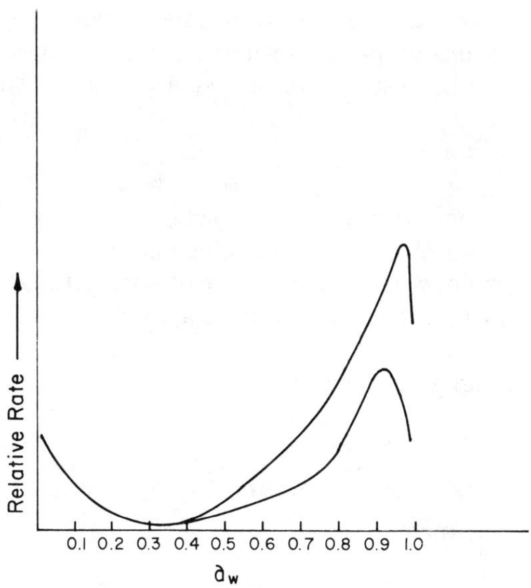

FIG. 3.10. EFFECT OF ∂_w RATE

Upper curve for rancidity; lower curve for browning.

softness, hardening, and caking. The gain or loss of moisture for a food held at constant temperature and exposed to a given external relative humidity can be predicted from simple engineering relationships as reviewed by Labuza *et al.* (1972). The basic equation for rate of moisture gain or loss is:

$$\frac{dw}{d\theta} = \frac{k}{x} A(P_{out} - P_{in}) \tag{29}$$

where $\frac{dw}{d\theta}$ = g water gained or loss per day

$\frac{k}{x}$ = film permeability

P_{out} = vapor pressure outside the package

P_{in} = vapor pressure inside the package, i.e. the vapor pressure of water from the food

A = package surface area

As with temperature acceleration, an increase in external humidity conditions can be used to accelerate the time it would take for a given packaged dry food to reach the undesirable moisture content. The factors that would be needed to predict this time include:

(1) The moisture sorption isotherm as in Fig. 3.9. For simplification the isotherm can be assumed to be a straight line of the form:

$$m = b\,a + c_o \tag{30}$$

where m = moisture in g H_2O/g solids

a = water activity at a given point

b = slope of straight line isotherm through initial moisture

c_o = intercept on m axis at $a_w = 0$

(2) The package film permeance $\frac{k}{x}$:

where $k = \frac{\text{g } H_2O \cdot \text{thickness}}{\text{days} \cdot \text{area} \cdot \text{pressure driving force}}$

and x = thickness

Manufacturers usually list a range of values for a given packaging film; however, actual values can be obtained by simple tests.

TABLE 3.5
VAPOR PRESSURE OF WATER BELOW 100 °C
(Pressure of aqueous vapor over water in mm Hg for temperatures from −15.8 to 100 °C).

Temp. °C	0.0	0.2	0.4	0.6	0.8
−15	1.436	1.414	1.390	1.368	1.345
−14	1.560	1.534	1.511	1.485	1.460
−13	1.691	1.665	1.637	1.611	1.585
−12	1.834	1.804	1.776	1.748	1.720
−11	1.987	1.955	1.924	1.893	1.863
−10	2.149	2.116	2.084	2.050	2.018
− 9	2.326	2.289	2.254	2.219	2.184
− 8	2.514	2.475	2.437	2.399	2.362
− 7	2.715	2.674	2.633	2.593	2.553
− 6	2.931	2.887	2.843	2.800	2.757
− 5	3.163	3.115	3.069	3.022	2.976
− 4	3.410	3.359	3.309	3.259	3.211
− 3	3.673	3.620	3.567	3.514	3.461
− 2	3.956	3.898	3.841	3.785	3.730
− 1	4.258	4.196	4.135	4.075	4.016
− 0	4.579	4.513	4.448	4.385	4.320
0	4.579	4.647	4.715	4.785	4.855
1	4.926	4.998	5.070	5.144	5.219
2	5.294	5.370	5.447	5.525	5.605
3	5.685	5.766	5.848	5.931	6.015
4	6.101	6.187	6.274	6.363	6.453
5	6.543	6.35	6.728	6,822	6.917
6	7.013	7.111	7.209	7.309	7.411
7	7.513	7.617	7.722	7.828	7.936
8	8.045	8.155	8.267	8.380	8.494
9	8.609	8.727	8.845	8.965	9.086
10	9.209	9.333	9.458	9.585	9.714
11	9.844	9.976	10.109	10.244	10.380
12	10.518	10.658	10.799	10.941	11.085
13	11.231	11.379	11.528	11.680	11.833
14	11.987	12.144	12.302	12.462	12.624
15	12.788	12.953	13.121	13.290	13.461
16	13.634	13.809	13.987	14.166	14.347
17	14.530	14.715	14.903	15.092	15.284
18	15.477	15.673	15.871	16.071	16.272
19	16.477	16.685	16.894	17.105	17.319
20	17.535	17.753	17.974	18.197	18.422
21	18.650	18.880	19.113	19.349	19.587
22	19.827	20.070	20.316	20.565	20.815
23	21.068	21.324	21.583	21.845	22.110
24	22.377	22.658	22.922	23.198	23.476

continued . . .

TABLE 3.5 (*continued*)

Temp. °C	0.0	0.2	0.4	0.6	0.8
25	23.756	24.039	24.326	24.617	24.912
26	25.209	25.509	25.812	26.117	26.426
27	26.739	27.055	27.374	27.696	28.021
28	28.349	28.680	29.015	29.354	29.697
29	30.043	30.392	30.745	31.102	31.461
30	31.824	32.191	32.561	32.934	33.312
31	33.694	34.082	34.471	34.864	35.261
32	35,663	36.068	36.477	36.891	37.308
33	37.729	38.155	38.584	39.018	39.457
34	39.898	40.344	40.796	41.251	41.710
35	42.175	42.644	43.117	43.595	44.078
36	44.563	45.054	45.549	46.050	46.556
37	47.067	47.582	48.102	48.627	49.157
38	49.692	50.231	50.774	51.323	51.879
39	52.442	53.009	53.580	54.156	54.737
40	55.324	55.91	56.51	57.11	57.72
41	58.34	58.96	59.58	60.22	60.86
42	61.50	62.14	62.80	63.46	64.12
43	64.80	65.48	66.16	66.86	67.56
44	68.26	68.97	69.69	70.41	71.14
45	71.88	72.62	73.36	74.12	74.88
46	75.65	76.43	77.21	78.00	78.80
47	79.60	80.41	81.23	82.05	82.87
48	83.71	84.56	85.42	86.28	87.14
49	88.02	88.90	89.79	90.69	91.59
50	92.51	93.5	94.4	95.3	96.3
51	97.20	98.2	99.1	100.1	101.1
52	102.09	103.1	104.1	105.1	106.2
53	107.20	108.2	109.3	110.4	111.4
54	112.51	113.6	114.7	115.8	116.9
55	118.04	119.1	120.3	121.5	122.6
56	123.80	125.0	126.2	127.4	128.6
57	129.82	131.0	132.3	133.5	134.7
58	136.08	137.3	138.5	139.9	141.2
59	142.60	143.9	145.2	146.6	148.0
60	149.38	150.7	152.1	153.5	155.0
61	156.43	157.8	159.3	160.8	162.3
62	163.77	165.2	166.8	168.3	169.8
63	171.38	172.9	174.5	176.1	177.7
64	179.31	180.9	182.5	184.2	185.8
65	187.54	189.2	190.9	192.6	194.3
66	196.09	197.8	199.5	201.3	203.1
67	204.96	206.8	208.6	210.5	212.3
68	214.17	216.0	218.0	219.9	221.8
69	223.73	225.7	227.7	229.7	231.7

continued . . .

TABLE 3.5 (*concluded*)

Temp. °C	0.0	0.2	0.4	0.6	0.8
70	233.7	235.7	237.7	239.7	241.8
71	243.9	246.0	248.2	250.3	252.4
72	254.6	256.8	259.0	261.2	263.4
73	265.7	268.0	270.2	272.6	274.8
74	277.2	279.4	281.8	284.2	286.6
75	289.1	291.5	294.0	296.4	298.8
76	301.4	303.8	306.4	308.9	311.4
77	314.1	316.6	319.2	322.0	324.6
78	327.3	330.0	332.8	335.6	338.2
79	341.0	343.8	346.6	349.4	352.2
80	355.1	358.0	361.0	363.8	366.8
81	369.7	372.6	375.6	378.8	381.8
82	384.9	388.0	391.2	394.4	397.4
83	400.6	403.8	407.0	410.2	413.6
84	416.8	420.2	423.6	426.8	430.2
85	433.6	437.0	440.4	444.0	447.5
86	450.9	454.4	458.0	461.6	465.2
87	468.7	472.4	476.0	479.8	483.4
88	487.1	491.0	494.7	498.5	502.2
89	506.1	510.0	513.9	517.8	521.8
90	525.76	529.77	533.80	537.86	541.95
91	546.05	550.18	554.35	558.53	562.75
92	566.99	571.26	575.55	579.87	584.22
93	588.00	593.00	597.43	601.89	606.38
94	610.90	615.44	620.01	624.61	629.24
95	633.90	638.59	643.30	648.05	652.82
96	657.62	662.45	667.31	672.20	677.12
97	682.07	687.04	692.05	697.10	702.17
98	707.27	712.40	717.56	722.75	727.98
99	733.24	738.53	743.85	749.20	754.58
100	760.00	756.45	770.93	776.44	782.00
101	787.57	793.18	798.82	804.50	810.21

(3) The ratio of the package area (A) to dry weight (W_s) contained:

$$A/W_s = m^2/g \text{ solids}$$

(4) The initial moisture content m_i and critical moisture m_c above or below which one should not go.

(5) The relative humidity and temperature to which the product will be subjected. From this and the isotherm equation, m_e, the moisture content the food would achieve if it had no package, can be found. In addition the value of p_0 at the temperature of the test can be obtained from standard tables such as Table 3.5.

Given these values, eq (32) and (33) can be found, which give the time (θ) to reach a certain moisture content m. The exponential term of these equations plotted vs time gives a straight line as in Fig. 3.11.

$$\theta_{gain} = \frac{\ln\left[\frac{m_e - m_i}{m_e - m}\right]}{\left[\frac{k}{x}\,\frac{A}{W_s}\,\frac{p_o}{b}\right]} \tag{32}$$

$$\theta_{loss} = \frac{-\ln\left[\frac{m - m_e}{m_i - m_e}\right]}{\left[\frac{k}{x}\,\frac{A}{W_s}\,\frac{p_o}{b}\right]} \tag{33}$$

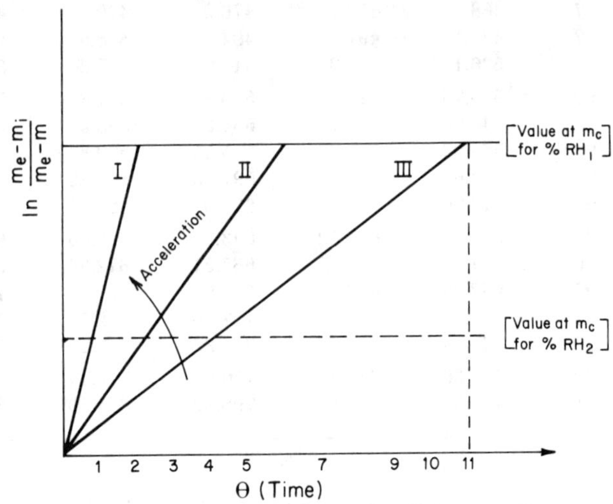

FIG. 3.11. MOISTURE GAIN

As indicated in Fig. 3.11, if condition III were the actual food/package/environment, then storage under condition I would decrease the time to reach a critical moisture content by a factor of 11/2 or 5.5 times. This can be done by using a more permeable film (k/x of 5.5 times greater). This is usually difficult to do, since very few films are available for use in foods, and most labs like to test the food in the actual film that will eventually be used. Another method for achieving the same acceleration is by storage at a temperature which would raise the vapor pressure of water (P_o) by 5.5 times. Table 3.5 gives the vapor pressure of water as a function of temperature. For the temperatures possible for dry foods, the vapor pressure ranges from about 17 mmHg (at 20 °C) to 72 mmHg (at 45 °C). Thus, an acceleration of only about 4.5 times could be achieved without adversely affecting the food itself. If the food could withstand 50 °C the acceleration could be done. Of course, a combination of both package change and higher temperature could be used. A third method would be to test the food in a package of smaller size. Since A/W_s decreases by 1/3R (R is the mean radius) this would mean that a package of about 1/5 the radius would have to be used, a very impractical method to achieve a 5.5 × acceleration.

The most often used acceleration method is a combination of a higher humidity (% RH) and temperature (T) than the food would normally be subjected to. Most food processors suggest, for dry foods, that the average temperature/humidity is 70 °F at 50% RH so that to accelerate shelf-life for moisture gain 100 °F at 90% RH can be used. The way the % RH change affects the moisture gain is to increase the driving force ($P_{out} - P_{in}$) in eq (29). For the moisture gain (eq 32) the effect is on m_e, since m_e is the value of the moisture content in the external test atmosphere if the food had no package. For example, if:

$$m_i = 1$$

$$m_c = 4$$

$$\text{and at 50\% RH, } m_e = 6$$
$$\text{and at 90\% RH, } m_e = 20$$

then:

at 50% RH

$$\ln\left[\frac{m_e - m_i}{m_e - m_c}\right] = \ln\left[\frac{6 - 1}{6 - 4}\right] = 0.92$$

and at 90% RH

$$\ln\left[\frac{m_e - m_i}{m_e - m_c}\right] = \ln\left[\frac{20 - 1}{20 - 4}\right] = 0.17$$

If the study only involved a humidity change from 50 to 90% RH, the decrease in time for the same package would be 5.4 times, achieving the desired goal. If the storage study was done at 100 °F (37.8 °C) instead of 70 °F (21.2 °C) the ratio of vapor pressures would give an additional 2.63× factor (49.2 ÷ 18.7) so the total acceleration would be 14.2 times. Humidity and temperature acceleration can be used easily to greatly accelerate the moisture gain or loss as compared to normal storage.

Using this method, the shelf-life θ_s of a food for which the mode of deterioration is moisture gain or loss can be predicted if the external conditions of distribution and marketing are presumed to remain constant. However, in the real world the humidity can vary as well as the temperature. Fluctuating temperature effects were discussed previously. In general, higher humidities are associated with higher temperature but no exact pattern of correlation exists.

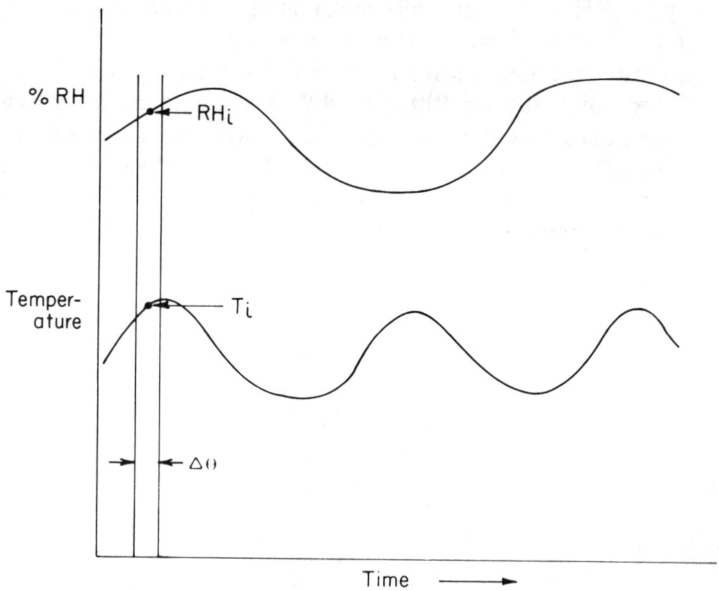

FIG. 3.12. STORAGE CONDITIONS

If a T/%RH distribution were known, as in Fig. 3.12, the time θ to reach a given change in moisture would have to be calculated by breaking up total time in small $\Delta\theta$ parts. For each θ_i, a T_i and % RH_i could be read off the graph. Then, to get the change in moisture for that segment of time (i.e. starts at m_i and ends at m_{i+1}) one must:

(1) Get a new p_o from Table 3.5 at T_i.

(2) Derive a new m_e from the isotherm for the new external % RH_i. If m_e is less than m_i at $\Delta\theta_i$, the loss equation would be used; if it is greater than m_i, the gain equation is used.

From these steps the value of m as a function of time could be calculated and θ_s could be found. These calculations, in fact, could be used to predict the net weight losses of cereals and flour under given variable external conditions. This could easily be solved by computer methods.

Constant Weight Loss Prediction

Two situations exist in which a more simplified version of weight loss can be derived: (1) loss of moisture from frozen foods; and (2) loss of moisture from fresh produce such as meats, fish, vegetables and fruits. In both cases a constant external humidity and constant temperature are assumed, based on the fact that either frozen or refrigerated storage is used. The solution for both situations is based on eq (29).

$$\frac{dW}{d\theta} = \frac{k}{x} A(p_{in} - p_{out}) = \frac{g\ H_2O}{day} \tag{34}$$

Given that k/x, the area A, external humidity, and p_{out} are constant, the question is to determine if p_{in} is constant. By definition, p_{in} is the vapor pressure of water in the food. For a frozen food p_{in} is determined solely by the temperature that pure ice would have at the storage temperature and could be read from a standard table. Since fresh products have moisture contents in the range of 60 to 98% and the loss of weight to produce an unacceptable quality is not large, the vapor pressure p_{in} is equivalent to that for liquid water at the storage temperature (Fig. 3.9). Thus eq (29) becomes:

$$\frac{\Delta W}{\Delta\theta} = \frac{k}{x} A\ \Delta p = \text{constant} \tag{35}$$

If m_c is the critical moisture content and m_i is the initial moisture for a package containing W_s g of dry solids of a food, the time to reach end of shelf-life is:

$$\theta_s = \frac{(m_i - m_c)W_s}{\left[\frac{k}{x}\ A\ \Delta p\right]} \tag{36}$$

To accelerate this loss in shelf-life testing would require storing the product at a humidity below that which would occur in normal storage, since the only logical accelerating factor is Δp. The larger the Δp, the shorter is the time to reach end of shelf-life. For example: for a vegetable like celery, in a package for which we would want 12 weeks before it lost enough water to lose crispness, at refrigerated storage of 5 °C (41 °F) the following conditions would prevail:

$$p_{in} = 6.54 \text{ mmHg}$$
$$p_{out} \simeq 80\% \text{ RH} \times 6.54 = 5.23 \text{ mmHg}$$
normal condition of storage
$$\therefore \Delta p = 1.31 = 6.54 - 5.23$$

To accelerate by a factor of three times the external humidity for the test would be as follows:

$$\Delta p = 1.31 \times 3 = 3.93$$
$$3.93 = p_{in} - p_{out} = 6.54 - p_{out}$$
$$p_{out} = 2.61$$

$$\therefore \text{external RH} = \frac{2.61}{6.54} = 40\%$$

In fact, the highest acceleration would be with $p_{out} = 0$, an absolutely dry atmosphere, which would increase the rate by five times to reach θ_s, or in this case 2.4 weeks.

Thus, rapid tests can be made for moisture loss in these two situations; the only problem is in defining some critical moisture content. Of course in real life, both temperature and humidity vary, so an iterative procedure as described earlier must be used, based on a constant weight loss by eq (34) for each of these periods.

Moisture Change with Simultaneous Reaction for Constant External Conditions

In a classic research endeavor, Karel and Labuza (1969), developed the mathematical techniques which combined the equations for prediction of moisture change with the reaction kinetics of various modes of deterioration as a function of water activity. These theories were tested in detail by Mizrahi *et al.* (1970a,b), for the prediction of loss of shelf-life of dehydrated cabbage undergoing nonenzymatic browning by a zero order mechanism. The results were extremely satisfactory.

The basic steps needed to be able to predict end of shelf-life under these conditions are:

(1) Store the dehydrated product at constant temperature and various relative humidities and measure extent of degradation with time. Data like this can be found in the literature for dehydrated foods, especially concerning vitamin loss. At least three humidities (a_ws) are required. The reaction order must be determined. The product is stored without a package.

(2) Decide what extent of degradation is considered to be unacceptable. Plot the log of the time to reach this extent vs the water activity of the product as in Fig. 3.13. Generally, a straight line above the monolayer water activity should be obtained at constant temperature.

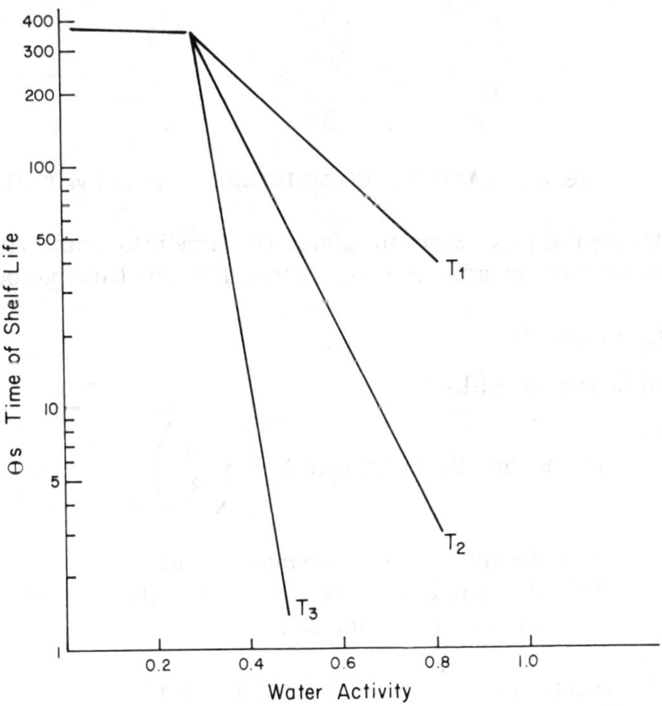

FIG. 3.13. SHELF-LIFE AS A FUNCTION OF a_w AND TEMPERATURE

(3) Using either the moisture gain or loss equation and proceeding step by step as previously described, predict the moisture content change as a function of time for some constant external temperature and humidity (Fig. 3.14).

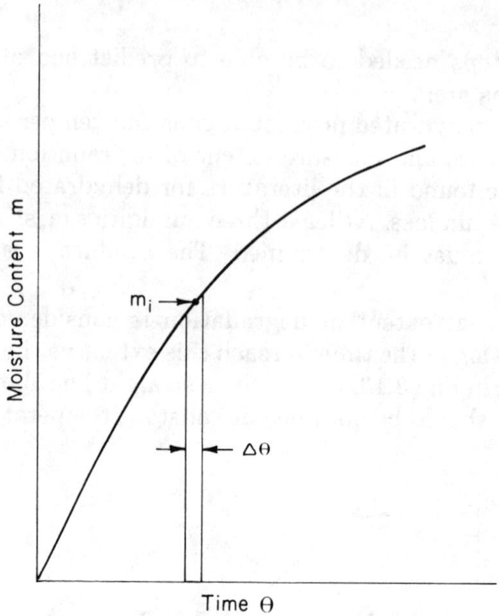

FIG. 3.14. CALCULATED MOISTURE CONTENT vs TIME

(4) Using the m vs θ graph, divide the time into small $\Delta\theta$ segments and measure the average moisture content in this time period. Then:

Zero Order Reaction

(a) Loss of Shelf-Life

$$\text{Fraction shelf-life consumed } f_c = \left(\frac{\Delta\theta}{\theta_s}\right)_{a_n} \tag{37}$$

$\Delta\theta$ = time for interval at some moisture m_N
θ_s = shelf-life from Fig. 3.13 at the water activity (a_w) corresponding to the moisture content m_N

The total fraction consumed would then be summed up and the shelf-life left at some constant temperature and humidity predicted by:

$$\theta_{left} = f_R \cdot (\theta_s)_{a_e} = \left[1 - \sum f_c\right](\theta_s)_{a_e} \tag{38}$$

where $(\theta_s)_{a_e}$ is the total shelf-life at the assumed final temperature T_e and water activity a_e from Fig. 3.13.

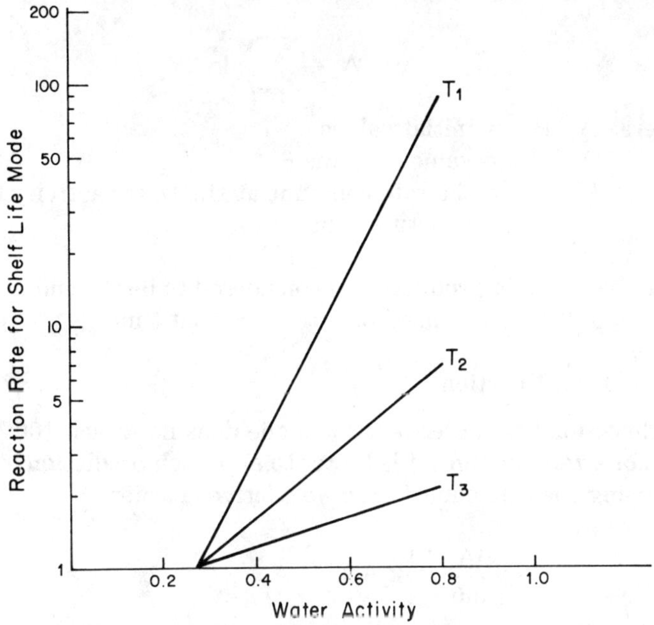

FIG. 3.15. REACTION RATE AS A FUNCTION OF a_w AND TEMPERATURE

(b) Production/Loss of Desirable Component

In many cases, a rate plot as in Fig. 3.15, rather than shelf-life plot may be more applicable, such as in production of nonenzymatic browning pigments. Thus:

$$\text{Rate of browning} = \frac{dB}{d\theta} = k \tag{39}$$

B = brown pigment
k = rate or rate constant at constant temperature and water activity

Proceeding as above in (a):

production

$$B = B_o + \sum (k_a \Delta\theta)_a \tag{40}$$

loss:

$$A = A_o - \sum (k_a \Delta\theta)_a \tag{41}$$

where A_o, B_o = initial values
A, B = values at time θ
k_a = the rate constant at the water activity (a_w) for moisture content m_N

If a given loss or production is considered to be the end of shelf-life, eq (40) or (41) can be used to determine that time.

First Order Reaction

Since for first order reactions, one does not reach 100% completion or a zero amount, it is better to approach prediction of shelf-life by using the rate equation as was derived earlier:

$$-\frac{dA}{d\theta} = k_a A \tag{7}$$

In integrated form, and using the approach as above for changing moisture content with time, this becomes:

$$\ln A/A_o = -\sum (k_a \Delta\theta)_a \tag{42}$$

where k_a is the rate constant at the a_w of the product, given its moisture m_N from Fig. 3.15 and $\Delta\theta$ is the time period chosen. To determine the time for end of shelf-life, some extent of degradation (ln A_E/A_o must be previously chosen. Mizrahi and Karel (1977) have recently shown that this procedure can be simplified by storing the food in a very permeable material at a given high relative humidity. The time to reach end of shelf-life for either zero or first order and for any other film material is then simply:

$$(\theta_s)_2 = \frac{K_1}{K_2} \quad (\theta_s)_1 \tag{43}$$

where $(\theta_s)_2$ = the predicted time to reach desired end-point for condition (2)
$(\theta_s)_1$ = the actual time to reach desired end-point for test condition (1)

K_2 = film condition for condition (2)

K_1 = film condition for test condition (1)

$$= \frac{k}{x} \frac{A}{W_s} p_o$$

As in the above solutions, this assumes constant external temperature and humidity.

Simultaneous Reaction with Moisture Change under Variable Temperature and Humidity Conditions

The previous section described the prediction of the loss of shelf-life for constant external conditions. The same procedures can be used to calculate the extent of reaction for variable temperature and humidity conditions, applying the kinetic derivations as a function of temperature as discussed previously. The first step would be the calculation of the moisture content as a function of time for a variable time/temperature/humidity distribution as previously shown. Then, applying either zero or first order kinetics, the extent of degradation is calculated for small time segments knowing the moisture content, a_w, temperature and external relative humidity at that point.

Although this is the real world situation, no literature exists which has tested this idea, so it is not known how good the predictions would be for estimation of a shelf-life date. Even more critical is the fact that the external humidity distribution is even less well known for food systems, and is not as easily predicted as is the external temperature distribution. Therefore, only rough estimates can be made of the actual loss of shelf life. Of course another way that this could be controlled would be by using a pouch with a very low water permeability, and thereby eliminating the moisture change problem. This could extend food shelf-life, but at the expense of using more precious raw materials (petroleum, aluminum, etc.) and at a greater cost to the consumer. It is this trade-off that the consumer must make: a longer guaranteed shelf-life at a greater cost, or a possible out-of-date food at lower cost.

Oxygen Effects on Shelf-Life

Introduction. — Oxygen availability is another factor that can affect the time to reach end of shelf-life and the open date put on a food package. Several reactions can be analyzed with respect to oxygen availability including:

(1) microbial growth, (2) senescence of fruits/vegetables, (3) browning of fresh meat, (4) rancidity (lipid oxidation), and (5) vitamin C degradation.

Very little information is available on the use of shelf-life prediction equations as has been done with respect to temperature and moisture content. Karel (1974) has reviewed this area, and a further reading list is provided at the end of this chapter. Part of this is due to the difficulty in designing simple equipment to control oxygen levels during experiments which utilize oxygen as one parameter, as well as measurement and control of oxygen in a food package.

Fruit and Vegetable Senescence. — Once fresh produce is harvested, it continues its biological processes, calling upon the internal starch and sugar stores for an energy supply. This will continue until the supplies are depleted or the buildup of breakdown products affects the tissue in such a way that spoilage or microbial attack occurs. This rate of biological reactivity is a function of oxygen availability in terms of oxygen pressure as shown by Fig. 3.16. As seen, the lower the oxygen

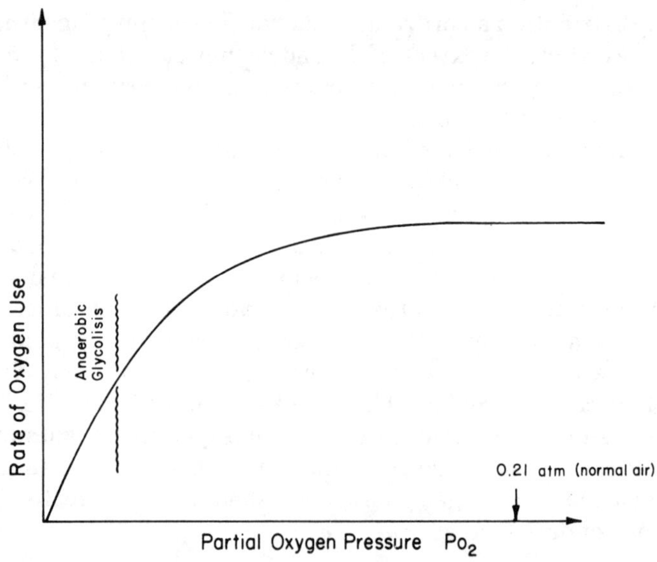

FIG. 3.16. SENESCENCE RATE AS A FUNCTION OF O_2

pressure (p_{O_2}) the lower is the rate of oxygen uptake via respiration or conversely, the lower is the rate of loss of stores. A low p_{O_2} will give a longer shelf-life. Unfortunately, below a certain p_{O_2} level an anaerobic process of incomplete breakdown occurs in which acids and alcohols are produced which also destroy the food quality. Thus, a lower limit exists. Some fresh produce is preserved using this principle of limiting oxygen availability by: (1) holding under partial vacuum (hypobaric storage); (2) flushing the truck or storehouse with nitrogen to force out the oxygen; or (3) flushing and sealing in a semi-permeable pouch. In addition, carbon dioxide (CO_2) may also be added. This also slows the rate of oxidation by mass action since it is a product of the respiration process. Jurin and Karel (1963) have done some of the classic work in this area. They showed that shelf-life in a pouch can be predicted graphically.

Basically, to solve for the shelf-life, a graph such as Fig. 3.16 must be constructed from data of respiration rates. Then the equation for gas transport into the pouch is:

$$\frac{dO_2}{d\theta} = \frac{k\,A}{x\,W_s}\,(p_{out} - p_{in}) \tag{44}$$

where $\frac{dO_2}{d\theta}$ = rate of oxygen permeation into package in cc/day/unit weight of food

$\frac{k}{x}$ = oxygen permeance of film

A = package area

p_{out} = outside oxygen partial pressure = 156 mm Hg oxygen

p_{in} = inside package oxygen partial pressure

Since the external oxygen pressure p_{out} remains constant, and if one fixes p_{in} at some value, the rate of permeation is a constant. The rate as a function of p_{in} is a straight line which can be superimposed over the oxygen uptake graph, as in Fig. 3.17. Lines A and B represent two different films of different oxygen permeability.

Figure 3.17 can be used to illustrate what would happen if a product were packaged in a film with a permeability described by A, and at an initial oxygen partial pressure p_i. Initially oxygen flow into the pouch is greater than uptake, so oxygen pressure rises which slows the flow and increases the uptake. At some point the two are equal and the flow rate just matches the reaction rate. Then the package will remain at some constant oxygen level P_* and the uptake will be a constant R^* cc/g/day. If the total oxygen uptake (V_T) to reach end of shelf-life is known then the shelf-life is:

$$\theta_s = \frac{V_T}{R^*} \tag{45}$$

FIG. 3.17. RESPIRATION RATE AND PERMEATION RATE AS A FUNCTION OF O_2

To increase shelf-life, all one has to do is lower the film permeability (k/x) such as for B ensuring that the new oxygen level is not below the point where anaerobic glycolysis occurs. This method has been put into practice with much success, but few film types are available with sufficiently low oxygen permeance to be able to control shelf-life to the desired value. Most oxygen impermeable films also retain moisture, which tends to induce mold growth on the product surface. In addition, most data are taken at a single temperature. Since the Q_{10} for respiration is about 2—3, data must be analyzed as a function of temperature also, utilizing the techniques described previously.

Rancidity. — Labuza (1971a) reviewed the relationship of oxygen to stability of foods, with respect to rancidity. A similar situation exists with respiration in that the oxygen uptake follows the same pattern. However, there is no lower oxygen critical limit; i.e. the lower the better, and CO_2 does not slow the reaction.

Simon *et al.* (1971) were the first to apply this to oxidation of a dehydrated shrimp product using the same type of mathematical and graphical analysis. Karel and Quast (1972) did a more in-depth study in which moisture was also simultaneously diffusing into the package for potato chips stored at constant temperature and external humidity. Very elegant computer-based solutions were presented; however, the time to develop the necessary data for equation development for most foods would be far in excess of that desirable in shelf-life testing or product development.

Basically, it can be stated that methods can be developed to predict the end of shelf-life when caused by oxygen sensitive reactions which also depend on a_w and temperature.

REFERENCES

BYRNE, C. 1976. Temperature indicators — The state of the art. Food Technol. *30* (June), 66.

CECIL, S.R., and WOODROOF, J.G. 1962. Long term storage of military rations. Ga. Exp. Sta. Tech. Bull. *25*.

FARQUHAR, J.N. 1977. Time temperature indicators in monitoring the distribution of frozen foods. J. Food Qual. *1*, 119.

GUTSCHMIDT, J. 1974. The storage life of frozen chicken with regard to temperature in the food chain. Lebensmittlen Forschung and Technol. *7*, 137.

HAYAKAWA, K., and WANG, Y. 1974. Performance of frozen food indicators subjected to time variable temperatures. ASHRAE J. *16* (4), 44-48.

HICKS, E.W. 1944. Note on the estimation of the effect of diurnal temperature fluctuation on reaction rates in stored foodstuffs and other materials. J. Counc. Sci. Ind. Res. *17*, 111.

HU, K. 1972. Time temperature indicating system writes status of product shelf life. Food Technol. *26* (8), 56.

JURIN, V.A. and KAREL, M. 1963. Studies on control of respiration of McIntosh apples by packaging methods. Food Technol. *17*, 104.

KAREL, M. 1974. Quantitative analysis of food packaging and storage stability problems. Food Technol. *28* (8), 50.

KAREL, M. and LABUZA, T.P. 1969. Optimization of protective packaging of space foods. Air Force Contract F 41-609-68-C-0015, Feb.

KAREL, M. and QUAST, D.G. 1972. Computer simulation of storage life of foods undergoing two interacting mechanisms. J. Food Sci. *37*, 679.

KNIGHTLY, W. 1977. Staling of bread. Bakers' Digest *51* (5), 52.

KRAMER, A. and FARQUHAR, J. 1976. Testing of time-temperature indicating and defrost devices. Food Technol. *30* (2), 53.

LABUZA, T.P. 1971a. Nutrient losses during drying and storage of dehydrated foods. Crit. Rev. Food Technol. *3*, 355.

LABUZA, T.P. 1971b. Water and food stability. Proc. 3rd International Congress of Food Science and Technology. IFT Press, Chicago.

LABUZA, T.P. 1979. A theoretical comparison of losses in foods under fluctuating temperature sequences. J. Food Sci. *44*, 1162-1168.

LABUZA, T.P. 1980. The effect of water activity on reaction kinetics of food deterioration. Food Technol. *34* (1), 36.

LABUZA, T.P., MIZRAHI, S. and KAREL, M. 1972. Mathematical models for the optimization of flexible film packaging of foods for storage. Trans. ASAE *15*, 150.

LEE, Y.C., KIRK, J.R., BEDFORD, C.L. and HELDMAN, D.R. 1977. Kinetics and computer simulation of ascorbic acid stability of tomato juice as functions of temperature, pH and metal catalyst. J. Food Sci. *42,* 640.

LENZ, M. and LUND, D. 1977a. The lethality Fourier number method: Experimental verification of a model for calculating temperature profiles and lethality in conduction heating foods. J. Food Sci. *42,* 989.

LENZ, M., and LUND, D. 1977b. The lethality Fourier number method: Experimental verification of a model for calculating average quality factor retention in conduction heating canned foods. J. Food Sci. *42,* 997.

LENZ, M. and LUND, D. 1977c. The lethality Fourier number method: Confidence intervals for calculated lethality and mass average retention of conduction heating canned foods. J. Food Sci. *42,* 1002.

MIZRAHI, S. and KAREL, M. 1977. Accelerated stability tests of moisture sensitive products in permeable packages by programming rate of moisture content increase. J. Food Sci. *42,* 958.

MIZRAHI, S., LABUZA, T.P. and KAREL, M. 1970a. Computer aided prediction of extent of browning in dehydrated cabbage. J. Food Sci. *35,* 799.

MIZRAHI, S., LABUZA, T.P., and KAREL, M., 1970b. Feasibility of accelerated tests for browning in dehydrated cabbage. J. Food Sci. *35,* 804.

OLLEY, J. 1976. International Institute of Refrigeration, Australian National Committee, Joint Meeting of Commissions, Melbourne, Sept.

POWERS, J.J., LUKASZEWICZ, W., WHELLER, R., and DORNSETTER, T.P. 1965. Chemical and microbial activity ratio under square wave and sinusoidal temperature fluctuations. J. Food Sci. *30,* 520.

SCHUBERT, H. 1977. Criteria for the application of TT-I indicators to quality control of deep frozen food products. Proceedings IIF-IIR Commissions C1/C2, Ettlingen, Germany, 407.

SCHWIMMER, S., INGRAHAM, L.L. and HUGES, H.M. 1955. Temperature tolerance for frozen food processing. Effective temperatures in thermally fluctuating systems. Ind. Eng. Chem. *27* (6), 1149.

SIMON, I.B., LABUZA, T.P. and KAREL, M. 1971. Computer predictions of food storage stability: Oxidation deterioration of shrimp product. J. Food Sci. *36,* 280.

SING, R.P., KIRK, J. and HELDMAN, D.R. 1976. Kinetics of quality degradation: Ascorbic acid oxidation in infant formula. J. Food Sci. *41,* 304.

TOMPKIN, R.B. 1973. Refrigeration temperature. Food Technol. *27* (12), 54.

USDA. 1960. Conference on Food Quality. USDA Agric. Res. Service, Albany, CA., Nov. 4.

VILLOTA, R., SAGUY, I. and KAREL, M. 1980. Storage stability of dehydrated food: Evaluation of the literature. J. Food Qual. *3,* 123.

FURTHER READING

Effect of Oxygen on Microorganisms

ADAMS, J.R. and HOFFMAN, D.L. 1972. Effect on controlled gas atmosphere and temperature on quality of packaged pork. J. Food Sci. *37,* 869.

APPLING, J.W. 1946. Microorganisms in paper. Modern Packaging. *19.*

CURDA, D., MARKYTAN, J. and SILANKOVA, L. 1966. Influence of oxygen accessivity on the growth of molds under packaging materials. Inst. Chem. Techn. Sci. Papers. Prague, Ell.

DEBEVERE, J. and VOETS, J. 1971. Microbiological changes in prepackaged cod fillets in relation to the oxygen permeability of the film. J. Appl. Bacteriol. *34,* 507.

DEMPSTER, J.F. 1972. Vacuum packaged bacon, effects of processing and storage temperature and shelf-life. J. Food Technol. *7,* 271.

GRIFFIN, R.G., NOSRATI, M., LAMPI, R. and SZCZEBLOWSKI, J. 1967. Bacterial resistance of films. Modern Packaging *40* (14), 164.

LANDERS, K.E., DAVIS, N. and DIENER, U. 1967. Influence of atmospheric gases on aflatoxin production by *Aspergillus flavus* in peanuts. Phytopathology *57,* 1086.

O'NEILL, R.D. 1964. The microbial significance of food packaging materials. J. Milk and Food Technol. *27,* 116.

RONSIVALLI, L., BERNSTEINS, J. and TINKER, B. 1966. Method for determining bacterial permeability of plastic films. Food Technol. *20,* 98.

SANBORN, J.R. 1940. Microbiological content of paper-board used in the packaging of foods. Am. J.P.H. *30,* 247.

Effect of Oxygen Pressure on Fresh Foods

BIALE, J.B. 1960. Post-harvest biochemistry of tropical and subtropical fruits. Adv. Food Res. *10,* Academic Press, New York.

BIALE, J.B. 1964. Growth, maturation and senescence in fruits. Science *146.*

HARDENBERG, R. *et al.* 1958. Polyethylene film for fruit. Modern Packaging *31* (6), 135.

JURIN, V. and KAREL, M. 1963. Studies on control of respiration of McIntosh apples by packaging methods. Food Technol. *17,* 104.

KIDD, F. and WEST, C. 1945. Respiratory activity and duration of life of apples. Plant Physiol. *20,*467.

PLATENIUS, H. Effect of oxygen concentration on the respiration of carbon dioxide on quality of apples stored in controlled atmosphere. Can. J. Plant Sci. *46,* 317.

PROUDFOOT, F.G. 1966. Sealed cryovac and polyethylene case liners for preservation of hatching eggs. Poultry Sci. *45,* 105.

SMITH, W. 1963. Use of Carbon Dioxide in the Transport and Storage of Fruits and Vegetables. Adv. Food Res. *12,* Academic Press, New York.

TAYLOR, M. and HELBACKA, N. 1966. Evacuated packaging of fresh broiler chickens. Poultry Sci. *45,* 1207.

TOLLE, W.E. Film permeability requirements for storage of apples. USDA Tech. Bull. No. 1257. U.S. Govt. Printing Office, Washington, D.C.

TOMKINS, R.G. 1965. Changes in the concentrations of CO_2 and O_2 produced within sealed plastic packages by fruits and vegetables. Ditton Lab. Memorandum No. 32.

VEERAJU, P. and KAREL, M. 1966. Controlling atmosphere in a fresh fruit package. Modern Packaging *40,* 68.

CHAPTER 4

SHELF-LIFE DATA OF CEREAL GRAINS AND FLOUR

INTRODUCTION

Very little information is available in the literature on storage of cereal grains prior to processing. Recently, Fellers and Bean (1977) published a review of wheat-based foods which included some data on the grain itself.

SHELF-LIFE DATA

Fellers and Bean (1977) reported data on time to reach end of shelf-life of wheat grain based both in microbiological and enzymatic deterioration. The data are plotted in Fig. 4.1. The figure shows the importance of

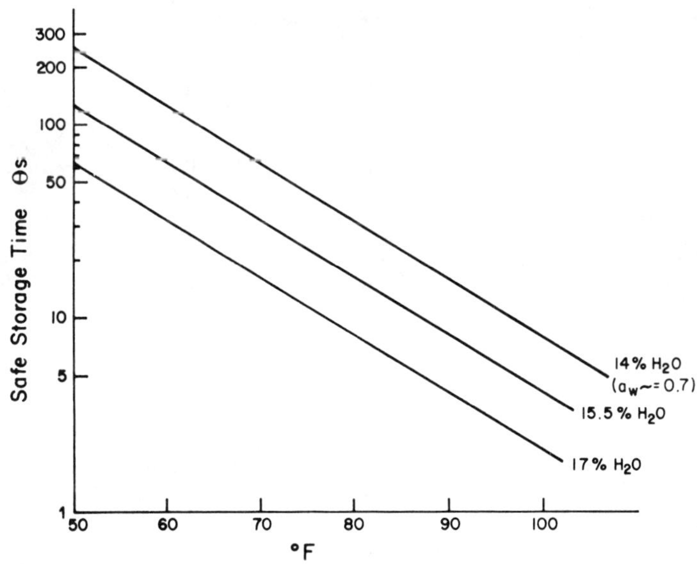

FIG. 4.1. SHELF-LIFE OF WHEAT GRAIN

drying the grain. A drop of 3% H_2O from 17 to 14% increases shelf-life by a factor of 4. The Q_{10} of the reaction for deterioration is about 3.5, which is quite high, but is indicative of microbiological growth.

As indicated for all grains including barley, oats, wheat and rye, the moisture content as well as the storage temperature is critical in the loss of shelf-life based on time to visible mold growth. In Table 4.1 (Kreyger 1974) the activation energies and therefore the temperature coefficient, Q_{10} for visible mold growth decreases significantly as moisture content increases. The lower activation energies at higher moisture contents in-

TABLE 4.1
TIME TO VISIBLE MOLD DEVELOPMENT OF SEVERAL CEREAL GRAINS

Moisture Content %	Storage Life in Weeks at 10°C	E_a Kcal/mole	Q_{10}
Barley			
16.6	120	30.7	6.5
17.2	50	31.0	6.6
18.3	20	23.7	4.2
19.4	9	19.2	3.2
20.7	5	14.1	2.4
22.7	5	14.1	2.4
Oats			
16.0	35	30.2	6.3
16.7	10	25.2	4.6
17.5	4.5	14.3	2.4
18.6	3	11.2	2.0
20.0	2	10.1	1.9
22.0	1.5	5.4	1.4
Wheat			
17.1	30	39.5	11.1
17.6	6	29.7	6.1
18.4	2.5	12.9	2.2
19.6	1.5	7.0	1.5
21.0	1	7.0	1.5
23.0	1	9.3	1.8
Rye			
17.0	30	39.5	11.1
17.9	6	29.7	6.1
19.0	2.5	12.9	2.2
20.3	1.5	7.0	1.5
22.1	1	7.0	1.5
24.4	1	9.3	1.8

From Kreyger (1972).

TABLE 4.2
TIME TO LOSS OF GERMINABILITY OF SEVERAL CEREAL GRAINS

Moisture Content %	Storage Life in Weeks at 10°C	E_a Kcal/mole	Q_{10}
Barley			
11	240	27.9	5.5
12	170	26.4	5.0
13	100	27.1	5.2
14	65	26.4	5.0
15	40	25.5	4.7
16	20	26.4	5.0
17	10	23.6	4.2
19	4	20.1	3.4
23	1	22.8	4.0
Oats			
11.0	160	24.2	4.4
11.5	110	23.5	4.2
12.5	70	22.6	3.9
13.0	45	21.3	3.7
14.0	26	21.3	3.7
15.0	15	21.7	3.7
17.0	7.5	20.8	3.6
19.0	3.5	18.0	3.0
22.0	1	18.0	3.0
Wheat			
12.0	100	21.2	3.6
13.0	75	20.6	3.5
13.5	50	20.1	3.4
14.5	30	18.9	3.2
15.5	20	17.6	2.9
16.5	12	17.2	2.9
17.5	6	18.8	3.1
19.5	3	18.0	3.0
23.0	1	18.0	3.0
Rye			
11.5	50	15.0	2.5
12.5	34	14.3	2.4
13.0	23	14.1	2.4
14.0	16	10.8	1.9
15.0	10	12.4	2.1
16.0	6.5	13.1	2.2
18.0	4	12.9	2.2
20.0	2	11.4	2.0
24.0	1	11.3	2.0

From Kreyger (1972).

dicate that temperature of storage is more critical in extending shelf-life at low moisture contents than at high ones. For example, at 17.6% moisture wheat can be stored 15 times longer at 50 °F than at 77 °F, while at 19.6% and higher the grain has a shelf-life only two times longer at 50 °F than at 77 °F. This suggests that the moisture content (a_w) is very important to microbial storage. Therefore, drying grain prior to storage is a useful means of extending shelf-life without having to resort to refrigerated storage in warm climates.

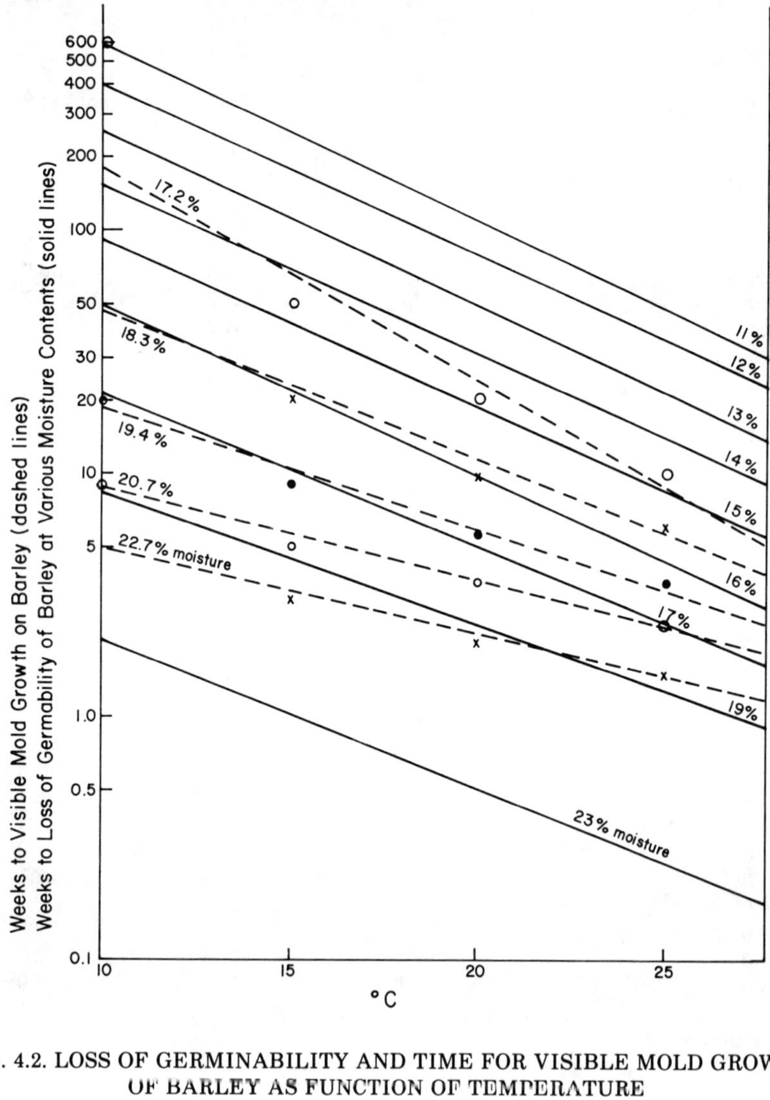

FIG. 4.2. LOSS OF GERMINABILITY AND TIME FOR VISIBLE MOLD GROWTH OF BARLEY AS FUNCTION OF TEMPERATURE

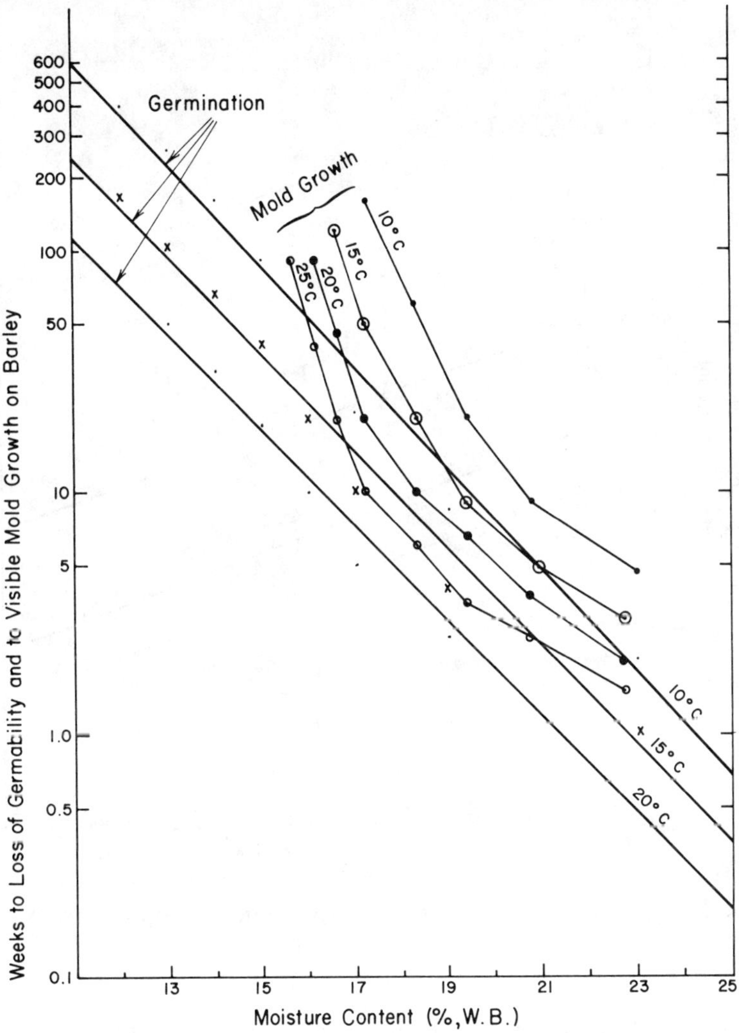

FIG. 4.3. LOSS OF GERMINABILITY AND TIME FOR VISIBLE MOLD GROWTH OF BARLEY AS FUNCTION OF MOISTURE

Loss of germinability of barley, oats, wheat and rye is also dependent upon both moisture content and storage temperature as seen in Table 4.2 (Kreyger 1972). The effect of moisture content upon activation energies is much less than for microbial growth. It should be noted that loss of germination ability has little effect on the use of the grain for food, but has a great effect on food production. The data for barley are shown in Fig. 4.2 and 4.3 as a function of moisture content and temperature.

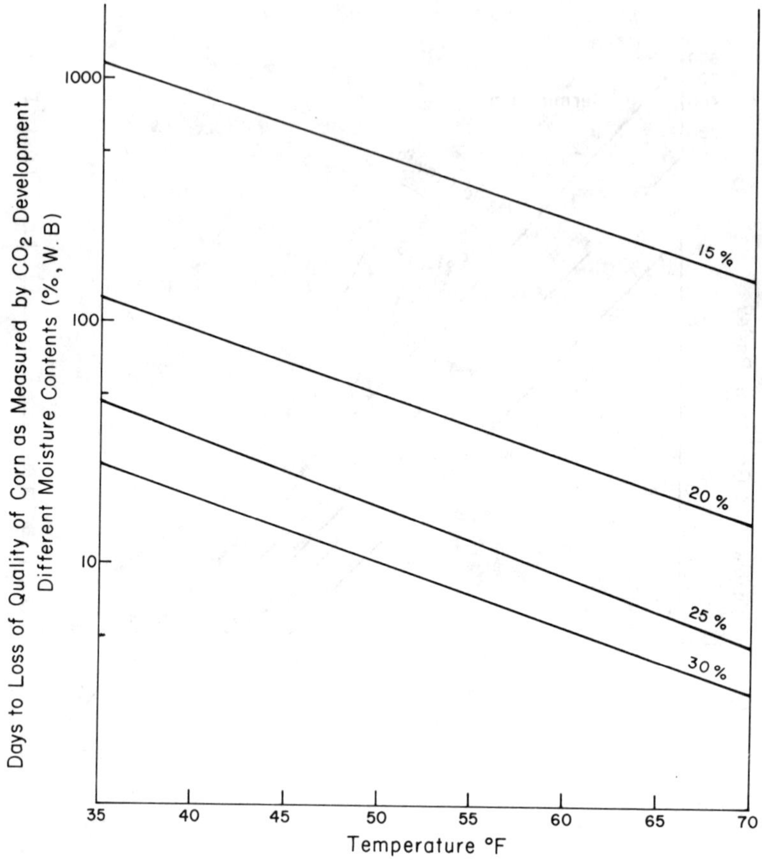

FIG. 4.4. TIME FOR LOSS OF QUALITY OF CORN AS MEASURED BY CO_2 DEVELOPMENT

Data from the USDA (1968) (also cited in Brooker *et al.* 1974) for loss of quality in corn with storage as measured by CO_2 development and loss of dry matter indicate that both storage air temperature and moisture content are critical to shelf-life. At each of the four different moisture contents tested, shelf-life at 35 °F was about ten times as long as at 75 °F. The activation energies at each moisture content and Q_{10}s were very similar to each other as seen in Table 4.3. At each of the nine different temperatures the shelf-life was about 50 times longer at 15% moisture content than at 30% moisture content, as seen in Fig. 4.4.

Fellers and Bean (1970) also discuss storage of flour indicating a similar improvement in shelf-life with a decrease in moisture content.

TABLE 4.3
CORN: LOSS IN GERMINATION QUALITY ABILITY

Moisture Content %	E_a Kcal/mole	Q_{10}
Corn		
15	7.4	1.59
20	7.4	1.60
25	7.8	1.62
30	8.3	1.69

From USDA (1968); cited in Brooker *et al.* (1974).

TABLE 4.4
TIME IN WEEKS FOR A 15% LOSS OF LOAF VOLUME IN FLOURS STORED AT 37.8°C

Flour Type	Flour % Moisture in Storage			
	3	6	10	14
Patent	50	57	38	5
1st clear	48	52	28	2
Whole wheat	32	10	3	1

From Fellers and Bean (1970).

Table 4.4 from their paper shows significant losses in loaf volume as flour moisture increased, a problem that would occur in humid environments. Fellers and Bean (1977) also reported some industry shelf-life factors. One company uses six weeks at 100°F/70% RH to be equivalent to one year at normal temperature and humidity, which is an accelerating factor of 8.6, much like that calculated for moisture changes in Chapter 3.

OPEN DATING

Consumers themselves rarely buy whole grain products, so open dating seems irrelevant for these products, especially based on the way in which grain is marketed in the U.S. Flour, however, is a normal consumer market product. No data are available regarding the temperature effect on baking character, but moisture gain severely decreases baking quality. Shelf-life generally increases with reduced moisture unless it goes below 3%, which would only occur in very hot, dry or frigid, dry environments. Thus, basing shelf-life on moisture loss does not seem useful. The shelf-life equations developed earlier, however, can be used to predict time for some critical moisture loss based on net weight regulations.

REFERENCES

BROOKER, D.B., BAKKER-ARKEMA, F.W. and HALL, C.W. 1974. Drying Cereal Grains. AVI Publishing Co., Westport, Conn.

FELLERS, D.A. and BEAN, M.M. 1970. Flour blend A. 2. Storage studies. Bakers Dig. *44* (6), 42.

FELLERS, D.A. and BEAN, M.M. 1977. The storage life of wheat based foods: A review. J. Food Sci. *42*, 1143.

KREYGER, J. 1972. Drying and storing grains, seeds and pulses in temperate climates. Bull. 205, Institute for Storage and Processing of Agricultural Produce, Wageningen, The Netherlands.

KREYGER, J. 1974. *Cited by* D.B. Brooker *et al.* Drying Cereal Grains. AVI Publishing Co., Westport, Conn.

USDA. 1968. Guidelines for mold control in high moisture corn. Farmers' Bull. 2238.

FURTHER READING

AGRICULTURAL STABILIZER AND CONSERVATION SERVICE, USDA. 1975. Purchase of wheat-soy blend for use in export programs, Announcement WEB-5, ASCS Commodity Office, P.O. Box 8377, Shawnee Mission, KS 66208.

ANDERSON, R.A. and PFEIFFER, V.F. 1970. Stability of vitamin A in wheat flour. Northwest. Miller, *3*, 14.

ANDERSON, R.H., MAXWELL, O.L., MULLEY, A.E. and FRITSCH, C.W. 1976. Effects of processing and storage on micronutrients in breakfast cereals. Food Technol. *30*(5), 110.

ANDERSON, R.H., MORAN, D.H., HUNTLEY, T.E. and HOLAHAN, J.L. 1963. Responses of cereal to antioxidants. Food Technol. *17*, 1587.

BAILEY, J.E. 1974. Whole grain storage. *In* Storage of Cereal Grains and Their Products. C.M. Christensen (Editor). Am. Assoc. Cereal Chemists, St. Paul.

BAKER, D., NEUSTADT, M.H. and ZELENY, L. 1957. Application of fat acidity test as an index of grain deterioration. Cereal Chem. *34*, 226.

BEAN, M.M., HANAMOTO, M.M., MECHAM, D.K., GUADAGNI, D.G. and FELLERS, D.A. 1976. Soy-fortified wheat flour blends. 2. Storage stability of complete blends. Cereal Chem. *53*, 376.

BEAN, M., HANAMOTO, M.M., NISHITA, K.D., MECHAM, D.K. and FELLERS, 1977. Soy-fortified wheat flour blends. 4. Storage stability with several surfactant additives. (In preparation).

BEAN, M.M. and NISHITA, K.D. 1976. Protein fortification. Baking with weak flours: Low protein or storage deteriorated. Paper presented at Spring Technical Conference, Milling and Baking Division, Am. Assoc. Cereal Chemists, Minneapolis, May 6-7.

BUSHUK, W. and WINKLER, C.A. 1957. Sorption of water vapor on wheat flour, starch and gluten. Cereal Chem. *34*, 73.

CHRISTENSEN, C.M. 1974. Storage of Cereal Grains and Their Products. Am. Assoc. of Cereal Chemists, St. Paul.

CORT, W.M., BORENSTEIN, B., HARLEY, J.H., and SCHEINER, J. 1976. Nutrient stability of fortified cereal products. Food Technol. *3*(4), 52.

CUENDET, L.S., LARSON, E., NORRIS, C.G. and GEDDES, W.F. 1954. The influence of moisture content and other factors on the stability of wheat flours at 37.8 °C. Cereal Chem. *31*, 362.

DAFTARY, R.D. and POMERANZ, Y. 1965. Changes in lipid composition in wheat during storage deterioration. Agric. Food. Chem. *13*, 442.

FELLERS, D.A., MECHAM, D.K. BEAN, M.M. and HANAMOTO, M.M. 1976a. Soy-fortified flour blends. 1. Composition and properties. Cereal Foods World *21*, 75.

FELLERS, D.A., MOSSMAN, A.P., JOHNSTON, P.H. and WHEELER, E.L. 1976b. Mechanical debranning of whole-kernal wheat. 3. Composition, cooking characteristics and storage stability. Cereal Chem. *53*, 308.

FELLERS, D.A., SHEPHERD, D.A., BELLARD, N.J., MOSSMAN, A.P., JOHNSTON, P.H. and WESSERMAN, T. 1966. Protein concentrates by remilling of wheat milling feeds. Cereal Chem. *43*, 715.

FERRIGAN, M. and W.F. GEDDES. 1958. The distribution of lipase in the commercial mill products from hard red spring wheat. Cereal Chem. *35*, 422.

FIFIELD, C.C. and ROBERTSON, D.W. 1959. Milling, baking and chemical properties of Marquis and Kanred wheat grown in Colorado and stored 25 to 33 years. Cereal Sci. Today *4*, 179.

GREENWOOD, C.T. 1975. Cereal science in the U.K. — Achievements and prospects. Cereal Foods World *20*, 23.

HARRIS, N.E., WESTCOTT, D.E., RAHMAN, A.R., KLUTER, R.A. and ROBERTSON, M.M. 1976. Bulgur — shelf life studies. Presented at the First International Congress on Engineering and Food; Boston, Aug. 9-13.

HARRISON, B.N., PLA, G.W., CLARK, G.A. and FRITZ, J.C. 1976. Selection of iron sources for cereal enrichment. Cereal Chem. *53*, 78.

KEAGY, P.M., STOKSTAD, E.L.R. and FELLERS, D.A. 1975. Folacin stability during bread processing and family flour storage. Cereal Chem. *52*, 348.

LAMOUR, R.K., HULSE, J.H., ANDERSON, J.A. and DEMPTSTER, C. 1961. Effect of package type on stored flour and farina. Cereal Sci. Today *6*, 158.

LUCHSINGER, W.W., CUENDET, L.S., BOYER, P.D. and GEDDES, W.F. 1955. A sensitive method for measuring lipase activity and its application to wheat products. Cereal Chem. *32*, 395.

MARNETT, L.F., TENNEY, R.J. and BARRY, V.D., 1973. Effects of storage times and temepratures on the baking characteristics of 12% soy-fortified wheat flour blends. Cereal Sci. Today *18*, 53.

MECHAM, D.K., HANAMOTO, M.M., BEAN, M.M. and FELLERS, D.A. 1976. Soy-fortified wheat flour blends. 3. Storage stability of ingredients and incomplete blends. Cereal Chem. *53*, 405.

MECHAM, D.K. and MOSSMAN, A.P. 1974. Titratable acidity in water-saturated n-butyl alcohol and petroleum ether extracts of some stored wheat products. Cereal Chem. *51*, 478.

NEUFELD, C.H.H., WEINSTEIN, N.F. and MECHAM, D.K. 1957. Studies on the preparation and keeping quality of bulgur. Cereal Chem. *34*, 360.

NIMMO, C.C. and FELLERS, D.A. 1975. Fortification of flour and flour products with ferripolyphosphate. U.S. Patent 3,876,813.

PAULSEN, T.M. 1960. U.S. Patent 31,100,709.

POMERANZ, Y. 1971. Composition and functionality of wheat flour components. *In* Wheat Chemistry and Technology. Am. Assoc. Cereal Chemists, St. Paul.

POMERANZ, Y., SHOGREN, M.D. and FINNEY, K.F. 1969. Improving breadmaking properties with glycolipids. 1. Improving soy products with sucroesters. Cereal Chem. *46*, 503.

STUCKEY, B.N. 1955. Increasing shelf life of cereals with phenolic antioxidants. Food Technol. *9*, 585.

TSEN, C.C., HOOVER, W.J. and PHILLIPS, D. 1971. High-protein blends. Use of sodium stearoyl-2-lactylate and calcium stearoyl-2-lactylate in their production. Bakers Dig. *45*(2), 20.

WALLACE, J.M. and WHELLER, E.L. 1972. Lipoxygenase inactivation in wheat protein concentrate by heat-moisture treatments. Cereal Chem. *49*, 92.

WHEELER, E.L. and WALLACE, J.M. 1973. Self-catalyzed destruction of lipoxygenase in wheat mill fractions. Food Sci. Technol. *6*(6), 205.

CHAPTER 5

SHELF-LIFE OF BREAKFAST CEREALS

INTRODUCTION: PROCESSING METHODS FOR BREAKFAST CEREALS

Uncooked breakfast cereals constitute one large segment of the cereals food group, Farina being the most popular. They are produced from various portions of the grain kernel. Two general steps are involved. First is the reduction of particle size and second is the elimination of the unwanted portion of the kernel, usually the bran and the germ. Processing losses here depend on how much of the kernel is removed, as most nutrients are in the bran and the germ. Table 5.2 shows the loss of various nutrients that occurs in milling (Schroeder 1971). This type of processing will primarily extend shelf-life by removing the germ. Mechanical disintegration has little effect on degradation.

The cooked and further processed cereals make up the largest segment of this food group. They can be subdivided into four major groups: flaked, puffed, shredded and granulated.

Flakes are the simplest of these to make. The process involves (1) cooking; (2) flaking; and (3) toasting. Figures (5.1a, b, c) show the effect of cooking and toasting on storage stability of wheat, corn and oat flakes at several temperatures (Anderson *et al.* 1963). In all three cereals, stability is decreased due to more rapid development of rancidity by cooking, probably due to breakdown of cellular structure which allows better contact between reactants. The graph also shows that toasting restores shelf stability to the cereal. This would probably be a result of lowering the water activity of the product to the monolayer.

Extrusion and/or puffing can also follow cooking instead of toasting. This is really similar to toasting, in that the cereal is cooked, shaped, and then dryed, and similar shelf stability is also achieved.

Shredding is quite different, in that it uses whole grain without removing the germ or bran (Matz 1970). Processing, however, is the same as for flakes, involving cooking, shaping and then drying. The overall heat treatment is much less than for flakes. This, coupled with the fact that the germ is not removed, causes unique packaging and storage difficulties which will be discussed in the next section.

Grape-Nuts is currently the only granulated cereal on the market. It is made from a very well baked stiff wheat dough. Storage stability is similar to flakes and puffs.

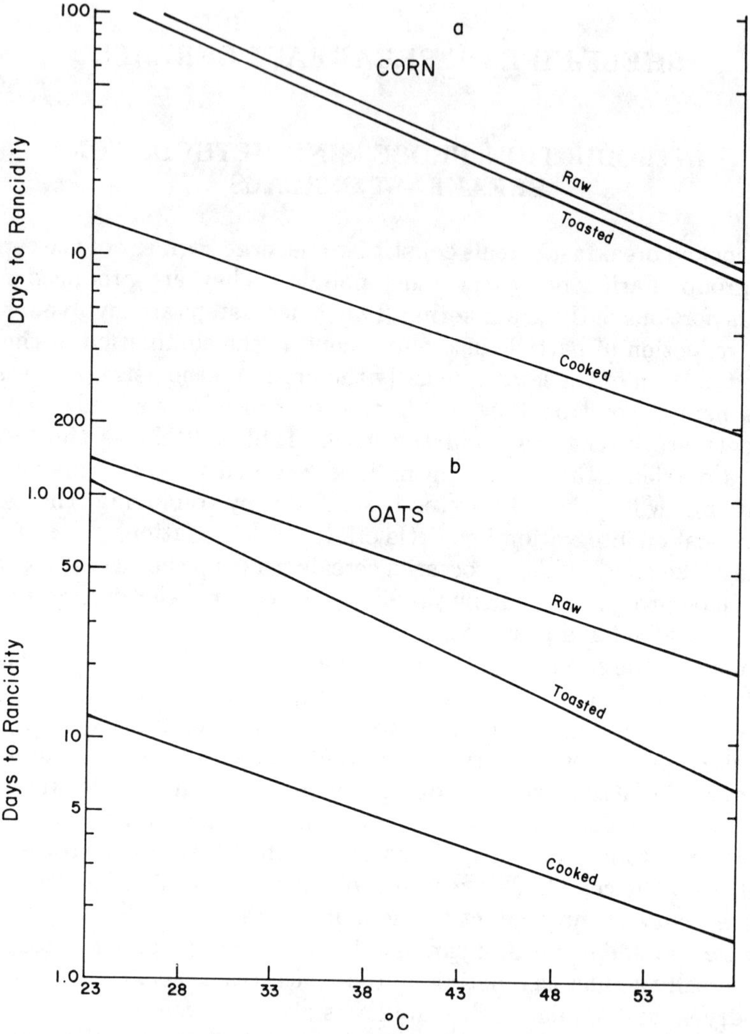

FIG. 5.1a,b. EFFECTS OF COOKING AND TOASTING ON STORAGE STABILITY OF: a — CORN; b — OATS

(Anderson *et al.* 1963)

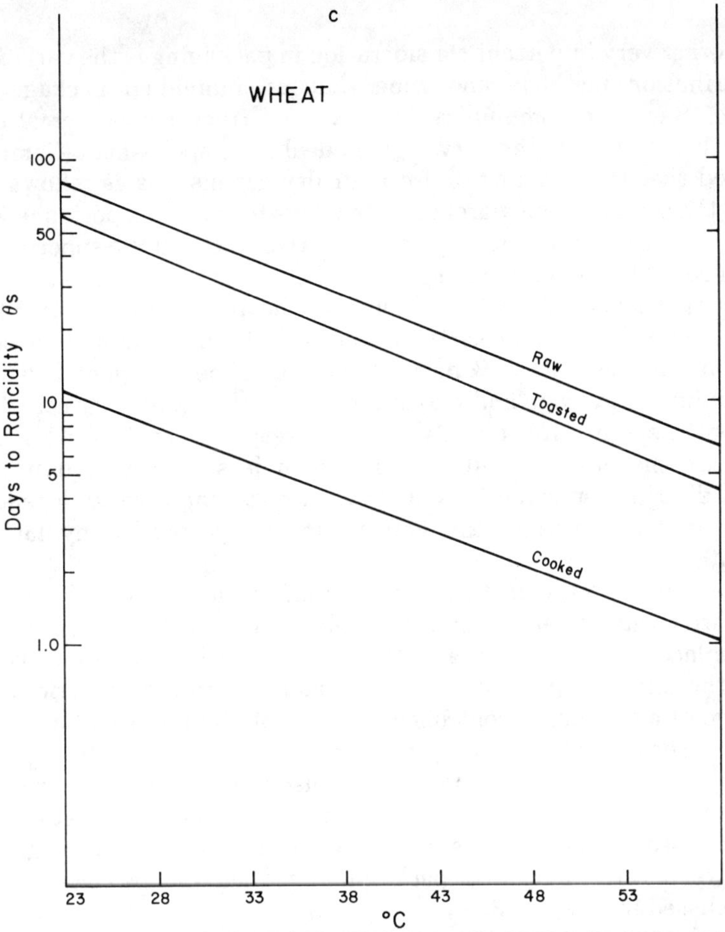

FIG. 5.1c. EFFECTS OF COOKING AND TOASTING ON STORAGE STABILITY OF: c — WHEAT

(Anderson *et al.* 1965).

MODES OF DETERIORATION: GENERAL SHELF-LIFE CONSIDERATIONS

There are four modes of deterioration to be considered when packaging and storing dry cereals. They are:

(1) Moisture gain, resulting in loss of crispness.
(2) Lipid oxidation, resulting in rancidity and off-flavors.
(3) Loss of vitamins, resulting in the nutritional labeling being incorrect.
(4) Breakage, resulting in an aesthetically undesirable product.

One other very important consideration in packaging is the variability of distribution methods and time that an individual package will undergo. Based on communications received from several cereal companies, distribution times vary a great deal. One spokesman (Company A) stated that the distribution for their dry cereals was as follows: one week in the process plant warehouse, ten days for rail transport, one week in the main distribution center and one to two weeks in the supermarket warehouse. This gives an average distribution time of five to six weeks. Another spokesman (Company A) felt that the average distribution time could actually be as long as three months, the maximum time being about nine months, with 98% being sold in that time. Company B reports their minimum, average and maximum distribution times for cereals as one month, six months and 24 months, respectively. The 24 month cereals are the preprocessed ones stored in jars with a vacuum seal. General distribution conditions are given as varying greatly depending on geography and time of year. This would be expected for any national distributor.

Packaging of dry cereals has characteristically been in fiberboard boxes with a wax coated glassine liner. More recently the glassine liner is being replaced by various more costly plastic materials as manufacturers realize the effect of packaging has on reducing product deterioration. Breakage of a product is controlled very simply by the use of a heavier gauge fiberboard box with proper handling. A product such as puffed wheat can be packaged just in a bag because breakage is not a problem.

Losses of vitamins, especially vitamin C, can occur as moisture content increases. Minerals are stable and are not lost. Moisture gain is directly related to the type of packaging used and can be calculated as was discussed in Chapter 3.

In the past, a two pound wax coated glassine liner was felt sufficient for most cereals, but recently, as distribution chains get longer and required shelf-lives are lengthened some cereal companies have gone to polyethylene and other films to protect their crispier products. Insufficient reported data are available on moisture gain in cereals; however, it can be estimated that a 2 to 3% moisture gain would be critical from a crispness standpoint.

Felt (1945) used the following equation for calculating moisture gain for shelf-life:

$$\text{moisture gain} = (\text{permeance})(\text{area})(\text{time})(\text{driving force})$$

The results of his study in comparison to actual data are shown in Table 5.1. This method has one major drawback, in that it does not use the integrated form derived in Chapter 3. In addition, the method also assumes

TABLE 5.1
COMPARISON OF CALCULATED AND OBSERVED SHELF-LIFE[1]

	Weeks to Reach Moisture Limit			
	Corn Cereal		Oat Cereal	
Location	Observed	Calculated	Observed	Calculated
Control cabinet	5.0	5.0	3.9	4.4
Houston, Texas	4.5	5.0	4.5	4.0
Jacksonville, Florida	5.5	6.0	4.5	5.0
Oklahoma City, Oklahoma	8.5	8.0	7.0	7.0
Kansas City, Missouri	10.5	8.0	9.0	8.0
Baltimore, Maryland	11.5	9.0	9.5	8.0
Chicago, Illinois	14.0	11.0	11.0	10.0
Providence, Rhode Island	12.5	11.0	12.5	10.0
Buffalo, New York	10.0	10.0	9.5	10.0
Minneapolis, Minnesota	11.0	11.0	11.0	10.0
Portland, Oregon	17.0	13.0	12.0	11.0
San Francisco, California	19.0	11.0	16.5	10.0
Ogden, Utah[2]	—	—	—	—

[1]Field test started in April, Felt (1945).
[2]The vapor pressure in Ogden reaches a maximum of 0.15 psi in July and August when the mean temperature is 80 °F and 75 °F respectively. Under these conditions, the cereal products cannot reach the critical moisture level. This was confirmed by observation, the products being tested in Ogden did not attain this level even after 24 weeks of observation.

that all cereals have the same isotherm. The overall agreement between calculated and experimental values does not appear to be that good in Table 5.1, although Felt thought it was quite good. Part of the problem could have been the unusual isotherm of high sensitivity he found at low a_ws.

The problem of prevention of moisture gain is not as simply solved in shredded cereals. Rancid odors tend to accumulate if shredded wheat is stored in an airtight container, due to the higher unsaturated fat content in this cereal. Therefore the product is usually sold in breather boxes without outer or inner linings. When so packaged, the product is just as stable as any other prepared cereal, except that moisture absorption can take place much more readily. The net effect is a reduction in shelf-life of these products (Matz 1970).

The last mode of deterioration that packaging must deal with is oxidative rancidity. A package itself cannot prevent rancidity, but it can inhibit the reaction or at least prevent the reaction from being accelerated by:

(1) Excluding light.
(2) Excluding oxygen (although oxygen is almost never rate limiting it may help in some cases).

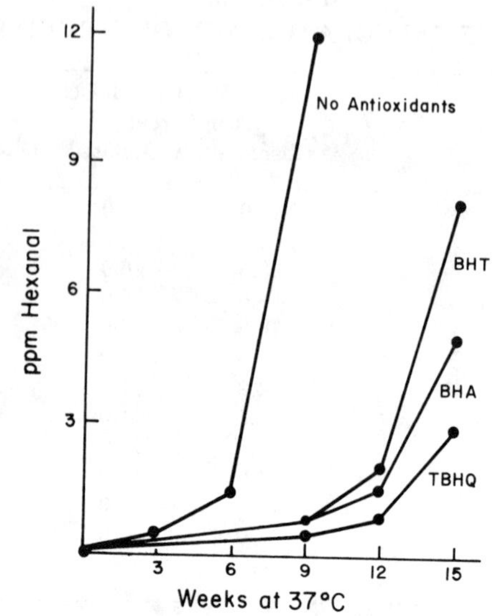

FIG. 5.2. EFFECT OF ANTIOXIDANTS ON STABILITY OF A WHEAT CEREAL

(Fritsch and Gale 1977)

(3) Being free of all trace metals.

(4) Containing antioxidant.

Figure 5.2 shows the results of a stability study on a wheat cereal conducted by Company A when three different antioxidants were added to the packaging material. The effect of the antioxidants is to extend the induction period to about twice what it is without the antioxidant. This would be equivalent to doubling the shelf-life since the induction period is considered equivalent to shelf-life (Fritsch and Gale 1977).

Exclusion of light is usually accomplished by a fiberboard box. However, for those cereals packaged solely in a bag, an opaque film should be used.

Excluding oxygen may help, but since the effect is minimal and cost is increased, most companies do not bother with gas-proof packaging. Many packages, as was mentioned for shredded wheat, do the opposite, allowing the product to "breathe" and thereby letting rancid odors to escape as they are formed.

To summarize packaging requirements, four factors are of primary importance:

(1) Use of a fiberboard box to exclude light and prevent breakage.

(2) Use of a liner that gives the required moisture barrier to preserve freshness.
(3) Use of an antioxidant in the liner to inhibit oxidative rancidity.
(4) Consideration for varying distribution times and conditions may require the use of a different package in summer than the one used in winter.

VITAMIN LOSSES

TABLE 5.2
LOSS OF NUTRIENT IN MILLING OF WHEAT

Nutrient	Whole Wheat ($\mu g/g$)	Flour ($\mu g/g$)	Loss Flour (%)	Germ ($\mu g/g$)
Thiamin	3.5	0.8	77.1	22
Riboflavin	1.5	0.3	80.0	5.5
Niacin	50	9.5	80.8	80
B_6	1.7	0.5	71.8	12
Pantothenic acid	10	5	50.0	25
Folacin	0.3	0.1	66.7	1.5
α-Tocopherol	16	2.2	86.3	125
Betaine	844	650	22.8	4825
Choline	1089	767	29.5	3002
Fat (%)	1.61	0.87	46.0	8.03
Starch (%)	57.21	68.66	+20.0	18.05
Protein (%)	10.50	10.71	+ 2.0	24.82

TABLE 5.3
EFFECT OF CEREAL PROCESSING ON VITAMIN LOSSES

Food Item	Biotin (μg)	Folacin (μg)
Corn	—	265
Corn flakes	—	55
Brown rice	120	200
Dry rice cereal	13	76

Vitamin and mineral fortification is very common in the cereal industry, so consideration must be given to loss of these nutrients. As the data in Table 5.2 show, there are moderate losses of some nutrients when milling grains. Table 5.3 presents further evidence of losses of nutrients in producing cereals (Schroeder 1971). These losses have stimulated the fortification of breakfast cereals. Two other factors have increased fortification: the ease with which the nutrients can be applied without influencing the product stability or flavor, and the low cost of fortification. In 1941 the cost of enriching 100 lb of flour at the mill was 17 cents; in 1967 it was two cents (Brooke 1968). With the increased trend towards nutritional labeling, this small cost becomes insignificant.

TABLE 5.4
MICRONUTRIENT CONTENT OF WHOLE WHEAT

Micronutrient	Level in Whole Wheat Flour
Folic acid (mg/100 g)	0.06
Paotothenic acid (mg/100 g)	0.94
Biotin (μg/100 g)	9.3
Magnesium (mg/100 g)	119
Phosphorus (mg/100 g)	362
Zinc (mg/100 g)	2.6
Manganese (mg/100 g)	2.4
Selenium (mg/100 g)	0.007

TABLE 5.5
EFFECT OF STORAGE ON LOSSES OF MICRONUTRIENTS IN WHEAT-BASED CEREAL

Micronutrient in 1 oz of Cereal	Initial Value	3 Months at 104°F	6 Months at 72°F
Vitamin A (IU)	5450	4745	5525
Vitamin C (mg)	74	69	70
Thiamin (mg)	1.7	1.7	1.8
Riboflavin (mg)	2.0	2.1	1.9
Niacin (mg)	26	24	25
Vitamin D (IU)	480	440	470
Vitamin E (IU)	14	14	13
Vitamin B_6 (mg)	2.4	2.5	2.3
Folic acid (mg)	0.5	0.4	0.5
Vitamin B_{12} (μg)	6.1	5.9	5.9
Pantothenic acid (mg)	12	11	11

TABLE 5.6
STABILITY OF VITAMIN A AND VITAMIN C IN A FORTIFIED CEREAL DURING STORAGE[1]

Vitamin A Added (IU/oz)	Vitamin C Added (mg/oz)	3 Months at 104°F Vitamin A	Vitamin C
2280	26.1	1922	22.0
2606	0	975	—
2581 + 22 ppm BHT	31.7	2050	26.7
2450 + 33 ppm BHT	0	1450	—

[1]Anderson *et al.* (1976).

Tables 5.4 and 5.5 from Company A show normal micronutrient levels in a whole wheat cereal, initial levels in a fortified cereal and loss of the nutrients under accelerated shelf-life testing (Anderson *et al.* 1976). The results in Table 5.5 clearly indicate that the only vitamin with any significant loss is vitamin A (about 14%). Further tests were done on this vitamin and the results are presented in Table 5.6 (Anderson *et al.* 1976). It shows that the addition of an antioxidant along with vitamin C will minimize the loss of vitamin A. Vitamin A, however, would still have to be overfortified, as some is still lost. Unfortunately not enough data exist to develop kinetic values for the loss of this vitamin.

The cereals were also tested in a weather room, where temperature and humidity were cycled to simulate day and night in a warm coastal city according to Fig. 5.3. The results were not published but the following statement was made about them: "stabilities of vitamins in the 'weather room' in our tests was [sic] good" (Anderson *et al.* 1976).

The data for vitamin C loss in the above study are somewhat contradictory to the findings of Vojnovich and Pfeifer (1970), who studied vitamin C destruction in a mixed cereal blend at various water contents. The data are presented graphically in Fig. 5.4. According to their data, one could expect 50% loss of vitamin C at 104°C and 5% moisture content (a_w 0.4) to take about 35 days. This is much greater loss than the 7% loss shown in the Anderson *et al.* (1976) study of 3 months at 104°F. Anderson *et al.* (1976) offer the following explanation for the 7% loss:

> Since cereals are of low moisture content, the lactone ring of ascorbic acid is not readily hydrolyzed to diketogulonic acid. Consequently, most of the ascorbic acid lost remains in the cereal as dehydroascorbic acid which has at least 90% of the vitamin C activity of ascorbic acid, so there is actually an insigificant loss of vitamin C activity during storage of most breakfast cereals.

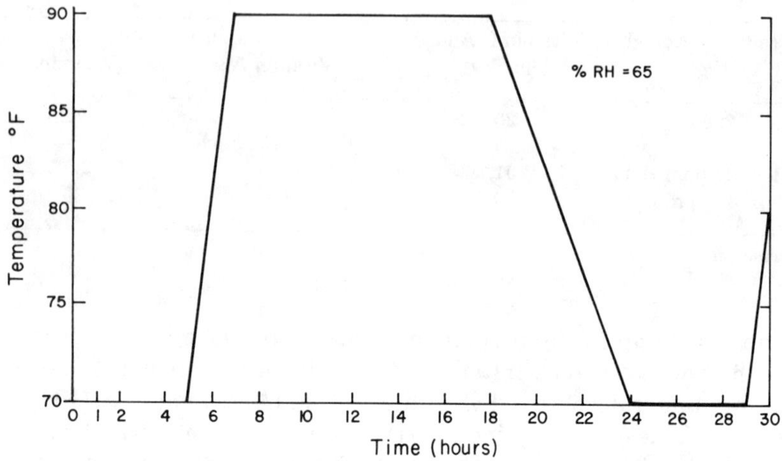

FIG. 5.3. WEATHER ROOM CONDITIONS (Anderson *et al.* 1976)

They further state that stabilities of vitamin C and A are adversely affected by moisture contents over 6% but by then most cereals are judged organoleptically unacceptable. The moisture content of their test cereals is not stated but would be expected to be around 3% ($a_w < 0.3$) which is the normal level for most cereals. This would explain much of the discrepancy between the data in the two articles.

The conclusion that can be drawn from this work is that micronutrient loss may not be a major mode of deterioration in dry cereals. Even vitamin A survives six months at room temperature with no measurable loss. Since average distribution time is only six months, micronutrient loss would not be a major factor in determining the shelf-life of dry cereals.

OXIDATIVE RANCIDITY

The primary mode of chemical deterioration in dry cereals is lipid oxidation. The reason for this is twofold. First of all, the water activity of dry cereals is at or below the monolayer, which essentially stops all other types of deteriorative reactions. Secondly, unsaturated fats are required in lipid oxidation and the grains used in cereals have a high ratio of unsaturated to saturated fats.

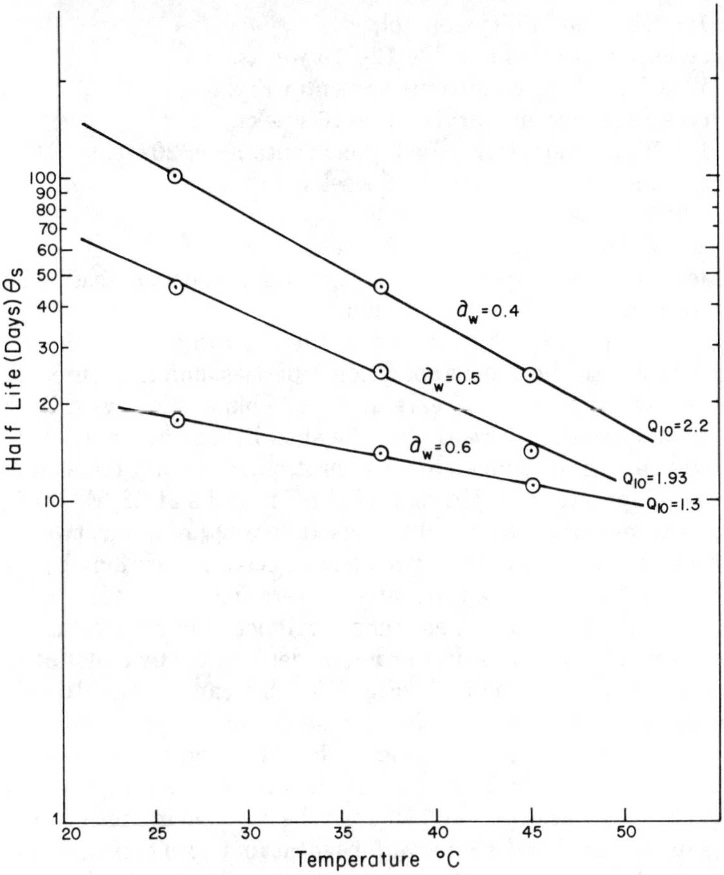

FIG. 5.4. TIME FOR LOSS OF 50% OF VITAMIN C IN INFANT CEREAL
(Vojnovich and Pfeifer 1970)

Accelerated shelf-life testing by industry is done by two methods: increased temperature and increased humidity. Increased humidity, however, is a bad choice for accelerating lipid oxidation for two reasons. (1) If the original moisture content is below the monolayer, an increase in humidity may actually show a decrease in oxidation. (2) Increasing moisture content above the monolayer will quickly show a change in mechanism to nonenzymatic browning as the primary mode of deterioration.

Company A gives this summary of accelerating conditions to measure oxidative rancidity development in cereals.

(1) 100 °F: no humidity control;
cereals should all survive 12—16 weeks.
(2) Weather room: conditions shown in Fig. 5.3;
cereals should all survive 12—16 weeks.
(3) 115 °F: packaged in sealed glass containers; 20—25% RH;
cereals should survive 3—4 weeks.
(4) 140 °F: packaged as in No. 3;
cereals should survive 1—2 weeks.

Conditions 1 and 2 are tested organoleptically, while conditions 3 and 4 are tested by n-hexanal determination.

Company B reports that they use 98 °F storage as their only accelerating factor to check organoleptic properties, and that three months at 98 °F is equivalent to two years at 70 °F. This would give a Q_{10} of 3.8, which would appear to overestimate the shelf-life considerably if lipid oxidation was the primary mode of deterioration. Rancidity development is much less temperature sensitive, and three months at 98 °F is probably equivalent to nine months at 70 °F, based on a Q_{10} of about two.

The best study of oxidative rancidity in cereals was done by Fritsch and Gale (1977). They used hexanal determination, which is an intermediate in lipid oxidation, as a chemical means of measuring rancidity. Production of hexanal is first order, as determined by a plot of ln hexanal concentration vs time as in Fig. 5.5. This can be used to calculate rate constants for the reaction in various cereals as presented in Table 5.7. Measurements were also done at four temperatures for corn and wheat cereals, as seen in Table 5.8. The k values when plotted to determine the activation energies and Q_{10}s for the reaction in these two cereals gave E_as of 14.5 kcal and 19.9 kcal for wheat and corn cereal, respectively. These are fairly consistent with those normally found for lipid oxidation.

TABLE 5.7
HEXANAL CONCENTRATION VS TIME IN STORAGE AT 37 °C

Time (Weeks)	ln Hexanal Oat	Corn	Wheat A	Wheat B
0	0.31	0.37	0.03	0.05
6	1.26	1.72	0.87	0.08
9	2.07	4.62	2.47	0.11
12	3.85	8.01	15.39	0.24
Rate constant K = weeks^{-1}	.211	.339	.522	.119

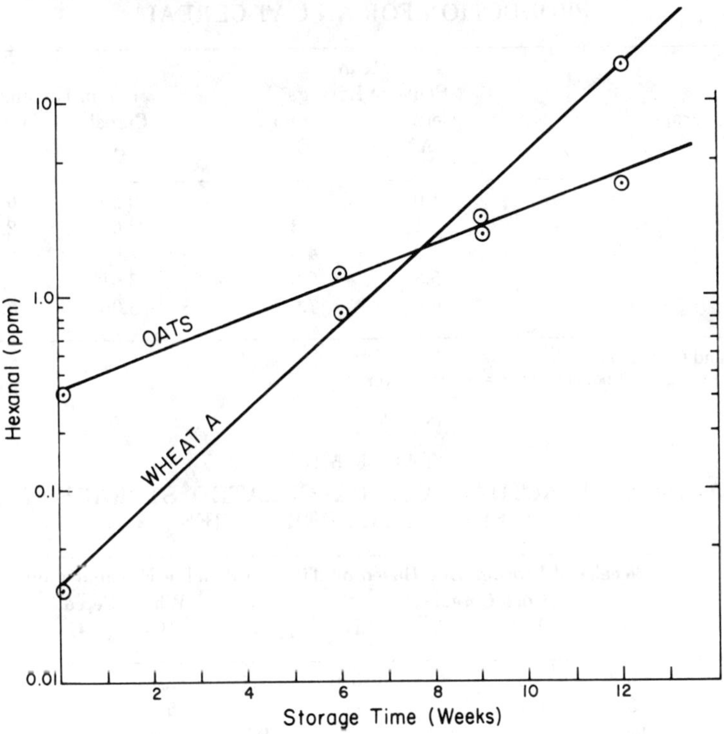

FIG. 5.5. STORAGE OF CEREALS — FIRST ORDER PLOT

TABLE 5.8
RATE CONSTANTS FOR HEXANAL PRODUCTION IN TWO CEREALS

Storage Temperature °C	Weeks^{-1} Corn	Weeks^{-1} Wheat
55	.836	1.874
45	.443	.974
37	.252	.541
21	.075	.146
E_a Kcal/mole	19.9	14.5
Q_{10}	2.78	2.10

TABLE 5.9
CORRELATION BETWEEN SENSORY EVALUATION AND HEXANAL PRODUCTION FOR AN OAT CEREAL[1]

Weeks Storage at 37°C	Mean Sensory Ratings[2] Cereal A	Cereal B	ppm Hexanal Cereal A	Cereal B
0	1.0	1.0	0.30	0.23
3	3.1	3.3	2.09	2.02
6	4.0	4.0	2.98	2.81
9	5.3	5.6	3.61	3.71
12	6.9	7.6	5.06	5.00

[1]Fritsch and Gale (1977).
[2]Sensory ratings — 9 point scale; 8 = rancid flavor.

TABLE 5.10
COMPARISON OF ACTUAL AND CALCULATED STORAGE-LIFE AT DIFFERENT TEMPERATURES

Storage	Weeks of Storage Life Based on Time to Reach a Hexanal Value of 5							
	Corn Cereal				Wheat Cereal			
°C	A	B	C	D	A	B	C	D
55	3.2	3.2	—	3.1	2.7	2.7	—	2.6
45	6.1	6.1	—	—	5.3	5.3	—	—
37	10.7	10.7	10.4	—	9.5	9.6	9.1	—
29	—	19.2	18.3	19.3	—	17.9	16.4	17.6
21	35.7	35.6	33.3	36.1	35.0	34.5	30.3	33.7

A — Experimentally determined results from rate constant for hexanal.
B — Based on k values from arrhenius plot.
C — Based on extrapolation of 45° and 55°C data.
D — Based on extrapolation of 45° and 37°C data.

Fritsch and Gale (1977).

The hexanal determination was then compared with a sensory evaluation as seen in Table 5.9. For oat cereal a hexanal value of about 5 ppm, or a sensory value of about 8 was indicative of rancidity. Other cereals gave a hexanal value between 5 and 10 ppm for a sensory rating of 8. The correlation coefficient between hexanal and sensory ratings was 0.99. A comparison of various methods for shelf-life predictions is shown in Table 5.10. It shows that using the actual k values to calculate an expected shelf-life vs that from a shelf-life plot gives about the same results.

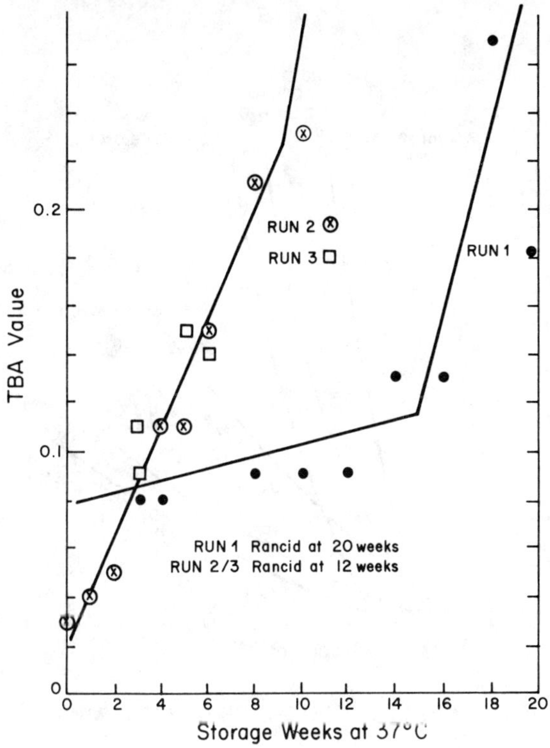

FIG. 5.6. STORAGE OF OAT CEREAL (Caldwell and Grogg 1955)

TABLE 5.11
STABILIZING CEREALS BY BLENDING ANTIOXIDANTS[1]

Cereal	Temperature	Average Stability in Days at: 145°F	74°F
Cream of corn	Control	12	60
	0.01% Tenox II antioxidant	28	77
	0.05% Tenox II antioxidant	33	78
Cream of oats	Control	40	90
	0.01% Tenox II antioxidant	50	175+
	0.05% Tenox II antioxidant	60	175+
Cream of rice	Control	12	50
	0.01% Tenox II antioxidant	21	70
	0.05% Tenox II antioxidant	22	75
Cream of barley	Control	20	80
	0.01% Tenox II antioxidant	25	175+
	0.05% Tenox antioxidant	35	175+

[1]Stuckey (1955).

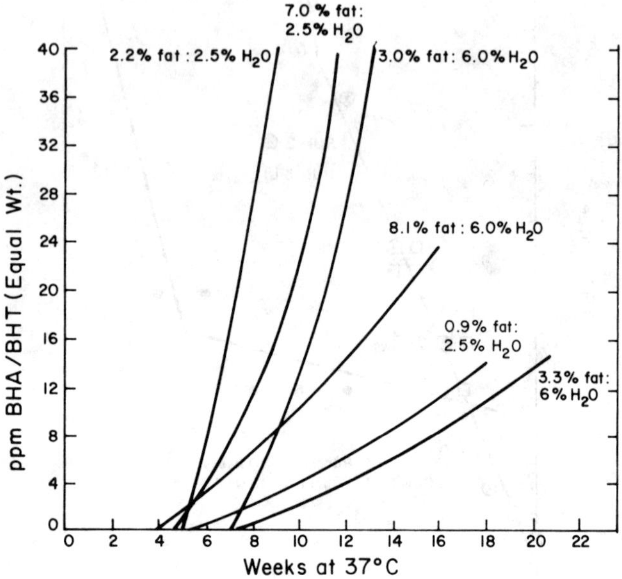

FIG. 5.7. CEREAL SHELF-LIFE IMPROVEMENT

TABLE 5.12
STABILIZING CEREALS BY ATOMIZING AN EMULSION OF ANTIOXIDANTS[1]

Product	Treatment	Average Stability in Days at: 145°F	74°F
Brown rice	Control	13	45
	0.025% Tenox VII antioxidant	200+	
	0.025% Tenox IV antioxidant	69	200+
	0.07% Tenox VI antioxidant	77	200+
Rice bran	Control	5	42
	0.025% Tenox VII antioxidant	17	200+
	0.025% Tenox IV antioxidant	18	135
	0.07% Tenox VI antioxidant	35	200+

[1]Stuckey (1955).

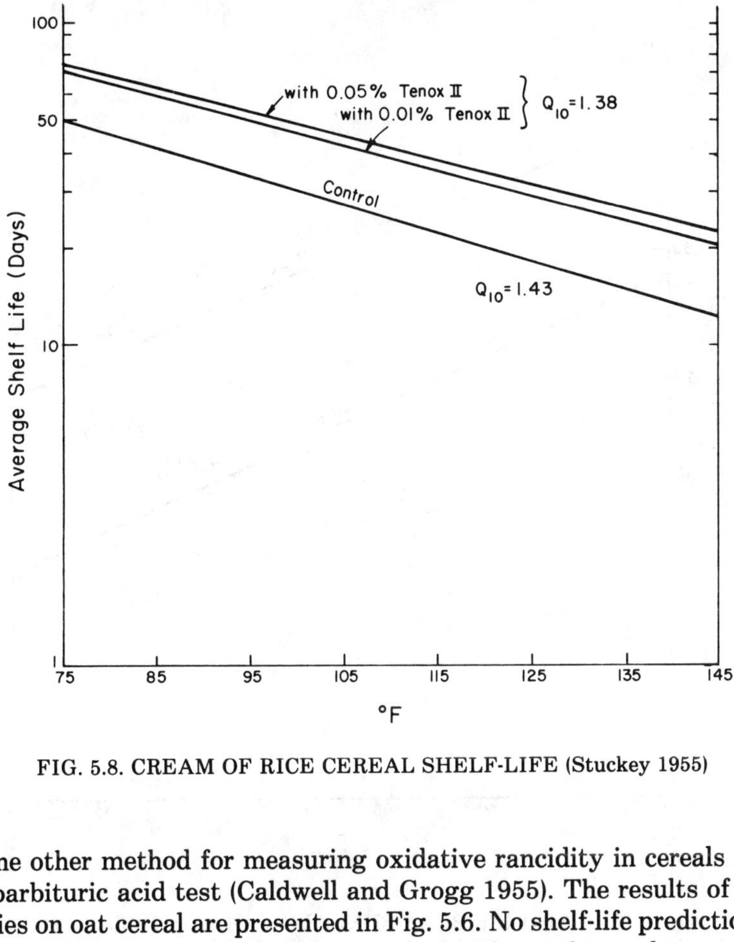

FIG. 5.8. CREAM OF RICE CEREAL SHELF-LIFE (Stuckey 1955)

One other method for measuring oxidative rancidity in cereals is the thiobarbituric acid test (Caldwell and Grogg 1955). The results of these studies on oat cereal are presented in Fig. 5.6. No shelf-life predictions or correlations with sensory ratings were made. The work was done at 37 °C, so an activation energy could not be determined. Figure 5.7 shows the effect of antioxidants on stability of cereals with various fat and moisture levels. There apperas to be a difference in the protective affect of BHA and BHT on different systems, but these differences are not determined by fat or moisture level alone.

An additional organoleptic shelf-life study on use of the antioxidants to improve shelf-life of cereals by addition of antioxidant to cereals was done by Stuckey (1955). Table 5.11 shows the stabilization of an antioxidant mixture that was blended with the cereal. Tenox II contains 20% BHA, 6% propyl gallate and 4% citric acid in propylene glycol. Figure 5.8 is a graphic presentation of the data for cream of rice cereal from

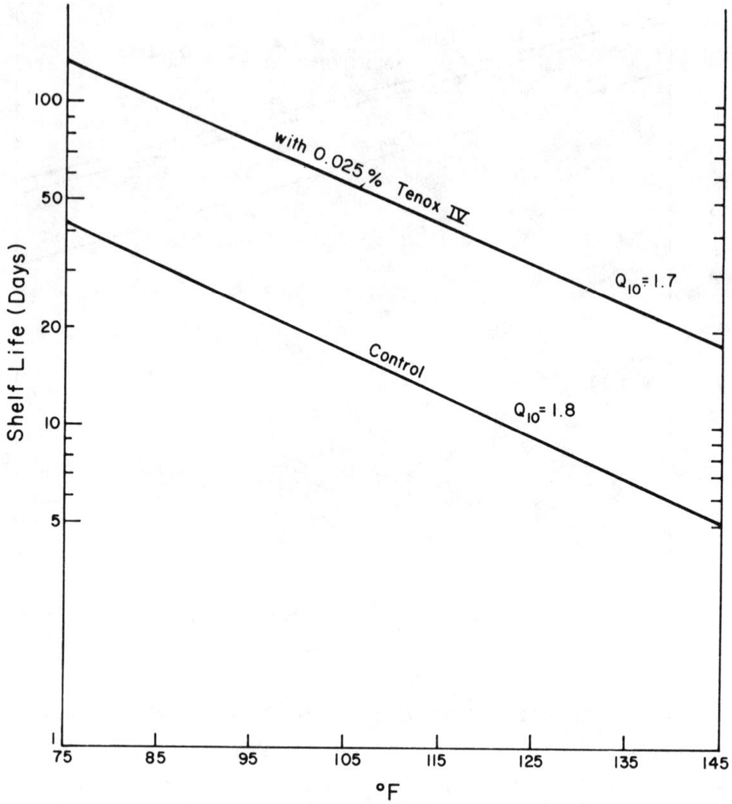

FIG. 5.9. RICE BRAN SHELF-LIFE (Stuckey 1955)

Table 5.11. The antioxidant affects Q_{10} very little, but does increase the shelf-life. Table 5.12 shows the results of stabilizing the cereal by spraying a mist of antioxidant mixture onto the cereal. Figure 5.9 shows the data for rice bran control and rice bran with Tenox IV, which is 0.005% BHA and 0.005% BHT in a water emulsion. Again the shelf-life is extended, but the Q_{10} is nearly unaffected. In all these cases the Q_{10} is less than two, indicating that both natural (produced by toasting) and added antioxidants are increasing shelf-life. In these studies the shelf-life was measured by organoleptic means.

OPEN DATING

Open dating probably has more potential for dry cereals than it does for many other processed foods due to the relatively long shelf-life of these products and its low abuse potential if storage is controlled. However, like all foods, there are some serious drawbacks to open dating of cereals.

The first consideration is what type of date could be used for cereals. The basic conclusion is that it should be "best if used by" or "use by" rather than a "pack" or "sell by" date. There is far more variation in shelf-lives of cereals than the average consumer would expect. Each type of cereal must be studied individually for any significant information to be derived on how long it will be acceptable. One important point is that the temperature sensitivity Q_{10} is low (about 1.5 to 2.5), so that slight abuses will not drastically affect the shelf-life. This is not the case with most foods, especially frozen ones. Therefore, a "best if used by" or "sell by" date would give some meaningful information to the consumer as long as storage conditions are noted on the package. Other benefits include:

(1) Easier to control stock rotation
(2) Easier to control overage pick-ups
(3) Satisfies consumers and consumer groups
(4) Gets the company "off the hook" if the product is overage.

However, when considering the benefits against the risks, the worth of open dating of cereals may be doubtful. The biggest reason against it is that it may be an unnecessary expense. The average shelf-life for dry processed cereals is somewhere between 6 and 12 months, which means that about 98% of all cereals are sold before they reach the end of their shelf-life. For 2% of the product open dating seems a little unnecessary, since to give a meaningful date, adequate temperature/humidity conditions must be obtained for all distribution systems. In any case, probably 2% of the product will end up being abused anyway. There are two other drawbacks to open dating of cereals:

(1) The problem of people picking only the freshest product thereby increasing the amount of overage product.
(2) There will always be abuses of some product, meaning that the date must be understated for most products, which again increases losses.

REFERENCES

ANDERSON, R.N., MORAN, D.H., HUNTLY, T.E. and HOLAHAN, J.L. 1963. Responses of cereal to antioxidants. Food Technol. *17*, 1587.

ANDERSON, R.H., MAXWELL, O.L., MULLEY, A.E. and FRITISCH, C.W. 1976. Effects of processing and storage on micronutrients in breakfast cereals. Food Technol. *30*(5), 110.

BROOKE, C.L. 1968. Enrichment and fortification of cereals and cereal products with vitamins and minerals. J. Agric. Food Chem. *16*, 163.

CALDWELL, E.F. and GROGG, B. 1955. Application of the thiobarbituric acid test to cereal and baked products. Food Technol. *9*, 185.

FELT, C.E. 1945. Shelf-life of packaged cereals. Cereal Chem. *22*, 261.

FRITSCH, C.W. and GALE, J.A. 1977. Hexanal as a measure of oxidative deterioration in low fat foods. J. Am. Oil Chemists Soc. *54*, 225.

MARTZ, S.A. 1970. Cereal Technology. AVI Publishing Co., Westport, Conn.

SCHROEDER, H.A. 1971. Losses of vitamins and trace minerals resulting from processing and preservation of foods. Am. J. of Clin. Nutr. *24*, 562.

STUCKEY, B. 1955. Increasing shelf-life with phenolic antioxidants. Food Technol. *9*, 585.

VOJNOVICH, C. and PFEIFER, V.F. 1970. Stability of ascorbic acid in blends with wheat flour, CSM and infant cereals. Cereal Sci. Today *15*, 317.

CHAPTER 6

SHELF-LIFE OF PASTA PRODUCTS

INTRODUCTION

The general product classification of pasta can be subdivided into two categories. The first, macaroni, has come to represent a generic family of foods in the United States. It includes over 140 items: products such as spaghetti, macaroni and vermicelli. This class of products is made from semolina (usually milled from durum wheat), water and, in most cases, added vitamins and minerals. With the exception of oil-dried products (i.e., ramen) macaroni products contain about 1.5% fat.

The second broad category of pasta is noodles. These products contain the same ingredients as macaroni as well as added egg solids (minimum level ~ 5.5%). The egg solids are usually in the form of yolks (to enhance color) and therefore the lipid content of noodles is about 4.6%. Noodles may also contain additional protein from sources such as soy flour.

All pasta products sold in America are covered by Standards of Identity. Over 85% of the products manufactured in the U.S. follow the standard's guidelines for enrichment (B complex vitamins and iron) and much of the noodle production is fortified with alternate protein sources. As a food source, therefore, pasta compares favorably with other staples such as rice, potatoes and enriched bread.

Pasta consumption in the U.S. in 1977 was 9.5 lb per person (Brown 1977). This level is double that of five years ago and industry projects consumption levels to double again by 1985 (Anon. 1977a). The increasing consumption trends and the high nutrient levels (up to 50% USRDA per 4 oz serving of the B vitamins and significant protein) makes pasta an important source of nutrients in the American diet.

PRESERVATION METHOD

Pasta is preserved in three major ways: by air drying and oil frying followed by packaging in cardboard boxes, cellophane or cellophane/polyethylene; by freezing; and by canning when it usually is combined with other ingredients. This chapter will deal exclusively with the first method of preservation. On the American market all canned and most frozen pasta products are of the finished goods type (i.e. TV dinners) and represent other shelf-life problems.

Sales of dried pasta products are about equally divided between retail sales (product used by the homemaker as a base for a meal) and sales for remanufacture into finished goods such as canned spaghetti and TV dinners.

SHELF-LIFE DATA

The Rutgers Food Stability Survey (1971) has listed four major modes for pasta product failure. The first of these is moisture gain (or loss). The optimum moisture content for pasta storage is 10% to 11% (Anon. 1977b) corresponding to an a_w of 0.44. If the product is allowed to lose moisture to less than 6% it becomes too fragile and unacceptable in quality. Conversely, if it gains moisture, mold growth and starch recrystallization (retrogradation) occurs. This happens rapidly at a water content somewhere between 13% and 16%. Mold growth makes the product unfit for consumption. Retrogradation leads to an unacceptably tough product when cooked (Anon. 1977b; Kumar *et al.* 1974; Siegel *et al.* 1975). Also, under proper conditions, the product may check as it gains moisture, causing fragmentation upon cooking.

A second mode of deterioration, especially for noodle products, is color loss. Loss of color through oxidation of carotene pigments is a result of lipoxidase enzymes, found naturally in semolina flour, which oxidize lipids especially in the presence of light. The formed peroxides then attack the pigments. The third mode of failure mentioned in the Rutgers study is from undesirable flavors being absorbed from the packaging material. The final deterioration type listed in the study is staling which, although not very well defined, is most likely due to oxidation of the lipids in the product.

Lipid oxidation would be more severe for higher oil content products. Nutritional losses may also occur, including losses of the added B vitamins and possible lysine loss due to nonenzymatic browning.

The fact that pasta is generally used as a carrier of other ingredients in a meal is probably the reason that studies of nutrient losses have received so little attention in research labs.

Manufacturers of pasta claim shelf-lives of macaroni and spaghetti products ranging from six months to indefinite. Noodle shelf-life claims range from one to six months. The U.S. Army data (see Chapter 3) claim a shelf-life of one to six months for chow mein, nine to thirty-six months for noodles and 24 to 48 months for macaroni and spaghetti. The exact shelf-life depends upon storage temperature, relative humidity and package type which is not well defined. The modes of failure assumed in the Army data are probably staling and either moisture gain or loss. These two failure modes also seem to be the major ones considered by industry.

With the exception of the Army recommendations for shelf-life reproduced in the Congressional Record (Anon 1977c), little, if any, information exists in the literature in English concerning storage degradation of pasta products. There appears to be a large body of literature in both Italian and Polish concerning macaroni and noodle storage and Japanese literature seems to have a good deal of data concerning fried noodles. A problem exists, however, in that only a few of these journals are translated into English and then, generally, only the abstracts are reproduced.

Table 6.1 lists the calculated rate constants (k values), temperature coefficients (Q_{10}s), and activation energies (E_as) calculated from the literature for various products. The standard industry data for shelf-life of spaghetti as reported by Winston (1971) gives a Q_{10} of 2.39 and an activation energy of 15.2 kcal/mole. When this Q_{10} is compared to the Q_{10} value of 1.29 from the Army (Anon. 1977c) data for shelf-life, it can be seen that the industry uses a higher Q_{10} than the actual data. If in fact, the "real" Q_{10}s are lower, this will result in the prediction of significantly more loss of shelf-life for variable conditions than actually would occur at higher temperature, or a longer shelf-life than would occur at a lower temperature.

With the exception of work by Kumar *et al.* (1974), none of the articles which defined an end of shelf-life described the mode of failure. In their study, θ_s was defined by moisture tolerance for vermicelli. If these data are compared to the other data in Table 6.1 and Fig. 6.1, it can be seen that both the Q_{10} and E_a for moisture tolerance data are much higher, indicating that this mode of failure was probably not considered a quality loss factor in the Army study. Low Q_{10}s and E_as as found from the analysis of the end of shelf-life data are characteristic of lipid oxidation (Q_{10} generally from 1.5 to 2.0). The Army data also show that the lower fat content products have the longest shelf-life, reinforcing the assumption that the basic mode of failure is actually due to lipid oxidation.

Pasta manufacturers do not use antioxidants, even though studies have been done showing that the addition of BHT and/or BHA greatly increase pasta shelf-life (Okado and Koyama 1969; Okado 1971).

Pasta products are distributed in the U.S. through normal ambient temperature warehouse channels. Most manufacturers do not worry about distribution time, but, for inventory investment reasons, do try to keep the turnover rate at about 30 to 60 days. Of the manufacturers that have storage recommendations, all specify "for longer lasting quality keep in a cool, dry place," which is applicable to prevention of moisture gain and rancidity.

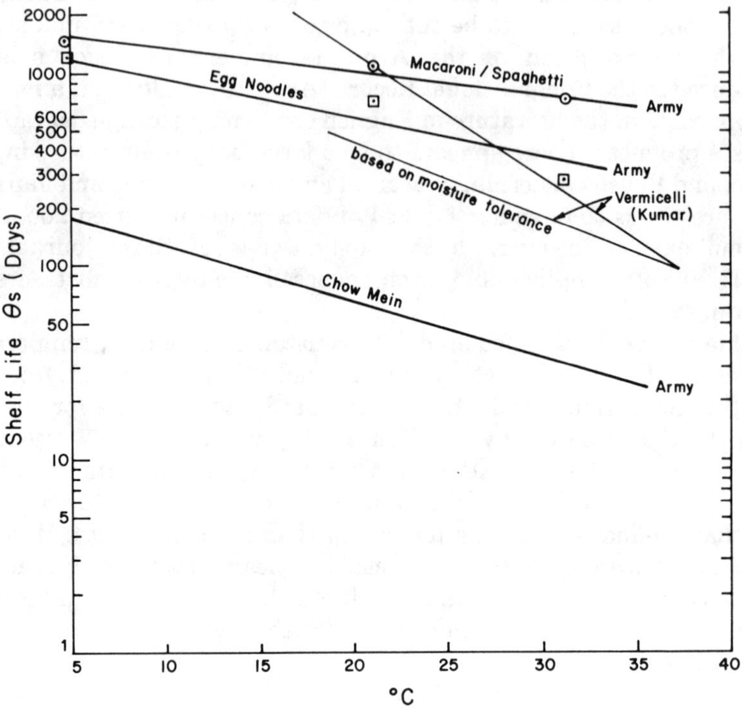

FIG. 6.1. SHELF-LIFE DATA OF PASTA PRODUCTS

Even though the quality of the protein found in pasta is low (P.E.R. = 0.8), at 13% protein pasta can be an important protein source in the diet. In fact, some pasta is currently fortified with protein which raises its P.E.R. to as high as 2.5 (Anon. 1976). As is shown in Fig. 6.2 and Table 6.1, the data of Fabriani and Fratoni (1972) indicate that protein quality loss in pasta is measurable at high temperature. A first order reaction for lysine loss was assumed. The Q_{10} calculated from the data is slightly higher than the end of shelf-life data and closer to the industry value. This raises the question of whether or not the shelf-life data accurately depict pasta nutritional quality losses. This becomes particularly significant in light of the fact that Fabriani's data (by chemical analysis) may overestimate the actual biological availability of lysine by 25 to 30%. Considering, however, that at 45 °C only a 30% loss occurs in 18 months (550 days) and the shelf-life (Army) is greater than this, the loss may not be important.

TABLE 6.1
KINETIC VALUES FROM PASTA LITERATURE

Product	Reference	Failure Mode	Rate Constant k	Q_{10}	E_a
Industry Standard	Winston (1971a)	ASLT data	7 days at 38 °C equivalent to 30 days at 21 °C	2.39	15.2 Kcal/mole
Enriched spaghetti/ macaroni	Anon. (1977a)	End of PSL[1]	0.021 mo^{-1} at 4.5 °C 0.028 mo^{-1} at 21 °C 0.042 mo^{-1} at 32.2 °C	1.29	4.48 Kcal/mole
	Kumar (1974)	End of PSL	0.0034 wk^{-1} at 25-30 °C 0.012 wk^{-1} at 38 °C	2.64—4.86	17.7-27.8 Kcal/mole
	Fabriani and Fratoni (1972)	Loss of available lysine	0.0192 mo^{-1} at 45 °C 0.046 mo^{-1} at 60 °C 0.104 mo^{-1} at 70 °C 0.147 mo^{-1} at 80 °C	2.12	13.3 Kcal/mole
Noodles (egg)	Anon. (1977a)	End of PSL	0.023 mo^{-1} at 4.5 °C 0.042 mo^{-1} 21 °C 0.111 mo^{-1} at 32.2 °C	1.67	9.03 Kcal/mole
Chow mein noodles	Anon. (1977a)	End of PSL	0.167 mo^{-1} at 4.5 °C 0.500 mo^{-1} at 21—C 1.00 mo^{-1} at 32.2 °C	1.88	11.2 Kcal/mole

[1]PSL — Practical shelf life.

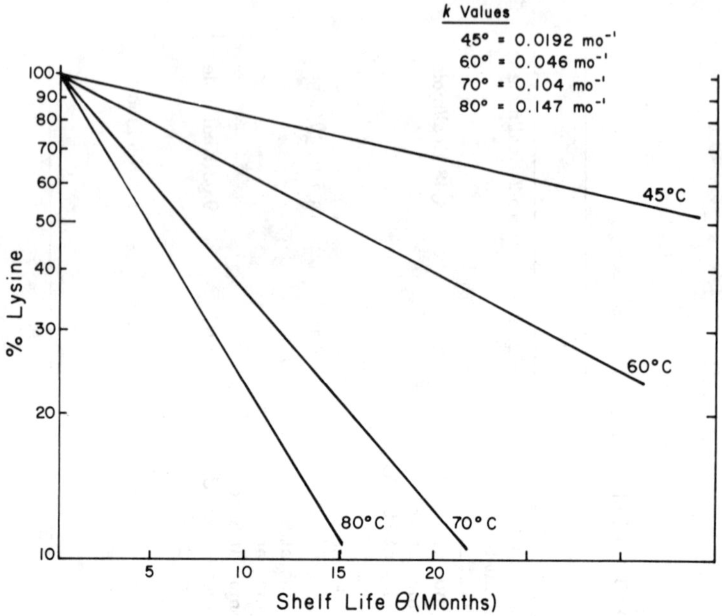

FIG. 6.2. LYSINE LOSS IN PASTA
(Fabriani and Fratoni 1972)

The fact that the shelf-life claims may slightly overestimate pasta nutritional quality is reinforced by the information available concerning vitamin losses. Chrzanowska (1974) has determined vitamin losses in enriched noodles stored at room temperature in paper or cellophane bags. He states that after 13 to 16 months, only thiamin content changed and only "slightly" when pasta was stored in opaque paper. However, when stored in cellophane and exposed to "diffuse sunlight" both riboflavin and pyridoxin decreased (with half lives of 19 and 62 days respectively) as seen in Fig. 6.3. The data for losses in bags have been supported by a number of other studies (Kwasniewska *et al.* 1972; Bunting 1965). In effect then, the B vitamins do degrade, especially when stored for long times in plastic bags. The amount lost can be significant as compared to the shelf-life. Also, numerous studies have shown that about one-half of the B vitamins are lost into the cooking water during preparation (Kwasniewska *et al.* 1972; Bunting 1965; and Ono and Niwa 1969).

In summary, pasta consumption in the U.S. is increasing rapidly, and becoming an important source of nutrients in the diet. Recognition of this fact is reflected in the pasta Standards of Identity which allow enrich-

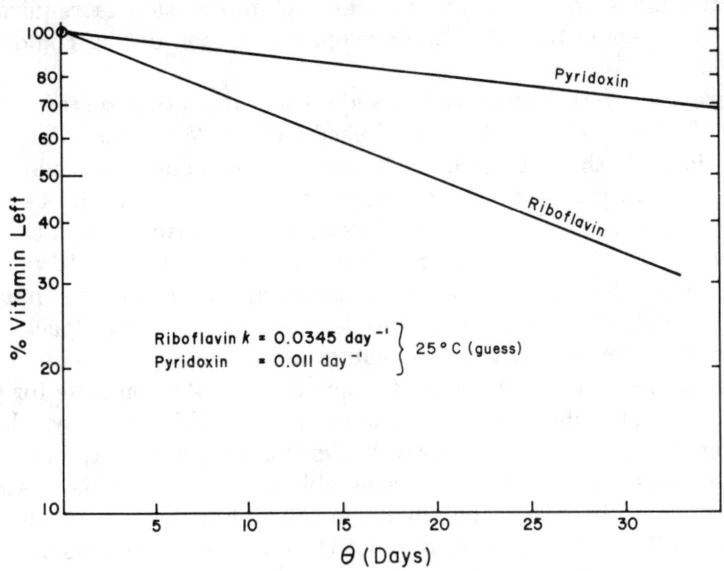

FIG. 6.3. VITAMIN LOSSES IN ENRICHED PASTA
(Chrzanowska 1974)

ment with B vitamins, iron and protein. Most American pasta is enriched and solid with nutritional labeling. Nutrient labeling is done even though there is no literature to support the claims. In fact, the Macaroni Journal published a list of permissable nutrient label levels "based upon approval obtained from the FDA as a result of a meeting in March by the members of the Standards and Nutrition Committee of the National Macaroni Manufacturers Association and the FDA" (Anon. 1974). This lack of information on kinetics of loss seems particularly important in light of the facts that the pasta protein has a low P.E.R. and that about one-half of the vitamin content is lost to the cooking water.

OPEN DATING

Both manufacturers and consumers seem to consider pasta as a foodstuff with an indefinite shelf-life. The few studies reported in English literature indicate that this is not true. There have not been enough data reported to forecast quality losses as a function of storage conditions and package type. There seems to be a real need for information about vitamin and protein quality losses in pasta. This information must come from storage study research. If shelf-life information is required for pasta, data would probably be developed and open dating could be instituted.

There are several recognized types of shelf-life dating systems: "pack date", "sell by date" and "best if used by" or "expiration date". The "pack date" is the data of manufacture of the product. A code of this type is currently used on most food products even though it is encoded and cannot be read by consumers. Because it is already in use, this data type would be the easiest for pasta manufacturers to use. It would be easy to teach the consumer what this date represents since a simple concept is involved. Two glaring problems exist with the "pack date" system, however. Initially, the consumer might have an extreme reaction against pasta products so labeled, since the distribution time for pasta products is somewhat longer than many realize. This perceived "lack of freshness" however, would probably dissipate rapidly as the consumer faith in industrial integrity was re-established. A second, more serious, problem would be that, even when the consumers understood the date, they would have to be educated about the expected shelf-lives of the different pasta products. This probably could be done but only with a massive educational effort.

Like the "pack date", if a "pull" or "sell by date" (date of last sale) were used, it would be very easy to educate the consumer about the concept of the date system, since many manufacturers of fresh products (i.e., dairy and bread) currently use this system. Since pasta has a low Q_{10}, the date would be quite representative of the products not severely abused. Most producers of pasta would have to collect distribution data, however, to give an adequate "pull date". Also, the time of acceptable quality remaining after the "pull date" would have to be standardized. This goes hand in hand with teaching the consumer how to apply the date during their day-to-day purchasing. Without some type of standardizing, only a massive educational effort on a product-by-product basis (much like that needed for the "pack date") would allow the consumer to fully understand how to use the "pull date". The question of simultaneous nutriet losses must also be considered with respect to the nutrient label.

With some form of expiration date or last day of high quality it would be easy to teach the consumer both the concept behind the date and how to apply it. Problems would result from the lack of data at the manufacturer's level and the fact that the consumer may perceive the food value of expired products as zero. This last problem could result in significant amounts of good food being discarded but the problem could be overcome by careful wording during the initial educational efforts (i.e., word the date as: "for highest quality consume by: ________ ").

In conclusion then, both producers and consumers need to be educated about the shelf stability of pasta. On the part of industry this will come about only through self-education. To the extent that open dating would force pasta manufacturers to recognize quality losses other than staling, it will provide a great benefit. The consumer will probably be best educated by storage information labeling. This is currently being done by some pasta manufacturers and distributors.

REFERENCES

ANON. 1974. Food value of macaroni products. Macaroni J. *55*(11), 15.

ANON. 1976. Whey fortified macaroni. Macaroni J. *58*(4), 30.

ANON. 1977a. Industry survey. Macaroni J. *58*(10), 5.

ANON. 1977b. Moisture in Macaroni. Macaroni J. *58*(7), 32.

ANON. 1977c. Blind dates. State of N.Y. Consumer Protection Board, NY.

BROWN, R. 1977. How high the pasta barrier? Staff and Welfare Caterer, February 24—25, 27.

BUNTING, W.R. 1965. The stability of pyridoxine added to cereals. Cereal Chem. *42*, 569.

CHRZANOWSKA, H. 1974. The determination of the maximum storage period for enriched pasta in 3-layer paper bags. Biul. Cent. Lab. Technol. Przetworstwa Przechow. Zboz Warsawie *18* 3/4.

FABRIANI, G. and, FRATONI, A. 1972. Bibliotheca Nutritia et Dieta, *17*, 196-202.

KUMAR, K.R., MAHADEVAIAH, B. and BALASUBRAMANYM, N. 1974. Package design for moisture sensitive product — vermicelli. J. Food Sci. Technol. India *11*, 4.

KWASNIEWSKA, I., NODOLNA, I., TRZEBSKA-JESKE, I. 1972. Use of dried yeast and dried skim milk for improving nutritional value of pasta products. Rocz. Panstw. Zakl. Hig. *23*(2), 205—215.

OKADO, Y. 1971. Storage of instant ramen. V. Antioxidant stability of common ramen. J. Food Sci. Technol. Japan *181*,9.

OKADO, Y. and KOYAMA, Y. 1969. Studies on storage of instant ramen. J. Food Sci. Technol. Japan *16*(8), 359—364.

ONO, M. NIWA, S. 1969. Studies on the method of enrichment of "Udon" III. Vitamin B_1 content of common enriched spaghetti. Jpn. J. Nutr. *27*,1.

RUTGERS UNIVERSITY. 1971. Food stability survey. Rutgers University Department of Food Science, for the State of New Jersey Department of Health. In cooperation with the U.S. Department of Agricultural/Economic Research Service.

SATTERLEE, L.D., KENDRICK, J.G. and MILLER, G.A. 1977. Rapid in vitro assays for estimating protein quality. Nutr. Rep. Intl. *16*(2), 187.

SIEGEL, A. *et al.* 1975. Development, acceptability and nutritional evaluation of high protein soy supplemented rice noodles for Thai children. Cereal Chem. *52*(6), 801.

WINSTON, J.J. 1971a. Macaroni, Noodles, Pasta Products. In Publishing Corp., New York.

WINSTON, J.J. 1971b. Iron investigation in macaroni products. Macaroni J. *53*(12), 22.

CHAPTER 7

SHELF-LIFE OF FRIED SNACK FOODS

INTRODUCTION

Fried snack foods can consist of many different ingredients. Of all the cereal ingredients available, popcorn and cornmeal are the most widely used. Large quantities of whole corn have also found their way into snack foods in tortilla-style products. Dehydrated cheese and cheese powders are used as flavors for crackers, corn collets, and popcorn. The popularity of nuts (particularly peanuts), potatoes, and other plant snack foods is manifested by the large quantities of these snacks consumed either by themselves or in combination with other ingredients. They are made by toasting, baking, extrusion and deep-fat frying.

Common to all of these snacks is fat applied as a processing agent (heat transfer medium) and/or as an important ingredient. In potato chips, for example, it functions as both. As a consequence, it is the presence of fat which frequently establishes the limit on snack shelf-life.

MODES OF DETERIORATION

All fats are subject to deterioration by oxidative and hydrolytic rancidity leading to the formation of objectional odors and flavors. Hydrolytic rancidity is responsible for the development of "soapy" flavors and for facilitating deterioration by direct oxidation (Matz 1976). Oxidative rancidity results in food spoilage associated with fat deterioration, i.e. the presence of pungent or acrid odors. With respect to food acceptability, fat oxidation is the most important of the two mechanisms and the susceptibility of a food to it depends on the type of fat and the number of unsaturated bonds in the fatty acid moiety. The more unsaturated a fat, the more sensitive and prone it is to oxidation.

Preservation of foods from hydrolytic rancidity can be achieved by control of processing and storage conditions. Moisture and enzymes cause the lipolysis of the triglyceride molecule into glycerol and free fatty acids. Temperatures in the neighborhood of 100°F accelerate this reaction. Therefore, it is recommended that enzymes be denatured and inactivated by sterilization, final moisture levels in the finished product be kept low, and storage temperatures be kept low. Most snacks are subjected to high process temperatures which greatly helps control hydrolytic rancidity through inactivation of the lipase enzymes.

Control of oxidative rancidity requires a means of protecting the unsaturated portion of fatty acids from oxygen attack. Heat, light, and trace quantities of metal ions, iron and copper in particular, will accelerate the free radical reaction. Preservation of fats, therefore, necessitates the protection from the above mentioned factors, plus the addition of phenolic-type antioxidants.

Lard is an animal fat used in baked snack goods. It does not have the quantity of natural antioxidants that the majority of vegetable fats and oils have. Therefore, rancidity in this fat is retarded by adding one or more of the antioxidants permitted by regulations of the USDA. Vegetable fats and oils contain various quantities of natural antioxidants such as the tocopherols. However, antioxidants are usually added to them to help make snack products more shelf stable. Some commercially important antioxidants are the following: butylated hydroxyanisole (BHA), butylated hydroxytoluene (BHT), tertiary butylhydroquinone (TBHQ), propyl gallate (PG), and nordihydroguaiaretic acid (NDGA).

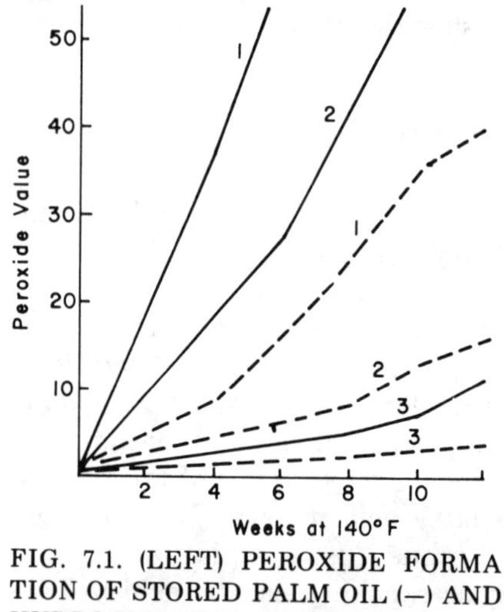

FIG. 7.1. (LEFT) PEROXIDE FORMATION OF STORED PALM OIL (—) AND HYDROGENATED COTTONSEED OIL (---) TREATED WITH NO ANTIOXIDANTS (1), WITH 100 PPM EACH OF BUTYLATED HYDROXYANISOLE AND BUTYLATED HYDROXYTOLUENE (2), AND WITH 100 PPM TERTIARY BUTYLHYDROQUINONE (3).
(Fritsch *et al.* 1975)

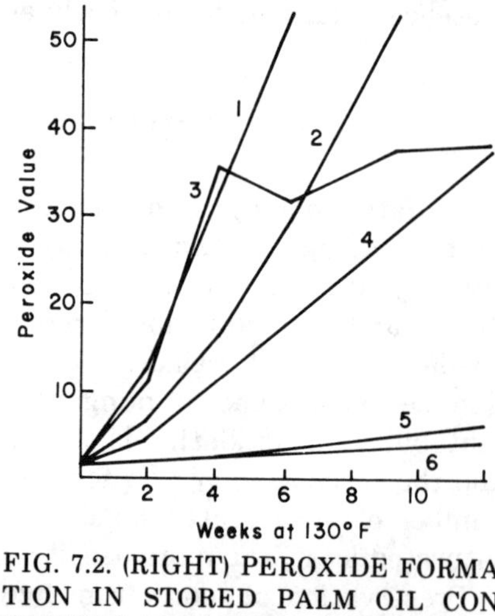

FIG. 7.2. (RIGHT) PEROXIDE FORMATION IN STORED PALM OIL CONTAINING NO ANTIOXIDANTS (1), 81 PPM BUTYLATED HYDROXYANISOLE (BHA) AND 106 PPM BUTYLATED HYDROXYTOLUENE (BHT) (2), 190 PPM BHA (3), 229 PPM BHT (4), CA. 100 PPM TERTIARY BUTYL HYDROQUINONE (TBHQ) (5), AND CA. 200 PPM TBHQ (6).
(Fritsch *et al.* 1975)

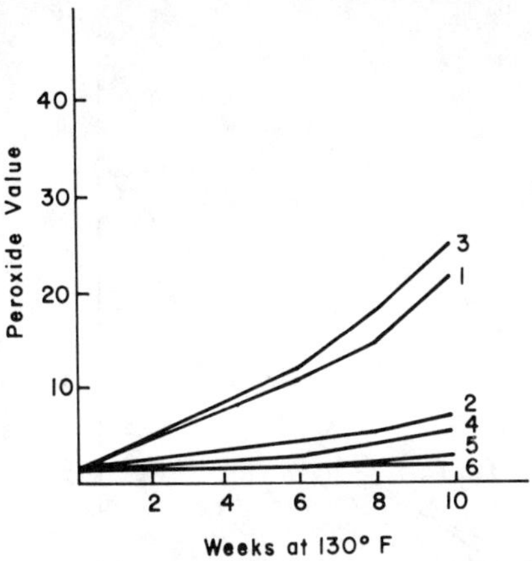

FIG. 7.3. (LEFT) PEROXIDE FORMATION IN STORED HYDROGENATED COTTONSEED OIL CONTAINING NO ANTIOXIDANTS (1), 90 PPM BUTYLATED HYDROXYANISOLE (BHA) AND 97 PPM BUTYLATED HYDROXYQUINONE (BHT) (2), 173 PPM BHA (3), 187 PPM BHT (4), CA. 100 PPM TERTIARY BUTYLHYDROQUINONE (TBHQ) (5), AND CA. 200 PPM TBHQ (6).
(Fritsch *et al.* 1975)

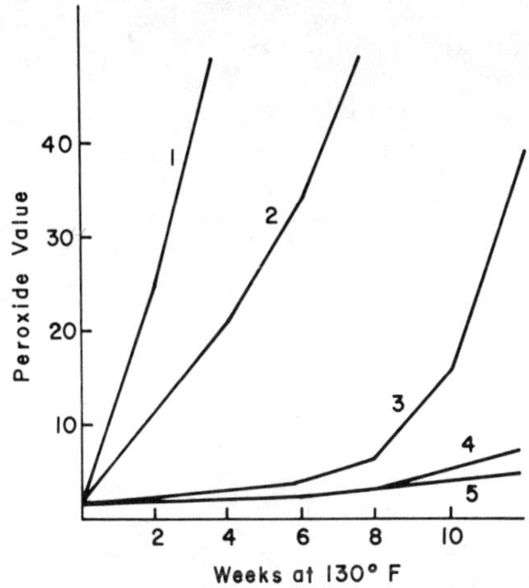

FIG. 7.4. (RIGHT) PEROXIDE FORMATION IN STORED PALM OIL CONTAINING NO ANTIOXIDANTS (1), 98 PPM BUTYLATED HYDROXYANISOLE (BHA) AND 122 PPM BUTYLLATED HYDROXYTOLUENE BHT (2), CA. 50 PPM TERTIARY BUTYLHYDROQUINONE (TBHQ) (3), CA. 100 PPM TBHQ (4), AND CA. 200 PPM TBHQ (5)
(Fritsch *et al.* 1975)

All of these have been found to be suitable antioxidants for the potato chip industry. The concentration of the antioxidant(s) in the food product must not exceed .02% of the weight of the total amount of fat and oil present (including essential oils) which applies to one or more antioxidant compounds used together.

Figures 7.1 through 7.4 show the effects of different antioxidants on peroxide formation when added to palm oil and cottonseed oil (Fritsch *et al.* 1975). Both BHT and TBHQ reduced the rate of oxidation in the oils. BHA was not effective in reducing the PV value at 54 °C, and from Fig. 7.3 it appears the antioxidant slightly accelerated the rate of peroxide decomposition for a period of time.

TBHQ is one of the newer antioxidants approved by the FDA for foods. Figures 7.5 and 7.5a show the effectiveness of different concentrations of this antioxidant in cereals, as opposed to BHA. It is somewhat more effective than BHA in extending the shelf-life of cereals and it is assumed it would have a similar effect in snack foods. Fritsch and coworkers (1975) fried a snack product in palm oil and cottonseed oil with different antioxidants including TBHQ. Figures 7.6, 7.7 and 7.8 show

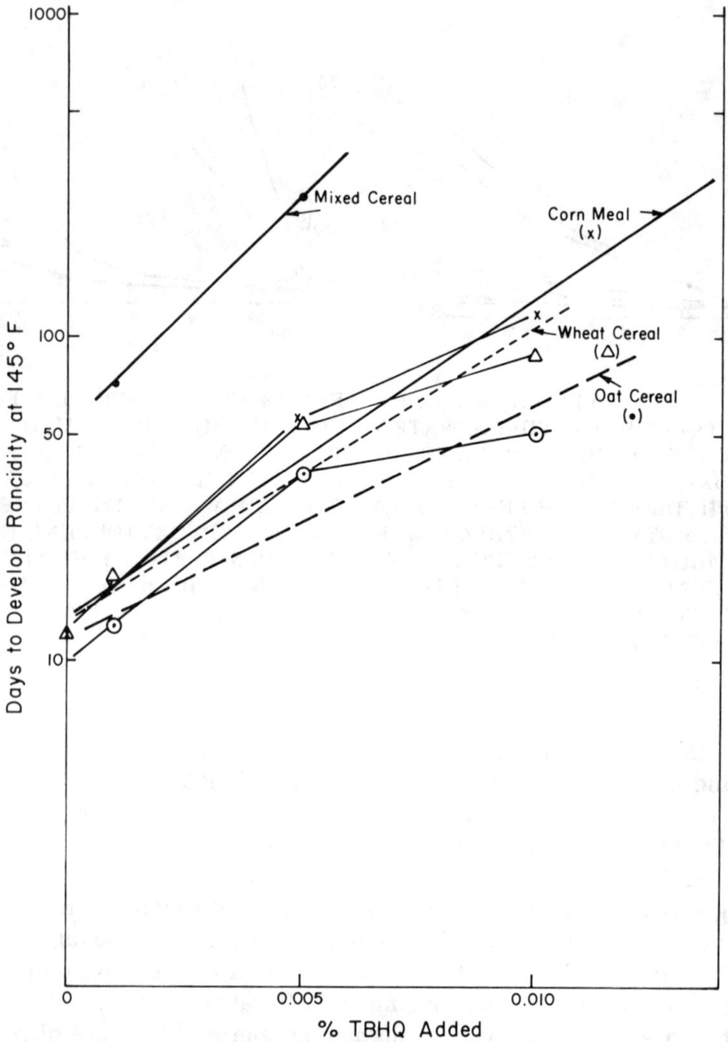

FIG. 7.5. EFFECTIVENESS OF TBHQ IN DRY CEREALS
(Fritsch *et al.* 1975).

their results. They found TBHQ reduced peroxide formation at 54 °C very effectively. BHA had little effect. BHT was more effective than TBHQ when the snack product was fried under harsh conditions (Fig. 7.8).

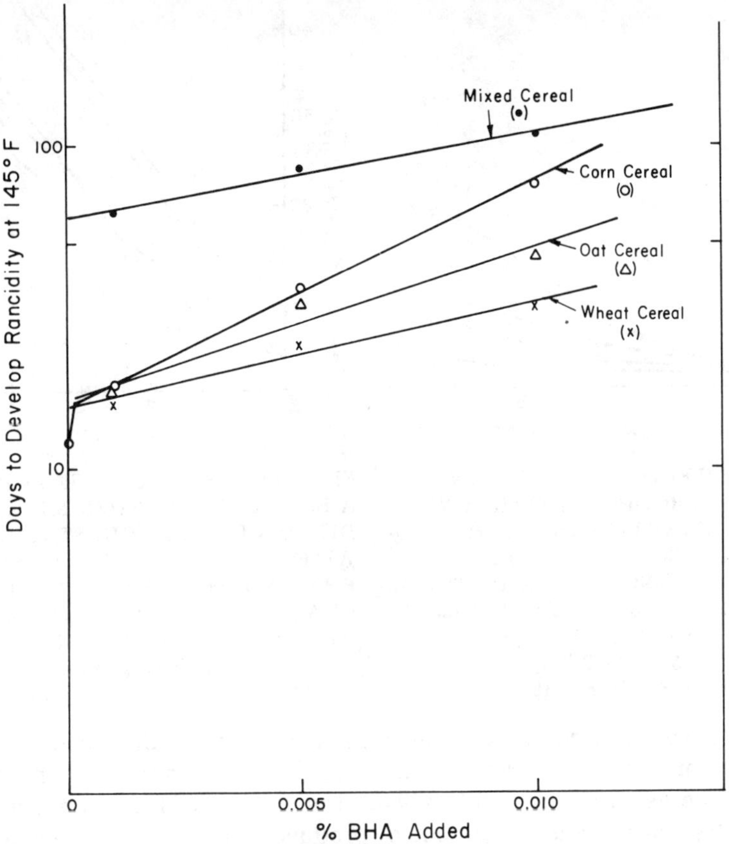

FIG. 7.5A. EFFECTIVENESS OF BHA IN DRY CEREALS (Fritsch *et al.* 1975).

BHA in combination with PG, hydroquinone, and a synergist such as citric acid has been found to be the best antioxidant for potato chips (Talburt and Smith 1967). The chips have their longest shelf-life when the above combination is used, without affecting the quality of taste of the chips as evaluated by a taste panel. BHA is also added to chips (and popcorn, nuts, etc.) by atomizing it onto the product as it is removed from the fryer. The most common method of addition is by adding the antioxidant directly to the oil. Package linings are frequently treated with antioxidants, so that oils which come in contact with and penetrate into the films or board will not become rancid as quickly as would otherwise occur.

When the shelf-life of a snack product is dependent on the rate of fat oxidation, it is important for processors to use oils and fats which have

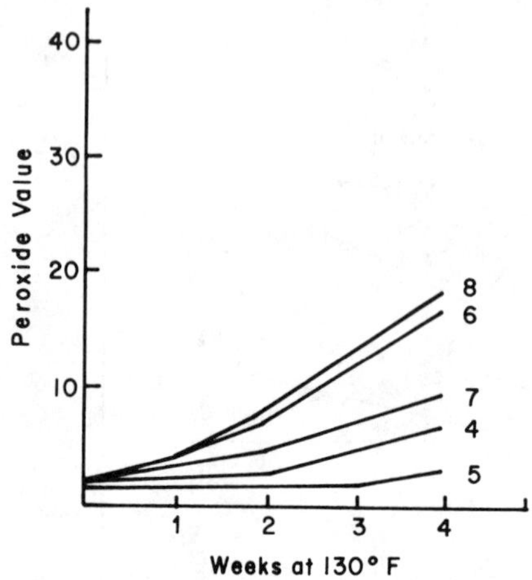

FIG. 7.6.(LEFT) INCREASE IN PV OF A SNACK PRODUCT FRIED UNDER MILD CONDITIONS IN HYDROGENATED COTTONSEED OIL STABILIZED WITH NO ANTIOXIDANTS (1), 100 PPM BHA & 110 PPM BHT (2), 150 PPM BHA (3), 140 PPM BHT (4), AND CA. 150 PPM TBHQ (5).
(Fritsch *et al.* 1975)

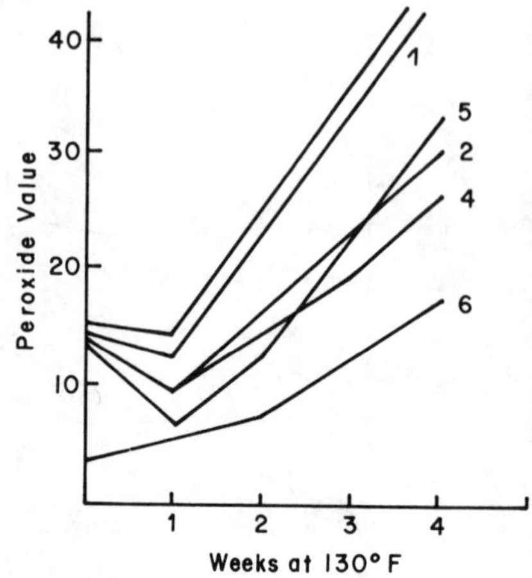

FIG. 7.7.(RIGHT) INCREASE IN PV OF A SNACK FRIED UNDER MILK CONDITIONS IN PALM OIL STABILIZED WITH NO ANTIOXIDANTS (1), 81 PPM BHA AND 106 PPM BHT (2), 190 PPM BHA (3), 229 PPM BHT (4), CA. 100 PPM TBHQ (5), AND CA. 200 PPM TBHQ (6).
(Fritsch *et al.* 1975).

not started to decompose. The resistance to rancidity development is an important characteristic of fats and oils. Tests on the fresh product, i.e., before use in frying, will indicate the amount of free fatty acids or peroxides present and the extent of product deterioration. The changes which can occur in a fat as it decomposes from being heated for long periods are the following: darkening of color; increase in the free fatty acid content; decrease in flavor — becoming more bland; decrease in the smoke point; and oxidation with rancidity development.

Oil stability to oxidative deterioration can be tested with the active oxygen method or AOM test. In the standard AOM test the fat is heated and held at 208 °F while air is bubbled through it. When a peroxide value of 100 meq per kg is reached, the product has reached the endpoint. Modifications of the test include setting different peroxide values which give better correlation to sensory perception of rancidity and heating the oil to higher temperatures because rancidity is known to be accelerated by increasing the temperature (Matz, 1976).

Another stability test used is the Schaal test. Here the fat or a sample of the product containing the fat is held at a specific temperature in an oven. Frequent examinations of the sample are made to determine the time required to reach a condition of detectable rancidity. Any interaction between product and package can also be tested with this method.

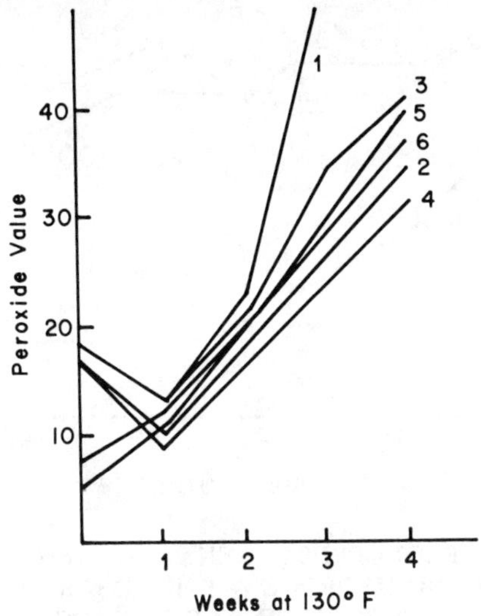

FIG. 7.8. INCREASE IN PEROXIDE VALUE OF SNACK FRIED UNDER HARSH CONDITIONS IN PALM OIL STABILIZED WITH NO ANTIOXIDANTS (1), 81 PPM BUTYLATED HYDROXYANISOLE (BHA) AND 106 PPM BUTYLATED HYDROXYTOLUENE (BHT) (2), 190 PPM BHA (3), 229 PPM BHT (4), CA. 100 PPM TERTIARY BUTYLHYDROQUINONE (TBHQ)(5), AND CA. 200 PPM TBHQ (6).
(Fritsch *et al.* 1975).

Ragnarsson and Labuza (1972) recently reviewed the ASLT tests for fats and showed the problems involved in extrapolating high temperature data to normal storage conditions. This was due both to a change in mechanism in which antioxidants are more pro-oxidant at high temperature, and the fact that antioxidant systems have a higher overall activation energy than systems without antioxidants.

Evans and coworkers (1973) evaluated commercially prepared and packaged soybean and cottonseed salad oils stored for 12 months. Oils were either canned or bottled, partially hydrogenated or unhydrogenated, packed under air or under nitrogen, and stored at 78° and 100°F. Control samples were held at 0°F for the storage period. Figures 7.9 and 7.10 show flavor results after long term storage under nitrogen and air. The nitrogen protected sample indicated excellent

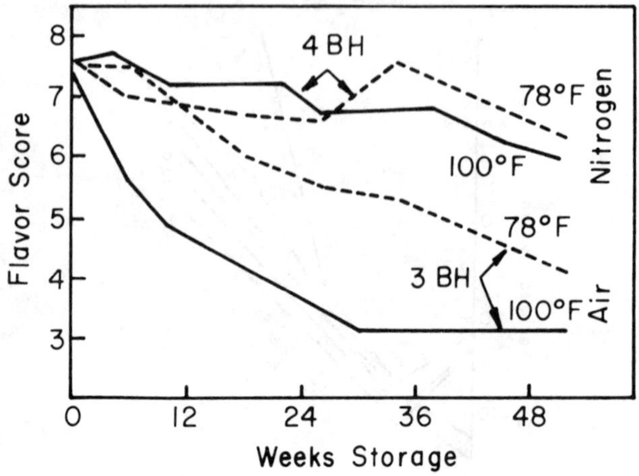

FIG. 7.9. EFFECT OF NITROGEN PACKAGING (SAMPLE 4 BOTTLED AND HYDROGENATED) CONTRASTED WITH AIR (SAMPLE 3 BOTTLED AND HYDROGENATED) ON FLAVOR SCORES OF HYDROGENATED-WINTERIZED SOYBEAN OILS STORED FOR 1 YEAR AT 78 AND 100F (Evans *et al.* 1973).

stability after 26 weeks, whereas the air packed sample was rancid after four weeks. The time to reach a flavor score of six, which was defined as rancid, is shown in Fig. 7.10B. As seen, nitrogen packaging plus hydrogenation gives a protection of 3 to 7 times in bottles and significantly reduces the sensitivity to temperature. The protection in tins is even greater.

Figure 7.11 shows the results of flavor loss of cottonseed oil stored at 100 °F. The value of using nitrogen for protection was evident from all of their evaluations; likewise the more hydrogenated the fat, the slower the development of rancidity. Flavor scores below six were described as rancid.

Sunflower oil used for frying potato chips has been found to be more resistant to oxidation than a commonly used commercial oil composed of a conttonseed-corn oil mixture (Robertson and Morrison 1977). Figure 7.12 shows results of the AOM test applied to commercial shortening and northern sunflower oil. Light hydrogenation of the sunflower oil made it less prone to oxidation after hours of heating. The commercial oil deteriorated three times faster than the hydrogenated sunflower oil. In addition, organoleptic evaluation of the potato chips made in this oil received higher flavor scores than chips fried in commercial oil.

Another form of deterioration for many snack products — potato chips

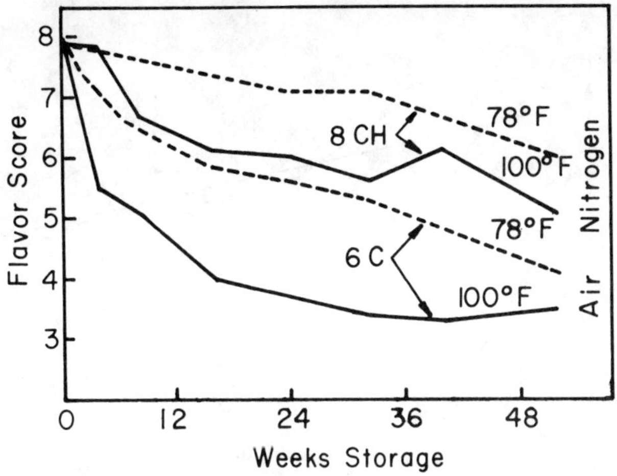

FIG. 7.10A. FLAVOR LOSS OF SOYBEAN OILS STORED IN CANS (C) AT TWO TEMPERATURES

(Sample (8-CH) hydrogenated winterized oil in gallon tins under nitrogen; (6-C) nonhydrogenated oil gallon tins packaged under air (Evans *et al.* 1973).

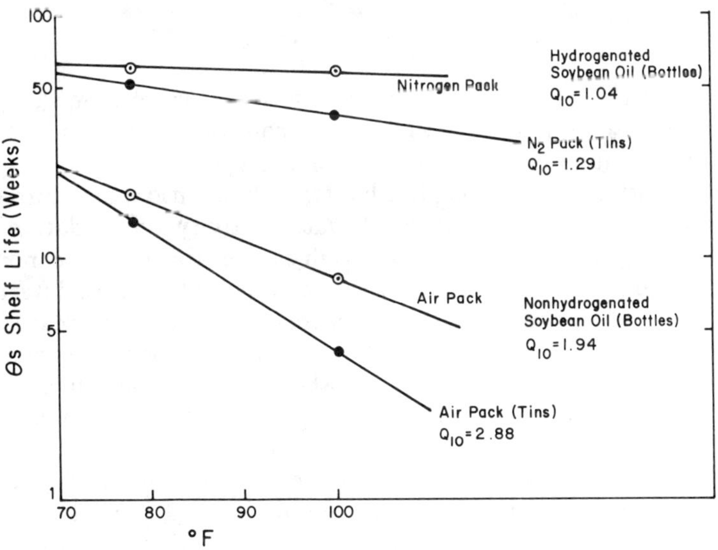

FIG. 7.10B. TIME TO REACH UNDESIRABLE FLAVOR SCORE OF 6 (Evans *et al.* 1973).

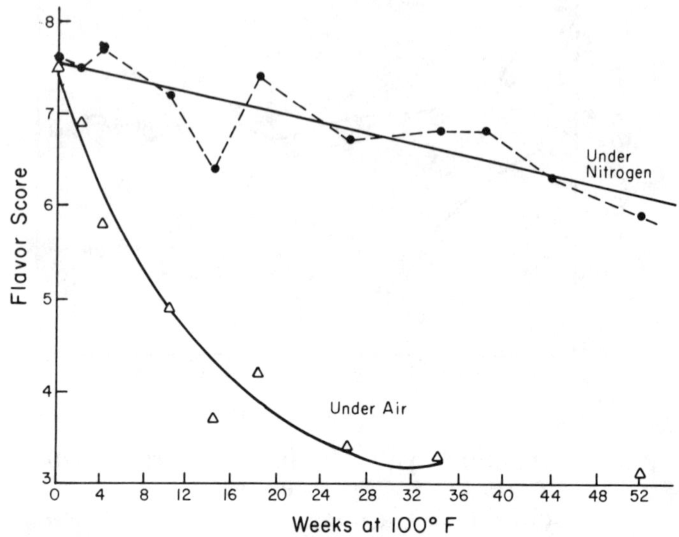

FIG. 7.11. EFFECT OF NITROGEN AND AIR PACKAGING OF BOTTLED, HYDROGENATED WINTERIZED SOYBEAN OIL STORED FOR 1 YEAR
(Evans *et al.* 1973).

in particular — is moisture gain leading to texture changes (sogginess), increased rate of oxidation, and loss of consumer acceptance. Moisture gain is a function of the package type and its permeability characteristics, as described in Chapter 3. In addition, moisture gain accelerates rancidity. The effect of water activity on oxidation rate is shown in Fig. 7.13. As the water activity increases above the monolayer, the reaction is slowed, up to the water activity where intermediate moisture foods begin. Here the water increase tends to increase the rate of oxidation. The effect on development of sogginess depends on the water activity at which the chips or other snacks are perceived as not being crips. No data exist for this, but it probably occurs at an a_w of 0.4 to 0.5. Isotherms of snack foods are also absent in the literature.

Problems with rancidity and moisture gain make packaging materials of critical importance in providing durability and protection from oxygen, moisture and light. Materials used and other processes applied such as nitrogen flushing must be chosen to meet the shelf-life needs of the product and not be so extensive that the cost of the item is affected.

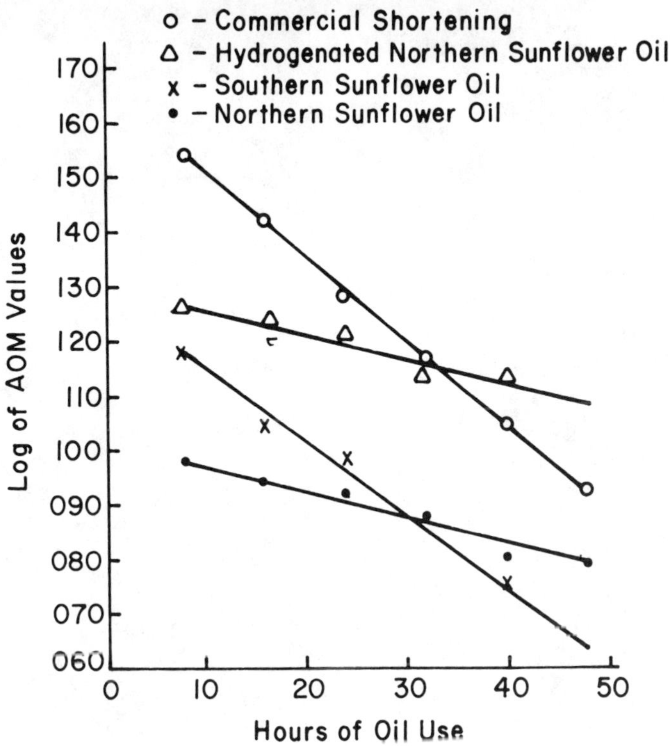

FIG. 7.12. CHANGE IN AOM VALUES WITH OIL USE (Robertson and Morrison 1977).

SHELF-LIFE DATA: CHIPS AND FRIED SNACKS

Potato chips are dried to a finished moisture level of 3% or less which is an a_w of about 0.2. Other snack foods such as cheese curls, puffs and sticks, corn chips, potato sticks, and tortilla chips are dried to less than 3%. From a study of potato chips a moisture content of 3.57% was the point at which a taste panel rejected the chip because of their texture deterioration (Talburt and Smith 1967). Texture changes can be prevented by the use of cellophanes coated with various moisture barriers. This is sufficient to give the chips a short (4—6 week) shelf-life at 70 °F.

Longer shelf-lives of up to six months can be obtained by using a combination of packaging materials (Fig. 7.14). Laminates usually consisting of materials such as aluminum foil, polyethylene waxed paper, polyvinyl-

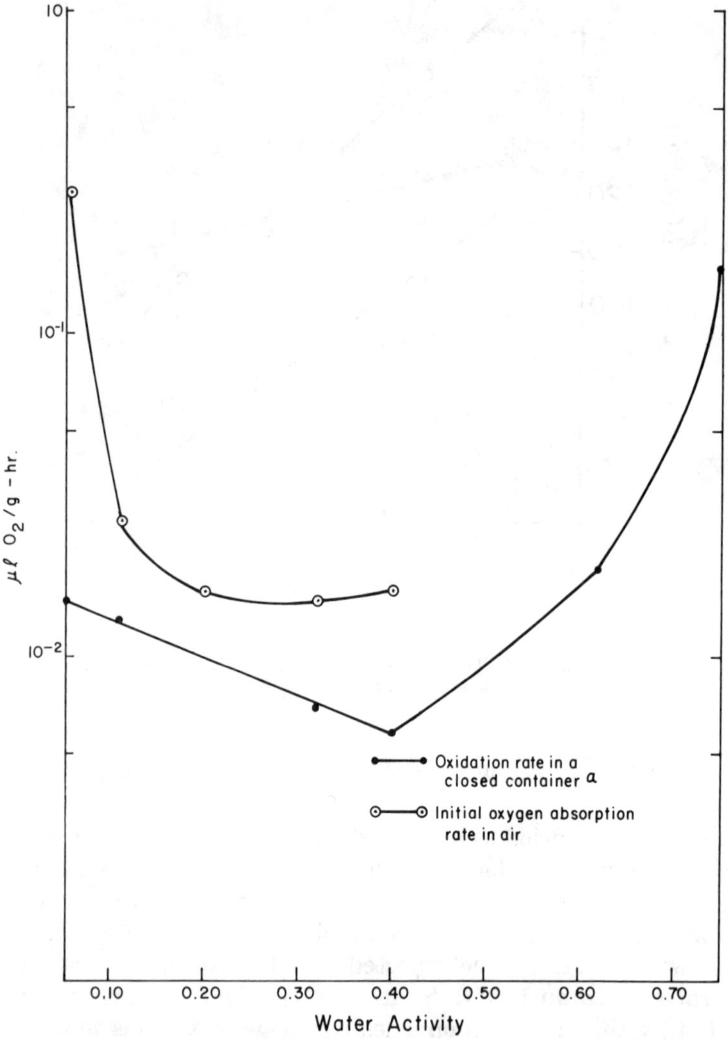

FIG. 7.13. EFFECT OF WATER ACTIVITY ON OXIDATION OF POTATO CHIPS STORED AT 37°C
(Graph Made from Table of Data in Quast and Karel 1979).

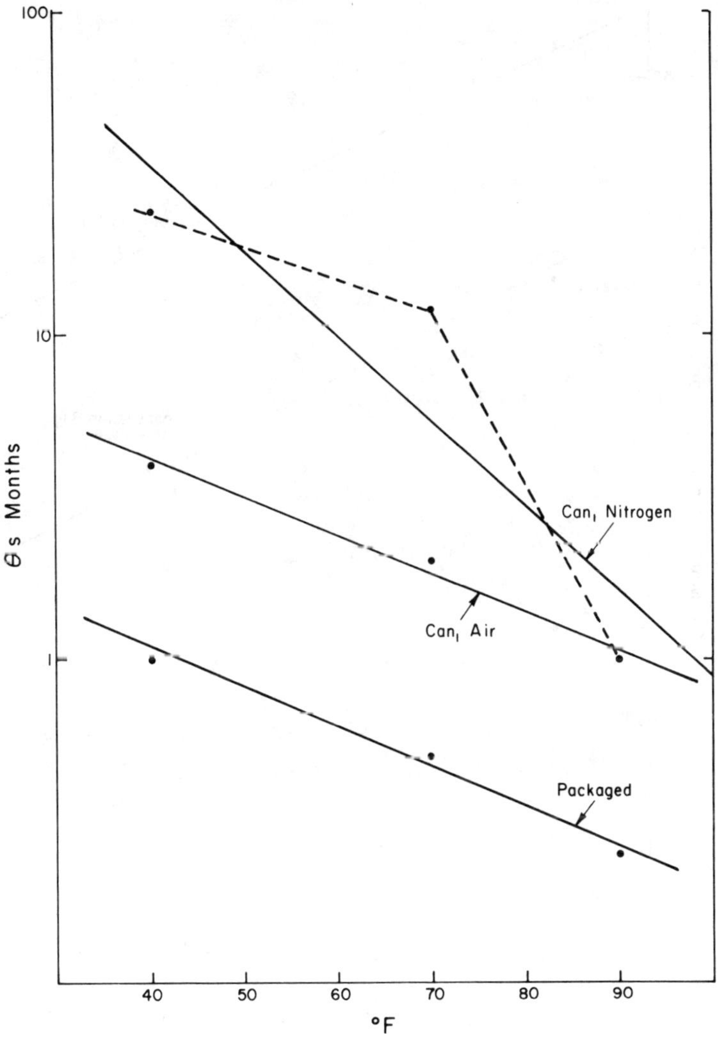

FIG. 7.14. STORAGE LIFE OF POTATO CHIPS
(Army Technical Manual 1971).

lidine chloride, and other materials including cans, are used for snack foods. Some products have had the air removed and are flushed with nitrogen gas. This not only protects against moisture absorption but, as discussed earlier, the presence of an inert gas helps to further retard

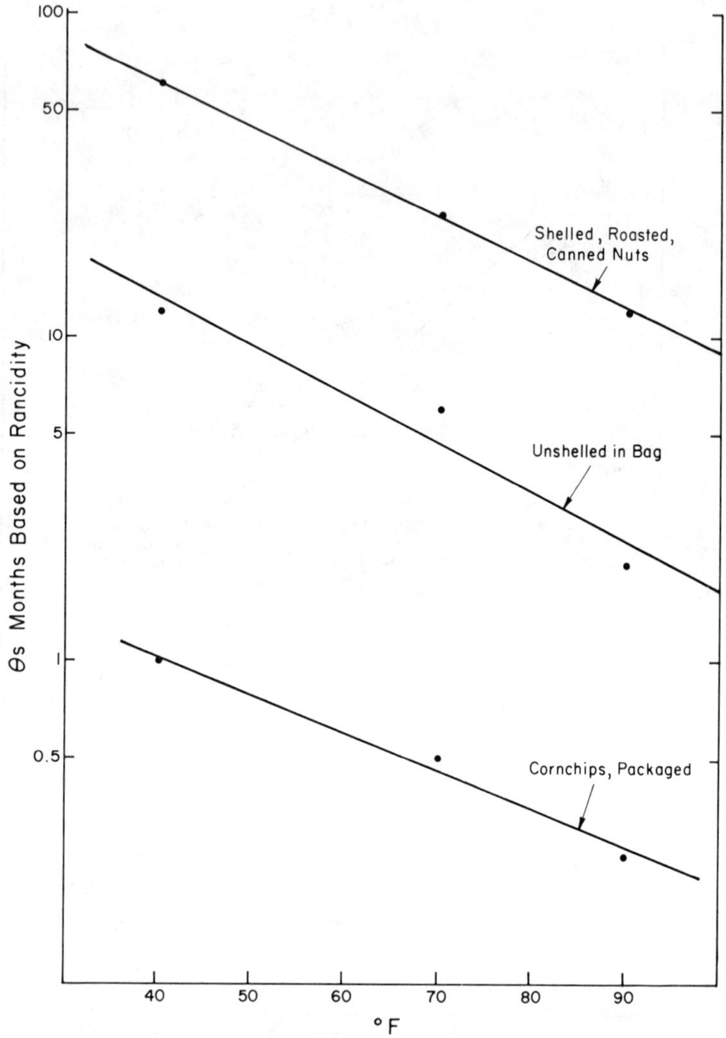

FIG. 7.15. SHELF-LIFE OF CORNCHIPS AND NUTS
(Army Technical Manual 1971).

rancidity development (Fig. 7.15). These measures allow for a shelf-life of six months at room temperature and normal humidity. If the products were stored in the refrigerator, they would last 2 to 4 times longer than they would at room temperatures.

To a certain extent, lamination must be tailored to fit the market area where some packages will be used because they may have a low cold weather resistance (Sacharow 1974). Examples here include cellophane and polymer-coated cellophane (PCC). PCC does offer good protection from oxygen permeation and fat rancidity, so these fairly economical bags are in common use for snacks.

Oriented polypropylene is an oriented crystalline polymer with good oxygen barrier properties, machineability, resistance to low temperatures, and increased stiffness.

Packaged snacks are held in an inner laminated liner of foil surrounded by an outer folded carton. The inner barrier provides the protection from oxygen and water moisture. The outer carton is composed of a printed clay coated cylinder board. The advantages to this material are its resistance to crushing and handling damage; it protects the product from light; it stacks on shelves better; and it is easier to open and close.

Prefabricated potato chips are packaged in foil-lined composite cans. Chips in unopened cans will stay crisp as long as a year but the cost of production, including the can, averages about 25% more than regular chips.

Light accelerates the rate of oxidation and the development of rancidity. Dornseifer and Powers (1965) studied the volatile changes in potato chips made from Kennebec potatoes by storing them under the following conditions and testing them organoleptically for rancidity up to five weeks: (1) 35 °C in the dark; (2) 60 °C in the dark; (3) room temperature in the light; and (4) a control of chips stored in a blast freezer. The chips stored in sunlight developed a rancid off-flavor in five days. Those in the dark at 60 °C were rancid by the fifth week and those in the dark at 35 °C were considered unchanged at the end of the fifth week. Butyric acid is known to increase during chip storage, particularly when the chips are exposed to light. Rancidity is accelerated with blue and invisible light such as red, while yellow has little effect. Therefore, opaque packaging materials may be of any visible color except blue (Morgan 1935). Foil laminates, pigmented pastics, and yellow transparent cellulose films are th epackaging materials of choice and are most utilized by the food service industry.

The delay of rancidity must also be considered when transporting and distributing oil and fat-based products. Considerations of temperature and moisture variations at different times of the year are important. Trucks should be insulated and well ventilated. For longer trips temperature controlled trucks or cars are necessary. Regular stock rotation in warehouses should be observed along with temperature control and a sanitary environment. The latter consideration may be the most abused condition in snack products' quality control programs. Information about this is not readily avalable.

SHELF-LIFE DATA: NUTS

Dry, roasted nuts are fried in oil so they, too, are subject to deterioration by rancidity which is accelerated by moisture, high temperatures, and light (Fig. 7.16). The storage life of these snacks, like potato chips, depends on the container used. Nuts stored in their shells at low temperature have the slowest rate of staling (Table 7.1). Shelled nutmeats are most susceptible to rancidity and can easily absorb off-odors from the environment (Matz 1976). Long term storage of fried nuts requires refrigeration. Refrigeration can increase the storage life of nuts 2 to 5 years (Matz 1976) maintaining natural texture, flavor, and color and retarding staleness and rancidity (ASHRAE 1966). For each 20° drop in temperature the shelf-life can be doubled or tripled.

TABLE 7.1
STORAGE LIFE OF SHELLED AND IN-SHELL PEANUTS[1]

Peanuts	Temperature (°F)	RH (%)	Expected Storage Life
In shell	32—50	65—75	9-24 months
Shelled	32	65—75	1 year
Vacuum or gas pack	32—50	—	1—2 years
Frozen	0	—	3 years

[1]Refrigeration Research Foundation (1961).

Nuts and nutmeats will have the longest shelf-life when stored in vacuum packed cans or under nitrogen (Table 7.1). Nuts in single film pouches will have a short shelf-life because of the exposure to light and air. The FDA permitted antioxidants used for other snack foods are also available for nut snack products. Antioxidants will extend the storage life of fresh nuts a few weeks or months but will not reverse deterioration which has already occurred. Table 7.2 gives the average composition of various nuts.

Of particular concern with peanuts (more so than with other snacks) is the presence or potential presence of aflatoxins. These compounds are produced by certain fungi in nature and are known to be carcinogenic. Nuts which appear moldy can contain aflatoxins but many which are not moldy in appearance can still have some present. Prevention of these toxic substances requires surveillance and inspection of commercial shipments by the Food and Drug Administration. "All reliable suppliers will have had their stocks analyzed for the contaminant but it is advisable for purchasers to specify that shipments must conform to USFDA standards" (Matz 1976).

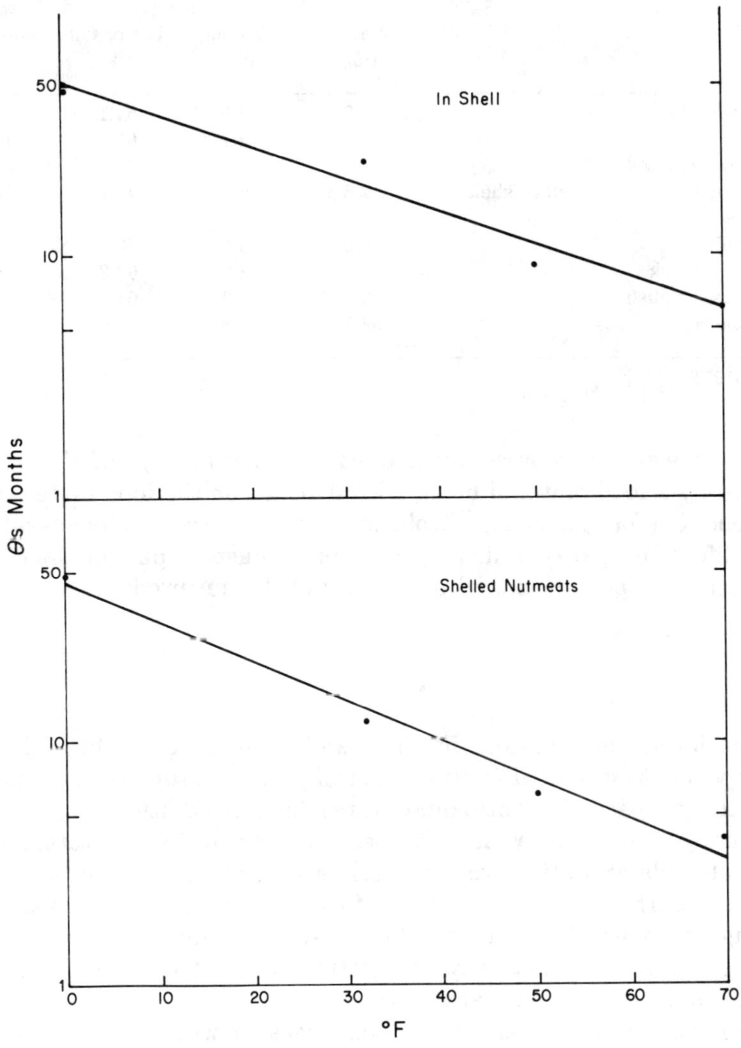

FIG. 7.16. RELATIVE STORAGE OF PEANUTS
(Rutgers Food Stability Survey 1971).

Peanut oil used for frying can contain this contaminant. Aflatoxin B_1 and B_2 were found up to .02 to .26 ppm in unrefined Indian peanut oil (Dwarankanath *et al.* 1969). When the oil was heated to 150 °C for 10 min,

TABLE 7.2
TYPICAL COMPOSITION OF NUTS[1]

Nuts	Water (%)	Protein (%)	Fat or Oil (%)	Total Carbohydrate (%)
Almonds	4.7	18.6	54.1	19.6
Brazil	5.3	14.4	65.9	11.0
Cashews, roasted	4.1	19.6	47.2	26.4
Peanuts, Virginia roasted in shell	2.6	26.9	44.2	23.6
Pecans	3.0	9.4	73.0	13.0
Pistachios	5.6	19.6	53.2	18.6
Walnuts, black	2.7	18.3	58.2	18.7
Walnuts, English	3.3	15.0	64.2	15.6
Chestnuts	53.2	2.8	1.5	41.5

[1]Matz (1976)

50% of the aflatoxin present was destroyed. The amount of aflatoxin absorbed by a food material being fried depends on the food material. The presence of aflatoxin is not a problem which can be solved by alteration of shelf-life or by package dating. Emphasis must be put on the culture, harvest, transportation, and processing of the nut products.

OPEN DATING

The development of rancidity in oil and fat products has been shown to be dependent on several factors, especially temperature, if the product is not nitrogen packed or antioxidants are added. In addition, moisture gain accelerates rancidity. Without proper attention to these factors, the rate of quality deterioration will be accelerated and the product's shelf-life shortened. Therefore, the benefits of using average industry values for dating packages will not be reliable for snack products. Consumers cannot be guaranteed that they are getting the best quality because the quality is dependent on many factors.

The "pull date" or "sell by date" on a package would probably be most helpful on the retail level as long as it is determined for the specific product. This could be used to encourage rotation of stock on the shelves. All snacks would benefit by being stored in a refrigerator until time to be displayed on the grocer's shelf. Once on display they should be protected from warm areas, direct sunlight and artificial light. Most snack product produders consider their products high or fast turnover items, so long term storage is not a critical concern.

Consumers would benefit most from having the package display the optimum means of storing the different products at home or have a "best if used by date". However, without a knowledge of the storage history from processing to purchase time, expiration dates would be meaningless and could actually cause a product to be discarded before the end of the shelf-life.

From shelf-life plots, potato chips packaged in bags can be expected to have a shelf-life of less than one month when stored at room temperature, moderate humidity, and in the dark. Those canned with air in the headspace would be stable for about two months; those canned in an inert gas would be stable for approxiamtely six months at room temperatures. Other snack products stored in bags at room temperature would behave like the potato chips in bags. They would remain fresh for 15 days or less. Nuts, on the other hand, if packaged in bags or cans would be stable for a year or more. All snack products should be protected from heat, light, and high relative humidities as much as possible.

REFERENCES

ANON. 1969. A move to metal. Snack Food *58*, 45-47.

ANON. 1972. Longer shelf life for potato products. Food Processing *33*, 32.

AMERICAN SOCIETY OF HEATING, REFRIGERATION AND AIR-CONDITIONING ENGINERS, 1966. ASHRAE Guide and Data Book, Appli cations for 1966 and 1967. New York.

BERGER, K.G. 1971. Practical applications of an accelerated stability test to rancidity problems in food processing. J. Food Technol. *6*,253.

DORNSEIFER, T.P. and POWERS, J.P. 1965. Volatile constituents of potato chips and changes during storage. Food Technol. *19*, 195.

DWARAKANATH, C.T., SREENIVASAMURTHY, V. and PARPIA, H.A.B. 1969. Aflatoxin in Indian peanut oil. J. Food Sci. Technol. *6*, 107.

EVANS, C.D., LIST, G.R., MOSER, H.A. and COWAN, J.C. 1973. Long term storage of soybean and cottonseed salad oils. J. Am. Oil Chemists Soc. *50*, 218.

FRITSCH, C.W., WEISS, V.E. and ANDERSON, R.H. 1975. Effect of antioxidants on refined palm oil. J. Am. Oil Chemists Soc. *52*, 517.

FULLER, G., GUADAGNI, D.G., WEAVER, M.L., NOTTER, G. and HORVAT, R.J. 1971. Evaluation of oleic safflower oil in frying of potato chips. J. Food Sci. *36*, 43.

MATZ, S.A. 1976. Snack Food Technology, AVI Publishing Company, Westport, Conn.

MORGAN, W.L. 1935. Retarding rancidity; Colored transparent cellulose wrapper. Ind. Eng. Chem. *27*, 1287.

POMINSKI, J., PEARCE, H.M. Jr., VIX, H.L.E. and SPADARO, J.J. 1975. Improvement of shelf life of partially defatted peanuts by intromission of nitrogen into the interstices of the peanuts. J. Food Sci. *40*, 192.

QUAST, D.G. and KAREL, M. 1972. Effects of environmental factors on the oxidation of potato chips. J. Food Sci. *37,* 584.

REFRIGERATION RESEARCH FOUNDATION 1961. Commodity Storage Manual. Nuts and nut meats. Washington, DC.

ROBERTSON, J.A. and MORRISON, W.H. III. 1977. Effect of heat frying on sunflower oil stability. J. Am. Oil Chem. Soc. *54,* 77A.

RAGNARSSON, J. and LABUZA, T.P. 1977. Accelerated shelf-life testing for oxidative rancidity in foods: A review. J. Food Chem. *2,* 292.

ROCK, W.A. and VALLEROY, G.J. 1972. Potato Snack Product. U.S. Patent 3,681,084.

RUTGERS UNIVERSITY, 1971.Food Stability Survey, Vol. II. Rutgers University Dept. of Food Science, for the State of New Jersey Dept. of Health. In cooperation with the U.S. Dept. of Agriculture/Economic Research Service.

SACHAROW, S. 1974. Packaging requirements for snack foods. Food Eng. *46,* 70.

STORAGE LIFE OF SEMI-PERISHABLE FOODS. 1971. Reprinted from the Congressional Record, The Technical Manual for Storage and Material Handling for the Departments of the Army, Washington, DC.

TALBURT, W.F. and SMITH, O. 1967. Potato Processing. AVI Publishing Co., Westport, Conn.

USDA, Food Safety and Quality Service 9CFR319.702. Regulations Governing Meat Inspection of the United States Dept. of Agriculture.

CHAPTER 8

SHELF-LIFE STUDIES ON POULTRY

INTRODUCTION

During the last two decades the United States poultry industry has become the most efficient producer of animal protein in the history of agriculture (Blaxter 1961). Poultry research has played a major role in this development. In the interval between 1910 and 1960, per capita consumption of chicken increased from 15.5 to 28.0 lb, to 43.3 lb in 1976, and although it has decreased recently, the publication of the U.S Dietary Goals may stimulate further increased poultry consumption.

Birds classified as poultry include chickens, turkeys, ducks, geese, guineas and pigeons. Most poultry marketed is in the ready-to-cook form: dressed poultry with blood, feathers, head, feet and viscera removed. Most ready-to-cook poultry is distributed in chilled form, although distribution of frozen poultry, especially turkeys, is increasing tremendously.

The following poultry product categories and varieties are found in the retail market: (1) Fresh, whole, eviscerated, (2) Frozen, whole, eviscerated, (3) Poultry parts, and (4) Processed poultry.

Before grading, poultry are divided into market classes according to their species, age and sex (Table 8.1). In some cases their age is limited to a span of several weeks, in other cases they may be classified simply as young or old.

Ready-to-cook poultry may be graded for class, condition and quality in that order and given an individual U.S. letter grade of A as top quality, B as second quality and C as third quality.

Grading for quality has been based on conformation, fleshing, fat covering, degree of freedom from pin feathers and vestigial hairs, and the degree of freedom from tears, cuts, disjointed and broken bones, discoloration of skin and flesh, blemishes and bruises of the skin and flesh and freezer burn.

PROCESSING POULTRY

General

Antimortem and postmortem inspections are required for interstate transportation of poultry and poultry products by the USDA. The major steps followed in processing are: slaughtering, carcass preparation, in-

TABLE 8.1
MARKET CLASS OF POULTRY

Species	Class	Sex	Age
Chicken	Cornish game hen	Either	5—7 weeks
	Broiler or fryer	Either	9—12 weeks
	Roaster	Either	3—5 weeks
	Capon	Unsexed male	under 8 months
	Stag	Male	under 10 months
	Hen or stewing	Female	over 10 months
	Cock	Male	over 10 months
Turkey	Fryer — roaster	Either	under 16 weeks
	Young hen	Female	5—7 months
	Young tom	Male	5—7 months
	Yearling hen	Female	under 15 months
	Yearling tom	Male	under 15 months
	Mature or old	Either	over 15 months
Duck	Broiler or fryer duckling	Either	under 8 weeks
	Roaster duckling	Either	under 16 weeks
	Matured duck	Either	over 16 weeks
Goose	Young	Either	
	Old	Either	
Guinea	Young	Either	
	Mature	Either	
Pigeon	Squab	Either	
	Pigeon	Either	

USDA (1971).

spection, packaging and shipping. Sanitation and health standards must be maintained during slaughtering. Bleeding has to be properly done, because incomplete bleeding is a direct cause of poor keeping quality, and undesirable flavor and appearance.

In conventional processing it is customary to sacrifice the birds and then to scald them with water at a temperature of about 123° to 140°F, to facilitate removal of feathers by mechanical plucking machines. Plucking is followed by cleaning, and then by evisceration of the birds. Chilling follows by placing the carcass in an ice-slush bath or water-chilling bath for about 20 min to 24 hours. This soaking operation results in hydration of the carcasses with up to a 7% increase in weight and is almost universally done for poultry. Poultry is unique in that this is the only food product treated in this manner. During processing, an increase in the number of microorganisms can occur due to the handling of the birds. Storage of the poultry generally results in flavor changes in two days and spoilage in about 5 to 7 days at 35° to 45°F. To increase the shelf-life of poultry, various procedures can be employed, such as the use of salts and/or surface drying.

Holding of Prepared Carcasses

Poultry meat is kept either in refrigerated or frozen storage. Refrigerated storage is considered to be storage at temperature above freezing usually in the range of 32° to 45°F (0° to 7.22°C). Crushed ice, mechanical refrigeration or a combination of the two are used as the source of refrigeration for cool storage and liquified gases, and mechanical refrigeration for frozen storage.

McCoy (1963) has summarized the proper refrigeration requirements as:

(1) Controlled temperatures
(2) Proper air circulation
(3) Proper moisture control and
(4) Some control of air composition.

These are required for preventing loss of quality caused due to fluctuating conditions. In addition, maintenance of constant temperature helps to control mold growth; to prevent loss of moisture; and to keep a product free of odors and undesirable gases.

Refrigerated Storage

The temperature at which poultry is held during storage determines, to a large extent, its shelf-life. Carcasses held at 32°F (0°C) will remain edible for several weeks, while those held at 60°F (15.5°C) will remain edible only for a matter of hours due to organoleptic changes.

Products stored and delivered in crushed ice are acceptable in freshness, keeping quality, and appearance, but they pick up water. Mechanical refrigeration is good; however, some sort of packaging is needed to prevent moisture loss.

Chicken broilers are typically distributed packed in crushed ice. This method of transport requires transportation of 30% additional weight in ice, and yields a product of relatively short shelf-life. The Texas Agricultural Technical Report examined the following four packagings and pretreatments:

(1) Ice pack:
Carcass halves were iced and held at 35°F for 2 days. They were packed in styrofoam trays, pliofilm sacks and heat sealed.

(2) Deep chill pack:
Each half of the styrofoam tray was filled and covered with pliofilm. The package was heat sealed and then blast frozen at —34 °F for 2½ hours, and was held in 28 °F storage for 2 days.

(3) Cool pack:
Carcass halves were placed at 28 °F for 24 hours, packed simultaneously and stored for 7 days at 28 °F.

(4) Frozen pack:
Carcass halves were packaged similar to the above, blast frozen at —14 °F for 15 hours, and then transferred to 0 °F storage for a total of 12 days.

All storage comparisons were then conducted at 35 °F. The results showed that there was no change in the microbial count for the frozen pack. It was considered acceptable for up to 12 days of retail storage. The other three methods yielded essentially similar microbial growth, but greater than the frozen. These data therefore suggest that the initial type of packing will significantly affect shelf-life. Thus, the consumer without this knowledge would not know which product is better, based on a "pack date" and the better processor will suffer. Similar results were found for weight loss and tissue moisture. However, the overall organoleptic evaluation (48 member panel) found no significant differences between all four methods.

Freezing Poultry

Poultry can be frozen in air or liquid, or on refrigerated plates, and can either be sharp or quick frozen. Rapid freezing consists of freezing at —10 °F or lower, without mechanical agitation of the air.

Considerable controversy still exists regarding the value of marketing fresh and frozen poultry. Proponents of merchandising frozen broilers argue that frozen broilers have a longer shelf-life, that equilibrating supply and demand is easier, and that freezing would create no problem for the housewife, since many already freeze broilers at home. Proponents of fresh poultry argue that freezing increases the cost, requires better packaging, requires handling in and out of storage and requires storage and transportation in the frozen state. Since broilers are no longer a seasonal commodity, frozen poultry brought from storage for sale must still compete with fresh poultry in the market. Recently a compromise between fresh and frozen poultry has been tried in which the cut-up parts have been held at temperatures just above freezing. Using this method with the aid of good packaging, the shelf-life and high quality of poultry can be maintained for several weeks.

Canning

Canning is applied to some poultry products such as chicken and rice, chicken vegetable soup, and cream of chicken.

Dehydrated Poultry

Moisture can be removed from poultry meat by freeze-dehydration, drum drying on heated rollers, air tunnel drying, oven drying or by dehydration at 212 °F in edible oil (Palmer and Bowers 1972).

Curing and Smoking

Curing involves use of sodium chloride, sugar and sodium nitrite and/or sodium nitrate. Smoking may be carried out by heat and smoke from a common source, or from temperature sources. A minimum internal temperature of at least 155 °F is needed. Recently there has been considerable interest and marketing of poultry substituted cured meat products.

MODES OF DETERIORATION

Only those changes occurring after death in animal or poultry tissue that affect its wholesomeness or fitness for food use are classed as deteriorative changes. Meat, being constantly acted upon by its enzymes, bacteria and their enzymes, and the environment in which it is held, is subject to loss of quality. The various modes of failure include: (1) pathogen growth, (2) microbial decay, (3) sensory quality changes, (4) chemical and enzymatic degradation (color, rancidity), and (5) physical decay (bruising, syneresis, moisture loss).

Fresh Poultry: Microbiological Concerns

Hundreds of different species of microorganisms have been reported to grow in poultry meat and may or may not be pathogenic. According to Galton and Arnstein (1960), in the United States, fowl foods were the most frequent vehicle of dissemination in outbreaks of foodborne infections, especially *Salmonella* infections. However, according to the CDC, poultry has now become a minor vehicle for food poisoning. Ingalls (1950) stated that at least 26 diseases which are reported to occur in poultry can

can cause disease to man. However, despite the large number of pathogenic organisms found in poultry which are transmissible to man as noted, poultry today plays a very minor role since it is eaten after cooking and the heat process destroys the organisms if present.

Walker and Ayres (1956) found that live poultry generally had from 60 to 8100 organisms/cm² of skin area and that after processing, they had 11,000 to 93,000 organisms/cm². Also, Walker and Ayres (1959) reported that live turkeys generally had from 750 to 41,000 organisms/cm². Spoilage is observed organoleptically when the log of the number of bacteria reaches about 6.5 to 8/cm². Slime formation occurs when the number of organisms reaches a log concentration of 7.5 to 9.0/cm². The rate of this reaction, Q_{10} and E_a are shown in Figs. 8.1 and 8.2. The study conducted by Ayres *et al.* (1950) in Fig. 8.3, shows the significant effect of initial organism load on shelf-life. Thus, the change in initial microbial count which could be very variable gives a large change in the shelf-life of the product held at constant temperature.

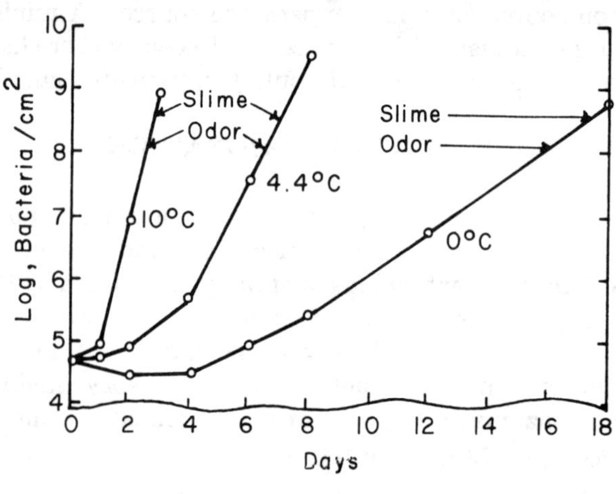

FIG. 8.1. EFFECT OF STORAGE TEMPERATURE ON GROWTH OF BACTERIA ON CHICKEN MEAT
(From Elliot & Michener (1965) U.S. Dept. of Agr. and Data of Ayres *et al.* (1950)).

One of the factors associated with microbial spoilage of meat during storage is increased water holding capacity. Other changes that occur during rigor mortis that directly or indirectly affect the development of microorganisms are autolysis, stopping of phagocytic action, decreased pH, accumulation of metabolites, production of actomysin, lowering of

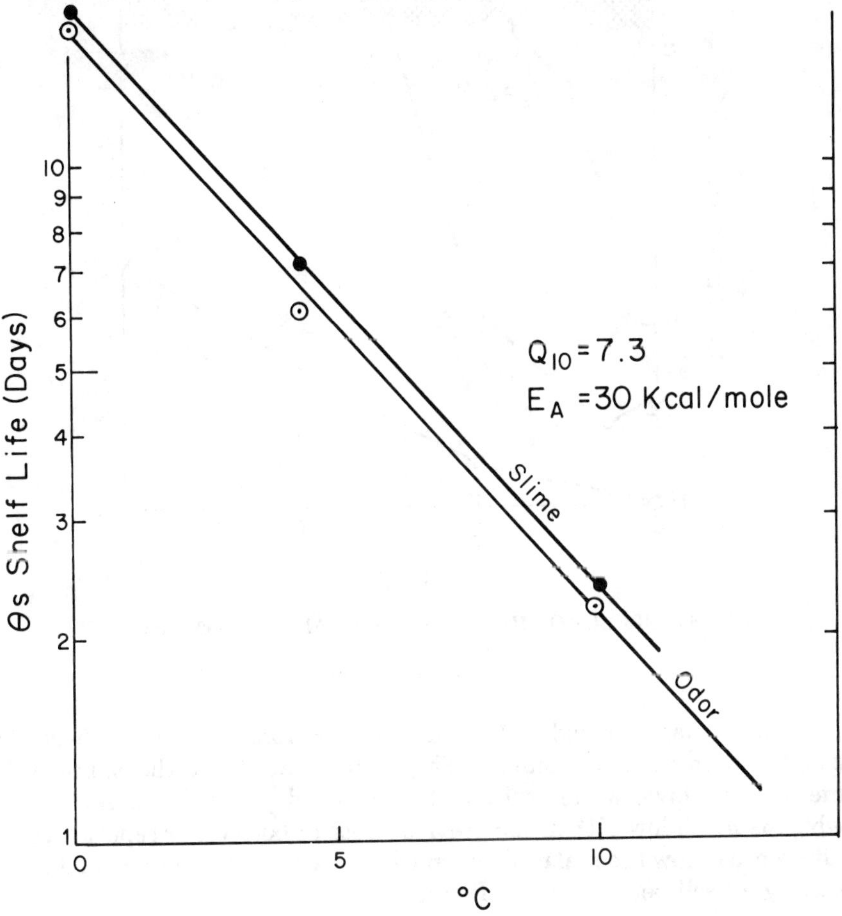

FIG. 8.2. CHICKEN SHELF-LIFE (BACTERIAL GROWTH)
(From Ayres *et al.* 1950).

oxidation-reduction potential, release of calcium and sodium, and absorption of potassium (Lillard 1977). A number of methods of delaying spoilage of poultry have been tested. Of these, low temperature remains the most dependable and widely used method.

A storage temperature study done by Dawson and Stadelman (1960), showed that at 32 °F the shelf-life was nine times that at 68 °F. This is a Q_{10} of three which is lower than the previous work. Barnes and Impey (1975) observed the bacterial counts on uneviscerated and eviscerated

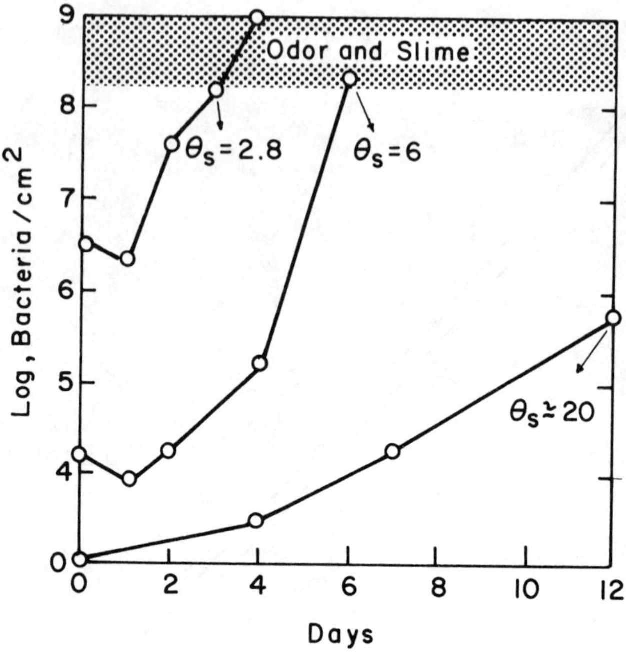

FIG. 8.3. EFFECT OF INITIAL BACTERIAL LOAD ON CHICKEN SHELF-LIFE @4.4 °C
(Ayres *et al.* 1950).

chicken carcasses stored at 10 °C and 4 °C. Before storing, the bacterial count of both were very similar. They found that at 4 °C the end of shelf-life was six days, while at 10 °C it was four days, giving a Q_{10} of two, which is much lower than the previous data of both other reports. These differences show the real problem in dealing with fresh poultry, and make setting a "sell before date" difficult.

Effect of Freezing on Microbes

Clostridium botulinum has never been reported to grow below 40 °F, and to produce toxin it must grow. The same is the case for *Staphylococcus aureus.* Usually, *Salmonella* will not cause infection unless they are present in large numbers. The growth of *Salmonella* below 4 °F has not been reported. Microbial growth however, can occur in frozen foods at temperatures above 20 °F, and occasionally down to 14 ° or 10 °F. In view of this information, it would seem that the danger of microbial deterioration in food stored below 10 °F would be infinitesimal, but that the danger of microbial deterioration and spoilage becomes increasingly great as temperature rises above this point, as could happen in fluctuating storage.

Cotterill *et al.* (1977) studied the microbial content of unfrozen and frozen ground turkey meat (GTM) in the retail market. The unfrozen product had an average total aerobic count of 53×10^4 cells/g. These counts reduced slightly when held in a display case for one day at 1—2 °C.

Lillard (1977) studied the effect of freezing on incidence and levels of *Cl. perfringens* in mechanically deboned chicken meat (vegetative cells and spores) before and after 4—6 weeks at —23 °C. He found that after that particular frozen period, which is a common industrial practice with good food handling practices, *Cl. perfringens* should not pose any undue hazards. According to Lillard (1977), freezing to —10 °C kills 50% of the spores. Gunaratne and Spencer (1974), evaluated the effect of certain freezing methods upon microbes associated with chicken meat, using liquid nitrogen spray (—196 °C), nitrogen (—51 °C) and air blast at (—29 °C). Statistical analysis showed that there was no significant difference between the methods.

Thus, freezing reduces the microbial population of foods but considerable numbers usually survive even prolonged frozen storage. Reduction of storage temperature increases survival. In addition, food poisoning bacteria have not been reported to grow below 40 °F but they survive freezing. For example, some fecal indicators can grow at 32 °F. The studies show that temperature for growth of some psychrophiles is probably between 10—14 °F but growth slightly above this minimum takes many months to become evident. Foods with high counts spoil faster and this can adversely affect quality even at temperatures below freezing.

Texture Effects

de Fremery (1966) studied the relationship beween the chemical properties of muscle and tenderness of poultry. Chickens were subjected to severe mechanical feather plucking, immediately postmortem (to induce toughness). The disappearance of ATP, the chemical reaction most closely linked with the onset of rigor mortis, was accelerated. Other pre-rigor treatments that accelerated ATP and glycogen disappearance as well as the onset of rigor mortis, also induced toughness that was only partially reversed by prolonged aging. When postmortem glycolysis was minimized by epinephrine injections, sodium iodoacetate injections, or rapid cooking, the meat was tender without aging. Since these treatments accelerate rigor mortis, it is the acceleration of portmortem glycolysis, not the acceleration of rigor mortis, which induces toughness. Figures 8.4 and 8.5 show the effect of freezing and thawing fresh muscle on the rate

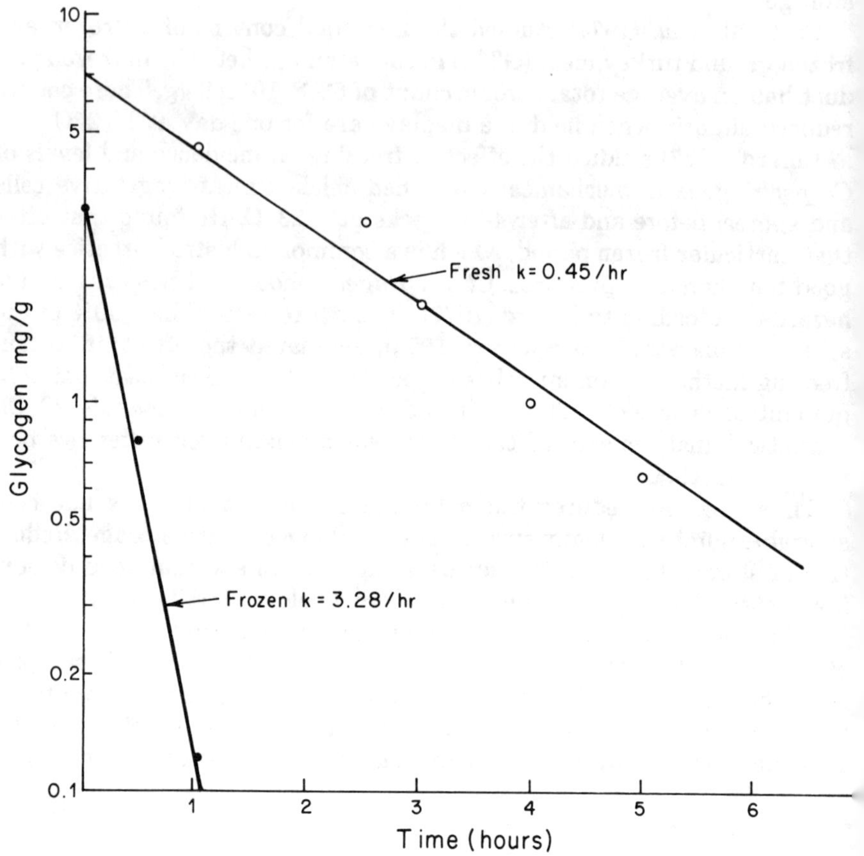

FIG. 8.4. GLYCOGEN BREAKDOWN AFTER STORAGE OF CHICKEN (de Fremery 1966).

of ATP disappearance and glycogen breakdown. The thawing temperature was 13—14 °C and the freezing temperature was —23 °C. It is obvious that the rate of glycogen breakdown is seven times faster, and for ATP disappearance it is ten times faster for frozen as compared to fresh muscle. Thus, acceleration of postmortem glycolysis in young poultry increases the toughness of fully aged meat.

Miller and May (1965) studied the effect of the rate of freezing, storage time and temperature on poultry. They found that the rate of freezing had no effect on tenderness. The data for shelf-life were insufficient for kinetic analysis.

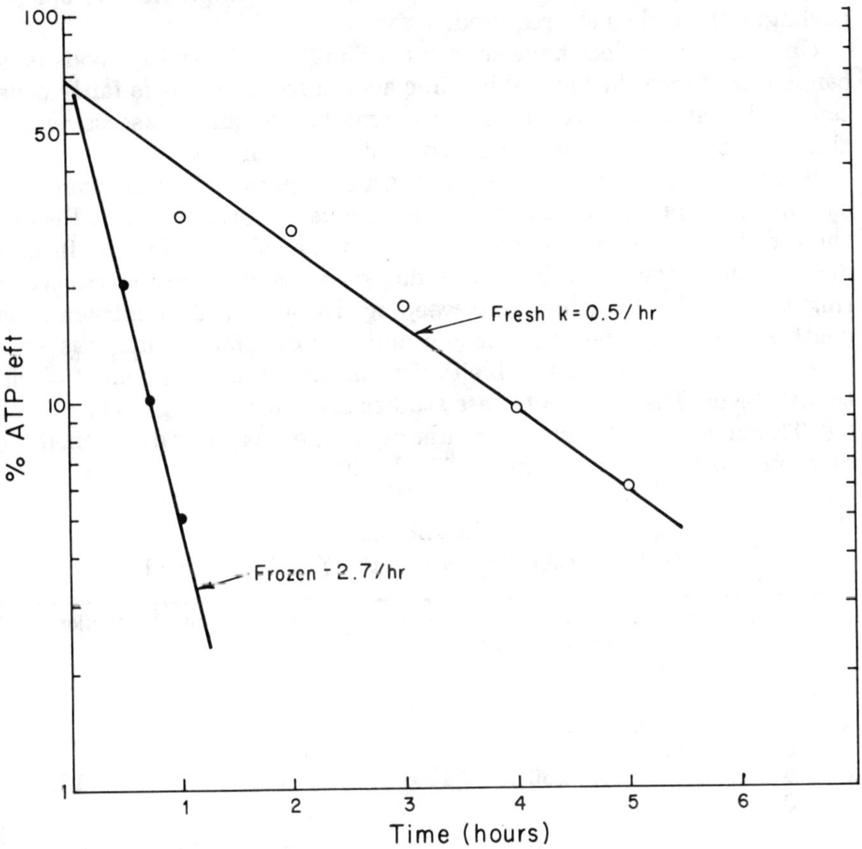

FIG. 8.5. ATP LOSS AFTER STORAGE OF CHICKEN
(From de Fremery 1966).

Flavor Changes

Although considerable work has been carried out on the flavor of poultry, a number of problems remain unsolved.

Age, sex, and quality do affect flavor. Change in glycogen and acid contributes to flavor change. Increase in hypoxanthene lessens natural flavors and causes an unacceptable flavor, as does an increase in bacterial count. The environment and surroundings also change the flavor, as does an increase in bacterial count. The environment and surroundings also change the flavor of chickens. Fat contributes to desirable aroma but is also a source of rancidity. Poultry, especially turkey, is very high in unsaturated fatty acids, so moisture-proof, oxygen-impermeable, opaque packaging materials are required.

One factor that does have an influence on flavor of poultry foods is inosinic acid. Since the level of inosinic acid in fresh muscle is fairly constant and related to flavor, an objective method of quality assessment of chicken meat based on inosinic acid content is feasible.

Khan *et al.* (1968) studied degradation of inosinic acid in chicken muscle during aseptic storage and its possible use as quality index. Results showed that measurements of the amounts of inosinic acid would furnish direct information on freshness and flavor and would reflect losses occurring as a result of leaching and weeping. Inosinic acid in chicken after death slowly degrades into inosine and hypoxanthine which has been associated with loss of desirable flavor and with the development of bitter off-flavor. The results of these studies are shown in Figs. 8.6, 8.7 and 8.8. The time to reach a given amount of change was plotted as a shelf-life plot and the results are shown in Table 8.2.

TABLE 8.2
BIOCHEMICAL CHANGES IN POULTRY MEAT

	Inosinic Acid Loss			Hypoxanthine Production		
Temp. (°C)	k weeks^{-1}	Q_{10}	E_a Kcal/mole	k mg/g/wk	Q_{10}	E_a Kcal/mole
0	0.426			0.09		
5	0.56	2.80	15.8	0.13	3.3	17.5
10	0.85			0.24		

Gutschmidt (1974) applied the zero order TTT equation based on organoleptic shelf-life to determine the extent of degradation in each part of the storage chain. The results are in Table 8.3. This table gives the quality loss for different possible cold chains in Norway. As seen, the major losses occur before the product has reached the consumer. The results compared very well to actual shelf-life. The shelf-life plot is shown in Fig. 8.9 and has a Q_{10} of 3.73.

Effect of Packaging on Deterioration

The packaging of poultry products is done for both aesthetic and utilitarian purposes. Uncooked products are packed in many forms such

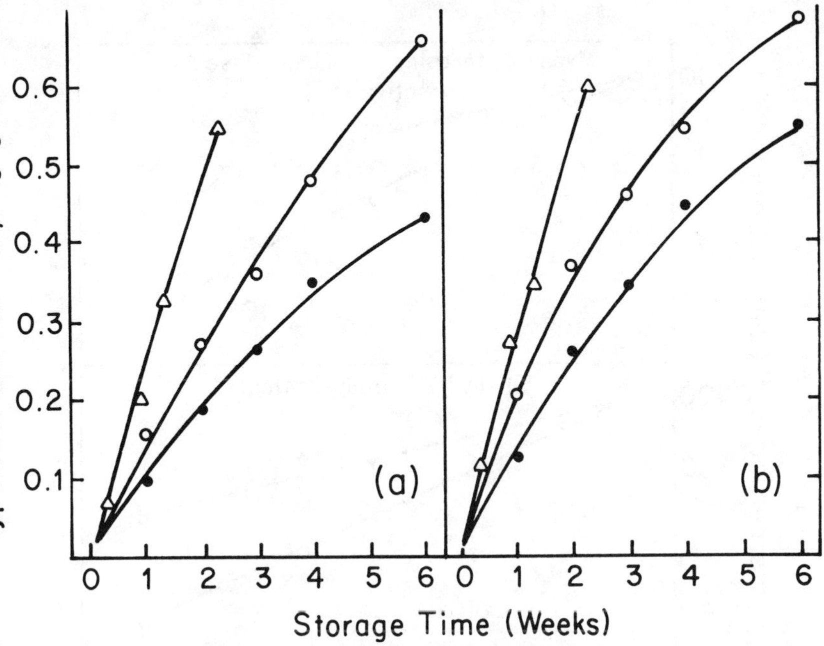

IG. 8.6. EFFECT OF STORAGE ON HYPOXANTHINE CONTENT OF CHICKEN MUSCLE: a, PECTORALIS MAJOR: b, BICEPS FEMORIS; ●, STORED AT 0°C; ○, STORED AT 5°C; Δ, STORED AT 10°C

(From Khan 1966).

TABLE 8.3
TTT APPLICATION TO FROZEN CHICKEN[1]

old Chain	Mean Storage Temp. (°C)	Practical Storage Life (days)	Quality Loss (%/day)	Mean Storage Time (days)	Quality Loss (%)
roducer	−23	540	0.180	40	7.5
ransport	−20	420	0.239	2	0.5
Vholesaler	−22	520	0.196	190	37.1
ransport	−16	370	0.370	1	0.4
etail	−20	420	0.239	30	7.2
op Layer	−14	210	0.476	3.1	1.4
ransport	−7	60	1.67	1/6	0.3
onsumer	−12	150	0.666	14	9.3
Total				280	63.7

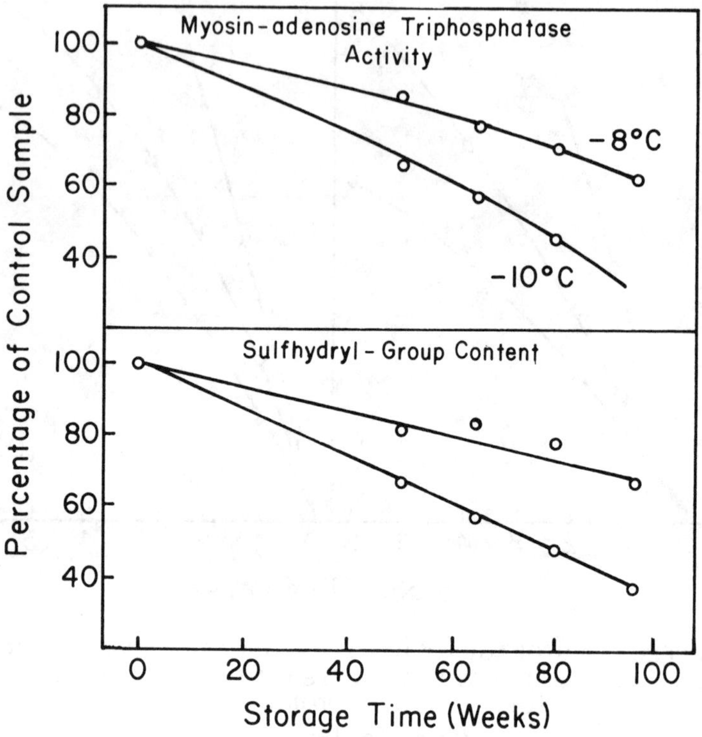

FIG. 8.7. EFFECT OF FROZEN STORAGE ON MYOSINE-ADENOSINE TRIPHOSPHATASE ACTIVITY AND SULFHYDRYL GROUP CONTENT OF CHICKEN BREAST MUSCLE
(From Kahn *et al.* 1968).

as refrigerated ice pack, dry pack, whole, parts, cut-up, and deboned. Frozen poultry is packed as whole, parts, cut-up or deboned.

Arafa and Chen (1976) studied the quality characteristics of convenience chicken products as related to packaging and storage. Precooked and prefried chicken products were prepared and packed by three methods, using commercial polyester pouches, polyethylene laminate pouches, and oil resistant papers. No permeability values were reported. The effect of frozen storage on weight loss, TBA value, peroxide value, acid value, and organoleptic qualities of the prepared products were studied. Vacuum packed samples had lower weight losses. The results are shown in Fig. 8.10 for weight loss, which would be essentially water.

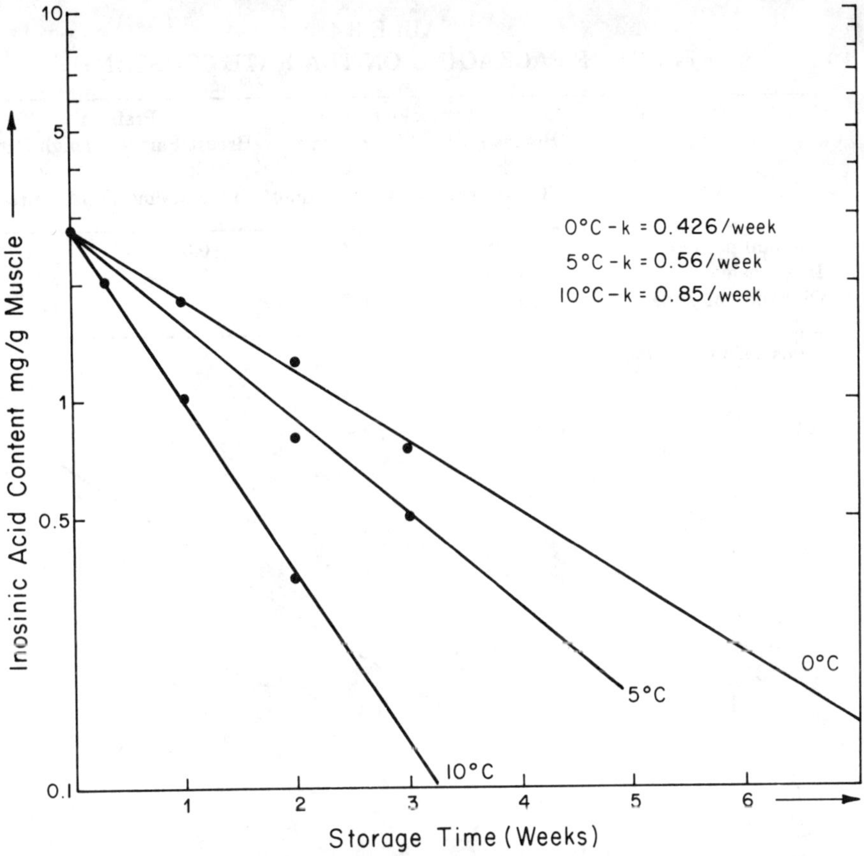

FIG. 8.8. EFFECT OF STORAGE TIME ON INOSINIC ACID CONTENT OF MEAT

(From Khan *et al.* 1968).

As seen, a straight line exists which justifies the equations developed in Chapter 3. Thus, one cut-off could be based on weight loss.

Vacuum packed samples also had lower TBA values and the rate of gain of TBA was also lower. A zero order reaction was assumed and a rate constant was calculated. The results are presented in Table 8.4.

Vacuum packed samples also had a very low peroxide value which increased insignificantly over a period of one month, and then leveled off. The heat sealed and oil resistant paper samples increased in peroxide value over four months and then leveled off. The overall flavor scores (1 = excellent, 9 = totally undesirable) seen in Fig. 8.11 supported the chemical data as a function of packaging. Again, these data present the dilemma in the use of a "pack date", since the more expensive package might be considered equivalent to the poorer package by the consumer.

TABLE 8.4
EFFECT OF PACKAGING ON TBA RATE CONSTANT[1]

	Precooked		Prefried	
	Breast Part k (TBA units/mo)	Thigh Part k (TBA units/mo)	Breast Part k (TBA units/mo)	Thigh Part k (TBA units/mo)
Vacuum packed	0.36	0.4	0.3	0.32
Heat sealed	0.61	0.57	1	0.5
Oil resistant paper	0.5	0.57	1	0.5

[1]Arafa and Chen (1976).

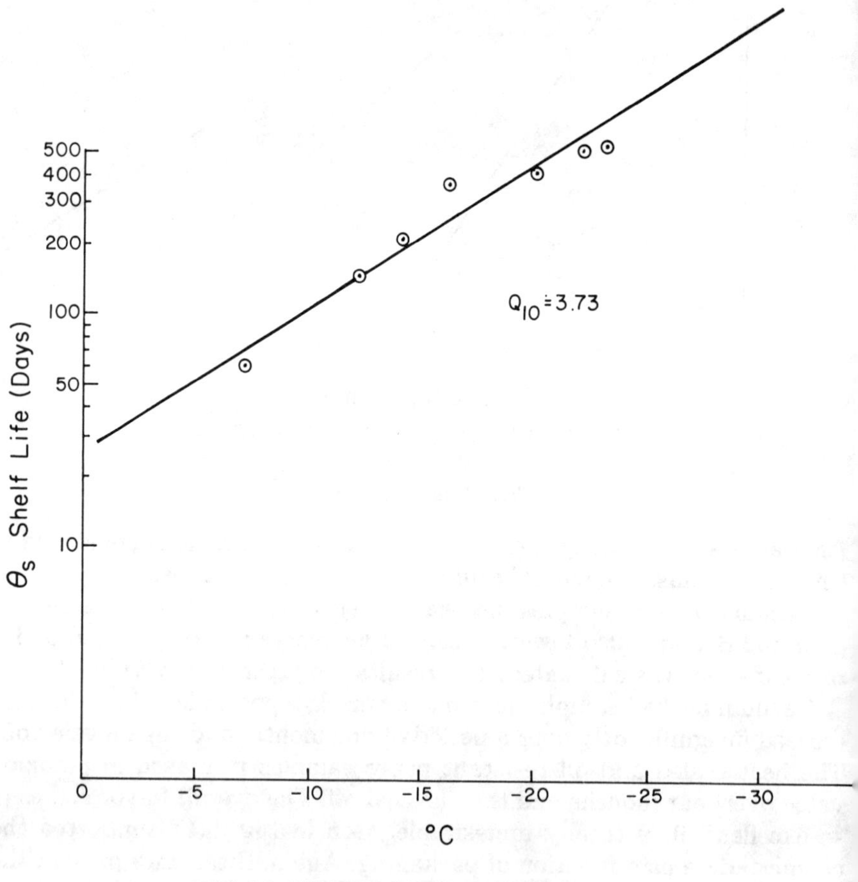

FIG. 8.9. FROZEN CHICKEN SHELF-LIFE
(Gotschmidt 1974).

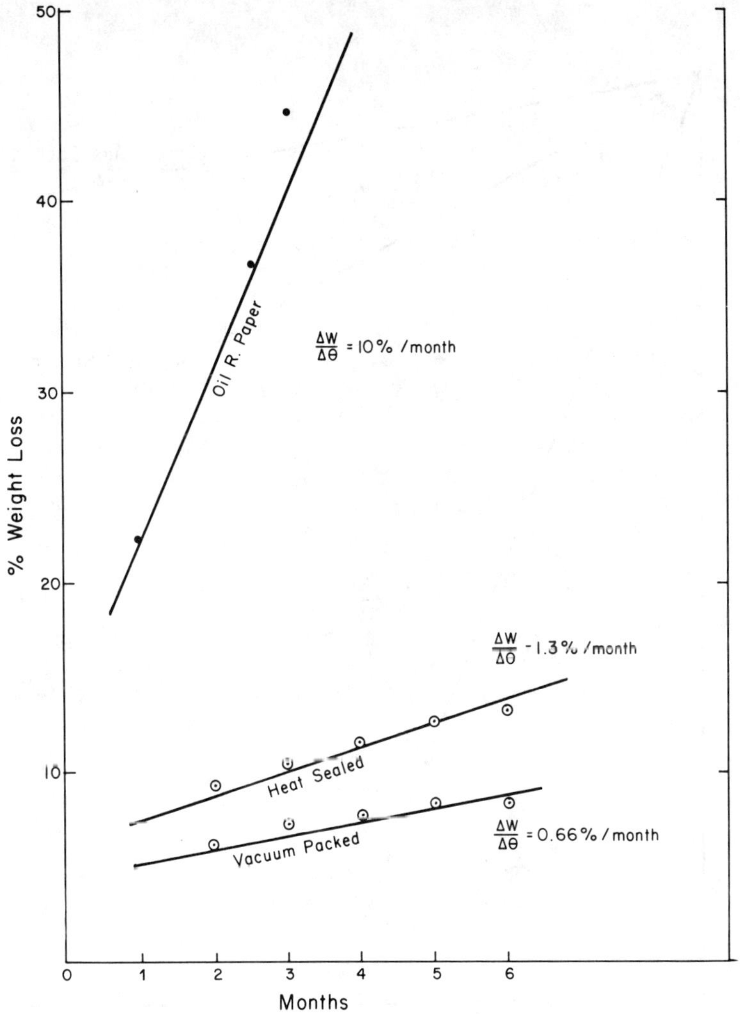

FIG. 8.10. PERCENT WEIGHT LOSS OF FROZEN CHICKEN AT −18°C (Arafa and Chen 1976).

SHELF-LIFE DATA

Data presented by Ayres *et al.* (1950) for fresh poultry at higher temperature, taking the end of shelf-life as the time when an unacceptable odor developed was shown earlier in Fig. 8.1. The calculated Q_{10} was about seven. Figure 8.12 shows shelf-life data comparisons of three groups. As seen, the data do not make a very good straight line on linear

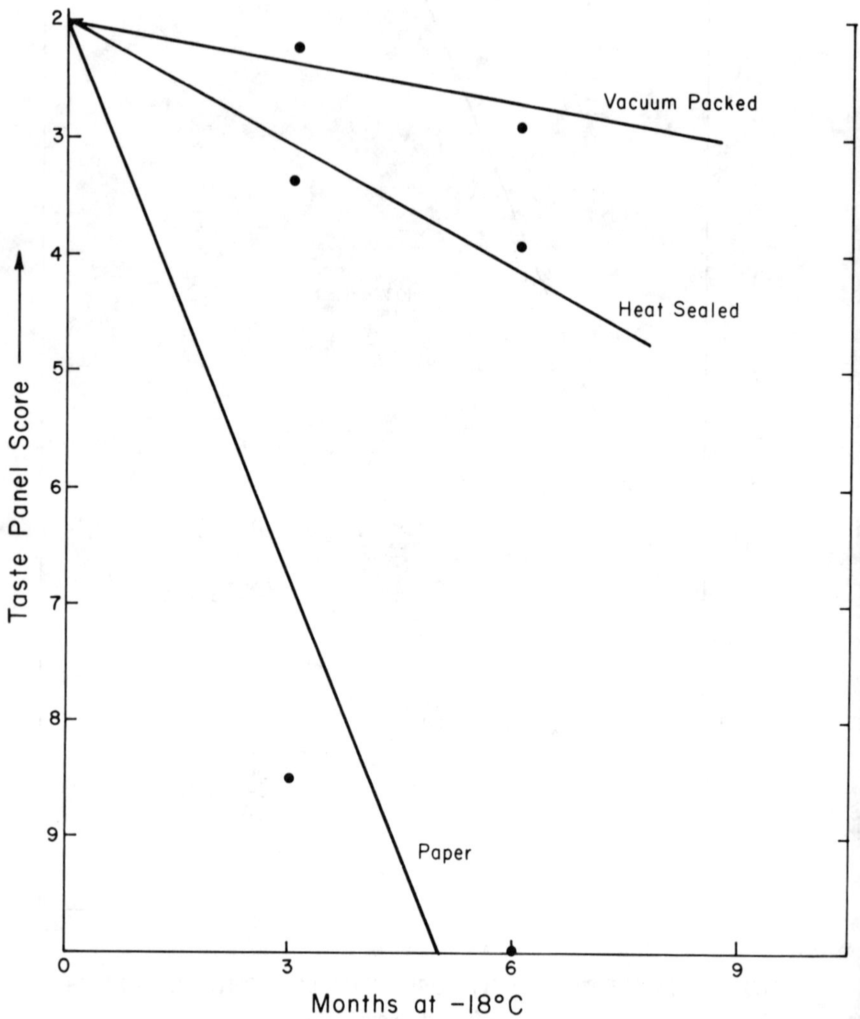

FIG. 8.11. FLAVOR PANEL SCORES
(Arafa and Chen 1976).

paper, but when graphed as a log θ_s plot the data are quite straight between 30 and 45 °F (Fig. 8.13) with a Q_{10} of about 4.5 if all the data are averaged. Below 30 °F for frozen storage, the data of lockhead and Landerkin (1935) give a Q_{10} of about 20, which is typical for frozen foods.

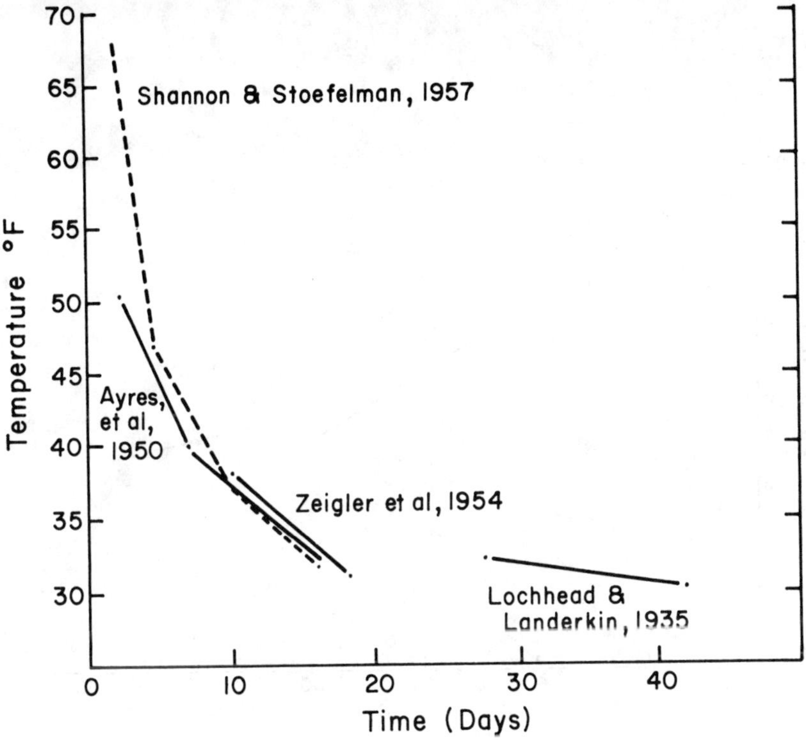

FIG. 8.12. EFFECT OF TEMPERATURE ON SHELF-LIFE OF CHILLED POULTRY (Elliot and Michner 1960).

TABLE 8.5
SHELF-LIFE DATA FOR FRESH POULTRY

Author	Shelf-Life (days)	Temperature (°C)	Q_{10}	E_a Kcal/mole
Ayres *et al.* (1950)	15.5	0		
	6.5	4.4	7.3	27.5
	2.5	10		
Shannon and Stadelman (1957)	12	0		
	9	4.4	2.7	15.8
	5.5	10		
Lockhead and Londerkin (1935)	30	0		
	8	4.4	21	45.8
	1.5	10		
Dawson and Stadelman (1960)	18	0	5.2 (0-2 °C)	
	11	2	3 (0-20 °C)	31.47
	2	20		

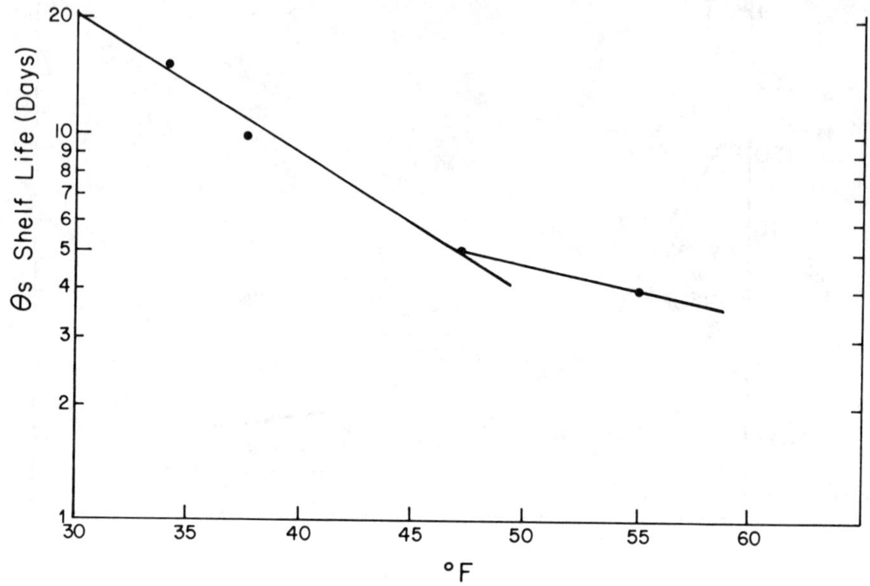

FIG. 8.13. EFFECT OF TEMPERATURE ON SHELF-LIFE OF CHILLED POULTRY
Data of Fig. 8.12 graphed as a log θ_s plot versus temperature (°F).

Dawson and Stadelman (1960) reported the data in Fig. 8.14. These data give a Q_{10} for refrigerated storage of three, if all the data are considered. However, based on the same problem as in Fig. 8.13, if the 20 °C (68 °F) point is neglected the Q_{10} is 5.2. The results of all these studies for fresh poultry are summarized in Table 8.5.

Shelf-life data for frozen poultry presented by Ristic (1975) were based on 38 quality criteria. These data are presented in Fig. 8.15. The line was drawn based on an assumption of linearity of the Arrhenius plot. The Q_{10} of the data is quite low, being only 2.3.

Other shelf-life data are summarized in Table 8.6 and Fig. 8.16. Again, the variation can be seen as was found for fresh poultry. This can best be seen in Table 8.7 where the shelf-lives stated at various temperatures are

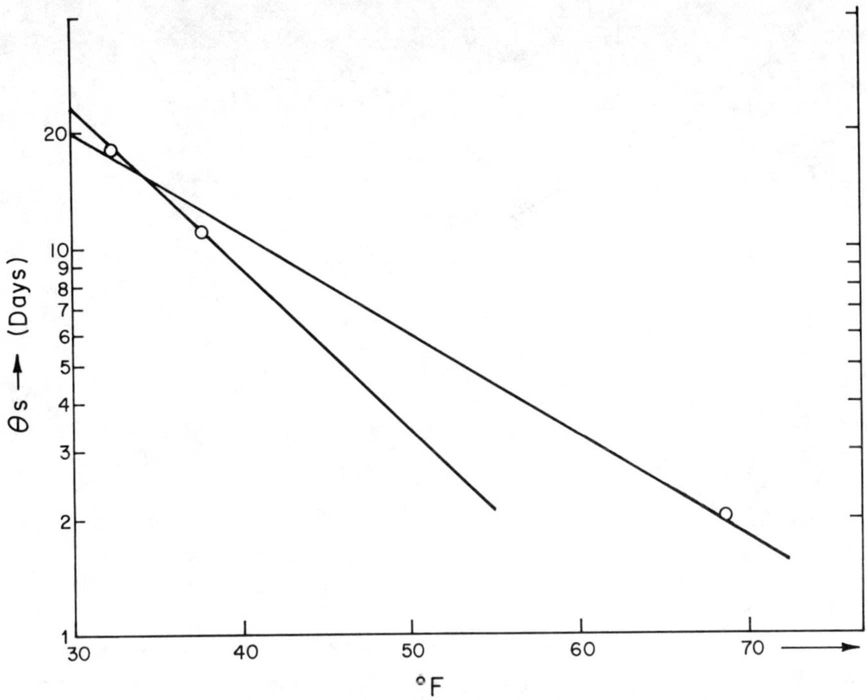

FIG. 8.14. SHELF-LIFE OF POULTRY
(Dawson and Stadelman 1960).

TABLE 8.6
SHELF-LIFE OF FROZEN POULTRY

Product	Shelf-Life (months)	Temperature °C	Q_{10}	E_a (Kcal/mole)
Whole chicken	4—6	−10		
	10—12	−15	2.3	10.7
	12—15	−20		
	18	−30		
Ready-to-cook frozen	1—6	− 7		
cut-up	3—10	−12	4.78	20.2
	6	−18		
Giblets	1	− 7.2		
	3—5	−17.7	3.9	19.4
	8—10	−23		
Roasts	4	− 7.2		
	8—10	−17.7	2.1	10.6
	12—15	−23		
Well packaged parts	12	−17.7		
	6	−12.2	3.53	19.2
	3	− 6.1		
Comminuted poultry meat	6	−25		

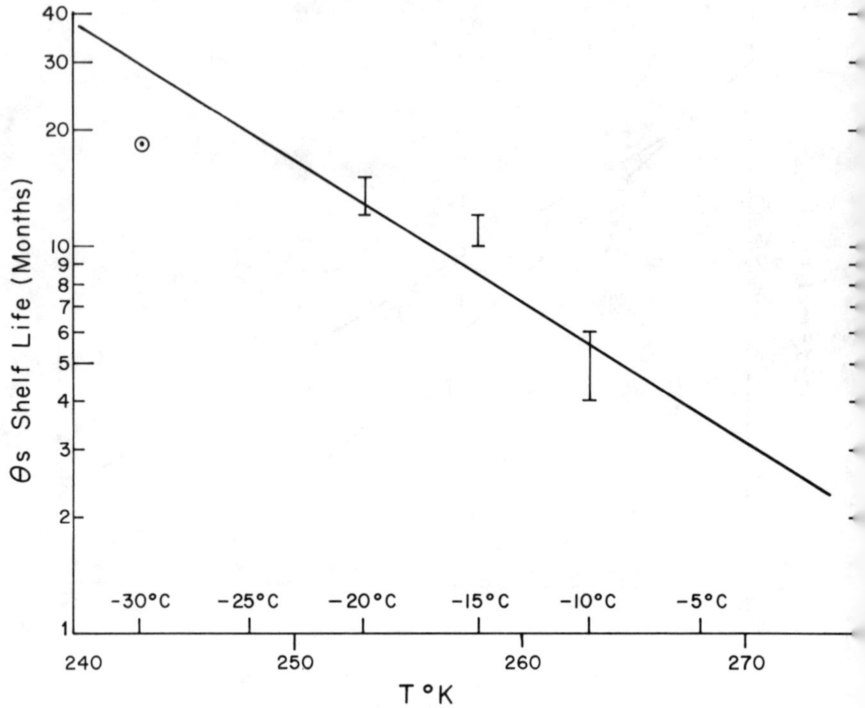

FIG. 8.15. FROZEN POULTRY SHELF-LIFE (Ristic 1975).

TABLE 8.7
COMPARISON OF VARIOUS PREDICTIONS OF SHELF-LIFE FOR POULTRY

Temperatures °C	Various Predictions of Shelf-Lives (days)
−32	360
−30	540
−23	270
−25	180
−20	390
−17	360, 120
−15	330
−12	180, 50
−10	150
− 7	90, 30
− 6	90
0	30, 15.5, 12, 18
2	11
4.4	9, 8, 6
10	5.5, 2.5
20	2

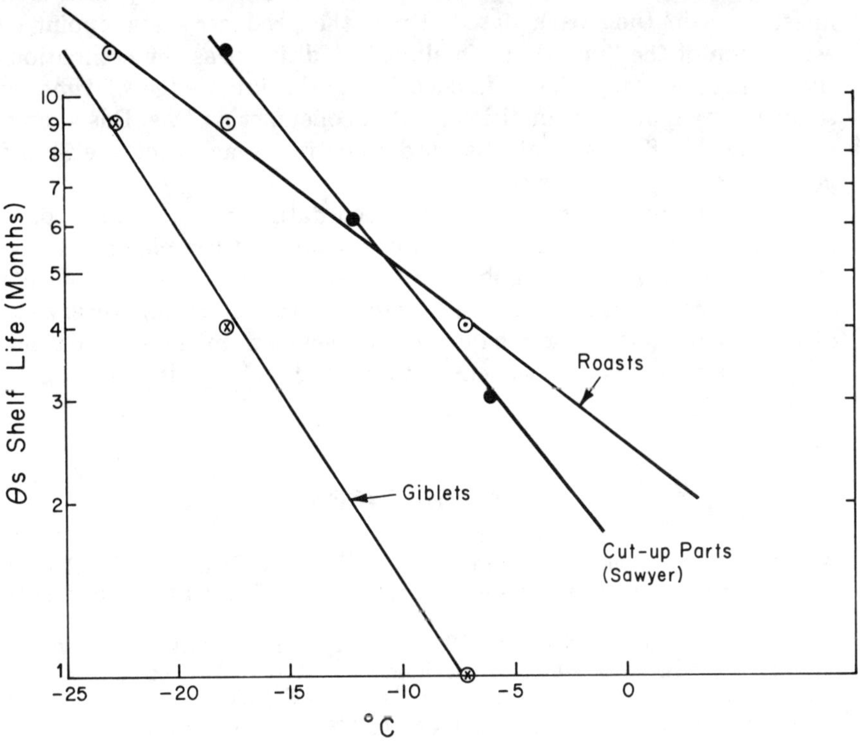

FIG. 8.16. POULTRY SHELF-LIFE
(Tressler *et al.* 1957).

compared. It is obvious that the preprocessing steps have a very significant effect on shelf-life and will thus make open dating difficult.

OPEN DATING

With a product such as poultry which has a short shelf-life, a "pack date" if done at retail or in a process center would be a useful data if it is close to the date of slaughter. However, temperature abuse would lead to an improper guess by the consumer as to the quality of the product.

The "pull date" or "sell by date" is the date after which the product should not be sold. The estimation of "pull date" requires the knowledge of shelf-life at various temperatures and a knowledge of the distribution system, including the retail store. The "pull date" would provide some help to the consumer for poultry, but the exact information regarding how long after the "pull date" the product could be safely used is still missing as in the "pack date". From the producer's standpoint, the estimation of the "pull date" is almost as difficult as the estimation of the expiration date, the difference being the knowledge of time, and temperature/humidity conditions at the consumer's home. Based on the data in Table 8.7, it would be hard to estimate an exact shelf-life for poultry as the product is so variable.

From a producer's point of view, open dating may provide a proper safeguard and may lead to a reduction of consumer complaints. It would certainly require a considerable expenditure of money to collect the required information. In addition, different methods for the grocery store display of products might have to be developed unless a "pack date" were used, in which case the customers could make their own judgment as to quality.

REFERENCES

ANON. 1965. Storage of frozen foods at 0°F or below. Congress OAL Record — The technical manual for storage and material handling for the Department of the Army.

ARAFA, A.S. and CHEN, T.C. 1976. Quality characteristics of convenience chicken products as related to packaging and storage. J. Food Sci. *41*, 18-22.

AYRES, J.C., OGILVY, W.S. and STEWART, G.F. 1950. Post-mortem changes in stored meats. I. Microorganism associates with development of slime on eviscerated cut-up poultry. Food Technol. *4*, 199.

BARNES, E.M. and IMPEY, C.S. 1975. The shelf life of uneviscerated and eviscerated chicken carcasses stored at 10°C and 4°C. Br. Poul. Sci. *16*, 319-326.

BENJAMIN, E.W., PIERCE, H.C. and TERMOHLEN, W.D. 1949. Marketing Poultry Products, 4th Ed. John Wiley & Sons, New York.

BLAXTER, K.L. 1961. Efficiency of food conversion by different classes of livestock in relation to food production. Fed. Am. Soc. Exp. Bioo. Med. *20*(1), 268-274.

COTTERILL, O.J., GLAUERT, H.P. and RUSSELL, W.D. 1977. Microbial counts and thermal resistance of *Salmonella oranienburg* in ground turkey meat. Poult. Sci. *56*, 1889-1892.

DAWSON, L.E. and STADELMAN, W.J. 1960. Microorganisms and their control on fresh poultry meat. WCM-7 Tech, Bull. 278, Michigan State University.

DE FREMERY, D. 1966. Relationship between chemical propeties and tenderness of poultry muscle. J. Agric. Food Chem. *14*, 214.

DE FREMERY, D. and POOL, M.F. 1963. Influence of post-mortem glycolysis on poultry tenderness, J. Food Sci. *28*, 173.

DE FREMERY, D. and SAYRE, R.N. 1968. Poultry: characteristics and stability of frozen products. *In* The Freezing Preservation of Foods, 4th Ed., Vol. 2, D.K. Tressler, W.B. Van Arsdel and M.J. Copley (Editors). AVI Publishing Co., Westport, Conn.

DHILLON, A.S. and MAURER, A.J. 1975. Stability study of comminuted poultry meats in frozen storage. Poult. Sci. *54*, 1407-1414.

ELLIOTT, R.P. and MICHENER, H.D. 1960. Review of microbiology of frozen foods. Conference on Frozen Food Quality, USDA Agric. Res. Serv., ARS 74-21, Albany, Calif., Nov. 4-5.

ELLIOTT, R.P. and MICHENER, H.D. 1961. Microbiological standards and handling loads for chilled and frozen foods. A review. Appl. Micro. *12*, 452-468.

FISHWICK, M.J. 1968. Changes in the lipid of turkey muscle during storage at chilling and freezing temperatures. J. Sci. Food Agric. *19*, 440-445.

FANELLI, M.J. and AYRES, J.C. 1959, Methods of detection and effect of freezing on microflora of chicken pies. Food Technol. *13*(6) 294-300.

GALTON, M.M. and ARNSTEIN, P. 1960. Poultry diseases in public health, review for epidemiologists. U.S. Dept. HEW Public Health Service Publ. 767. Communicable Disease Center, Atlanta, Georgia.

GUNARATNE, K.W.B. and SPENCER, J.V. 1974. Effect of certain freezing methods upon microbes associated with chicken meat. Poult. Sci. *53*, 215-220.

GUTSCHMIDT, J. 1974. The storage life of frozen chicken with regard to temperature in the cold rain. Lebensm. Wiss. Technol. *7*, 137.

HULTIN, H.O. 1976. Characteristics of muscle tissue. *In* Principles of Food Science. O.R. Fennema (Editor). Marcel Dekker, New York.

INGALLS, W.L. 1950. The public health aspects of poultry diseases. Proc. Am. Vet. Med. Assoc. 282-291.

JANTAWAL, P.P. and DAWSON, L.E. 1977. Stability of broiler pieces during frozen storage. Poult. Sci. *56*, 2026-2030.

JONES, M.R. 1963. Proceedings of the 11th International Congress on Refrigeration, Munich.

KAESS, G. and WEIDEMANN, J.F. 1969. Freezer burn of animal tissue. Temperature influence on development of freezer burn in liver and muscle tissue. J. Food Sci. *34*, 392.

KHAN, A.W. 1966. Cryochemistry of animal tissue. Cryobiology. *3*, 224-228.

KHAN, A.W. and DERG, V.D. 1967. Biochemical and quality changes occurring during freezing of poultry meat. J. Food Sci. *32*, 148-150.

KHAN, A.W., DANDEK, J. and LENTZ, C.P. 1968. Degradation of inosinic acid in chicken muscle during aseptic storage and its possible use as an index of quality. J. Food Sci. *33*, 25-26.

KLOSE, A.A., POUL, M.F., CAMPBELL, A.A. and HAWSON, H.L. 1959. Time temperature tolerance of frozen foods. XIX. Food Technol. *13*, 477.

LIBBY, J.A. 1975. Meat Hygiene, 4th ed. Lea & Febiger, Philadelphia.

LILLARD, H.S. 1977. Effect of freezing on incidence and levels of *Cl. perfringens* in mechanically deboned chicken meat. Poult. Sci. *56*, 2052-2055.

LOCKHEAD, A.G. and LANDERKIN, G.B. 1935. Bacteriological studies on dressed poultry. Can. J. Agric. Sci. *15*, 765-70.

MARION, J.E., BOGGESS, T.S., Jr. and WOODROOF, J.G. 1964. Pretreatment and processing methods for canned whole chickens. Poult. Sci. *43*, 1097-1101.

McCOY, D.C. 1963. Refrigeration in food processing. *In* Food Processing Operations. M.A. Joslyn and J.L. Heid (Editors). AVI Publishing Co., Westport, Conn.

MILLER, W.O. and MAY, K.N. 1965. Tenderness of chicken as affected by rate of freezing. Storage time and temperature and freeze drying. Food Technol. *19*(5), 147-150.

MOUNTNEY, G.J. 1976, Poultry Products Technology, 2nd Ed. AVI Publishing Co., Westport, Conn.

PALMER, H.H. and BOWERS, J. 1972. Poultry and fish. *In* Food Theory and Application, P.C. Paul and H.H. Palmer (Editors). John Wiley and Co., New York.

PETERSON, D.W. and CRAWFORD, L. 1975. Vitamin E and fishy off-flavor in turkey meat. The quality of poultry meat (lect.), p. 31A (1—8). University of California, Davis, CA.

PETERSON, D.W., SIMONE, M., LILYBLADE, A.L. and MARTIN, R. 1959. Some factors affecting intensity of flavor and toughness of chicken muscle. Food Technol. *13*, 204.

PETERSON, J. 1974. Poultry industry in the United States. *In* Encyclopedia of Food Technology series, Vol. 2. AVI Publishing Co., Westport, Conn.

POULTRY and Egg Situation, ERS, U.S. Dept. of Agriculture, June, 1977.

RISTIC, M. 1975. Gerfrierlagerung von schlactgeflugel. Kalte *28*(4), 133.

RUTGERS UNIVERSITY, 1971. Food Stability Survey. Rutgers University Department of Food Science, for the State of New Jersey Department of Health. In cooperation with the U.S. Department of Agriculture Economic Research Service.

SAWYER, F., MIDURA, T. and VONDELL, R.M. 1960. Handling and merchandising frozen food. Coop. Extn. Serv., University of Massachusetts.

SCOTT, M.L. 1956. Composition of turkey meat. J. Am. Diet. Assoc. *32*, 941-944.

SHANNON, W.G. and STADELMAN, W.J. 1957. The efficacy of chlorotetracycline at several temperatures in controlling spoilage of poultry meat. Poult. Sci. *36*, 121.

SPECK, M.L. and RAY, B. 1977. Effects of freezing and storage on microorganisms in frozen foods. A Review. J. Food Protection *40*, 333-336.

STEPHENS, J.F. 1977. Consumer acceptance of turkey cooked from frozen state in roasting bag. Poul. Sci. *56*, 563-570.

TEXAS AGRICULTURAL MARKET RESEARCH AND DEVELOPMENT CENTER. Product quality and consumer preference as affected by alternative methods of handling and packaging chicken. Technical Report MRC-71-2. Texas Agricultural Market Research and Development Center. Department of Agricultural Economics and Sociology.

TOMPKIN, R.B. 1973. Refrigeration temperatures. Food Technol. *27*, 54-58.

THOMPSON, J.E. COX, N.A. and BAILEY, J.S. 1976. Chlorine, acid and heat treatment to eliminate salmonella on broiler carcasses. Poult. Sci. *55*, 1513-1517.

TRESSLER, D.K. and EVERS, C.F. 1957. The Freezing Preservation of Foods. AVI Publishing Co., Westport, Conn.

USDA. 1971. Agriculture Handbook No. 31, Poultry Grading Manual.

WALKER, H.W. and AYRES, J.C. 1956. Incidence and kinds of organism associated with commercially dressed poultry. Appl. Microbiol. *4*, 345-349.

WALKER, H.W. and AYRES, J.C. 1959. Microorganism associated with commercially processed turkeys. Poul. Sci. *38*, 1351-1355.

WANG, P.L., DAY, E.J. and CHEN, T.C. 1976. Microbial quality of frozen fried chicken product obtained from retail store. Poult. Sci. *55*, 1290-1293.

WEISS, G.H. 1971. Poultry Processing. Noyes Data Corporation, Parkridge, NJ.
WINTER, A.R. and FUNK, E.M. 1951. Poultry Science and Practice, 4th Ed. R.W. Gregory (Editor). J.B. Lippincott Co., Chicago, Philadelphia, New York.
ZIEGLER, F., SPENCER, J.V. and STADELMAN, W.J. 1954. A rapid method for determining spoilage in fresh poultry meat. Poult. Sci. *33*, 1253.

CHAPTER 9

SHELF-LIFE OF FRESH MEAT

INTRODUCTION

According to the Food Stability Survey (Rutgers University 1971) beef constitutes 32% of the meat department sales, while fresh pork constitutes 15% and lamb only 1%. If data available on shelf-life for a particular meat were broken down to percentages, the breakdown would follow a pattern similar to that given for sales. The preponderance of information published in this country deals with either beef or pork. This chapter will not go into poultry shelf-life as it is covered in Chapter 8.

PACKAGING AND DISTRIBUTION

Following slaughter, beef is generally aged from 5—10 days under refrigeration (2 °C). During this time the carcass loses weight through evaporation, and enzyme systems tenderize the meat. The carcass is then either shipped whole or cut into wholesale pieces, and shipped to the retail outlet under refrigeration, where it is cut into consumer portions and packaged. Pork and lamb follow similar patterns, although lamb is aged for 7—10 days.

Proper sanitation during distribution and packaging is very important in assuring normal shelf-life, as is maintenance of proper temperature. These factors are particularly important during the preparation of chopped and hamburger meats. Equipment and personal sanitation affect these products much more than sliced meat.

SHELF-LIFE DATA

There are essentially two modes of spoilage for fresh meat: bacterial growth and loss of appropriate color. Consumers associate the characteristic red color of fresh meat with quality and freshness. This red color occurs when red oxymyoglobin is formed due to the oxidation of purplish myoglobin. Exposure of fresh meat to air and light changes the red fresh meat to brown, generally within 24 h (Table 9.1). This color change does not signify bacterial spoilage, with the resulting off-odor and flavor. The organoleptic shelf-life of fresh meat is generally 3—4 days

TABLE 9.1
SHELF—LIFE DATA FOR BEEF, PORK AND LAMB

Product	How θ_s Determined	Spoilage Mode	θ_s at 5°C	Q_{10}	E_a (Kcal/mole)	Reference
Beef round (air)	odor	bacterial growth	6 days	3.2	18	Clark and Lentz (1972);
Beef round (air)	color	color	17 h	33.3	54	Snyder (1964)
Beef fillet	color	color	20 h	750	101	MacDougall and Taylor (1975)
Beef rump	color	color	26 h	17.7	44	MacDougall and Taylor (1975)
Beef sirloin	color	color	736 h	—	—	MacDougall and Taylor (1975)
Beef ground	color	color	24 h	—	—	Rutgers University (1971)
Beef ground	organoleptic	bacterial growth	3-4 days	1.7	8	Al-Delaimy and Stiles (1975)
Meat (except ground beef, lamb, or fresh pork)	—	—	3 days	—	—	Rutgers University (1971)
Pork	bacterial counts	bacterial	4 days	6	27	Patterson and Edwards (1975)
Lamb	—	—	24 h	—	—	Rutgers University (1971)

TABLE 9.2
EFFECT OF O_2—CO_2 MIXTURES ON ODOR AND COLOR SHELF-LIFE OF PREPACKAGED FRESH BEEF[1]

Atmosphere	Odor θ_s (days)	Color θ_s (days)
Air	6	5
15% CO_2 — air	16	8
15% CO_2 — 50% O_2 (balance, N_2)	17	12
15% CO_2 — 70% O_2 (balance, N_2)	19	14
15% CO_2 — 85% O_2	19	14

[1]From Clark and Lentz (1973).

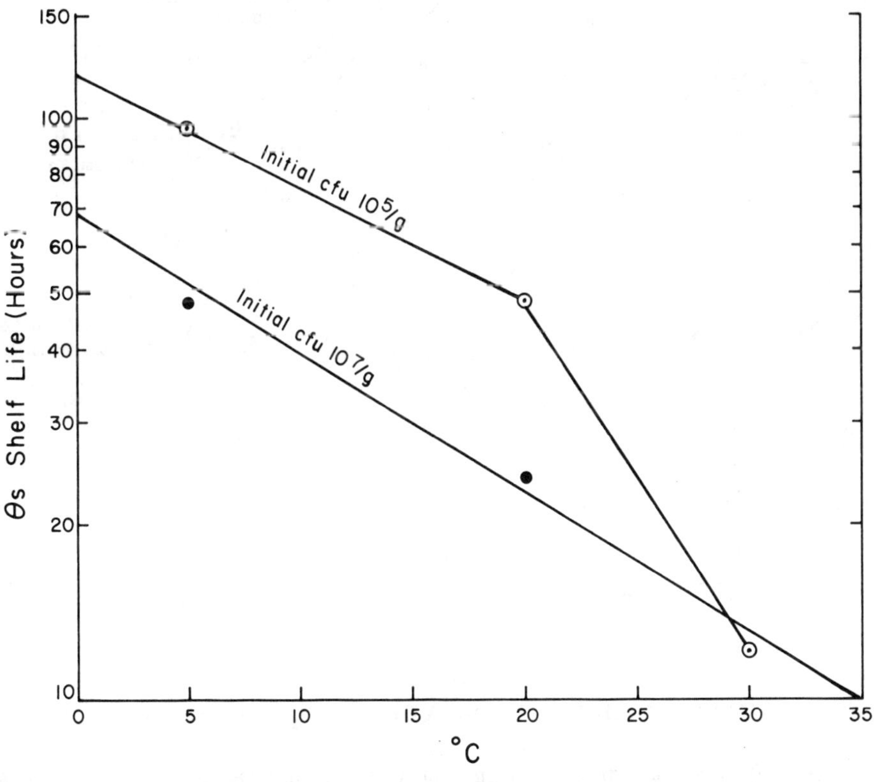

FIG. 9.1. ORGANOLEPTIC SHELF-LIFE OF GROUND BEEF (Al-Delaimy and Stiles 1975).

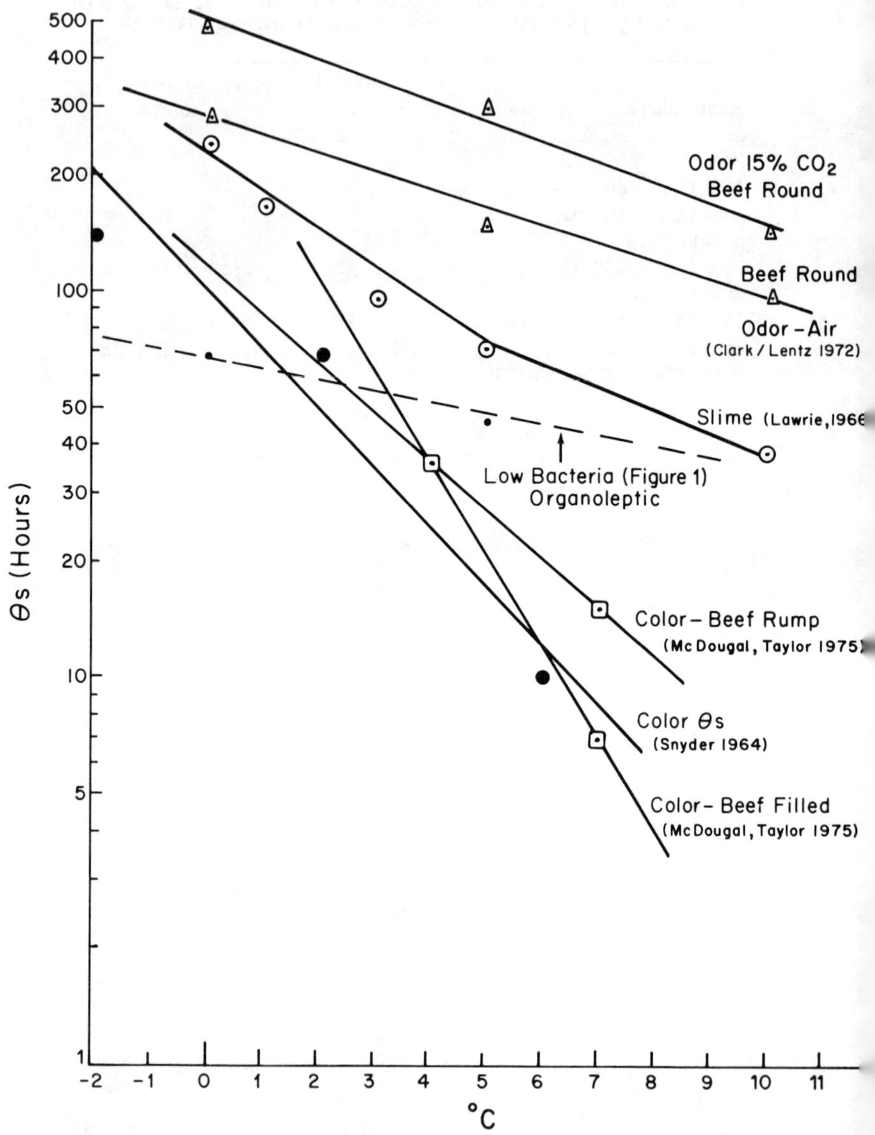

FIG. 9.2. SHELF-LIFE DATA OF VARIOUS CUTS OF BEEF

(Table 9.1), a considerably longer time than that required for off-colors. The oxymyoglobin color change can be delayed by packaging with an O_2 atmosphere (Table 9.2). The Q_{10} data in Table 9.1 also indicate that this reaction is extremely temperature-sensitive. It is a first order reaction which increases as temperature increases (Adams and Huffman 1972).

Bacterial spoilage is due mainly to psychotrophs, and with the exception of ground beef, is primarily a surface problem yielding slime and off-colors, as well as off-colors. The critical factors for bacterial spoilage are: (1) maintenance of proper temperature since the Q_{10}s are relatively high (Table 9.1); and (2) keeping the original bacterial load low. Figure 9.1 demonstrates that at 5 °C ground beef with an original load of 10^5 cells/g has two more days of shelf-life than ground beef with an original load of 10^7 cells/g. Here again the atmosphere of packaging can drastically affect shelf-life (Table 9.2), as a CO_2 atmosphere will lower the pH of the meat surface and retard growth. It can also be seen that, for the high load, the shelf-life line is not straight, indicating a change in mode. Additional shelf-life data on beef, as well as pork and lamb, can be found in Table 9.1.

Additional shelf-life data are presented in Fig. 9.2 for comparison. Near 0 °C color changes occur the fastest although the product is still acceptable. The next fastest reaction is overall organoleptic change, which has a low Q_{10} compared to other reactions, so slime or odor formation could actually limit shelf-life.

OPEN DATING

The debate over open dating of fresh mat is unique since almost all fresh meat is packaged by the retailer. The retailer deals with the public directly, and it is to the retailer's benefit to provide his customers with some form of shelf-life data. Since carcasses of properly handled beef are internally essentially sterile it is the packaging procedure that initiates color and bacterial spoilage. Hence, the date of packaging is critical in determining shelf-life. This date is probably of more use to the retailer than the consumer. The retailer can use such a date to remove old stock although this is easily represented by the color change. This date is probably useful to the consumer if some form of holding time is given. Thus, if fresh meats were labeled "use or freeze by a particular date," and also labeled with a pack date, the retailer could monitor his product, and the consumer would be able to estimate shelf-life.

REFERENCES

ADAMS, J.R. and HUFFMAN, D.L. 1972. Effect of controlled gas atmosphere and temperatures on quality of packaged pork. J. Food Sci. *37*, 869-872.

AL-DELAIMY, K.S. and STILES, M.E. 1975. Microbial quality and shelf-life of raw ground beef. Can. J. Publ. Health *66,* 317-321.

CLARK, D.S. and LENTZ, C.P. 1972. Use of carbon dioxide for extending shelf-life of pre-packaged beef. Can. Inst. Food Sci. Technol. J. *5,* 175-178.

CLARK, D.S. and LENTZ, C.P. 1973. Use of mixtures of carbon dioxide and oxygen for extending shelf-life of prepackaged fresh beef. Can. Inst. Food Sci. Technol. J. *6,* 194-196.

INGRAM, M. 1972. Meat presentation — Past, present, and future. Roy. Soc. Health J. *92,* 121-130.

MACDOUGAL, P.B. and TAYLOR, A.A. 1975. Color retention in fresh meat stored in oxygen — A commercial scale trial. J. Food Technol. *10,* 339-347.

PATTERSON, R.L.S. and EDWARDS, R.A. 1975. Volatile amine production in uncured pork during storage. J. Sci. Food Agric. *26,* 1371-1373.

RUTGERS UNIVERSITY. 1971. Food Stability Survey. Rutgers University Department of Food Science, for the State of New Jersey Department of Health. In cooperation with the U.S. Department of Agriculture/Economic Research Service.

SNYDER, H.F. 1964. Measurement of discoloration in fresh beef. J. Food Sci. *29,* 535-539.

CHAPTER 10

SHELF-LIFE OF FISH

INTRODUCTION

Fish, particularly fresh fish, is not a main source of protein in the U.S. diet. Data on percentage of fish sales in supermarkets have not been collected. According to the Food Stability Survey (Rutgers University 1971) the following types of fish and shellfish are used in the U.S. market:

(1) New England: ground fish (haddock, cod, whiting, flounder, ocean perch), lobsters, clams, scallops and sardines.
(2) Middle and South Atlantic: menhaden, oysters, clams and blue crab.
(3) Gulf Coast: shrimp, oysters, red snapper, clams and mullet.
(4) Mississippi Valley and Great Lakes Region: lake herring, chubs, blue and yellow pike.
(5) Pacific Coast and Alaska: tuna, halibut, salmon, ground fish, king and dungeness crabs and oysters.

PACKAGING AND DISTRIBUTION

Fresh fish generally is not prepackaged for the consumer, but if this is done, it is at the retail level. Fresh fish is generally packed in ice, maintaining a temperature of 32 to 40°F. During distribution, fresh fish is also transported packed in ice. The Food Stability Survey (Rutgers University 1971) states that:

> The storage temperature should not be above 35°F. Ice on the fish serves a twofold function. The fish must not only be cooled and kept cold, but the surface of the fish must be constantly washed by water from the melting ice to prevent the concentration of bacteria in the slime from becoming too high. If the ice on the fish is prevented from melting by holding it in a storage room at or near the freezing point of water, the bacteria count in the slime will build up to a high level, and the fish will spoil or sour.

SHELF-LIFE DATA

Basically, the major mode of spoilage for fresh fish is bacterial decomposition. Factors thus affecting the keeping quality of fish are: (1) Environment (season, location, bacterial load of water, (2) Fish species, and

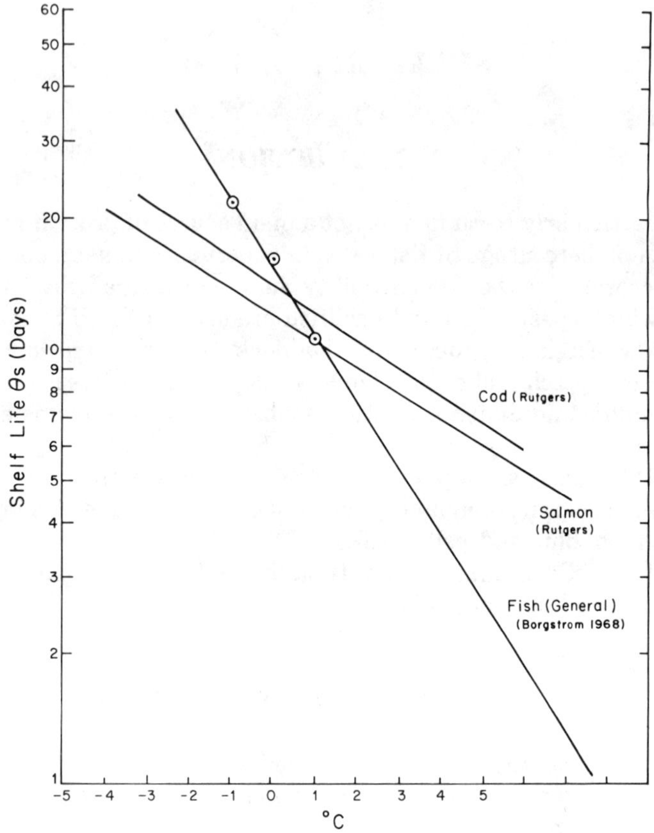

FIG. 10.1. SHELF-LIFE OF FISH

(3) Handling (temperature, sanitation). The same factors apply to shellfish. However, lobsters, clams, and crabs have the unique characteristic of being sold alive, and for these species proper temperature, particularly prevention of any rapid change in temperature, is important.

Tables 10.1 and 10.2 present shelf-life data for several common species of fish and shellfish. It appears that a typical marine fish such as cod has a shelf-life of approximately 14 days when stored on ice. The Q_{10} data shown in Fig. 10.1 indicate the importance of keeping fish properly chilled, since the values are from 4 to 6. Thus, even a small change in

TABLE 10.1
SHELF-LIFE DATA FOR MARINE FISH

Product	How θ_s Determined	Spoilage Mode	θ_s (days)	Q_{10}	E_a	Reference
Sovel	volatile base	bacterial	1 (16—19 °C)	—	—	Tomiyasu and Zenitani (1957)
Mackerel	volatile base	bacterial	1 (16—19 °C)	—	—	Tomiyasu and Zenitani (1957)
Yellow tail	volatile base	bacterial	1 (16—19 °C)	—	—	Tomiyasu and Zenitani (1957)
Cod	—	bacterial	14 (0 °C) 1 (16 °C)	4.4	2.3 Kcal	Rutgers University (1971)
Salmon	—	bacterial	12 (0 °C) 1 (16 °C)	4.7	24. Kcal	Rutgers University (1971)
Halibut	—	bacterial	14 (0 °C) 1 (16 °C)	4.4	23 Kcal	Rutgers University (1971)
Cod	—	bacterial	7-14 (0 °C)	—	—	Burt *et al.* (1975)
Fish — "general"	—	bacterial	21.5 (—1 °) 16 (0 °C) 10.5 (1 °C)	6.0	26 Kcal	Borgstrom (1968)
Cod	—	bacterial	12 (0 °C)	—	—	Huss *et al.* (1974)

TABLE 10.2
SHELF-LIFE DATA FOR SHELLFISH

Product	How θ_s Determined	Spoilage Mode	θ_s (days)	Reference
Crustaceans				
shrimp	—	bacterial	7 (°C)	Fieger and Novak (1961)
lobster	—	bacterial	6—16 (alive)	Fieger and Novak (1961)
crabs	—	bacterial	5 (alive)	Fieger and Novak (1961)
Mollusks				
oysters	—	bacterial	14-21 (4—6 °C)	Fieger and Novak (1961)
clams	—	bacterial	3 (alive)	Fieger and Novak (1961)
scallops	—	bacterial	8 (°C)	Thomsom *et al.* (1974)

TABLE 10.3
TEMPERATURE COEFFICIENTS OF GROWTH OF MARINE BACTERIAL OFTEN INVOLVED IN BACTERIAL SPOILAGE OF FISH[1]

Bacterial Species	Temperature Range	Q_{10}	E_a
Psuedomonas fluorescens	5 to 20	3.7	20 Kcal (5—15 °C)
	0 to 5	8.4	33 Kcal (0—10 °C)
	—3 to 0	9.3	34 Kcal (0—10 °C)
Flavobacterium deciduosum	20 to 37	1.2	3 Kcal (20—30 °C)
	5 to 20	1.2	3 Kcal (5—15 °C)
	—3 to 0	11.2	37 Kcal (0—10 °C)
Achromobacter sp.	7 to 25	1.86—2.84	10—14 Kcal (5—15 °C)
	—4 to 7	4.58—5.82	23—27 Kcal (0—10 °C)

[1]From Reay and Shewan (1949).

temperature has a drastic effect on keeping quality. Temperature coefficients of growth for typical spoilage bacteria are given in Table 10.3, and closely resemble the actual keeping quality data presented in Table 10.1. The date in Table 10.3 again illustrate the extreme importance of maintaining the proper temperature.

OPEN DATING

With an extremely sensitive product such as fish or shellfish, the benefits of open dating are obvious. Both the retailer and consumer should be given the date of catch. It is this date that is essential in determining shelf-life. Presenting the consumer with specific shelf-life data may be difficult because the shelf-life depends mainly on the species and handling from the instant the fish are caught. A specific pull date may be impossible to determine, but a pack date as is used for meat would be justifiable. It may be more appropriate to supply the consumer with the date of catch of the fish displayed, and guidelines as to the expected shelf-life for each species of fish. Then both the consumer and the retailer can make informed decisions on the quality of fish being purchased.

REFERENCES

BORGSTROM, G. 1968. Principles of Food Science, Vol. I, MacMillan and Co., New York.

BURG, J.R., GIBSON, P.M., JASON, A.C. and SANDERS, H.R. 1975. Comparison of methods of freshness assessment of wet fish. I. Sensory assessments of boxed experimental fish. J. Food Technol. *10,* 645-656.

FIEGAR, E.H. and NOVAK, A.F. 1961. Microbiology of shell fish deterioration. *In* Fish as Food. G. Borgstrom (Editor) Academic Press, New York.

HUSS, H.H., DALSGAARD, D., HANSEN, L., LODEFOGED, H., PEDERSON, A. and ZITTAN, L. 1974. The influence of hygiene in catch handling or the storage life of iced cod and plaice. J. Food Technol. *9,* 213-221.

REAY, G.A. and SHEWAN, J.M. 1949. The spoilage of fish and its preservation by chilling. *In* Advances in Food Research, Vol. 2. Academic Press, New York.

RUTGERS UNIVERSITY. 1971. Food Stability Survey. Rutgers University Department of Food Science, for the State of New Jersey Department of Health. In cooperation with the U.S. Department of Agriculture/Economic Research Service.

THOMSON, A.B., DAVIS, H.K., EARLY, J.C. and BURT, J.R. 1974. Spoilage and spoilage indicators in queen scallops (chlanys opercularis). I. Held in ice. J. Food Technol. *9,* 381-390.

TOMIYISU, Y. and ZENITANI, B. 1957. Spoilage of fish and its preservation by chemical agents. *In* Advances in Food Research, Vol. 7. Academic Press, New York.

CHAPTER 11

SHELF-LIFE OF DAIRY PRODUCTS (FLUID, PROCESSED, DRY)

INTRODUCTION: PROCESSING AND PRESERVATION

The main principle behind the preservation of milk and milk products is treatment to control natural pathogenic and spoilage microorganisms, usually by heating or adjustment of acidity (pH) levels to make the products safe for consumption.

Fluid Milk and Milk Products

Production of a safe milk supply begins with the maintenance of healthy dairy cows as established by various departments of health. Sanitary requirements for milking and subsequent storage and transportation of milk are contained in requirements of the various states and the Federal government. Presently, both bulk milk systems and the conventional 40-q cans for temporary storage are in use. Of utmost importance is rapid cooling of the raw milk to 40°F or lower. This milk is then generally pumped into insulated tank trucks which take it to a central processing plant.

Both on the farm and at the processing plant, the health and cleanliness of all animals, employees, handling and processing equipment may be required to conform to standards specified by state and local laws and/or regulations. A statistical sampling procedure employing bacterial counts and other quality tests (chemical components, adulterants, abnormalities and sensory characteristics) is generally used to monitor sanitation and product quality. Microbiological testing both at the farm (if possible) and processing plant is recommended to ensure high quality products for the consumer.

All fluid milk, except a small amount of "certified" raw milk, is pasteurized at either 145°F for 30 min (LTLT) or at 161°F for 16 sec (HTST) and is then quickly cooled to 40°F or below. Ultra-high temperature (UHT) milk is heated to 190—270°F for two sec. Temperatures over 270°F are used to produce a sterile product. The former heat treatments (HTST, LTLT, UHT) are designed to destroy microbes that produce disease and to reduce the number of spoilage microbes present. They do not sterilize the product (render it free of all microbes).

Separation of the milk results in skim milk and cream. The cream is then adjusted to various required percentages of butterfat for the consumer market. Most fluid milk, however, is homogenized immediately before or during pasteurization to disperse fat globules evenly in the milk. Milk may also be fortified with vitamins A and D. Established specifications must be met when milk is either homogenized or fortified.

Fluid milk products must be cooled to and maintained at 40 °F or below until delivered to the consumer. Temperatures as low as 35 °F are recommended, as this will slow the growth of psychrophiles and help minimize spoilage. From studies on the marketing of milk (Harkin *et al.* 1977), it has been shown that such temperatures are not readily maintained in channels of distribution, retail supply and during consumer use. It should be emphasized here that pasteurization significantly reduces the microbial population in milk and it is only through post-pasteurization contamination of the milk (especially with psychrophiles) that significant deterioration of milk quality will occur. Refrigeration will not cover up faulty sanitation and cleaning practices, nor will it keep milk from spoiling indefinitely. If proper sanitation procedures and adequate temperature controls are followed, a much longer shelf-life for fluid milk can be obtained. Exclusion of sun and fluorescent light will also maximize shelf-life.

Additional ingredients may be added to milk to make various flavored milks and dairy drinks. These products are then pasteurized and should be handled as specified above for fluid milk.

Cultured Products

Buttermilk, sour cream and yogurt are prepared by inoculating pasteurized milk or cream with a specific quantity and species of non-pathogenic lactic acid producing bacteria culture. The organisms are allowed to grow at a specified temperature for a specified time, during which lactic acid and other compounds are produced. The reaction is then stopped, and the product is cooled to 40 °F or below prior to packaging, shipment and sale. Yogurt is a cultured product containing added milk solids which is inoculated with a culture containing equal parts of *S. thermophilus* and *L. bulgaricus.* In all of these cultured products, refrigeration and acid production are the major modes of preservation.

Butter

Pasteurized cream is cooled to 50 °F or lower and churned to produce butter. It must contain at least 80% butterfat and may be either sweet (unsalted) or salted. Salt will inhibit the growth of many bacteria, but many molds are salt-tolerant and can grow well on the surface of butter. The butter is then packed automatically from the churn and is immediately stored under refrigeration. Spoilage, if any, is from proteolytic and lipolytic bacteria, yeasts and molds. However, butter is not a very good medium for their growth, especially at refrigeration temperatures.

Cheese

Cheese is made from milk curds which are precipitated by (1) coagulation by an enzyme, such as rennin, and/or (2) an acid, such as lactic. A starter culture of bacteria, or sometimes mold, is added and allowed to grow under specified time-temperature conditions, depending upon the variety of cheese being made.

Most cheeses are made from pasteurized milk. Those made from raw milk, which are not processed to high enough temperatures, are required by FDA cheese standards to be cured for no less than 60 days at not less than 35 °F. During this time sufficient lactic acid is produced to prevent the growth of pathogens. Any pathogens present should no longer be viable.

"Fresh" cheeses, such as cottage, are usually made from pasteurized milk by addition of a bacteria starter culture. They are not ripened or cured, and so must be handled as fresh dairy products, requiring constant refrigeration at 40 °F or below. Cream cheese is also unripened.

Processed cheeses and cheese spreads are melted at a temperature high enough to be equivalent to pasteurization, and are not further ripened. They are not federally graded, but may be inspected and hence bear an inspection stamp shield. These cheeses should be stored at refrigerated temperatures to preserve them.

Most cheese should not be frozen as low temperature may damage the texture and consistency. Table 11.1, which has been taken from the Rutgers University study (1971) lists ideal storage temperatures for most of the common varieties of cheese.

Ice Cream and Frozen Dessert Products

The composition of these products can vary considerably, but once the ingredients are blended, they are pasteurized at a higher temperature than that for milk, and are then quickly cooled to 45 °F or lower. Additional ingredients (fruits, nuts, etc.) are added after pasteurization, which preserves their flavor, texture and color. Unless these additional ingredients are of high quality and are handled sanitarily, they can significantly decrease the overall shelf-life of the product. The ice cream is frozen at 20—22 °F, either by continuous or batch process, during which time air is incorporated. It is then filled into containers and hardened at —20 to

TABLE 11.1
STORAGE OF COMMON TYPES OF CHEESE: IDEAL AND MAXIMUM TEMPERATURES[1]

Type of Cheese	Temperature (°F)	
	Ideal[2]	Maximum
Brick	30—34	50
Camembert	30—34	50
Cheddar	30—34	60
Cottage	32—34	45
Cream	32—34	45
Limburger	30—34	50
Neufchatel	32—34	45
Process American	40—45	75
Process brick	40—45	75
Process limburger	40—45	75
Process Swiss	40—45	75
Roquefort	30—34	50
Swiss	30—34	60
Cheese foods	40—45	55

[1]Source: ASHRAE (1967).
[2]For longest shelf-life.

—50°F. After hardening is complete ice cream is usually stored at about —10°F. It should never be held above 0°F, and fluctuations in temperature should be avoided as they adversely affect the texture, leading to a grainy, crystallized product.

Dried Milk Products

Whole milk and skimmed milk may be dried by either drum or spray drying to produce dried whole milk or nonfat dry milk solids (NFDM). The latter is quite stable if packed and sealed properly, and is normally marketed at room temperature. Packing it in an O_2 free (vacuum) or inert atmosphere greatly improves its shelf-life. Dried whole milk is much more susceptible to deteriorative reactions due to its high butterfat content. It is not sold in great volume in the U.S., but is frequently used in infant formulas. It should be refrigerated during storage, although this is often not the case; much of it is sold in drug stores. Packing under O_2 free atmosphere (or with an inert gas) also enhances its shelf-life.

Concentrated Milk

Concentrated milk refers to those products from which sufficient water is removed to concentrate the milkfat (MF) to ≥7.5% and total milk solids (TMS) to >25.5%. It is pasteurized to prevent spoilage, but not sterilized. It is preserved by refrigeration and is not widely sold at the retail level in the U.S.

Condensed milk generally refers to sweetened concentrated milks., The sugar present preserves sweetened condensed milk, and it is usually stored at room temperature.

Evaporated milk is made from homogenized milk by concentrating with heat and vacuum to obtain ≥7.5% MF and ≥25.5% TMS. Vitamin D is added and vitamin A addition is optional. It is generally sterilized in the can or before canning aseptically. UHT sterilized and aseptically canned evaporated milk has a much less carmelized flavor and is lighter in color. Evaporated milk can be stored at room temperature for several months without significant deterioration.

TYPES OF PACKAGING

Fluid Milk Products

Four basic types of packaging are used for fluid milk: plastic-coated paper; blow-molded plastic (returnable and nonreturnable); plastic bag in a box (generally for institutional use); and glass bottles. Plastic-coated paper cartons are also available with a thin layer of aluminum foil between the paper and inner layer of plastic. These are used for packaging sterile products and those with a long shelf-life because of the necessity to limit O_2 penetration. At least two companies presently fill plastic-coated paper cartons aseptically (Campbell and Marshall 1975).

In selecting packages for fluid products, the following factors should be considered: economy, convenience, appearance, disposability and ecology, safety, consumer preference, ease of filling and handling, durability and protection afforded. The major protection necessary for improved shelf-life is resistance to light penetration. Colored, rather than clear, glass bottles should be used, although this is often not the case. Another drawback of using glass bottles is that glass is comparably heavy, so higher inputs of energy are required for handling and transport. High energy inputs are also required for manufacture of glass. Detergents used in washing bottles must be diposed of with the potential for water pollution and additional demands for water. Raw materials for glass manufacture are not renewable, but supplies appear to be abundant (Campbell and Marshall 1975).

Raw materials for paper containers are renewable. The greatest problem in the manufacture of paper cartons is air pollution by sulfhydryl compounds in the vicinity of the plant. Paper containers are biodegradable, lightweight, easy to handle, and fairly opaque to light transmission.

Ethylene, the basic raw material for polyethylene, is stripped from natural gas, a limited nonrenewable resource. High energy inputs are required for manufacture and there is no significant waste accumulation, although air prollution may be a problem. Some plastic conainers are returnable; these are usually heavier in weight and involve increased transportation costs. Most plastic containers are not biodegradable, and are not very resistant to light transformation.

Glass, plastic and paper can be recycled, but for plastic and paper, recycling results in decreased quality. Therefore, one must weigh the benefits against the drawbacks to determine the most suitable package for the particular product, distribution and retailing system, and desired shelf-life. Economics also enter in, and it can be very costly to change from one type of package to another.

PACKAGING OF OTHER DAIRY PRODUCTS

Butter

Butter should be packaged in a material that affords protection against loss of moisture and absorption of foreign odors. It is presently packaged in waxed or plastic-coated paper which is suitable for short-term storage, but for long term storage it should probably be covered with yet another barrier (e.g., aluminum foil).

Canned Milks

These products are canned and retorted. Of great importance is an appropriate can lining (enamel) of good quality and proper thickness.

Dried Milk Products

Packaging for dried milk products should afford protection against air, light and moisture penetration, Thus, a laminate of paper, foil and plastic is probably most suitable. Most dried milk products are packaged under vacuum or after flushing with an inert gas. These treatments greatly increase shelf-life.

Cheese

Cheese is usually packaged in wax, plastic films or aluminum foil. Basically the package should be air and moisture impermeable. Packages are often sealed under vacuum or after flushing with an inert gas. Some cheese is packaged only for marketing and not for extended storage. This cheese should be repackaged by the consumer if extended storage is planned.

Cottage Cheese, Yogurt, Sour Cream

Generally, either molded plastic or plastic-coated paperboard cups are used. The packaging operation is the step in manufacture most likely to contribute to contamination of the product, so good manufacturing practices should be followed.

Frozen Dairy Products

More than 75% of frozen dairy products are packaged in half-gallon containers. Generally these are made of paper or plastic. Quarts are commonly packaged in round plastic or paper containers. Specialty items are usually packaged individually in paper wraps and then together (six-pack) in a paperboard box (often with a layer of foil).

DISTRIBUTION

Data on distribution times and temperatures of dairy products are difficult to obtain. Basically, the trend over the last three decades has been away from small processors and distributors, with an increase in other types of sales outlets such as supermarkets, dairy stores, convenience food stores, discount houses and vending machines. With the growth of these different sales outlets, the processor has become less in control of his market (Henderson 1971).

As late as 1930, 94% of all milk sold to Chicago consumers was distributed to homes. Presently, about 80% of the Chicago milk sales to consumers is through stores; for the entire U.S., the figure approximates 70%. Reasons for this trend include increased use of automobiles to purchase groceries, development of supermarkets with low milk prices, introduction of paper and plastic containers for easier handling, improved safety and keeping quality of milk, home refrigerators, and mechanized loading and unloading of milk in large quantities. Home delivery will probably remain viable in residential areas of cities, and deliveries will most likely be limited to once or twice weekly, with an increased need for better route planning to save money (Campbell and Marshall 1975).

A number of types of wholesale distribution are in use. These are: (1) trucks serving grocery stores and other outlets from the processing plant; (2) transport relays serving company branch depots in neighboring cities. Local retail and wholesale trucks operating out of the depot serve their immediate area; (3) delivery to warehouses of chain stores or to other large customers that can take truckload deliveries; and (4) platform or dock delivery. This system results in the lowest price to customers since a delivery charge is not involved. Large multiunit supermarkets may obtain an entire truckload of dairy products at the dock and then distribute to the other stores in the chain. Often the product may be packaged in containers bearing the brand of the chain (private label). There are many variations in types of wholesale service including full service, drop shipment and warehouse or platform delivery (Henderson 1971). The individual retailer must determine what services best suit his needs for the cost.

As of 1971, about 60% of milk sold, both retail and wholesale, was in half-gallon containers. Sales in quarts were on the decline, while sales of pints and half-pints were static (Henderson 1971). In 1972, sales in half-gallon, gallon and quart containers accounted for 41, 32 and 9%, respectively, of fluid milk sales in the U.S. (Campbell and Marshall 1975). Current trends are probably similar to this, although gallon containers seem to be increasing in use.

Of utmost importance in distribution of dairy products are maintenance of temperatures of 40 °F or below and proper rotation of stock. For retailers, the following recommendations can be made (Bernard 1974): (1) Place in cooler at ≤40 °F immediately after delivery; (2) fill the case in the refrigerated zone only; (3) do not block air ducts; keep air temperature ≤30 °F; (4) place no more than a two day supply in the dairy case; rotate stock; (5) maintain product temperature at ≤40 °F; (6) observe open coded dates; aim to sell within 3—5 days after processing; and (7) never use fluorescent lights in the dairy case as night lights. This leads to an oxidized, tallowy flavor. In a blown plastic container the shelf-life is less than 12 hours while in a more opaque paper container it is about 48 hours.

MODES OF DETERIORATION

Consumer acceptance of milk products is generally based on flavor and shelf-life (Barnard 1974). Bacteria are commonly associated with quality problems of milk. Control depends upon preventing their entrance, both before and after pasteurization and creating conditions unfavorable for their growth.

Psychrophilic (cold loving) bacteria are the primary group of microorganisms responsible for spoilage at refrigeration temperatures. Although the optimum temperature for their growth is between 68—86 °F, they also grow quite well at refrigeration temperatures (Packard 1967). Milk products are an ideal medium for their growth, and so when food is available to them, these microbes grow and alter the product quite rapidly.

Storage temperature greatly influences the growth of microbes. The higher the temperature, the shorter the generation time — time for one bacterial cell to divide to two — will be. Thus, at lower temperatures their growth is much slower, and the milk should maintain good quality longer. Other factors that influence the growth of psychrophiles (and other microbes) are water, type of food, O_2 and pH.

Growth of psychrophiles in milk can lead to a variety of off-flavors and defects. The milk can become bitter, fruity, rancid, stale, putrid or ropy. One problem associated with trying to establish standards for acceptable levels of various microbes in milk is that different species grow differently, producing compounds which lead to a variety of off-flavors and odors. Thus, to arbitrarily choose a level of microbial load such as 1×10^6 cfu/ml for end of shelf-life may not be correct. It may only require 1×10^4 cfu/ml of a particular species before off-flavors are noted, whereas another species may have to grow to levels of 1×10^7 cfu/ml before there is a noticeable change. The species and type (proteolytic, lipolytic, etc.) of bacteria present determines the type of spoilage and hence the level of microbes necessary to produce off-flavors. Table 11.2 lists some common psychrophiles and the levels in pasteurized milk associated with flavor changes (Punch *et al.* 1965).

Following pasteurization, it is generally only thermoduric (durable to heat) bacteria, some of which can be psychrophiles, which remain. Their numbers should be quite low and at low temperatures (32—35 °F) the milk should have a fairly long shelf-life. Thus, the best way to prevent spoilage is to prevent recontamination of the milk with bacteria following pasteurization. All surfaces and utensils that come in contact with the product should be clean and sanitary to prevent contamination with both psychrophiles and other microbes (e.g., coliforms).

Aside from microbial growth, there are other defects which can occur due to reactions of the lipids in milk, either by autoxidation or by the action of enzymes. Certain enzymes, such as lipase, hydrolyze the ester linkage (between fatty acids and glycerol) of triglycerides to yield free fatty acids. Many of the short chain fatty acids only need to be present at levels as low as parts per billion (ppb) to alter the flavor. These flavors

TABLE 11.2
POPULATION RANGE OF FIVE PSYCHROPHILIC SPECIES ASSOCIATED WITH A DEFINITE FLAVOR CHANGE IN PASTEURIZED MILK AT 6 AND 20°C
(Punch *et al.* 1965).

Species	Culture No.	Population Range Associated with a Definite Flavor Change 6°C	20°C
		(millions/ml)	
Chromobacterium sp.	0—2	4.1—5.7	4—17
Pseudomonas fragi	0—3	5.5—5.6	9—20
Pseudomonas fluorescens	14—A	5[2]	10—39
Pseudomonas sp.	108—A	3[2]	7.2—16
Aerobacter sp.	265—A	1.5—2.6	7.8—21

[1]A summary of the population levels of four trials for each culture at 6 and 20° embracing a decrease in flavor score of two or more points. The population range represents the highest population observed prior to a detectable change, and the lowest population level at the time a detectable change was observed. Controls did not exceed 150,000/ml and flavor did not change.
[2]An average value is given due to overlapping of upper and lower limits within the four trials.

and odors are collectively termed rancid. Factors which promote the development of rancidity include: (1) excessive agitation; (2) homogenization; (3) warming raw milk to 30°C and recooling; and (4) freezing and thawing. Lipase is generally inactivated by pasteurization, but certain microbes can produce it as they grow.

Oxidation of unsaturated fats and phospholipids can lead to off-flavors described as painty, nutty, grassy, tallowy, cardboard and fishy. The metallic or oxidized flavors vary with both product and cause. Sunlight, fluorescent light, copper and iron, small amounts of ascorbic acid, riboflavin, and excessive agitation favor or catalyze the oxidative reaction. Antioxidants, such as α-tocopherol prevent or retard it. Present U.S. standards do not allow the use of antioxidants in dairy products. Tocopherols are the only antioxidants known to be present naturally, although sulfhydryl groups produced during pasteurization also have antioxidant properties (Campbell and Marshall 1975).

Table 11.3 lists other defects of flavor and odor and their probable causes. Depending upon the milk itself, the microbial load, and the time-temperature conditions of distribution and storage, any of these defects could potentially determine the end of shelf-life.

The modes of deterioration and defects listed in Table 11.3 can be applied to most dairy products in general. For each specific product there are other appearance and textural changes that can also lead to end of shelf-life. For example, "wheying off" in cottage cheese is unacceptable and can generally be overcome with proper manufacture. Body defects in

TABLE 11.3
DEFECTS OF FLAVOR AND ODOR AND THEIR PROBABLE CAUSES

Flavor or Odor	Probable Cause
Acid	fermentation of lactose or other carbohydrate growth of microbes allowed by inadequate cooling
Bitter	protein breakdown by microbes and/or enzymes consumption of certain weeds by cows
Coarse	in cottage cheese — excessive diacetyl production in butter — too much acidity, lack of pleasant flavor
Cooked	heating leads to H_2S
Feed	most prevalent flavor detect — diet of cow
Flat/watery	low concentration of solids in milk
Foreign/disinfectant	absorption of odors or direct contamination with foreign materials or disinfectants
Fruity/fermented	bacterial growth, especially in cultured products
Garlic/onion	diet of cow
Lacks freshness	bacterial counts increase chemical reactions produce undesirable compounds and lead to loss of desirable compounds
Malty	streptococci produce aldehydes
Metallic/oxidized	lipid oxidation (autoxidation) (see above) homogenization retards light induced oxidation pasteurization enhances autoxidation, Cu induced oxidation
Musty	growth of molds and filamentous bacteria diet of cow
Unclean/old cream	growth of microbes producing enzymes (especially proteases)
Rancid	presence of lipase (see above)
Storage	absorption of odors change in chemical composition
Yeasty	growth of yeast; more common in acid products like cottage cheese

From Campbell and Marshall 1975.

sour cream are probably more noticeable than other defects; weak body can be caused by low nonfat milk solids, low fat, insufficient acid, and pumping, all of which could be corrected during manufacture. Textural changes in ice cream resulting in coarse, grainy crystals are often the result of temperature fluctuation, which could be prevented. Due to the low temperature of storage for ice cream, 10 to 0°F, microbial growth is inhibited almost entirely, and end of shelf-life will probably result from either textural changes or oxidation of lipids.

Although the principles discussed above apply in general, it can be seen that each product must be examined individually. Even within one product type, deterioration can vary tremendously depending upon formulation, processing, packaging and distribution times and temperatures. It is therefore unwise to generalize on modes of deterioration for a particular product (e.g., fluid milk) prepared under different conditions, because the mode of deterioration may be different for each brand of product and may change during handling and storage. It was noted by Webb *et al.* (1974) that with the improved bacteriological conditions of milk, the incidence of oxidized flavor in milk has increased. Thus, even the modes of deterioration present may influence which mode predominates.

Lastly, it should be noted that for all dairy products, further shelf-life studies should be conducted. Only with more accurate predictions of quality loss via different mechanisms can the most limiting mode of deterioration be clearly elucidated and predicted.

Nutrient losses can be another mode of degradation. Generally, although nutrients are lost in storage, the levels to which they drop are not severe. Usually, one of the other modes of degradation would result in end of shelf-life prior to a significant loss in nutritional value. The one exception to this might be loss of available lysine in NFDM during storage. Here significant loss could occur under high temperature, high humidity conditions, while the product would remain organoleptically acceptable.

SHELF-LIFE DATA

This section contains representative data on shelf-life of various products held at more than one temperature. The majority of the data in the literature is given for storage at one temperature only, and may not be indicative of changes in the mode of deterioration that may occur with changes in temperature. These data were analyzed using the techniques in Chapter 3. It can be seen that in general, the Q_{10}s for flavor changes are about 3 to 4 and are lower than the Q_{10}s for microbial growth which range from 6 to 30 for dairy products. This would indicate that for a 10 °C rise in temperature, the rate of change in flavor scores is much less than the rate of change in microbial growth. Thus, the microbes would grow much faster than the flavor changes that would occur and would become the predominating mode of failure. It should be noted that the dairy industry has developed a very standardized organoleptic scoring

TABLE 11.4
REPRESENTATIVE DATA ON SHELF-LIFE OF VARIOUS PRODUCTS

Product	Criteria for Determining End of Shelf-Life	Figure No.	Comments	E_a (Kcal/mole)	Q_{10}	Reference
Pasteurized homogenized milk	flavor score <37	11.1	plant A	17.7	3.13	Boyd *et al.* (1955)
	flavor score <37	11.1	Average of 4 plants	21.8	4.10	Boyd *et al.* (1955)
	microbial growth psychrophiles (PPC) >10^6 cfu	11.1	plant A	54.7	33.9	Boyd *et al.* (1955)
	microbial growth psychrophiles (PPC) >10^6 cfu	11.1	Average of 4 plants	30.1	6.95	Boyd *et al.* (1955)
	flavor score <37	11.2	Average	18.8	3.37	Boyd *et al.* (1955)
	microbial growth (PPC)	11.2	Average	39.1	12.48	Boyd *et al.* (1955)
	flavor score <37	11.3	N.Y. October milk	21.8	4.08	Dahlberg (1945)
	flavor score <35 SPC/PPC 10^6 cfu/ml	11.4	winter plant C	20.5	3.75	Finley *et al.* (1968)

continued . . .

TABLE 11.4 *Continued*

Product	Criteria for Determining End of Shelf-Life	Figure No.	Comments	E_a (Kcal/mole)	Q_{10}	Reference
Pasteurized homogenized milk	flavor score <35 SPC/PPC>10^6 cfu/ml	11.4	winter plant F	15.0	2.64	Finley *et al.* (1968)
	flavor score <35 SPC/PPC=10^6 cfu/ml	11.5	Average of 6 plants summer	35.3	9.76	Finley *et al.* (1968)
	flavor score <35 SPC/PPC=10^6 cfu/ml	11.5	Average of 6 plants winter	23.9	4.66	Finley *et al.* (1968)
	SPC≤1 × 10^6 cfu/ml	11.6	—	24.1	4.73	Smith (1968)
	flavor	11.7	plant A	31.0	7.38	Harmon *et al.* (1959)
	flavor	11.7	plant B	26.5	5.51	Harmon *et al.* (1959)
	TPC 10^6/ml	11.8	"good milk"	29.7	6.81	Harmon *et al.* (1959)
	lipolytic count 10^6/ml	11.8	"good milk"	13.8	2.44	Harmon *et al.* (1959)
	TPC 10^6/ml	11.9	"poor milk"	22.1	4.17	Harmon *et al.* (1959)
	uncertain	11.11	—	18.8	3.36	Randolph *et al.* (1965)
Sterlized whole milk	unknown	11.12	canned	8.5	1.71	Congressional Record (1977)
Sterilized chocolate milk	unknown	11.12	canned	8.5	1.71	Congressional Record (1977)
Chocolate milk (envelope)	unknown	11.12	—	9.8	1.88	Congressional Record (1977)
NFDM	unknown	11.12	can/drum	11.4	2.08	Congressional Record (1977)

continued

TABLE 11.4 *Continued*

Product	Criteria for Determining End of Shelf-Life	Figure No.	Comments	E_a (Kcal/mole)	Q_{10}	Reference
Whole dry milk	unknown	11.12	—	11.4	2.08	Congressional Record (1977)
Nonfat milk solids	25% loss of protein nutritive value	11.13	vacuum cans	5.1	1.39	Kramer (1974)
	25% loss of protein nutritive value	11.13	in bags 40% RH	5.4	1.33	Kramer (1974)
	25% loss of protein nutritive value	11.13	in bas 60% RH	5.2	1.31	Krmaer (1974)
	10% loss of protein nutritive value	11.14	vacuum cans	4.2	1.32	Kramer (1974)
	10% loss of protein nutritive value	11.14	in bags 40% RH	4.0	1.29	Krmaer (1974)
Nonfat milk solids	10% loss of protein nutritive value	11.14	in bags 60% RH	4.4	1.33	Kramer (1974)
NFDM	50% lysine loss	11.15	vacuum cans	3.4	1.25	Ben-Gera and Zimmerman (1972)
	50% lysine loss	11.15	40% RH	16.9	2.98	Ben-Gera and Zimmerman (1972)
	50% lysine loss	11.15	60% RH (missing 3rd data pt)	30.4	7.09	Ben-Gera and Zimmerman (1972)

continued . . .

TABLE 11.4 *Continued*

Product	Criteria for Determining End of Shelf-Life	Figure No.	Comments	E_a (Kcal/mole)	Q_{10}	Reference
NFDM	flavor	11.16	3% H_2O	7.8	1.65	Hall and Hedrick (1966)
	flavor	11.16	5% H_2O	11.0	2.03	Hall and Hedrick (1966)
	flavor	11.16	7.6% H_2O	43.1	16.1	Hall and Hedrick (1966)
Sweetened condensed milk	25% loss of thiamin	11.17	—	12.6	2.25	Kramer (1974
Concentrated milk	PPC = 1 × 10^6/ml	11.18	—	28.5	6.3	Olson *et al.* (1953)
Evaporated milk	50% loss of B_6	11.19	—	4.5	1.33	Gregory *et al.* (1964)
	30% loss of B_1	11.19	—	5.0	1.39	Gregory *et al.* (1964)
	20% loss of vitamin C	11.20	1st order reaction plant B	43.9	17.19	Bullock *et al.* (1968)
Evaporated milk	20% loss of vitamin C	11.20	1st order reaction plant C	41.3	14.54	Bullock *et al.* (1968)
	20% loss of vitamin C	11.21	zero under reaction plant B	12.4	2.23	Bullock *et al.* (1968)
Evaporated milk	20% loss of vitamin C	11.21	zero order reaction plant C	10.6	1.98	Bullock *et al.* (1968)
Pasteurized egg	time to reach flavor score = 2	11.22	1st order	26.1	5.37	Wood and Youngs (1969)
Spray-dried egg	60% loss of vitamin A	11.23	—	3.0	1.21	Harris and von Loesecke (1960)
Dehydrated egg	25% loss of vitamin A	11.23	no % RH specified	6.4	1.51	Kramer (1974)
	25% loss of thiamin	11.23	no % RH specified	5.4	1.42	Kramer (1974)
Whole dry egg	unknown	11.24	—	7.1	1.59	Congressional Record (1977)
Margarine	unknown	11.24	—	11.4	2.08	Congressional Record (1977)
	25% loss of vitamin A	11.25	—	10.0	1.91	Harris and von Loesecke (1960)

continued

TABLE 11.4 *Concluded*

Product	Criteria for Determining End of Shelf-Life	Figure No.	Comments	E_a (Kcal/mole)	Q_{10}	Reference
Refrigerated ice cream	SPC = 1 × 10^6/ml	11.26	not frozen	2.6	1.18	Nelson (1944)
Ice cream (powdered)	unknown	11.24	—	10.8	2.00	Congressional Record (1977)
Ice cream mix (paste)	unknown	11.24	canned	25.5	5.19	Congressional Record (1977)
UHT cream	time to P.V.=2	11.27	PV=2 may not be significant criteria	23.0	4.41	Downey (1969)
	time to TBA = .16	11.27	TBA=.16 may not be significant criteria	20.2	3.67	Downey (1969)
Processed cheese spread	O.D.=0.3	11.28	O.D.=0.3 may not be significant criteria	25.8	5.29	Thomas (1969)
Processed Cheddar cheese	unknown	11.29	canned	9.4	1.84	Congressional Record (1977)
Processed American cheese	unknown	11.29	dehydrated	10.8	2.00	Congressional Record (1977)
Grated cheese	unknown	11.29	—	11.0	2.03	Congressional Record (1977)
Coffee cream	unknown	11.29	—	7.7	1.64	Congressional Record (1977)
Whipping cream (30% fat)	unknown	11.29	—	15.1	2.65	Congressional Record (1977)

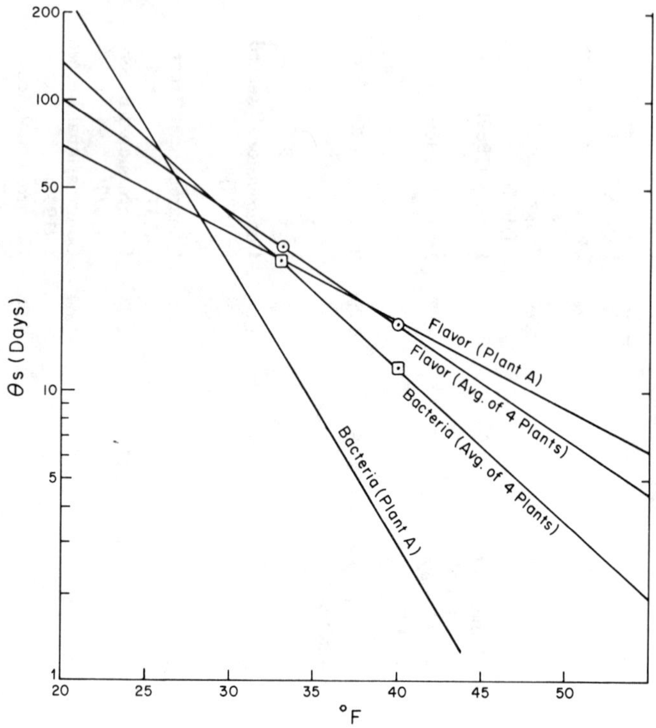

FIG. 11.1. PASTEURIZED HOMOGENIZED MILK SHELF-LIFE (Boyd *et al.* 1955).

method for flavor. A value of 40 is given as the initial score for milk, and when it drops to between 37 and 35 it is unacceptable. In some cases, since no endpoint was given for microbial growth, a level of 10^6 cfu/g was used as it was the common value reported for end of shelf-life in the other research papers.

More studies should be undertaken to determine suitable endpoints for the various products. Table 11.4 is a summary of the graphical data presented in these figures. The calculated Q_{10}s are based on the effect between 35 °F and 53 °F for fluid milk.

Figures 11.1 through 11.11 show data for homogenized pasteurized milk. As can be seen, depending on the data at any given temperature, in some cases flavor is the limiting mode of deterioration and in other cases bacterial count. In these cases the shelf-life lines cross over each other at some temperature as was illustrated kinetically in Chapter 3.

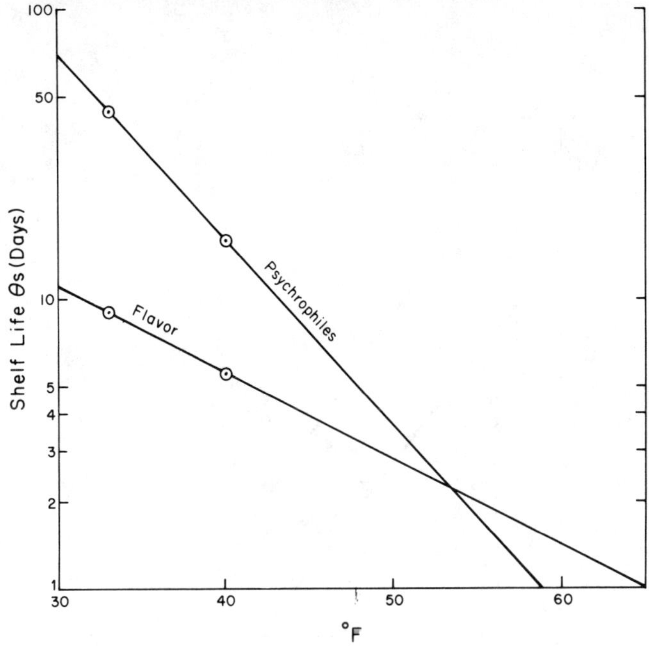

FIG. 11.2. SHELF-LIFE OF PASTEURIZED HOMOGENIZED MILK (Boyd *et al.* 1955)

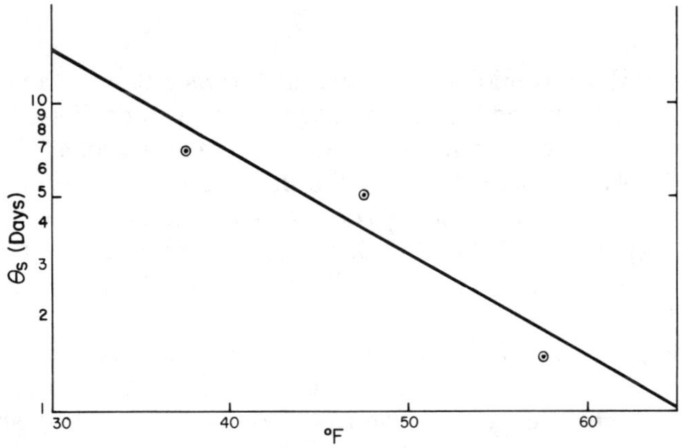

FIG. 11.3. PASTEURIZED HOMOGENIZED MILK (θ_s) DAYS TO REACH FLAVOR SCORE <37 (Dahlberg 1945).

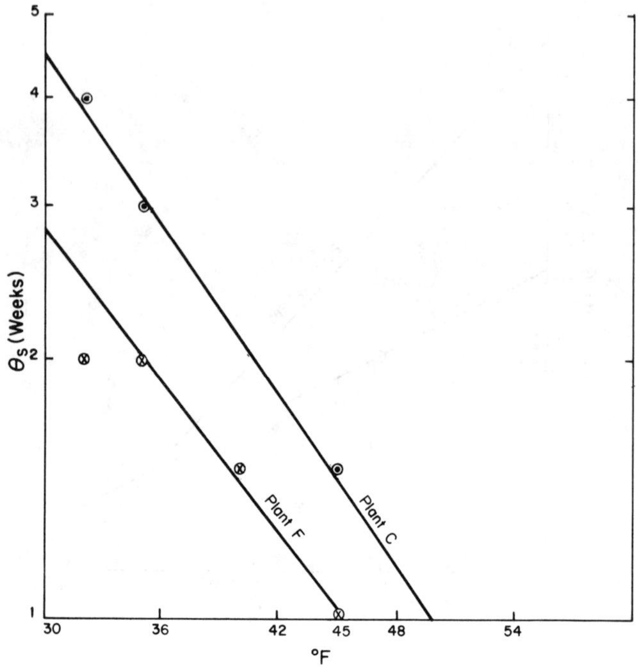

FIG. 11.4. SHELF-LIFE VS TEMPERATURE FOR WINTER MILK (PASTEURIZED AT 170°F FOR 16 SECONDS) FLAVOR SCORE AND PLATE COUNT (Finley *et al.* 1968).

At 35—40°F the shelf-life runs from as low as 3 days to as much as one month. It is also noted that different plots result for different plants (Fig. 11.1 and 11.4), and for milk obtained in different seasons (Fig. 11.5). It is also probably reasonable to use the flavor score as the major mode of deterioration since, as noted earlier, it is the result of microbial growth. As also seen in Fig. 11.8 and 11.9, the time to reach the limit of 10^6 cfu/ml depends on initial quality, poor milk reaching the limit about 2 to 3 times faster at 35 to 40°F.

Randolph *et al.* (1965) reported average keeping times of milk as represented in Fig. 11.11. Based on the Q_{10} of 3.36 it most likely is based on flavor score. The data are from 1965 and show a slightly shorter shelf-life than in the previous work described.

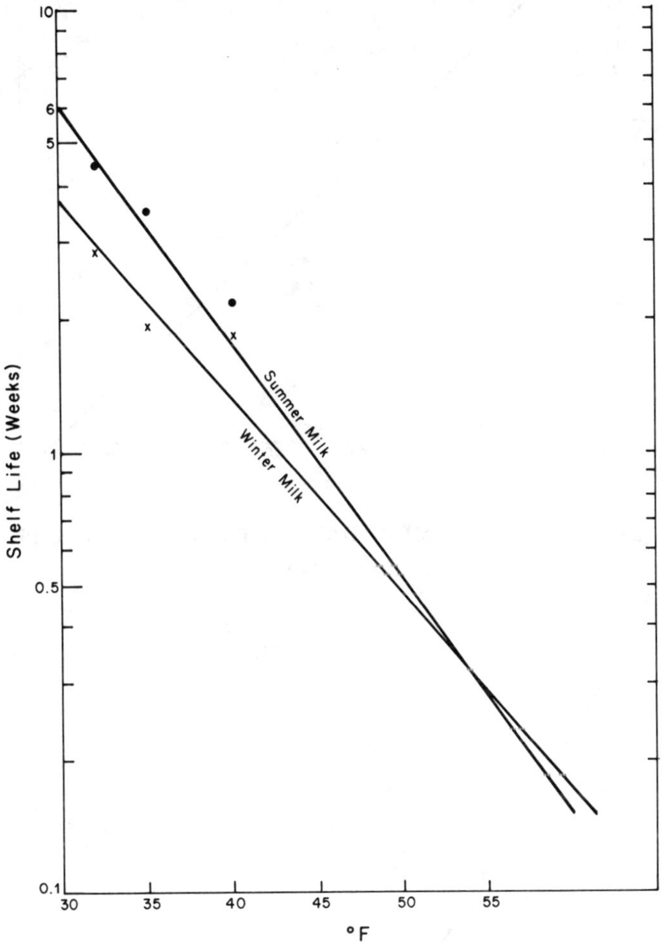

FIG. 11.5. EFFECT ON SEASON AND STORAGE TEMPERATURE ON SHELF-LIFE OF PASTEURIZED MILK (AVERAGE VALUES FOR SIX PLANTS)
(Finley *et al.* 1968).

As discussed in Chapter 3, the Army presented data on shelf-life of some foods. The figures are shown in Fig. 11.12. It is surprising that all the Q_{10}s are around two. No mode of deterioration is given. Figures 11.13 and 11.14 show results summarized by Kramer (1974) for quality loss in

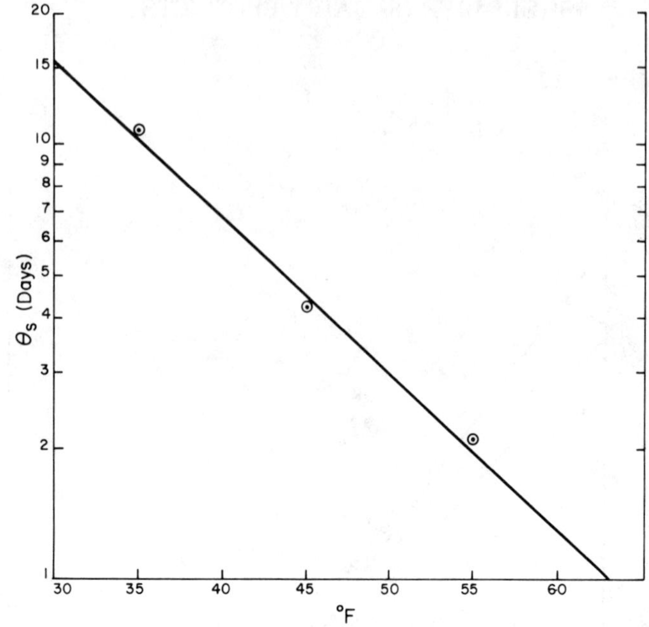

FIG. 11.6. PASTEURIZED MILK: DAYS (θ_S) TO REACH 10^6 CFU PER ML (Smith 1968)

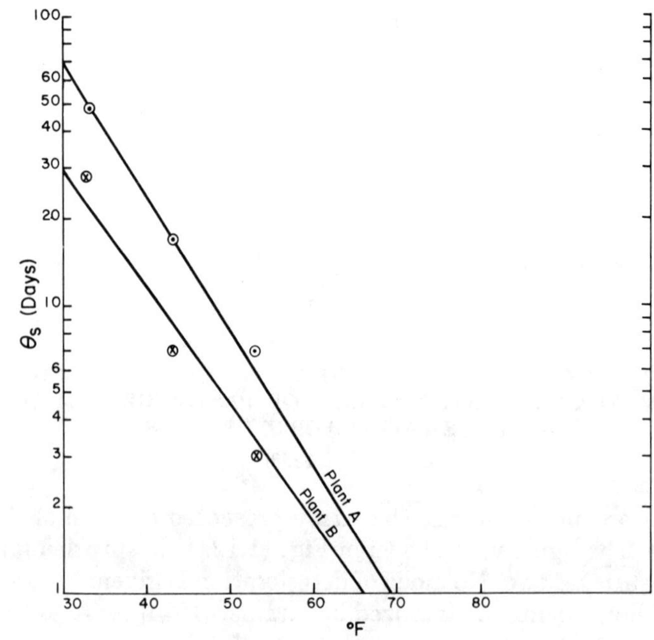

FIG. 11.7. QUALITY RATING: TIME TO REACH AN UNACCEPTABLE LIMIT FOR PASTEURIZED, HOMOGENIZED MILK (Harmon *et al.* 1959).

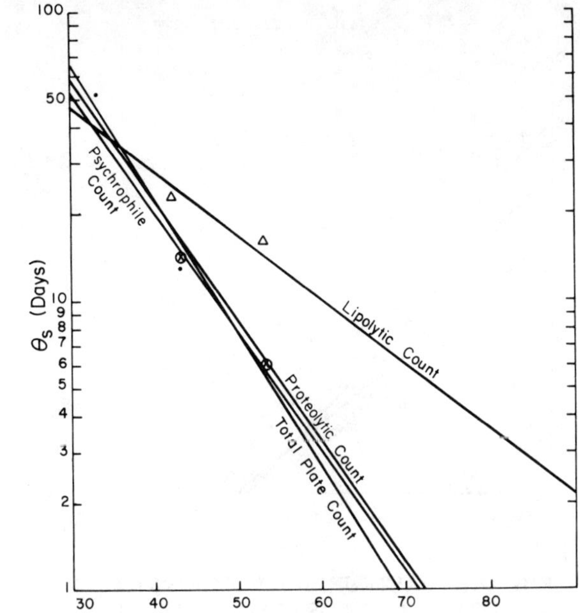

FIG. 11.8. GOOD MILK: TIME TO REACH 10^6 CFU PER ML (PASTEURIZED HOMOGENIZED MILK) (Harmon *et al.* 1959).

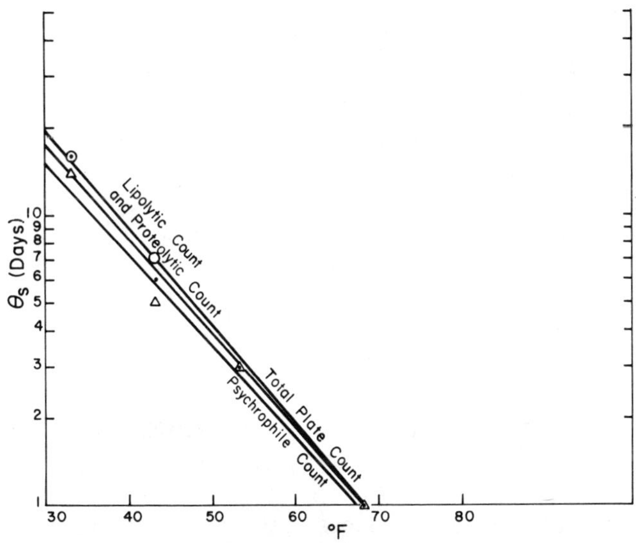

FIG. 11.9. POOR QUALITY MILK: TIME TO REACH 10^6 CFU PER ML (Harmon *et al.* 1959).

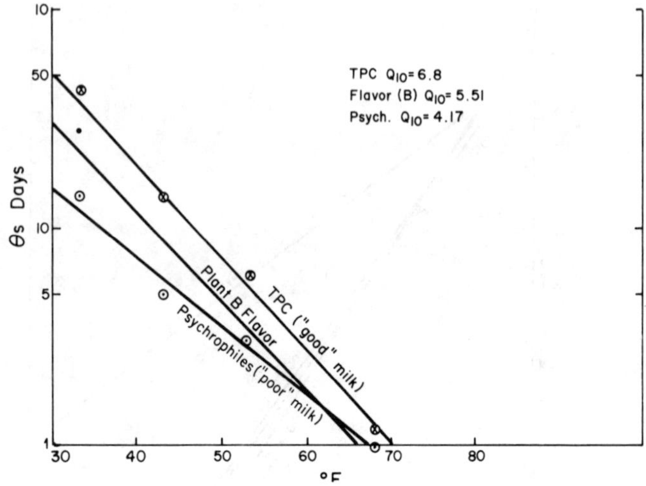

FIG. 11.10. PASTEURIZED HOMOGENIZED MILK: COMPARISON OF END OF SHELF-LIFE (Harmon *et al.* 1959).

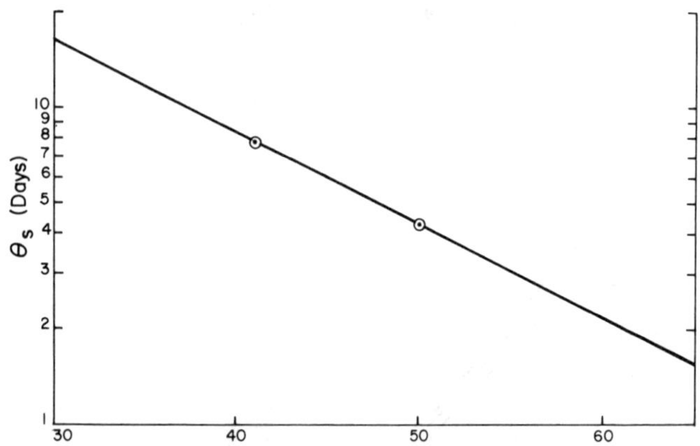

FIG. 11.11. PASTEURIZED WHOLE MILK SHELF-LIFE (Randolph *et al.* 1965).

nonfat dry milk. As seen, the loss of protein value depends on how it is packaged and on the a_w (% RH). As noted, the higher percent RH deteriorates the product faster, but the Q_{10}s are all similar. The low Q_{10} and activation energies (Table 11.4) make the data rather suspect since

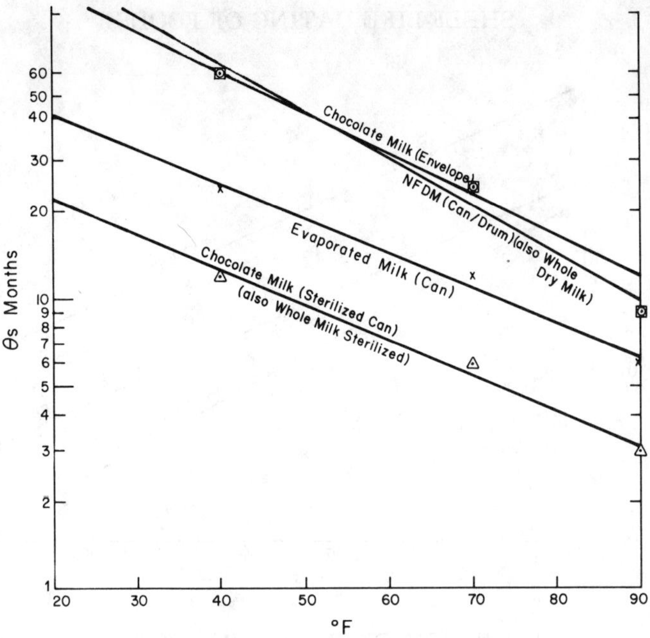

FIG. 11.12. U.S. ARMY SHELF-LIFE DATA OF VARIOUS DAIRY PRODUCTS (Congressional Record 1977).

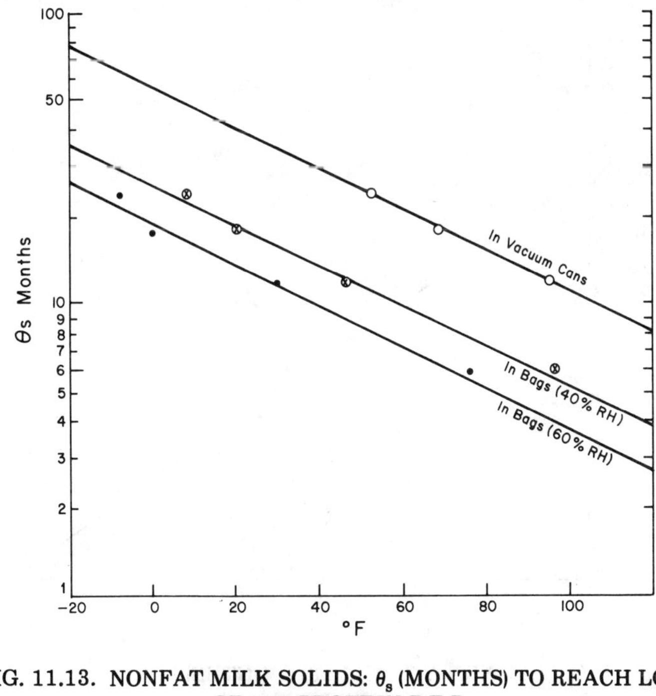

FIG. 11.13. NONFAT MILK SOLIDS: θ_s (MONTHS) TO REACH LOSS OF 25% PROTEIN P.E.R.

(Kramer *et al.* 1974).

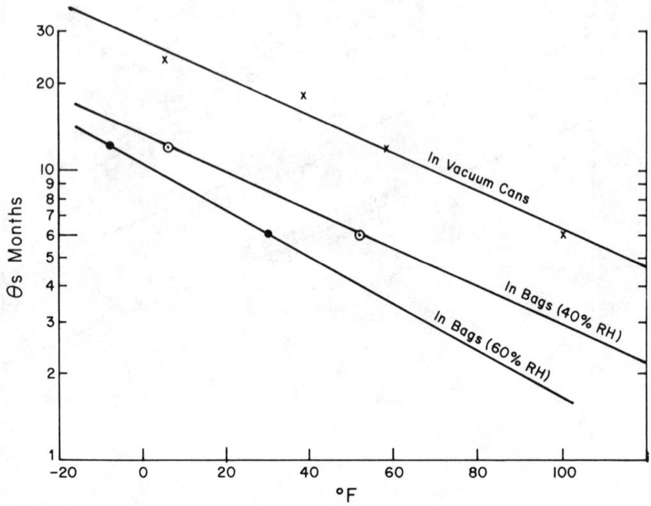

FIG. 11.14. NONFAT DRY MILK: θ_s (MONTHS) FOR 10% LOSS OF PROTEIN P.E.R.
(Kramer *et al.* 1974).

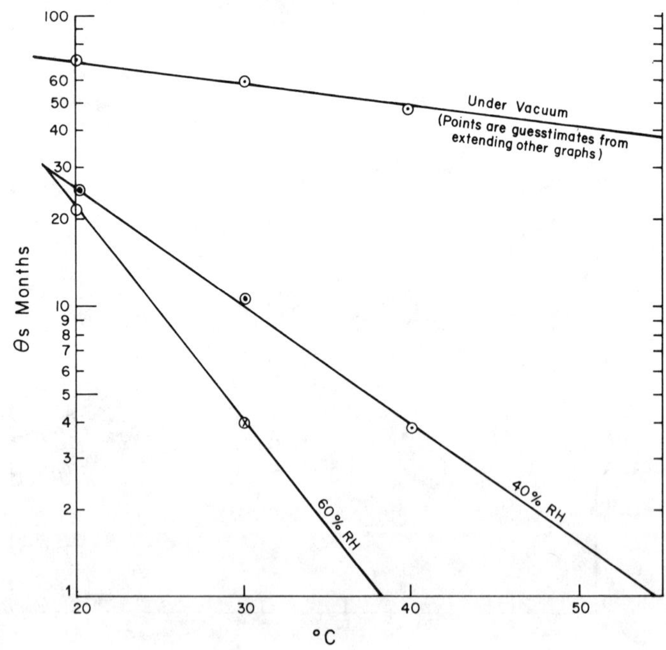

FIG. 11.15. NONFAT MILK: θ_s (MONTHS) FOR 50% LYSINE LOSS
(Ben-Gera and Zimmerman 1972).

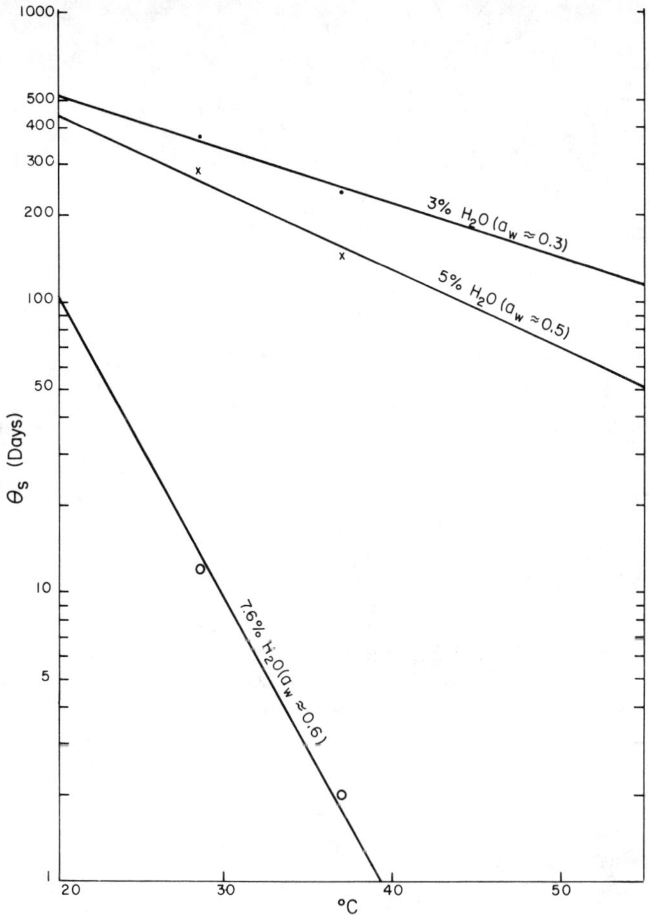

FIG. 11.16. NONFAT DRY MILK: TIME FOR UNACCEPTABLE FLAVOR (Hall and Hendricks 1966).

the reaction E_a should be around 20—30 Kcal/mole. The lines are paralleled at each a_w which also is questionable.

Ben-Gera and Zimmerman (1972) reported a similar study on lysine loss in nonfat dry milk at similar temperatures. Figure 11.15 shows the data at high RH (40/60%). The expected Q_{10}s and E_as are on the figure. As seen, at greater than 30 °C at 60% humidity, 50% or more lysine is lost in 6 months; at 40% RH, 50% or more is lost if the product is held above 35 °C. This suggests that low temperature and humidity are imperative for maintaining the protein quality of this product. The same effects of high percent RH and temperature affect flavor quality, as seen in

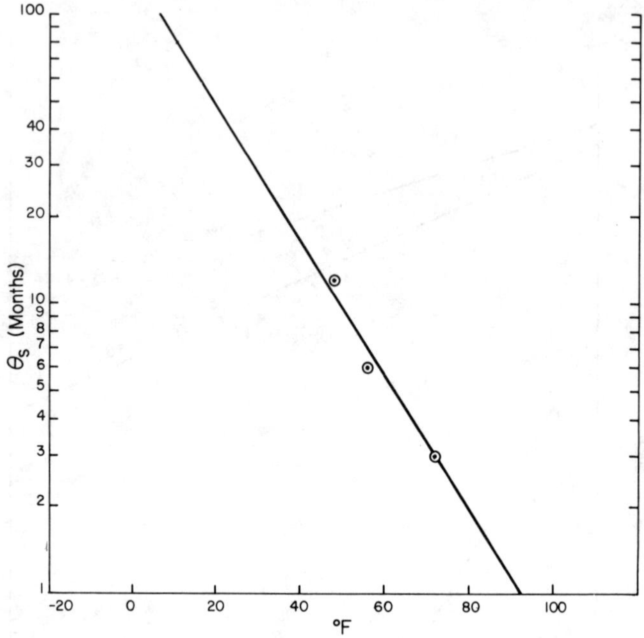

FIG. 11.17. CONDENSED MILK: θ_s (MONTHS) FOR 25% VITAMIN B_1 LOSS (Boyd *et al.* 1955).

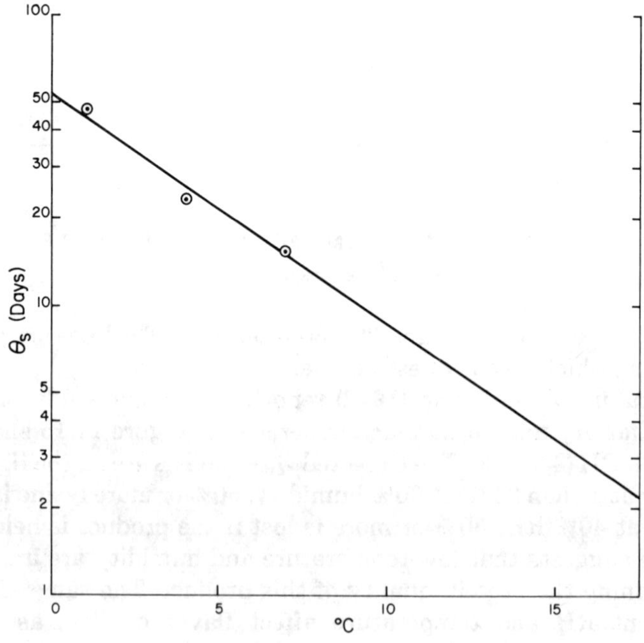

FIG. 11.18. CONCENTRATED MILK: θ_s (MONTHS) TO REACH 10^6 CFU PER ML (Olson *et al.* 1953).

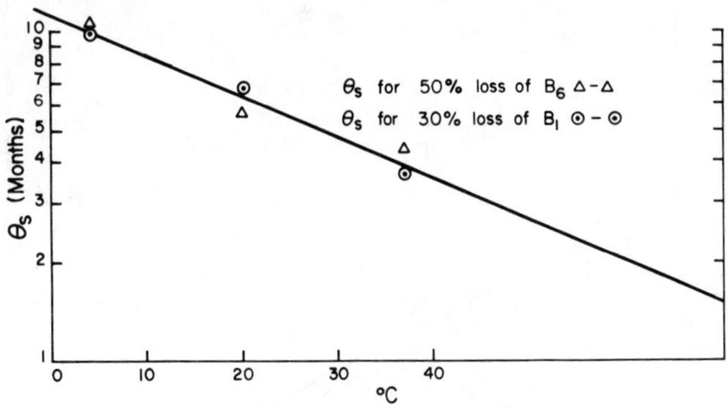

FIG. 11.19. EVAPORATED MILK
(Gregory *et al.* 1964).

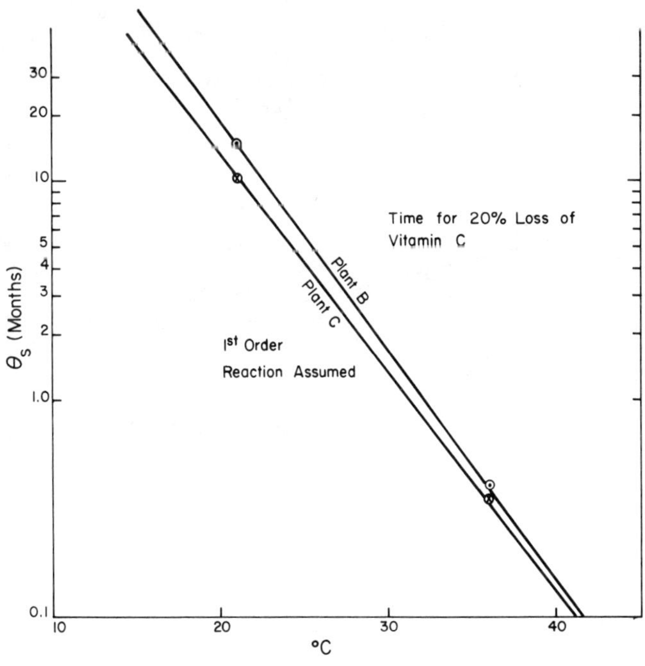

FIG. 11.20. EVAPORATED MILK
(Bullock *et al.* 1968).

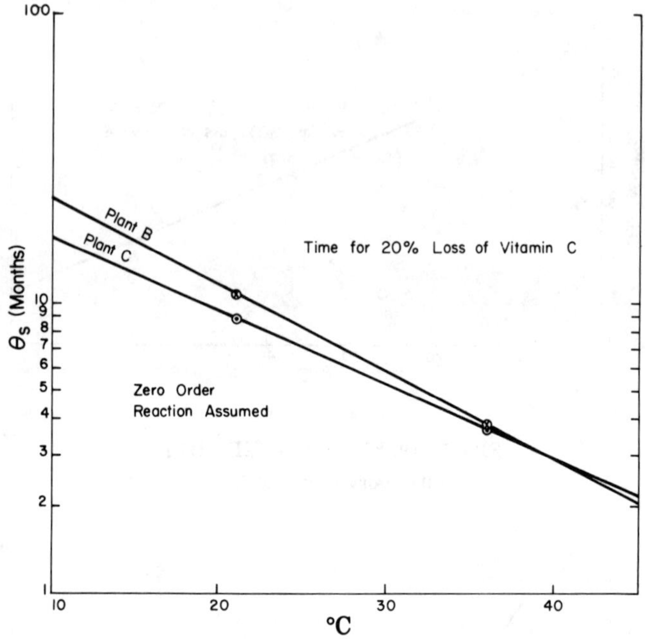

FIG. 11.21. EVAPORATED MILK (Bullock *et al.* 1968).

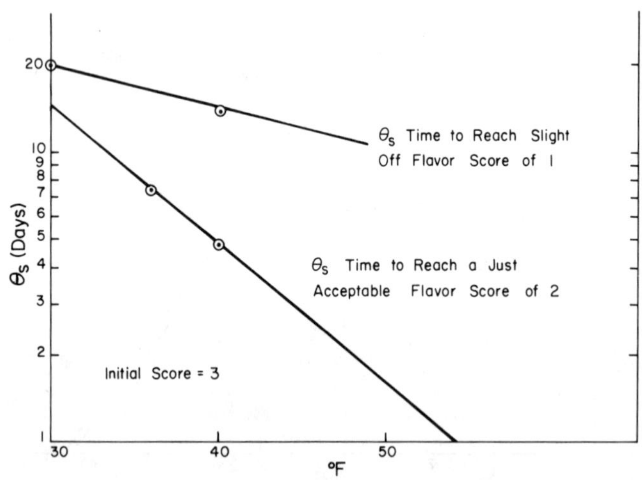

FIG. 11.22. PASTEURIZED EGG (Wood and Youngs 1969).

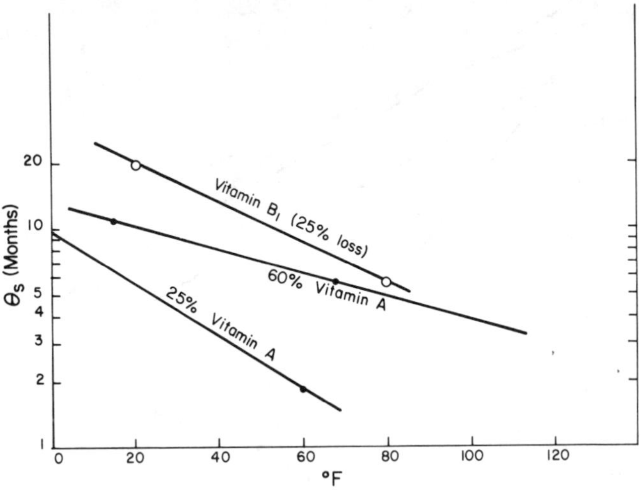

FIG. 11.23. TIME (MONTHS) FOR VITAMIN LOSS IN DEHYDRATED EGGS
(Kramer 1974).

Fig. 11.16. Milk kept near the monolayer moisture value ($a_w \approx 0.3$) will remain acceptable for nine months at 40 °C and below. The large change in Q_{10} must be related to a change in mode of deterioration. Probably lipid oxidation is occurring at low a_w and browning at the high a_w. In comparing the two studies at 25 °C (77 °F) Kramer (1974) reports 5.5 months and 7.5 months respectively for 60% and 40% RH as the time for 25% loss in protein quality which basically is lysine loss. Ben-Gera and Zimmerman (1972) report 9 and 16 months at the same percent RH for 50% loss. Assuming this is a first order reaction, the comparison is quite good for the two studies. Data for changes in concentrated milk products are shown in Fig. 11.17 through 11.21. Figure 11.18 shows that concentration alone does not preserve the milk, as counts reach 10^6 cfu/ml in several weeks at low temperature. As noted, concentrated milk is further preserved by sterilization and is used either for infant feeding or in desserts. Loss of vitamins would be critical in infant feeding. The figures show significant losses at normal storage temperatures. It should be noted that the data for vitamin C of Bullock *et al.* (1968) were analyzed both for first and zero order. Above 20 °C the first order analysis predicts a much more rapid loss of vitamin C. It is not known what the true order is since so few data points were taken.

Some data on processed egg products usually used on conjunction with dairy products is shown in Figs. 11.22 and 11.23. Pasteurized egg has a very short shelf-life and must be refrigerated. Figure 11.23 shows

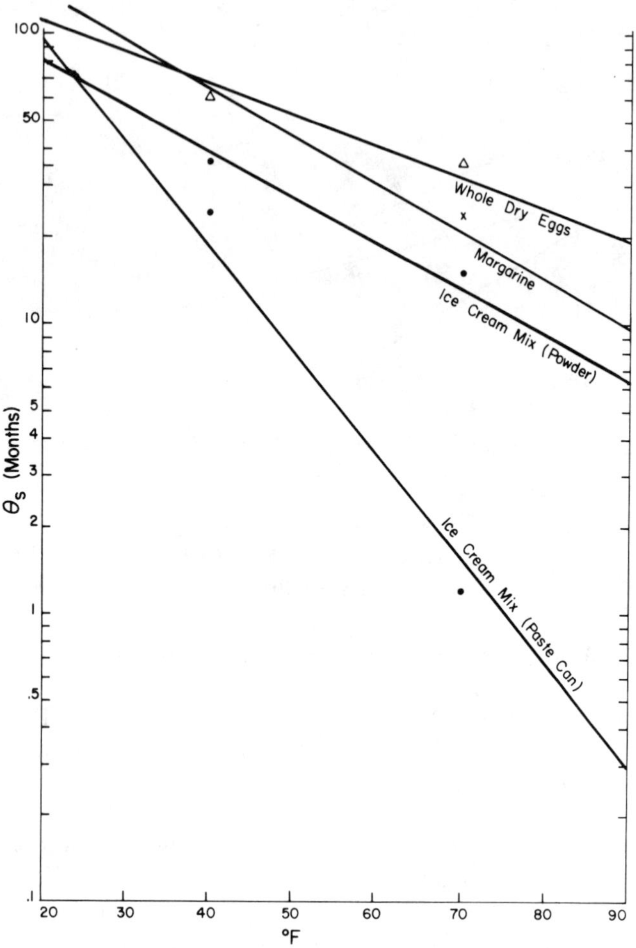

FIG. 11.24. U.S. ARMY SHELF-LIFE DATA FOR SOME PERISHABLE DAIRY FOODS (Congressional Record 1977).

that significant loss of vitamin A can occur in dry eggs, no percent RH was specified. The loss of thiamin was less below 80 °F.

Figure 11.24 shows some general shelf-life data for several other products along with dry eggs. It can be seen that at 80 °F the shelf-life of eggs is listed at 22 months. Based on the previous vitamin loss data, most of the vitamins would be lost if it were to be kept that long. The shelf-life thus should be questioned.

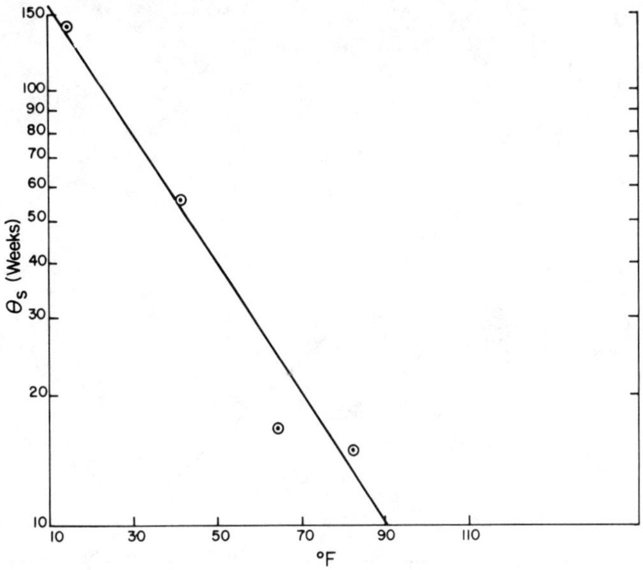

FIG. 11.25. TIME (WEEKS) FOR LOSS OF 25% VITAMIN A IN MARGARINE (Harris and von Loesecke 1960).

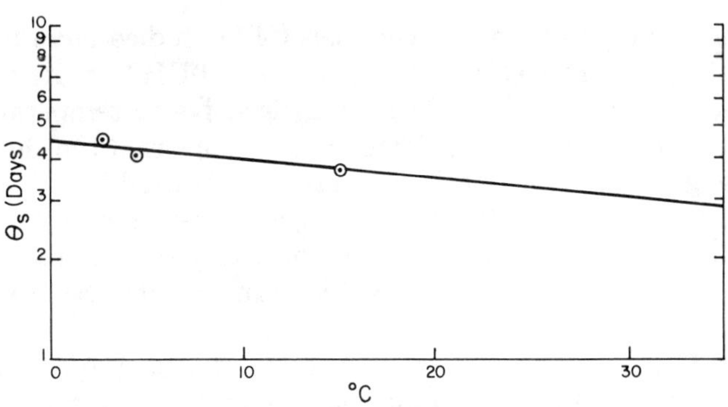

FIG. 11.26. TIME (DAYS) TO REACH 10^6 CFU PER ML REFRIGERATED ICE CREAM (Nelson 1944).

Figure 11.25 shows data for vitamin A loss in margarine. Given that the shelf-life is listed as 32 months at 45°F in Fig. 11.24, a substantial portion of the vitamin A could be lost. Fortunately the product is consumed much sooner.

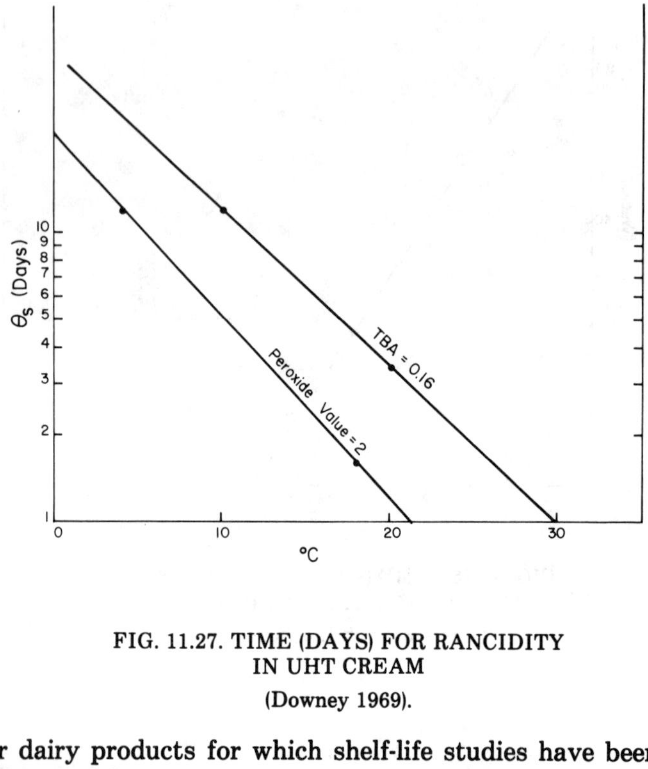

FIG. 11.27. TIME (DAYS) FOR RANCIDITY IN UHT CREAM

(Downey 1969).

Other dairy products for which shelf-life studies have been done include refrigerated ice cream in Fig. 11.26 and UHT cream in Fig. 11.27. As seen, the ice cream is relatively insensitive to temperature as compared to whole milk. The UHT cream data show that the shelf-life differs depending on what chemical index criterion is used.

Figure 11.28 gives data on browning of processed cheese. As expected, a high Q_{10} was found, making the product very sensitive to temperature. Figure 11.29 summarizes other Army data. As noted before, the E_as and Q_{10}s are in Table 11.4.

Table 11.5 contains general estimations for shelf-life of products. It should be noted that these values are general and cannot be considered absolute for any one product. Shelf-life will vary with the initial quality of the product and with its time-temperature pattern of distribution, retailing and home use as seen in the previous data.

TABLE 11.5
ESTIMATES OF SHELF-LIFE

Product	Package	Accepted Storage Temp. (°F)	Preferred RH %	Storage Time (days)	Reference
Butter					
Consumer packs	foil, plastic, paper	32—35	<55	42—56	Richardson (1976)
Patties	*	32—35	*	30	Congressional Record (1977)
Cheese					
Blue veined (natural)	*	32—35	70—75	135	Congressional Record (1977)
Cheddar (natural)	*	32—35	70—75	360	Congressional Record (1977)
Cottage	*	32—35	70—75	14	Congressional Record (1977)
Mozzarella (natural)	*	35	70—75	30	Congressional Record (1977)
Processed American					
loaf	*	32—35	70—75	240	Congressional Record (1977)
slice	*	35	70—75	180	Congressional Record (1977)
Parmesan (natural)	*	32—35	70—75	180	Congressional Record (1977)
Provolone (natural)	*	35	70—75	180	Congressional Record (1977)
Romano (natural)	*	32—35	70—75	180	Congressional Record (1977)
Swiss (natural)	*	32—35	70—75	360	Congressional Record (1977)
Cream					
Half and half	*	32—35	—	7	Congressional Record (1977)
Sour, cultured	*	32—35	—	14	Congressional Record (1977)
Table	*	32—35	—	10	Congressional Record (1977)
Whipping	*	32—35	—	10	Congressional Record (1977)
Whipping, sterilized	*	32—50	—	360	Congressional Record (1977)
Pasteurized	glass, plastic, plastic-lined paper	32—35	—	5— 8	Richardson (1976)

continued . . .

TABLE 11.5 *Concluded*

Eggs					
Shell	*	32	88—92	120	Congressional Record (1977)
Oil processed	*	32	88-92	180	Congressional Record (1977)
Cultured products					
Yogurt, sour cream, buttermilk	glass, plastic, plastic-lined paper	32—35	—	10—15	Richardson (1976)
Margarine					
Patties/prints	*	32—35	<55	60	Congressional Record (1977)
Polyunsaturated (table)	foil, plastic,	32—35	*	42	Richardson (1976)
Milk products					
Buttermilk	*	32—35	—	14	Congressional Record (1977)
Chocolate flavored	*	32—35	—	7	Congressional Record (1977)
Chocolate flavored (sterilized)	*	32—35	—	360	Congressional Record (1977)
Concentrated	*	32—35	—	6	Congressional Record (1977)
Fluid, pasteurized	*	32—35	—	7	Congressional Record (1977)
Fat, anhydrous	*	32—35	—	180	Congressional Record (1977)
Milk, pasteurized and/or homogenized	glass, plastic, plastic-lined paper	32—35	—	5— 8	Richardson (1976)
Evaporated	can	⩽77	—	180	Richardson (1976)
UHT pasteurized milk	can, plastic-lined paper	⩽77	—	90	Richardson (1976)
Infant's food (sterilized)	can	⩽77	—	120	Richardson (1976)
Sweetened condensed milk	can	⩽77	—	360	Richardson (1976)
Dry skim milk	can or plastic	⩽77	—	360	Richardson (1976)
Dry Infant's formula	can	⩽77	—	360	Richardson (1976)

*Conditions not specified

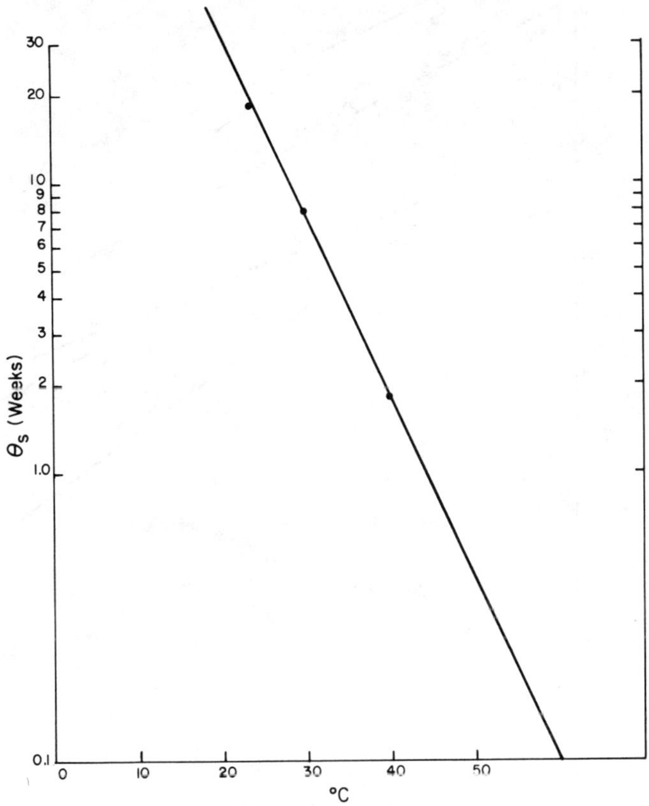

FIG. 11.28. PROCESSED CHEESE SPREAD: TIME (WEEKS) TO REACH BROWNING TO EQUAL TO 0.3 (Thomas *et al.* 1977).

BENEFITS/NONBENEFITS OF OPEN DATING OR OF LISTING SOME SHELF-LIFE ON PRODUCTS

Fluid Milk

It is clear that deterioration in the quality of milk and milk products is time-temperature dependent. It is also apparent that deterioration is dependent on the initial quality of the milk, especially the microbial quality. Thus, using a standard of 10 days after pasteurization, shelf-life

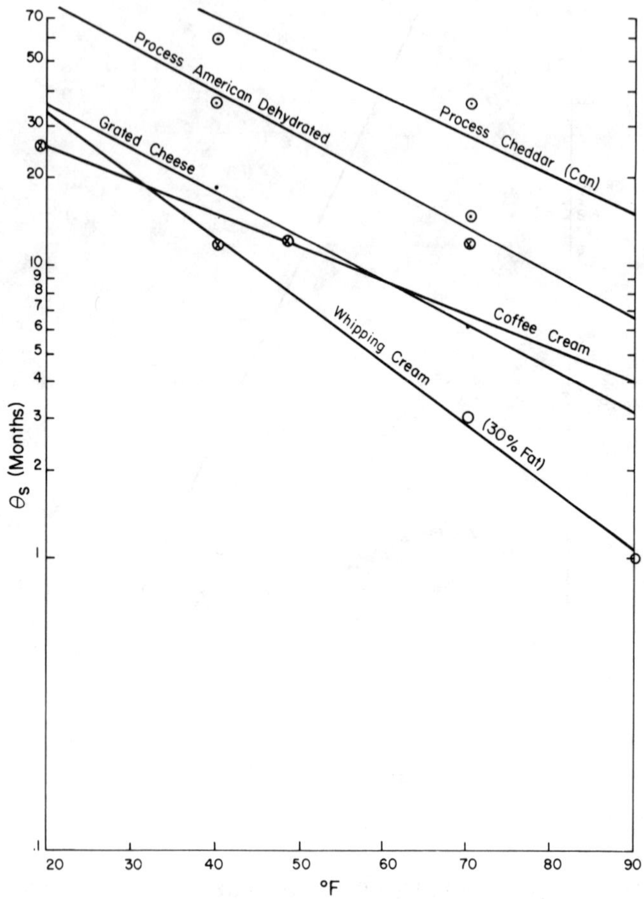

FIG. 11.29. U.S. ARMY SHELF-LIFE DATA FOR CHEESES AND CREAMS (Congressional Record 1977).

for all milk will not be meaningful for two reasons: (1) it says nothing of the time-temperature sequence the milk has been through. Hence if one carton was held below 40 °F for 10 days, while another had been above 40 °F, obviously they would not be of equal quality after 10 days. (2) Milk from a plant operating at borderline sanitary standards will be of lower quality than milk from a plant operating at high sanitary standards after 10 days. In both cases the milks would bear the same date. Thus, dating of fluid milk does not assure quality to the consumer. It can even lead to consumer rejection of a product that may still be good, although it may be a day or two past its pull date. It can also cause consumers to reject good milk with an earlier date in favor of good milk with a later date, thus allowing the former to spoil sooner than the latter might.

The Milk Industry: Foundation's Committee for Study of Milk Availability concluded the following (in part) (Glass and Butz 1970):

(1) Research does not support the premise that there is a meaningful relationship between age of pasteurized milk and quality.
(2) A dating regulation which includes an expiration date may discriminate against the product by implying a deterioration of quality which actually is not occurring.
(3) The age of milk offered for sale by stores is not significantly different between dating and nondating markets.
(4) Some method of inventory control through coding is necessary to insure proper rotation of milk in the store.
(5) Dating regulations do not necessarily assure rapid movement of milk through marketing channels.
(6) Properly pasteurized milk, free from post-pasteurization contamination, may be expected to show no increase in bacterial levels for at least 20 days (if the temperature is maintained at 40 °F or below).
(7) Psychrophilic and coliform organisms at the concentrations normally found in raw milk are destroyed by prescribed pasteurization procedures.
(8) Stores located in the six markets in which dating of milk is required generally receive more frequent delivery than stores located in contigous markets in which dating is not required.
(9) Volume of unsold milk returned by stores is higher in most dating markets than in markets where dating is not practiced.
(10) Elimination of milk dating could lead to more efficient and less costly systems of delivery to stores. Potential savings from elimination of milk dating range from 0.8 to a cent to 1.4 cents per quart.
(11) The practice of milk dating cannot be justified from public health, quality, or economic considerations.
(12) Processor coding is as effective as milk dating as a method of inventory control to assure proper rotation of stock.
(13) Dating deters the adoption of more efficient delivery practices and thus directly increases industry costs of delivering milk to stores. In the long run, these increased costs are borne by consumers.
(14) The committee concludes that improvements in distribution practices including in-store handling practices, would accomplish much more than milk dating in assuring consumers high quality fluid milk products.

The Rutgers survey team (Rutgers University 1971) is in agreement with these findings. However, if dating were voluntary, then a "sell by date" or "use by date" on the basis of the storage data would be useful in terms of better control of production and delivery. This would give the company doing this an advantage.

Another benefit would be a regulation to control the temperature of pasteurized milk to a maximum of 40 °F in storage after pasteurization, in distributor's transportation equipment, and in retail outlets. Eventually this temperature should be reduced to 34 °F, over a period of about five years, to allow distributors and retailers time to replace present equipment which may not attain such temperatures. By reducing temperature of storage the shelf-life of milk will be increased and the consumer will receive higher quality products. The question still exists, however, as to whether or not regulations should be established on a time-temperature basis for the length of time milk products should remain on public sale.

The Food Stability Survey (Ruters University 1971) pointed out that two opinions exist on this matter. First, milk producers could be allowed to withdraw old milk on a regular monitoring basis, since only they are aware of the true shelf-life of their product and the factors controlling it. Secondly, the Department of Health alone, or with the industry, should conduct studies to develop time-temperature specifications on microbiological and aesthetic milk qualities, and from these studies, establish a time limit for removal of products from the store shelf. These are the two possible means of resolving the dating problem and the feasibility of both must be more thoroughly examined.

It seems logical that, at least, producers should code date their products with date of pasteurization and reveal such codes to the public and regulators. It is also suggested that these codes be standardized to state the day and month of the year in numerical fashion. To assist the retailer in proper stock rotation, the implementation of a date of shelf display might also be done.

Other Dairy Products

Cultured Products and Cheese: — Since there are many variations in composition and storage conditions for these products, specific data must be collected on shelf-life before a shelf-life requirement could be made. A process date is recommended as an aid in monitoring products, as is a date of shelf display to assure proper rotation of stock. The possibility of establishing quality control (pH) levels for these products should be examined.

Frozen Dairy Products: — Once again, the quality of frozen products is determined by their time-tempeature holding pattern. Open dating with a "sell by date" does not appear to be the best alternative unless good temperature control can be achieved. The date of manufacture and of shelf display is recommended as a first step. The United Kingdom's three-star system for frozen foods should be considered by regulators. This system utilizes placards in retail outlets to illustrate the types of home freezers in common usage, their temperature of operation, and appropriate storage times at such temperatures. Home storage times for ice cream according to the U.K. system are: 21 °F, 1 day; 10 °F, 1 week; and 0 °F, 1 month. This could be coupled with a "sell by date".

As in the case of fluid milk, adoption of regulations for temperatures of distribution and retailing seems to be more useful than open dating. These temperatures should be set at 0 °F or lower, with −10 °F ideal. However, a "best if used by date" might be a viable alternative.

Dried Milk Products: — A "sell before date" or a "best if used by date" based on nutrient loss might be of value if good shelf-life data can be obtained for these products. The consumer should be educated on how to store the product as well.

Butter: — Dating of butter would not be meaningful because a packaging or distribution date would not reflect changes caused by temperature fluctuation or improper handling. Different storage conditions could readily account for different qualities at the time of sale of two lots of butter of equal age. Again, good temperature control is needed.

REFERENCES

ASHRAE. 1967. Guide and data book, Applications for 1966 and 1967. American Society for Heating, Refrigerating and Air Conditioning Engineers.

BARNARD, S.E. 1974. Flavor and shelf-life of fluid milk. J. Milk Food Technol. *37*(6), 346.

BEN-GERA, I. and ZIMMERMAN, G. 1972. Changes in the nitrogeneous constituents of staple foods and feeds during storage. I. Decrease in the chemical availability of lysine. J. Food Sci. Technol. (India) *9*(3), 113.

BLANKENAGEL, G. and HUMBERT, E.S., 1965. Observations on keeping quality of low bacterial count milk. Can. Dairy Ice Cream J. *44*(5), 16-18.

BOYD, J.C., SMITH, C.K. and TROUT, G.H. 1955. The role of psychrophilic bacteria in the keeping quality of commercially pasteurized and homogenized milk. J. Milk Food Technol. *18*(1), 32.

BULLOCK, D.H., SINGH, S. and PEARSON, A.M. 1968. Stability of vitamin C in enriched commercial evaporated milk. J. Dairy Sci. *51*(6), 921.

CAMPBELL, J.R. and MARSHALL, R.T. 1975. The Science of Providing Milk for Man. McGraw-Hill, New York.

CONGRESSIONAL RECORD. 1977. Technical manual for storage and material handling for the Department of the Army. US-GPO-D-295.

DAHLBERG, A.C. 1945. The keeping quality of pasteurized milk in the New York Metropolitan area during cold weather as determined by bacterial counts, presence of coliform bacteria and flavor score. J. Dairy Sci. *28*, 779.

DESROSIER, N.W. and DESROSIER, J.N. 1977. Technology of Food Preservation. AVI Publishing Co., Westport, Conn.

DOWNEY, W.K. 1969. Lipid oxidation as a source of off-flavour development during the storage of dairy products. J. Soc. Dairy Technol. *22*(3), 154.

FINLEY, P.D., WARREN, H.B. and HARGROVE, R.E. 1968. Storage stability of commercial milk. J. Milk Technol. *31*(12), 382.

FOLEY, J. and KING, J.J. 1975. Influence of pasteurization before and after separation of cream on the oxidative stability of ripened cream butter. J. Food Protection. *40*(7), 480-483.

GLASS, E.D. and BUTZ, W.T. 1970. Committee for Study of Milk Availability; Quality and Economic Considerations in the Dating of Milk. Special Report for the Milk Industry Foundation, Washington, D.C. (Feb.)

GREGORY, M.E., HENRY, K.M. and KON, S.K. 1964. Nutritive properties of freshly prepared and stored evaporated milks manufactured by a normal commercial procedure or by reduced thermal processes in the presence of nisin. J. Dairy Res. *31*, 113.

HALL, C.W. and HENDRICK, T.I. 1966. Drying Milk and Milk Products. AVI Publishing Co., Westport, Conn.

HARKIN, L., DILLMAN, W.F. and STEPHENS, G.R. 1977. Relation to code dates to quality of milk sold in retail markets. J. Food Protection. *40*(2), 116-19.

HARMON, L.G., TROUT, G.M. and HENDRICK, T.I. 1959. Relationship between storage temperatures and the rate of development of various organisms on the shelf life of homogenized milk. Milk Dealer. *48*(11), 40.

HARRIS, R.S. and VON LOESECKE, H. 1960. Nutritional Evaluation of Food Processing. AVI Publishing Co., Westport, Conn.

HENDERSON, J.L. 1971. The Fluid Milk Industry. AVI Publishing Co., Westport, Conn.

JEBSON, R.S., McDOWELL, A.K.R. and RUSSELL, R.W., 1974. The effect of storage temperature on the quality of salted sweet-cream butter. N.Z. J. Dairy Sci. Technol. *9*(4), 163.

KRAMER, A. 1974. Storage retention of nutrients. Food Technol. *28*(1), 50.

MELLOR, D.B., GARDNER, F.A. and CAMPOS, E.J. 1975. Effect of type of package and storage temperature on interior quality of shell treated shell eggs. Poult. Sci. *54*, 742.

NELSON, F.E. 1944. Changes in bacterial counts in stored ice cream mix. J. Dairy Sci. *27*, 460.

OLSON, J.C. Jr., NIELSEN, A.J., THOMAS, E.L. and MORRIS, H.A. 1953. Changes in bacterial counts and flavor of concentrated and recombined milks during storage at low temperatures. J. Dairy Sci. *36*, 817.

PACKARD, V.S. 1967. Bacteria in Milk. Univ. of Minn. Agric. Ext. Service Fact Sheet No. 10.

PUNCH, J.D., OLSON, J.C. Jr. and THOMAS, E.L. 1965. Psychrophilic bacteria. III. Population levels associated with flavor or physical change in milk. J. Dairy Sci. *48*(9), 1179.

RANDOLPH, H.E., FREEMAN, T.R. and PETERSON, R.W., 1965. Keeping quality of market milk obtained at retail outlets and at processing plants. J. Milk Food Technol. *28*(3), 92.

RICHARDSON, K.C. 1976. Shelf-life of packaged foods. CSIRO Food Res. Q. *36*(1), 1-7.

RUTGERS UNIVERSITY, 1971. Food Stability Survey. Rutgers University, Department of Food Science, for the State of New Jersey Department of Health. In cooperation with the U.S. Department of Agriculture/Economic Research Service.

SAMEL, R. and MUERS, M.M. 1962. The age-thickening of sweetened and condensed milk. J. Dairy Res. *29*, 269.

SMITH, A.C. 1968. The effect of filling temperature of milk on the keeping quality of the product. J. Milk and Technol. *31*(10), 306.

SMITH, A.C. 1971. The effects of storage temperatures on the keeping quality of half and half. J. Milk Food Technol. *34*(12), 574.

TASMA, A., KORTSON, A. and KURTZ, F.E. 1974. Relationships between volatile compounds, storage conditions, deodorization and flavor scores of milk fats and dry whole milks. J. Dairy Sci. *57*(10), 1143.

THOMAS, M.A. 1969. Browning reaction in cheddar cheese. Aust. J. Dairy Technol. *24*(4) 185.

THOMAS, M.A., TURNER, A.D., ABAD, G. and TOWNER, J.M. 1977. The influence of types of skim milk powder used and storage conditions on browning reaction in processed cheese spread. Milchwissenschaft *32*(1), 12-15.

WEBB, D.H., JOHNSON, A.H. and ALFORD, J.A. 1974. Fundamentals of Dairy Chemistry. AVI Publishing Co., Westport, Conn.

WOOD, E.C. and YOUNGS, M. 1969. The keeping quality of pasteurized egg. J. Appl. Bacteriol. *32*, 403-407.

CHAPTER 12

FRESH BAKERY PRODUCTS

INTRODUCTION

Bread is by far the most prevalent bakery product sold today, followed by cakes and bakery specialties. This discussion will concentrate mainly on bread and cakes.

Baking is similar to pasteurization in that enzymes and some microbes are destroyed. Because of this, it is possible to store bread at room temperature in spite of its high water activity ($a_w \approx 0.96$). By the time microorganisms do get a foothold and start to grow, the bread has usually been consumed or the shelf-life has ended for reasons other than microbial attack. Mold is the major microbe that will spoil bread. Often a mold inhibitor, the most common being calcium propionate, will be added to retard the growth of the mold.

Bread is baked and sent to the store for sale on the same day. Deliveries are made every day or every other day. Because of this frequent delivery, 350 miles is the maximum distance bread is delivered. The drivers of the trucks that deliver the bread are usually the ones who remove out-of-date loaves and stock shelves at the retail outlet. Some companies, such as the Continental Baking Co., then take out-of-date products and sell them at their "thrift stores" for a reduced price. Temperature during distribution of the product is very important, especially in the winter when the temperature is below freezing. Meisner (1953) found that during cold winter days the temperature of bread in uninsulated trucks could decrease to such a degree as to greatly affect the amount of staling during transport. The role of temperature and staling will be discussed later.

Bread is usually packaged in a moisture proof plastic bag. This helps retard one mode of deterioration in bread, that of moisture loss. This packaging has an interesting effect on the properties of the crust. Since moisture is not allowed to pass freely into the atmosphere, it tends to migrate from the crumb to the crust. This gives the crust a tough, leathery consistency. This crust staling is tolerated because it is not as bad as crumb staling and, unfortunately, the factors that decrease the rate of crust staling usually increase the rate of crumb staling. Some specialty breads, such as French and Italian, may be packaged in moisture permeable packages. This will help the crust remain crisp. In this case, high relative humidity in the air will promote crust staling.

MODES OF DETERIORATION

There are many modes of deterioration possible in bakery products. These include oxidative rancidity, nutritional losses, microbial growth, moisture loss, and staling. Each of these will be discussed in further detail.

Oxidative rancidity is not really a problem in bread. The shelf-life of the bread would be over before oxidation would have a chance to show its effects. Rancidity appears to be more of a problem in cakes. Kulp *et al.* (1959) did a study on white and yellow layer cakes. They canned cakes in oxygen and stored them at room temperature; a shelf-life of approximately 27 days was found. Cakes wrapped in foil and stored at room temperature had a shelf-life of only 14 days. This shows that oxidation of cakes is also not much of a factor in determining shelf-life, since they are usually consumed sooner than this time.

Nutritional losses in bread and baked products are also probably not of much concern during storage after baking. The actual baking process is where most of the nutritional losses occur (Pomeranz and Shellenberger 1971). A large portion of bread sold today is enriched. Enriched bread has 1.8 mg thiamin, 1.1 mg riboflavin, 15 mg niacin and 25 mg iron per pound of bread (Anon. 1976). As stated earlier, in the normal shelf-life of bread, losses of these nutrients are minimal. Another nutritional consideration would be destruction of lysine in the protein fraction of bread. Gluten is the major protein present in flour. Gluten is low in lysine, and further destruction of lysine would occur during baking. The major pathway of destruction of lysine is reaction of the ϵ-amino group with a reducing sugar and subsequent reactions associated with nonenzymatic browning. Again, after the baking process, loss of lysine during storage should be small. If gluten were the major source of lysine in the diet, every bit of lysine would be important because of the already low level of lysine in the gluten. Fortunately, this is generally not the case in the United States.

Microbial growth can be a major shelf-life problem. Bread has a water activity of 0.96 which will allow growth of many microorganisms. Mold is the major problem in bread, thus calcium propionate is commonly added to inhibit growth. Mold growth is usually not a problem because of the calcium propionate and the fact that staling will limit the commercial shelf-life before mold gets a chance to grow.

Moisture loss is a serious problem in breads and bakery products that are not wrapped in a moisture proof package. Kulp *et al.* (1959) found moisture loss to be the major mode of degradation in unwrapped white and yellow layer cakes. A shelf-life of 2—4 days was found at room temperature compared to foil wrapped cakes which had a room temperature shelf-life of 14 days. In cakes, moisture loss may be a major factor in the shelf-life and in the amount of staling which occurs.

Staling of bread is by far the major mode of deterioration. Maga (1975) states that most white bread in the United States has a commercial shelf-life of two days, after that it is no longer considered fresh because of the staling process.

Many consumers think that staling is associated with the loss of moisture from the bread. This is not necessarily so. It can be shown that bread will firm and stale with no loss of moisture. Waldt (1968) stated that in the broadest sense of the term, staling was related to all changes that take place after baking. Physical properties of bread affected by staling were summarized by Herz (1965). They included a change in taste and aroma, increased hardness of crumb, increased opacity of crumb, and increased crumbliness of crumb.

There are two major types of staling, crumb and crust staling. Crust staling, as discussed earlier, is the least objectionable, and since most measures employed to retard crust staling increase crumb staling, it is usually tolerated.

Crumb staling is the most important factor limiting the shelf-life of bread. From this point on, the term staling will refer to crumb staling.

Many factors affect the rate and extent of staling. Axford *et al.* (1968) found that as loaf volume increased, the rate of staling decreased. Bread from strong flours (high protein content) stales less rapidly than bread specific volume than weak flours (Elton 1969). Kim and D'Appolonia (1977a,b,c,d) found that pentosans have an effect on both rate of bread staling and rate of retrogradation in wheat starch gels. Pentosans, which are found in flour, decreased the rate of staling and retrogradation. Many factors before and during fermentation and baking have an effect on the rate of staling (Waldt 1968). Additives such as mono- and diglycerides also affect the amount of staling.

An interesting aspect of staling is that it has a negative temperature coefficient. As temperature increases the rate of staling decreases, up to 110 °F where the crumb begins to turn brown and becomes undesirable (Pomeranz and Shellenberger 1971). Staling rate passes through a maximum close to the maximum density point of water (4 °C). The rate of staling decreases as the temperature falls below that point. Another interesting fact is that stale bread can be refreshened by heating it near the baking temperature (Elton 1969). These two facts, along with changes in the x-ray diffraction pattern during staling, implicate the retrogradation of amylopectin as a major factor in bread staling.

It is generally agreed that retrogradation of the amylopectin portion of the starch plays a major role in the staling of bread. Willhoft (1971,

1973) claims that at temperatures above 35 °C (95 °F) a redistribution of moisture occurs with a transfer from gluten to the starch portion of the bread. He states at these temperatures, the moisture redistribution plays a major role in bread staling. Kim and K'Appolonia (1977c) found that bread stored at 35 °C (95 °F) followed a staling pattern that is characterized by retrogradation of starch.

Staling of bread can be accurately analyzed by the Avrami equation, as noted earlier. This analysis gives the rate of crystallization in a high polymer system. The rate is slow at temperatures just below the melting point of the crystal, and then increases as it is supercooled (Cornford *et al.* 1964). The equation used for this analysis is:

$$\frac{E_1 - E_\theta}{E_1 - E_o} = e^{-k\theta^n}$$

E is a linear measure of increasing degree of crystallinity.
E_1 = limiting modulus
E_o = initial modulus
E_θ = moisture at time θ
k = rate of constant (units:time^{-1})
θ = time
n = Avrami exponent

The Avrami exponent, n, is an integer from 1 to 4 and is characteristic of the type of crystallinity occurring. For bread it has been found that n = 1 (Cornford *et al.* 1964; Kim and D'Appolonia 1977b, c, d; Axford *et al.* 1968). An Avrami exponent equal to one is characteristic of rod-like growth from an instantaneous nuclei (McIver *et al.* 1968). The rate constant, k, is determined by graphing ln ($E_1 - E_\theta$) vs time. The slope of the line obtained is k.

The modulus, E, can be measured in different ways. It can be directly measured by the compressibility of the bread, or a cone indentor can be used and a standard equation used to give the compressibility of the bread. Another technique that has been successfully used is differential thermal analysis (McIver *et al.* 1968). As retrogradation increases, an endothermic peak is detected as the temperature is raised on the differential thermal analyzer. This peak is a measure of the degree of crystallinity of the starch.

SHELF-LIFE DATA

Meisner (1953) measured staling of bread by penetration at temperatures from 30 °F to 75 °F (1.1 °C to 24 °C). These penetration data were found to follow first order kinetics as in Fig. 12.1. The inverse Arrhenius plot as shown in Fig. 12.2 gave an activation energy (E_a) of —6.62 Kcal/mole and an inverse Q_{10} of 1.47. An inverse Q_{10} is the rate increase for a 10 °C decrease in temperature. It should be noted that the negative E_a is due to the negative temperature coefficient of staling. Unfortunately no data were given as to the penetration depth at which the bread is unacceptable. However, if some level is chosen then a shelf-life plot could be made and the time to reach staling as a function of variable temperature tested.

Pence and Standridge (1955) did a study on the effect of storage temperature on the firmness of bread (grams to cause a 4 mm compres-

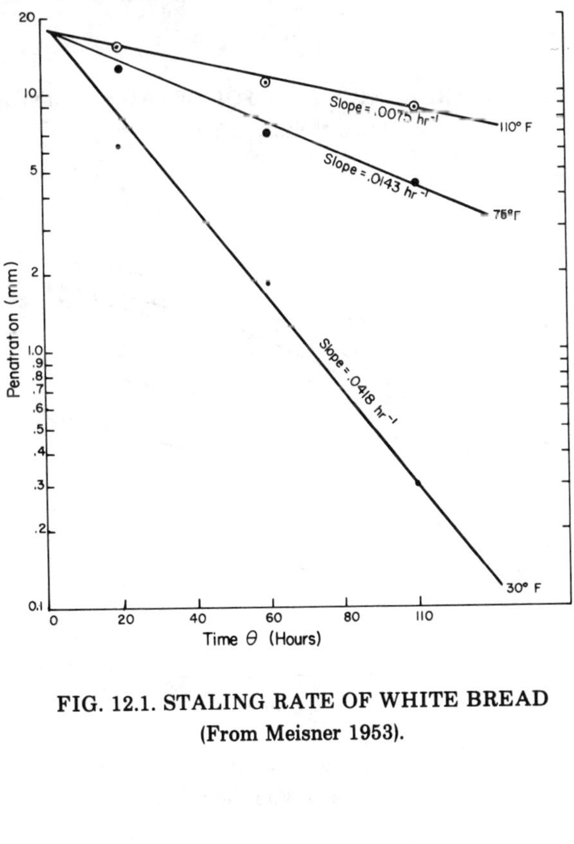

FIG. 12.1. STALING RATE OF WHITE BREAD (From Meisner 1953).

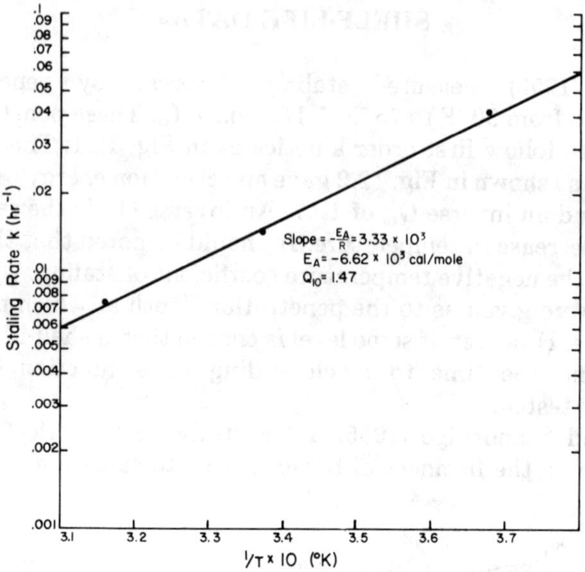

FIG. 12.2. ARRHENIUS PLOT FOR BREAD STALING (From Meisner 1953).

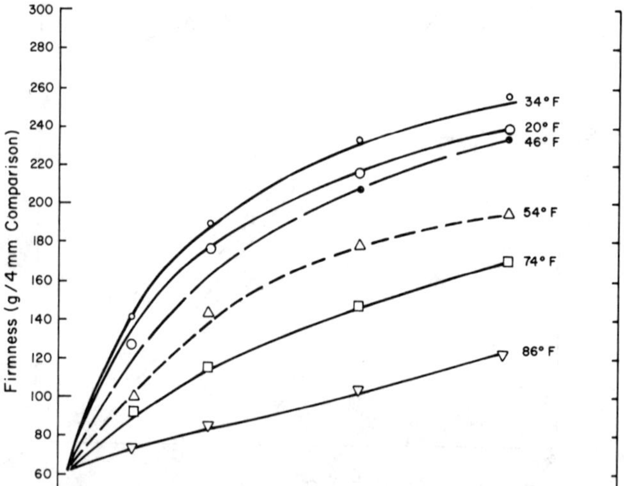

FIG. 12.3. BREAD FIRMNESS (From Pence and Standridge 1955).

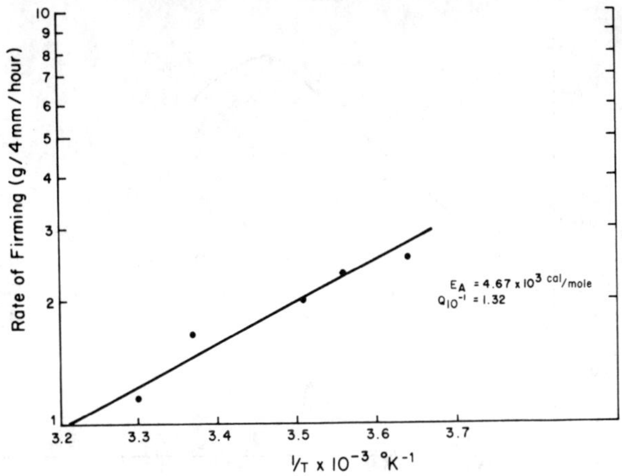

FIG. 12.4. ARRHENIUS PLOT
(From Pence and Standridge 1955).

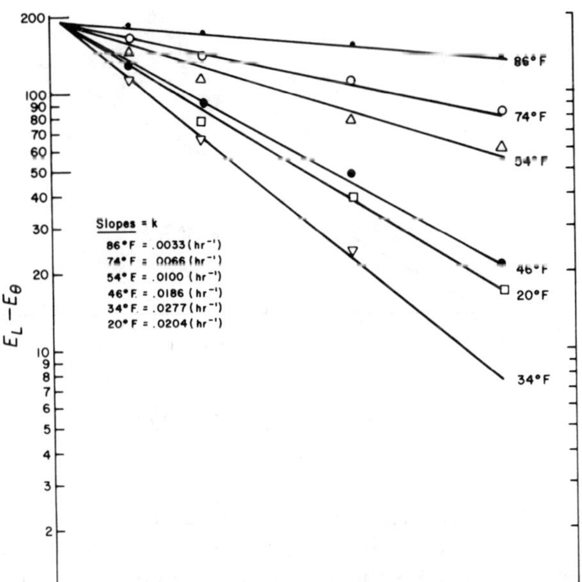

FIG. 12.5. AVRAMI PLOT
(From Pence and Standridge 1955).

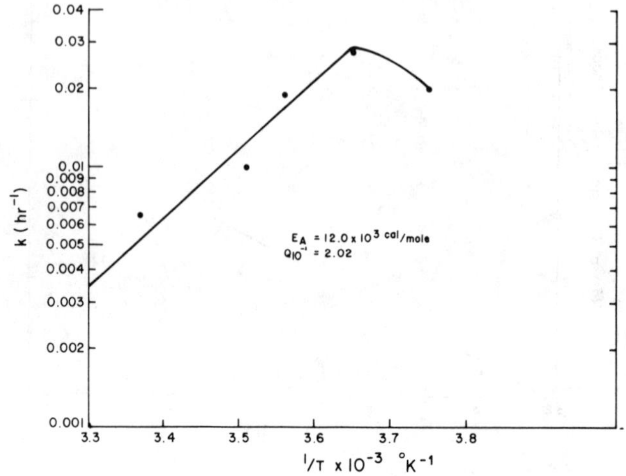

FIG. 12.6. ARRHENIUS PLOT FROM AVRAMI ANALYSIS
(From Pence and Standridge 1955).

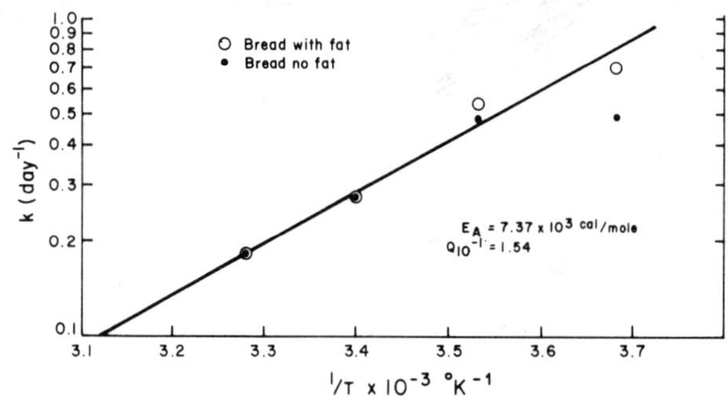

FIG. 12.7. ARRHENIUS PLOT
(From Cornford *et al.* 1964).

sion). Figure 12.3 shows the data they obtained. From these data they determined rates of staling by taking the most linear portion from Fig. 12.3. An Arrhenius plot for these data is shown in Fig. 12.4. E_a was equal to -4.67×10^3 cal/mole, which correspond to an inverse Q_{10} of 1.32. Since this measurement was basically the compressibility of bread, the Avrami analysis should give a better estimation of the rate of staling at different temperatures and therefore a better estimation of E_a and Q_{10}. The Avrami plot was made using an E_1 = 257 g/4 mm compressibility (Fig. 12.5). From this plot k's were determined and the Arrhenius plot was made. The

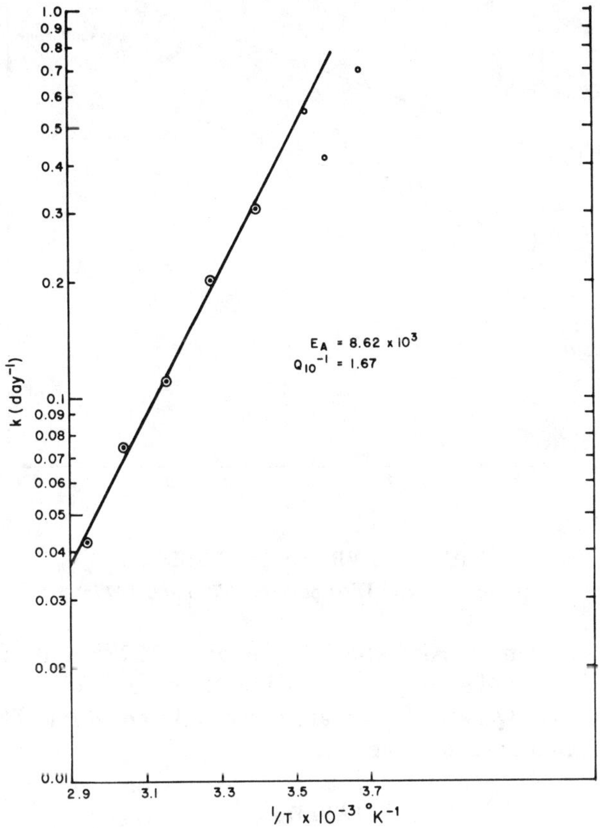

FIG. 12.8. ARRHENIUS PLOT FOR CHORLEYWOOD BREAD FROM AVRAMI ANALYSIS

(From Axford *et al.* 1965).

corresponding E_a was -12.0×10^3 cal/mole and the inverse Q_{10} was 2.2 (Fig. 12.6). This shows that the correct kinetic analysis is important to use. From this as before, the shelf-life plot can be made. It also shows that the Q_{10} is quite different depending on each study.

Cornford *et al.* (1965) did a study and found that fat had no effect on the rate of staling as seen in Fig. 12.7. Again the Q_{10}^{-1} is different. Figure 12.8 shows the Arrhenius plot for a loaf of bread with a higher specific volume than the bread in Fig. 12.7 from Axford *et al.* (1968). It can be seen that loaf specific volume has little or no effect on the E_a or Q_{10} of bread staling.

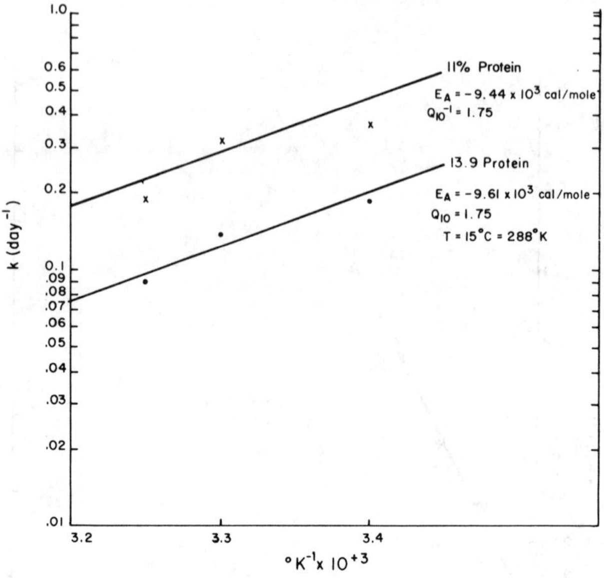

FIG. 12.9. AVRAMI ANALYSIS k's
(From Kim and D'Appolonia 1977b and 1977c)

Figure 12.9 is from Kim and D'Appolonia (1977b and 1977c). This shows that the rate of staling is affected by the amount of protein present in bread, but the Q_{10} and E_a remain essentially constant. The data for bread are summarized in Table 12.1.

TABLE 12.1
SUMMARY OF Q_{10}s AND E_as FOR STALING OF BREAD

Source	E_a (cal/mole)	Q_{10}^{-1}
Meisner (1953)	-6.62×10^3	1.47
Pence and Standridge (1955) (Avrami Analysis)	-12.00×10^3	2.04
Cornford *et al.* (1964)	-7.34×10^3	1.54
Axford *et al.* (1968)	-8.62×10^3	1.67
Kim and D'Appolonia 1977 (b,c)	-9.61×10^3	1.75
	mean value -8.84×10^3 cal/mole	$\overline{x} = 1.67$
	$s = 2.1 \times 10^3$	$s = 0.07$

all Q_{10}s calculated by formula:

$$\log Q_{10} \quad \frac{(2.19)(E_a)}{(T)(T+10)}$$

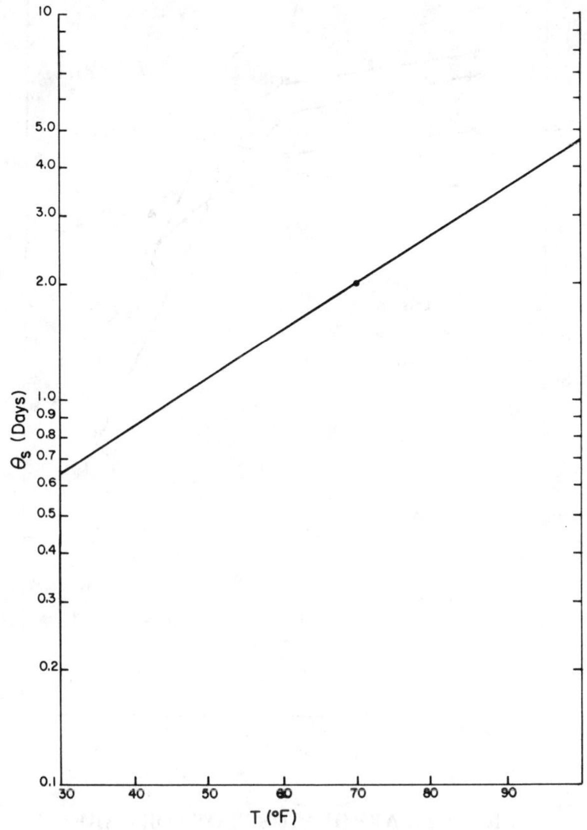

FIG. 12.10. SHELF-LIFE PLOT FOR WHITE BREAD
Assuming two days at 70 °F = θ_s; .60 = Q_{10}.

There are no specific shelf-life data in the literature. This is probably because the rate of staling varies with different constituents, additives, and treatments of the bread. Even though the rate of staling changes, its relationship to temperature is fairly constant, as shown in the summary of Q_{10}^{-1}s. With this knowledge, given the shelf-life of a certain bread at one temperature, predictions can be made for other temperatures. Maga (1975) stated that commercial shelf-life of bread is two days. If this is assumed to be at 70 °F (21 °C), a graph can be drawn to show shelf-lives at other temperatures as in Fig. 12.10.

A general shelf-life plot cannot be drawn for the staling of all bread because of the variability in formulation from company to company and

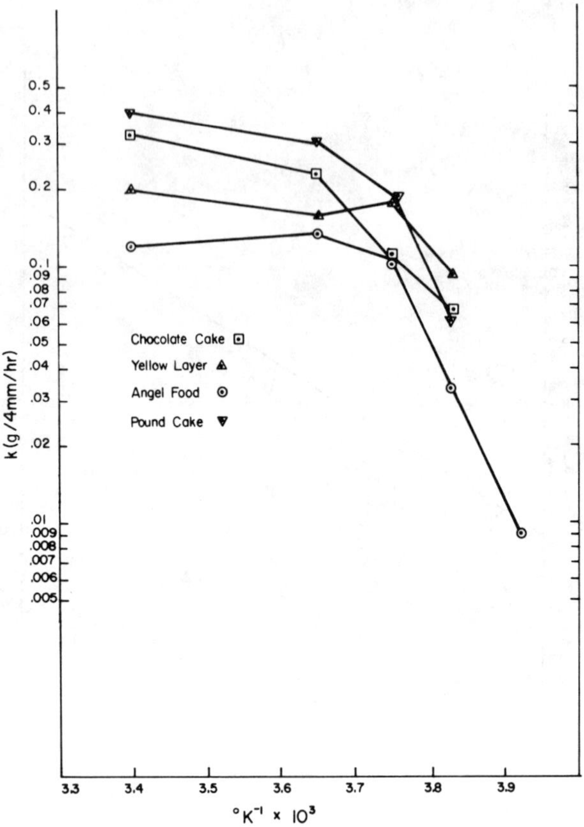

FIG. 12.11. ARRHENIUS PLOT FOR CAKES
(From Pence and Standridge 1958).

the effect these differences have on the rate of staling at one temperature. Figure 12.11 shows the data for staling for various types of cake. What is noticeable is that the rate decreases with decreasing temperature, opposite to that for bread. Why this occurs is not known, but suggests that cakes have a longer shelf-life if refrigerated.

OPEN DATING ANALYSIS

Open dating is definitely desirable in fresh bakery products. However, the type of open date that would be most beneficial needs to be looked at.

There are three basic types of open dates: "pack date", "pull or sell by date" and "expiration or best if used by date". The "pack date" would let the consumer know when the product was made. This would be acceptable for bakery products, although not the most desirable type of open date. With a "pack date" on the product, the consumer may expect bread to be fresh when it is in fact very close to staleness. On the other hand, for cakes, which have a shelf-life of approximately seven days, the consumer may feel the product is "too old" when in fact, there is considerable high quality shelf-life left.

An "expiration date" essentially says "don't consume after . . .". This would be unacceptable for fresh bakery products. This would lead the consumer to think that it is unsafe to eat staled bread. There is nothing wrong or dangerous about consuming stale bread or other staled bakery products. These staled products are safe to consume and can be sold if the consumer is aware that they are not buying a product of maximum freshness. From that standpoint a "best if used by date" would be more meaningful.

A "best if used by date" is probably the most desirable type of open date for fresh bakery products. This will tell the consumer that for maximum freshness to use it by then, without putting fear into them that if they do not use it by the date marked they must throw it away. This type of date would also be beneficial for bakeries. They could sell the products past that date at a reduced price and therefore would not have to dispose of them, as would be the case with an expiration date. Minnesota now uses this form of a "sell by date". They have found that consumers do tend to pick the freshest product, but this presents no real problem since deliveries are made every day or every other day. Continental Bakery has also found that it has no trouble selling the expired product in their thrift store.

REFERENCES

ANON. 1976. Federal Register *41*(30), 6247.

AXFORD, D.W.E., COLWELL, K.H., CORNFORD, S.J. and ELTON, G.A.H. 1968. Effect of loaf specific volume on the rate and extent of staling in bread. J. Sci. Food Agric. *19*, 95.

CORNFORD, S.J., AXFORD, D.W.D. and ELTON, G.A.H. 1964. The elastic modulus of bread crumb in linear compression in relation to staling. Cereal Chem. *41*(4), 216.

ELTON, G.A.H. 1969. Some quantitative aspects of bread staling. Baker's Dig. *43*(3), 24.

HERZ, K.O. 1965. Staling of bread — A review. Food Technol. *19*, 1828.

KIM, S.K. and D'APPOLONIA, B.L. 1977a. Effect of pentosans on retrogradation of wheat starch gels. Cereal Chem. *54*(1), 150.

KIM, S.K. and D'APPOLONIA, B.L. 1977b. Bread staling studies. I. Effect of protein content on staling rate and bread crumb pasting properties. Cereal Chem. *54*(2), 207.

KIM, S.K. and D'APPOLONIA, B.L. 1977c. Bread staling studies. II. Effect of protein content and storage temperature on the role of starch. Cereal Chem. *54,*(2), 216.

KIM, S.K. and D'APPOLONIA, B.L. 1974. Bread staling studies. III. Effect of pentosans on dough, bread, and bread staling rate. Cereal Chem. *54*(2), 225.

KULP, K., PONTE, Jr., J.G. and BECHTEL, W.G. 1959. Some factors that affect the staling of white and yellow layer cakes. Cereal Chem. *36*(2), 228.

MAGA, J.A. 1975. Bread staling. CRC Crit. Rev. Food Technol. *5*(4), 443.

McIVER, R.G., AXFORD, D.W.E., COLWELL, K.H., ELTON, G.A.H. 1968. Kinetic study of the retrogradation of genatinized starch. J. Sci. Food Agric. *19*, 560.

MEISNER, D.F. 1953. Importance of temperature and humidity in the transportation and storage of bread. Baker's Dig. *27,* 109.

PENCE, J.W. and STANDRIDGE, N.N. 1955. Effects of storage temperature and freezing on the firming of a commercial bread. Cereal Chem. *32*, 519.

PENCE, J.W. and STANDRIDGE, N.N. 1958. Effect of storage temperature on firming of cake crumb. Cereal Chem. *35*, 57.

POMERANZ, Y. and SHELLENBERGER, J.A. 1971. Bread Science and Technology. AVI Publishing Co., Westport, Conn.

WALDT, L. 1968. The problem of staling: Its possible solution. Baker's Dig. *42*(5), 64.

WILLHOFT, E.M.A. 1971. Bread staling. II. Theoretical study. J. Sci. Food Agric. *22*, 180.

WILLHOFT, E.M.A. 1973. Recent developments on the bread staling problem. Baker's Dig. *47*(6), 14.

ZOBEL, H.F. 1973. A review of bread staling. Baker's Dig. *47*(5), 52.

CHAPTER 13

SHELF-LIFE OF CANNED FRUITS AND VEGETABLES

INTRODUCTION

Canning, which began in the time of Napoleon because of military needs, is still one of the best ways to preserve foods. The term canned food includes preserved foods packed in glass containers as well as in conventional metal containers. The food may be eaten straight from the can with/or without preparatory heating, making it one of the earliest convenience foods (Rutgers University 1971).

In the nineteenth century and the first decade of the twentieth century, it was generally accepted that nutritive requirements of man and animals were supplied by proteins, fats, carbohydrates, and minerals. The influence of methods employed in producing, marketing, and preparing canned foods on nutritive values was of little interest during this period (Cameron 1955).

However, during the third through fifth decades of this century, a great deal of work was done to determine the retention of various vitamins in canned foods during processing and storage. The National Canners' Association was instrumental in obtaining and assembling much of this information.

More recently, there has been a resurgence of interest in overall acceptability of canned foods as well as nutrient retention during processing as a result of certain advances in the technology of processing. These studies center around the use of the new High Temperature Short Time (HTST) methods in retorting cans.

PRESERVATION BY CANNING

The basis for the preservation of canned foods is the application of enough heat for a long enough period of time to make the product commercially sterile and to prevent recontamination by adequate packaging. Commercial sterility is defined as the number of D values required to assure the death of *Clostridium botulinum* and to make the can safe from spoilage.

The processing of canned fruits and vegetables begins with a number of preprocessing steps. After the washing, pitting, cutting, trimming, sorting and peel removal steps, the fruits and vegetables are blanched.

During the blanching step, both temperature and time vary, depending on the food being processed.

After being blanched, the food is placed inside a container (can or glass jar), the air is removed by steam or vacuum, and the cans (glass jars) are hermetically sealed. The cans are then placed in a retort and sterilized with steam. After being retorted, the cans are quickly cooled, labeled, cased and stored in warehouses until shipped (Luh and Woodroof 1975a,b). When the product is filled into the containers before being sealed, it is usually topped with a liquid which can be juice water, or syrup with other ingredients which complement the flavor, texture, or color of the product being canned.

The retorting step varies in time with the product being processed. The end objective is to obtain a commercially sterile product in each case.

The rapid cooling step can be done by immersion in water or by rotary coolers with water sprays. This step is extremely important in assuring a stable product of good quality.

After being cooled, labeled, and cased, the canned products are stored in warehouses where the temperature should be kept below 80 °F. The warehouse optimally should be kept at 70—75 °F.

PACKAGING

Canned products may be packaged in various types of containers. These containers can vary in the degree to which they protect various components in the food product from deterioration. The most commonly used containers are metal containers and glass containers. The metal containers consist primarily of tin-coated steel which may or may not be coated with a lacquer or enamel for extra protection. Technology has permitted the use of better can coatings, and there have been studies comparing the quality of products in different containers.

In general, products in glass containers will be more susceptible to changes brought about by exposure to light. Products in tin cans, especially more acid fruits, will be susceptible to migration of tin into the product.

DISTRIBUTION

Since canned fruits and vegetbles are stable at room temperature, they are stored in warehouses which ideally should be kept at 72 °F and not exceed 80 °F. They are transported by rail to receiving warehouses of brokers or large supermarket chains where they may be stored again for up to one year. High temperature storage and transportation do not constitute health hazards, aesthetic quality changes can occur followed by nutrient losses (Rutgers University 1971).

MODES OF DETERIORATION

Components of canned fruits and vegetables deteriorate in the following order: (1) flavor; (2) color; (3) texture; and (4) (much later) nutritive loss. These changes are time and temperature dependent. They occur both during thermal processing and storage. In thermal processing, shorter times and high temperatures tend to reduce the amount of nutrient loss. During storage, lower temperatures tend to prolong the shelf-life of the products.

It is assumed that if good manufacturing practices are followed, deterioration of food components during processing will be small compared to those lost during storage and subsequent preparation in the home. In the storage studies presented, it was assumed that initial measurements were made on freshly canned products and that subsequent measurements of various components will reflect storage conditions, not thermal processing.

Clifcorn (1948) stated that several nutrients were sensitive to blanching and retorting. Early research had indicated that thiamin was more sensitive to blanching than ascorbic acid although many workers were using vitamin C as the indicator of heat sensitivity of canned products.

Table 13.1 shows canning losses in various vegetables of thiamin, riboflavin, vitamin C, and pyridoxine. As Lund (1975) pointed out, it is difficult to assume that these figures represent the norm for the canning industry. From Table 13.1 it seems apparent that, depending on the product, either thiamin or ascorbic acid is the most heat sensitive vitamin.

It is interesting to note that until recently, few studies in the published literature have utilized kinetics when evaluating the deterioration of canned fruits and vegetables during processing.

According to Lund (1975) there are significant losses of nutrients during processing which are dependent upon time, temperature, type of container and product. This observation does make the practice of basing nutrient labeling on products which have already been canned seem advisable.

Everson *et al.* (1964) found that thiamin retention was significantly greater in HTST products than in conventionally canned and retorted products. This effect was not as noticeable with pyridoxine, probably due to the fact that pyridoxine is not as temperature dependent as thiamin.

TABLE 13.1
LOSSES (%) OF NUTRIENTS DURING THERMAL PROCESSING[1]

Product	Thiamin	Riboflavin	Vitamin C	Pyridoxine
Asparagus	66.7	55.0	54.5	—
Asparagus	8.0[2]	10.0[2]	5.0[2]	—
Lima beans	83.3	63.6	78.9	—
Lima beans	42.0[2]	24.0[2]	28.0[2]	—
Green beans	62.5	60.0	70.0	—
Beets	66.7	—	—	—
Carrots	66.7	60.0	75.0	—
Corn	80.0	58.3	58.3	—
Mushrooms	80.0	45.6	33.3	—
Green peas	74.2	64.3	66.7	—
Green peas	45.0[3]	11.0[3]	73.0[3]	—
Spinach	80.0	50.0	72.5	—
Spinach	15.0[2]	12.0[2]	33.0[2]	—
Tomatoes	16.7	25.0	26.1	—
Strained lima beans (regular canned)	40.3	—	—	10.1
Strained lima beans (HTST canned)	15.8	—	—	9.5

[1]adapted from Lund (1975)
[2]adapted from Cain (1967)
[3]Guerrant and O'Hara (1953)

Table 13.2 lists the activation energies, k values, D values, and temperature of processing for the deterioration of various components in different fruits and vegetables. The data for fruits and vegetables have been grouped according to fruit or vegetable. In addition, the references where the data were obtained are included.

The D values for chlorophyll, time to acceptable texture, color, and time to organoleptic unacceptability are, in general, significantly smaller than the D values for thiamin degradation, indicating that these components are much more heat sensitive (have a larger Q_{10}) than for thiamin loss. It may be assumed that the other water soluble vitamins such as riboflavin and vitamin C will have D values of similar magnitude to thiamin based on the losses shown in Table 13.1.

These data indicate that attention should be given to basing critical losses of quality during thermal processing on color, texture, or overall organoleptic quality and probably not on nutrition loss.

Some caution should be exercised in making conclusions based on data as in the case of Lenz and Lund (1977) and Gold and Weckel (1959) who obtained extremely high D values for chlorophyll loss. Another difficulty with using kinetic data based on the older literature is that usually only one temperature and time for processing as well as the final percent loss

TABLE 13.2
KINETIC PARAMETERS FOR LOSS OF QUALITY IN CANNED FRUITS AND VEGETABLES DURING PROCESSING

Food Product	Food Component	Temp. Range °F	E_a (Kcal/mole)	D* min	k* min^{-1}	Temp.* °C	Reference
Peas	thiamin	220—270	21.2	164 min.	0.0140	121	Bendix *et al.* (1951)
Peas	thiamin	228—300	27	163 min.	0.0141	121	Fellicotti and Esselsen (1957)
Pea puree	thiamin	250—280	27.5	246.9 min.	0.0093	121	Mulley *et al.* (1975)
Puree Peas-in-brine	thiamin	250—280	27.0	226.7	0.0101	121	
Pea puree (blanched)	chlorophyll	240—280	16.1	14.0	0.1643	121	Gold and Weckel (1959)
Pea puree (unblanched)	chlorophyll	240—280	12.6	13.9	0.1655	121	Gold and Weckel (1959)
Pea puree (unblanched)	chlorophyll	175—280	22	113	0.0204	121	Lenz and Lund (1974) (adapted from Lund 1975)
Peas	color	175—300	15.0	25.0	0.092	121	Timbers (1971) (adapted from Lund 1975)
Peas	organoleptic quality	175—300	22.5	2.3	1.0	121	Timbers (1971) (adapted from Lund 1975)
Peas	texture	170—200	19.5	1.4 min.	1.64	121	Mansfield (1974) (adapted from Lund 1975)
Peas	overall quality	210—240	19.5	2.5	0.92	121	Mansfield (1974) (adapted from Lund 1975)
Peas	peroxidase	230—280	16.0	3.0	0.767	121	Adams and Yawger (1961)

*k and D value at indicated temperature

continued

TABLE 13.2 (continued)

Food Product	Food Component	Temp. Range °F	E_a (Kcal/mole)	D* min.	k* min^{-1}	Temp.* °C	Reference
Peas	thiamin	240	—	157.5	.0146	115.5	Fellers *et al.* (1940)
Peas, Alaska	thiamin	240	—	174.2	.0132	115.5	Clifcorn and Heberlein (1944)
Pea puree	thiamin	240-280	24	267	.0086	121	Lenz and Lund (1977)
Pea puree	chlorophyll	240-280	22	158.6	.0145	121	Lenz and Lund (1977)
Peas	thiamin	240	—	201.8	.0114	115.5	Clifcorn and Heberlein (1944)
Peas	thiamine	240	—	174.2	.0132	121	Guerrant *et al.* (1946)
Peas	thiamin	250	—	201.8	.0114	120.5	Clifcorn and Heberlein (1944)
Peas	thiamin	250	—	147.4	.0156	120.5	Heberlein *et al.* (1950)
Peas (immature)	thiamin	250	—	187.0	0.123	120.5	Heberlein *et al.* (1950)
Peas (immature)	thiamin	241	—	134.5	0.171	116	Guerrant and O'Hara (1953)
Peas (bottled)	thiamin	241	—	193.3	.0119	116	Guerrant and O'Hara (1953)
Peas	thiamin	240	—	174.2	.0132	115.5	Guerrant et al. (1946)
Spinach	thiamin	228-300	27	134.0	.0172	121	Feliciotti and Esselen (1957)
Spinach	chlorophyll a	260-300	15.5	13.0	.1769	121	Gupte *et al.* (1964)
Spinach	chlorophyll b	260-300	7.8	14.7	.1565	121	Gupte *et al.* (1964)
Spinach puree	chlorophyll	175-280	19	166	.0139	121	Gold and Weckel (1959)
Spinach	chlorophyll a	212-266	12.5	34.1	.0674	121	Hermann (1970)
Spinach	chlorophyll b	212-266	10.0	48.3	.0476	121	Hermann (1970)
Spinach	thiamin	252	—	87.1	.0264	122	Guerrant *et al.* (1946)
Carrott puree	thiamin	228-300	27	158	.0146	121	Feliciotti and Esselen (1957)

*k and D value at indicated temperature

continued

TABLE 13.2 (continued)

Food Product	Food Component	Temp. Range °F	E_a (Kcal/mole)	D* Min	k* min^{-1}	Temp.* °C	Reference
Carrots	overall cook quality (time to acceptability)	176-240	38	1.4	1.643	121	Mansfield (1974) (from Lund 1975)
Bean, green puree	thiamin	228-300	27	145	.0158	121	Feliciotti and Esselen (1957)
Bean, green							
Bean, green	chlorophyll	190-212	12	10.1	.2277	121	Feliciotti and Esselen (1957)
Beans, green cut	color	175-300	15.0	21.0	.1095	121	Timbers (1971) (from Lund 1975)
Beans, green cut	organoleptic (time to unacceptability)	175-300	22.0	4.0	.5750	121	Timbers (1971) (from Lund 1975)
Beans, green cut	overall cook quality	182-240	41.0	1.0	2.30	121	Mansfield (1974) (from Lund 1975)
Asparagus	color	175-300	14.0	17.0	.1353	121	Timbers (1971) (from Lund 1975)
Asparagus	thiamin	240	—	267.4	.0086	115.5	Fellers *et al.* (1940)
Asparagus	thiamin	250	—	63.01	.0365	120	Clifcorn and Heberlein (1944)
Whole kernel corn	organoleptic (time to unacceptability	175-300	19.5	6.0	.3833	121	Timbers (1971) (from Lund 1975)
Sweet corn	methyl methionine, Sulfonium bromide	178-212	31.6	4.5	.5111	121	Williams and Nelson (1974)
Whole kernel corn	overall code quality	212-250	16.0	2.4	.9583	121	Mansfield (1974) (from Lund 1975)
Corn cream style	thiamin	240	—	141.0	.0163	115.5	Fenster (1948) (from Lund 1975)

*k and D value at indicated temperature

continued

Table 13.2 (concluded)

Food Product	Food Component	Temp. Range °F	E_a (Kcal/mole)	D* min	k* min^{-1}	Temp.* °C	Reference
Corn cream style	thiamin	240	—	191.7	.0120	115.5	Fenster (1948) (from Lund 1975)
Corn cream style	thiamin	284	—	57.2	.0402	140	Fenster (1948) (from Lund 1975)
Tomatoes	methyl methionine	178-212	27.2	23.2	.0991	121	Williams and Nelson (1974)
Tomatoes	thiamin	212	—	697.0	.0033	100	Clifcorn and Heberlein (1944)
Broccoli	overall acceptable cook quality	212-250	13.0	4.4	.5227	121	Mansfield (1974) (from Lund 1975)
Squash	overall acceptance cook quality	182-240	25.0	1.5	1.533	121	Mansfield (1974) (from Lund 1975)
Potato	overall acceptable cook quality	161-240	27.5	1.2	1.917	121	Mansfield (1974) (from Lund 1975)
Beet puree	betanin	240-267	11.0	415.9	.00553	121	Lenz and Lund (1977)
Peas	color	175-300	18.1	13.52	.17	127	Hayakawa (1977)
Beans, green	color	175-300	19.8	8.51	.27	127	Hayakawa (1977)
Asparagus	color	175-300	15.2	11.5	.20	127	Hayakawa (1977)
Mushrooms	thiamin	266	—	33.43	.0688		Zhuk and Rod'Kina (1975)

*k and D value at indicated temperature

TABLE 13.3
KINETIC PARAMETERS FOR CANNED FRUITS AND VEGETABLES DURING STORAGE

Food Product	Basis for Shelf-Life	E_a (kcal/mole)	Q_{10} (70-88°F)	Figure No.	Reference
Apples, regular (cans)	overall quality	7.19	1.5	13.1	Congressional Record (1977)
Apples, baby food (jars)	overall quality	7.19	1.5	13.2	Congressional Record (1977)
Apple sauce	time to 50% loss color	21.71	3.4	13.3	Cecil and Woodroof (1963)
Apples, dietetic (cans)	overall quality	9.42	1.7	13.5	Congressional Record (1977)
Apples, junior food (jars)	overall quality	7.19	1.5	13.6	Congressional Record (1977)
Apricots	loss of 10% thiamin	19.49	3.0	13.7	Brenner *et al.* (1948)
Apricots	loss of 10% thiamin	15.33	2.4	13.8	Brenner *et al.* 1948)
Apricots, regular (cans)	overall quality	10.43	1.8	13.9	Congressional Record (1977)
Apricots, baby food (jars)	overall quality	7.19	1.5	13.10	Congressional Record (1977)
Apricots	loss of 20% vitamin C	20.07	3.1	13.11	Freed *et al.* (1949)
Apricots	loss of 20% thiamin	7.19	1.5	13.12	Freed *et al.* (1949)
Apricots	loss of 10% vitamin C	9.42	1.7	13.14	Kramer (1974)
Apricots	loss of 10% carotene	9.42	1.7	13.15	Kramer (1974)
Apricots, dietary (cans)	overall quality	9.42	1.7	13.16	Congressional Record (1977)
Asparagus	overall quality	10.43	1.8	13.17	Congressional Record (1977)
Asparagus	loss of 10% vitamin C	13.99	2.2	13.18	Kramer (1974)
Asparagus	loss of 10% thiamin	16.95	2.6	13.19	Kramer (1974)
Asparagus	loss of 10% carotene	8.34	1.6	13.20	Kramer (1974)
Asparagus	loss of 10% riboflavin	17.62	2.7	13.21	Kramer (1974)
Banana, baby food (jars)	overall quality	8.34	1.6	13.22	Congressional Record (1977)
Beans, green, baby food (jars)	overall quality	7.19	1.5	13.23	Congressional Record (1977)
Beans, green, regular (cans)	overall quality	9.42	1.7	13.24	Congressional Record (1977)
Beans, green, baby food (jars)	overall quality	7.19	1.5	13.25	Freed *et al.* (1949)
Beans, green	loss of 20% thiamin	10.57	1.9	13.85	Freed *et al.* (1949)
Beans, kidney (cans)	loss of 20% thiamin	9.42	1.7	13.26	Freed *et al.* (1949)
Beans lima	loss of 10% vitamin C	8.34	1.6	13.31	Kramer (1974)

continued

TABLE 13.3 (continued)

Food Product	Basis for Shelf-Life	E_a (kcal/mole)	Q_{10} (70-88 °F)	Figure No.	Reference
Beans, lima	loss of 20% thiamin	12.22	2.0	13.13	Freed *et al.* (1949)
Beans, sprouts	overall quality	9.42	1.7	13.27	Congressional Record (1977)
Beans, green	loss of 10% vitamin C	4.66	1.3	13.28	Kramer (1974)
Beans, green	loss of 10% thiamin	9.42	1.7	13.29	Kramer (1974)
Beans, green	loss of 10% riboflavin	20.07	3.1	13.30	Kramer (1974)
Beans, lima	loss of 10% riboflavin	5.97	1.4	13.32	Kramer (1974)
Beans, lima (cans)	overall quality	7.19	1.5	13.34	Congressional Record (1977)
Beets, baby food (jars)	overall quality	8.34	1.6	13.35	Congressional Record (1977)
Beets, regular (cans)	overall quality	10.43	1.8	13.36	Congressional Record (197)
Berries, black (cans)	overall quality	7.19	1.5	13.37	Congressional Record (1977)
Blueberries	overall quality	8.34	1.6	13.38	Congressional Record (1977)
Carrots, baby food and junior food (jars)	overall quality	7.19	1.5	13.39	Congressional Record (1977)
Carrots, regular and puree (cans)	overall quality	7.19	1.5	13.40	Congressional Record (1977)
Cherries, dietetic	overall quality	5.97	1.4	13.41	Congressional Record (1977)
Cherries, sweet, dark	overall quality	8.34	1.6	13.42	Congressional Record (1977)
Cherries, sweet, light	overall quality	9.42	1.7	13.43	Congressional Record (1977)
Corn, sweet	loss of 10% thiamin	19.49	3.0	13.44	Kramer (1974)
Corn, sweet	loss of 10% carotene	12.30	2.0	13.45	Kramer (1974)
Corn, whole	loss of 50% color	10.43	1.8	13.4	Cecil and Woodroof (1963)
Corn, sweet	loss of 10% vitamin C	10.43	1.8	13.33	Kramer (1974)
Corn, whole	degradation of 50% flavor	11.39	1.9	13.48	Cecil and Woodroof (1963)
Corn, cream and whole	overall quality	7.19	1.5	13.50	Congressional Record (1977)
Corn, sweet	loss of 10% riboflavin	10.43	1.8	13.46	Kramer (1974)

continued

TABLE 13.3 (continued)

Food Product	Basis for Shelf-Life	E_a (kcal/mole)	Q_{10} (70-88 °F)	Figure No.	Reference
Cranberry sauce	overall quality	8.34	1.6	13.51	Congressional Record (1977)
Figs	overall quality	8.34	1.6	13.52	Congressional Record (1977)
Fruit cocktail	overall quality	10.43	1.8	13.53	Congressional Record (1977)
Grapefruit segments	loss of 10% vitamin C	7.19	1.5	13.47	Kramer (1974)
Grapefruit, regular	overall quality	9.42	1.7	13.54	Congressional Record (1977)
Mushrooms	overall quality	9.42	1.7	13.55	Congressional Record (1977)
Mango squash	loss of 10% vitamin C	4.66	1.3	13.56	Sweed and Muvarak (1971)
Okra	overall quality	10.43	1.8	13.57	Congressional Record (1977)
Olives, green and ripe	overall quality	5.97	1.4	13.58	Congressional Record (1977)
Peaches, regular and dietetic	overall quality	8.34	1.6	13.59	Congressional Record (1977)
Peaches, baby food	overall quality	8.34	1.6	13.60	Congressional Record (1977)
Peaches	loss of 20% vitamin C	8.34	1.6	13.61	Clifcorn (1948)
Peaches	loss of 10% vitamin C	9.42	1.7	13.62	Kramer (1974)
Peaches	loss of 10% thiamin	27.46	4.7	13.63	Kramer (1974)
Peaches	loss of 10% carotene	8.34	1.6	13.64	Kramer (1974)
Pears, regular and dietetic	overall quality	10.43	1.8	13.66	Congressional Record (1977)
Pears and peas, baby food	overall quality	8.34	1.6	13.67	Congressional Record (1977)
Peas	loss of 10% vitamin C	9.42	1.7	13.65	Kramer (1974)
Peas	loss of 10% thiamin	17.62	2.7	13.68	Kramer (1974)
Peas	loss of 10% carotene	8.34	1.6	13.69	Kramer (1974)
Peas	loss of 10% riboflavin	20.64	3.2	13.70	Kramer (1974)
Peas, green and blackeyed	overall quality	7.19	1.5	13.72	Congressional Record (1977)
Pineapple	loss of vitamin C	4.66	1.3	13.71	Kramer (1974)
Pineapple, regular and dietetic	overall quality	10.43	1.8	13.73	Congressional Record (1977)
Prunes, baby food	overall quality	5.97	1.4	13.74	Congressional Record (1977)
Sauerkraut	overall quality	9.42	1.7	13.75	Congressional Record (1977)
Spinach	loss of 10% vitamin C	12.22	2.0	13.76	Kramer (1974)

continued

TABLE 13.3 (concluded)

Food Product	Basis for Shelf-Life	E_a (kcal/mole)	Q_{10} (70-88 °F)	Figure No.	Reference
Spinach	loss of 10% thiamin	13.99	2.2	13.77	Kramer (1974)
Spinach	loss of 10% carotene	26.29	4.4	13.78	Kramer (1974)
Spinach, baby and junior foods (jars)	overall quality	7.19	1.5	13.80	Congressional Record (1977)
Spinach, regular and puree	overall quality	8.34	1.6	13.81	Congressional Record (1977)
Summer squash	degradation of 50% of texture	7.19	1.5	13.82	Cecil and Woodroof (1963)
Summer squash	degradation of 50% flavor	7.19	1.5	13.83	Cecil and Woodroof (1963)
Tomatoes	degradation of 50% flavor quality	11.39	1.9	13.49	Cecil and Woodroof (1963)
Tomatoes	loss of 10% vitamin C	9.42	1.7	13.86	Kramer (1974)
Tomatoes	loss of 10% thiamin	11.39	1.9	13.87	Kramer (1974)

TABLE 13.4
SHELF-LIFES OF CANNED FRUITS AND VEGETABLES DURING STORAGE

Food Product	Shelf-Life	Temp. of Storage	Reference	Basis for Shelf-Life
Apple sauce	11 months	25 °C	Livingston *et al.* (1954)	loss of 25% of vitamin C
Baby foods	6 months	25 °C	Wodsak (1969)	overall quality
Baby foods	6-9 months	25 °C	Wodsak (1969)	20% loss of vitamins A,C,E and B_2
Grapefruit segments	3 months	15-29 °C	Ludin (1969)	Browning
Potatoes	6 months	25 °C	Von Elbe *et al.* (1974)	Los of 13% vitamin C
Carrots	6 months	25 °C	Von Elbe *et al.* (1974)	loss of 5% vitamin C

for a given component is given. This results in kinetic data based on end-point analysis as is the case with the references in Table 13.2, where there is no order of reaction provided.

Deterioration of various components during storage of fruits and vegetables is included in Tables 13.3 and 13.4. In Table 13.3 the activation energies and Q_{10}s for various fruits and vegetables are listed along with the references from which the data were obtained. The shelf-life plots of these data are at the end of this section. It should be noted, however, that in most cases for quality losses the Q_{10}s range from 1.5 to 2.5 which is quite low. Table 13.4 contains shelf-lives for fruits and vegetables where there was an insufficient amount of data in the reference to determine kinetic parameters of the deteriorative reaction in question.

Changes in flavor in canned fruits and vegetables during storage can be due to browning reactions, staling, and loss of flavor (flat taste). Browning reactions result in burned and bitter flavors in fruits, especially those canned in syrups, and to some extent in sweet potatoes. Many vegetables get a musty taste which could be described as "old." Products high in starch become stale tasting as staling of the starch takes place. This reaction can be accompanied by yellowing.

Changes in color during storage include fading of carotenoid-type pigments (red-orange) in red and green vegetables. Fruit and starchy vegetables generally turn dark or brown in color.

Changes in texture during storage include softening of some vegetables when stored at high temperatures. Extremely low temperature storage can disintegrate or break down the texture of many vegetables, especially potatoes, beans, squash, greens, peas and tomatoes. Other textural changes include a tendency toward lumping or clumping in beans and peas.

Changes or losses of different vitamins tend to occur more slowly than changes in flavor, color, and texture. In general, carotene or vitamin A may be said to be at least as stable as the overall quality of a given product (Cecil and Woodroof 1963) especially based on the Q_{10}.

Thiamin and ascorbic acid (vitamin C) may or may not remain at acceptable levels depending on the product, when compared to overall or organoleptic quality of canned fruits and vegetables, according to Cecil and Woodroof (1963). Enrichment of these vitamins will also have an effect on the length of time the vitamin is at an acceptable level in a given product.

Cecil and Woodroof (1963) suggested that acceptable levels of thiamin and vitamin C should be used as the shelf-life basis for canned foods which are significant sources of thiamin or vitamin C in the diet, such as beans and fruits.

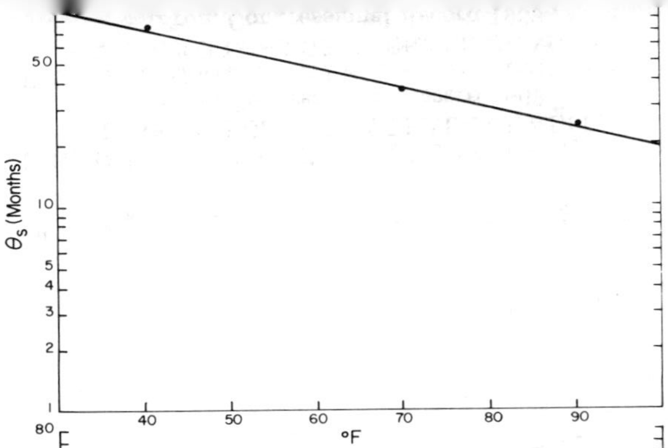

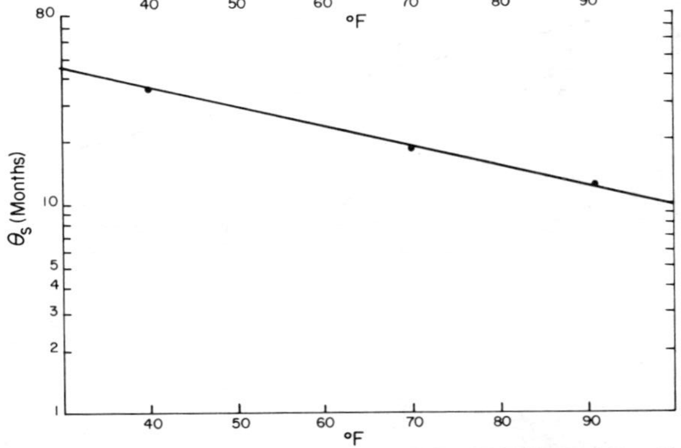

FIG. 13.1. (Top). APPLES (REGULAR CAN PACK)—TIME TO LOSS OF OVERALL QUALITY AS A FUNCTION OF TEMPERATURE
(From Congressional Record 1969).
FIG. 13.2. (Bottom). APPLES (BABY FOOD STRAINED, JAR)—TIME TO LOSS OF OVERALL QUALITY
(From Congressional Record 1969).

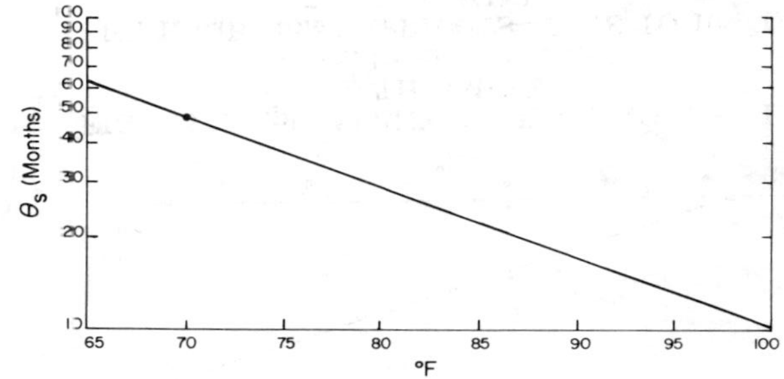

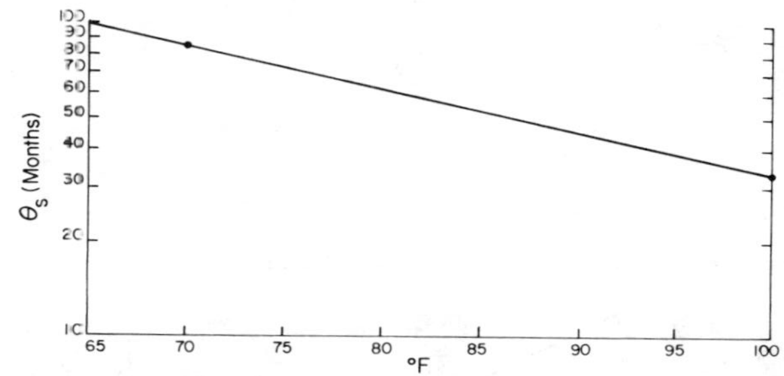

FIG. 13.3.(Top). APPLE SAUCE (DETROIT RED)—TIME TO 50% DEGRADATION OF COLOR
(From Cecil and Woodroof 1963).
FIG. 13.4.(Bottom). CORN (WHOLE GRAIN)—TIME TO 50% DEGRADATION OF COLOR
(From Cecil and Woodroof 1963).

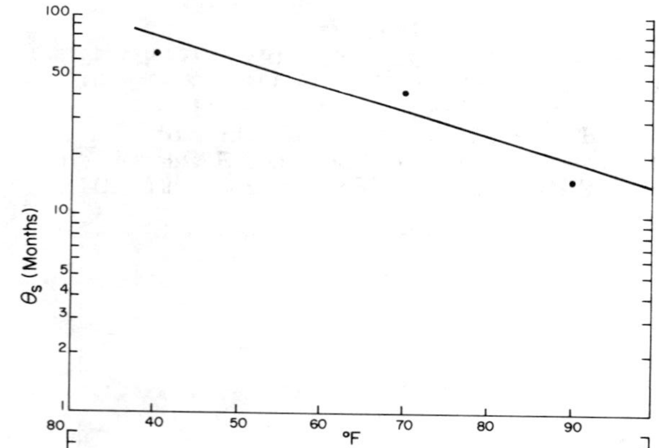

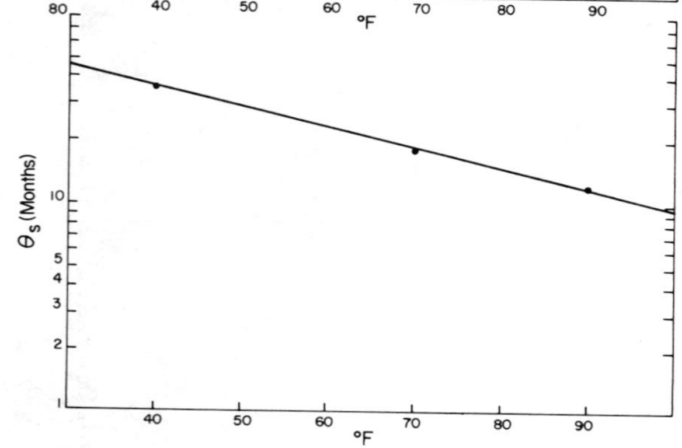

FIG. 13.5.(Top.) APPLES (DIETETIC PACK, CAN)—TIME TO LOSS OF OVERALL QUALITY
(From Congressional Record 1969).

FIG. 13.6.(Bottom). APPLES (JUNIOR FOOD)—TIME TO LOSS OF OVERALL QUALITY
(From Congressional Record 1969).

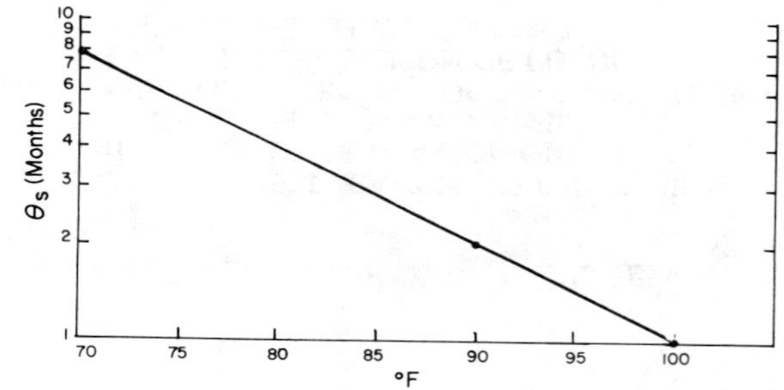

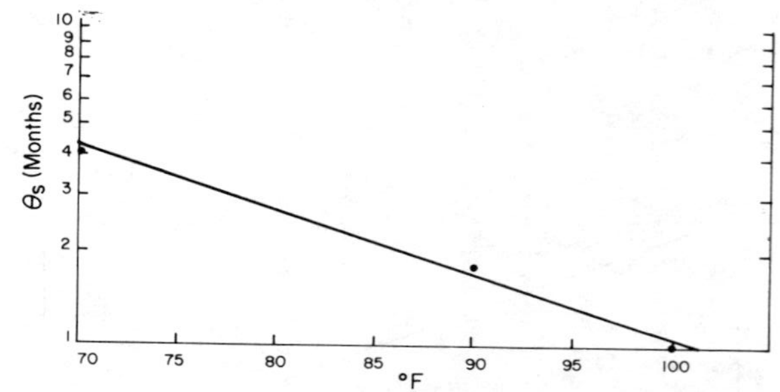

FIG. 13.7.(Top). APRICOTS—TIME TO 10% LOSS THIAMINE
(From Brenner *et al.* 1948).

FIG. 13.8.(Bottom.) APRICOTS—TIME TO 10% LOSS THIAMINE
(From Brenner *et al.* 1948).

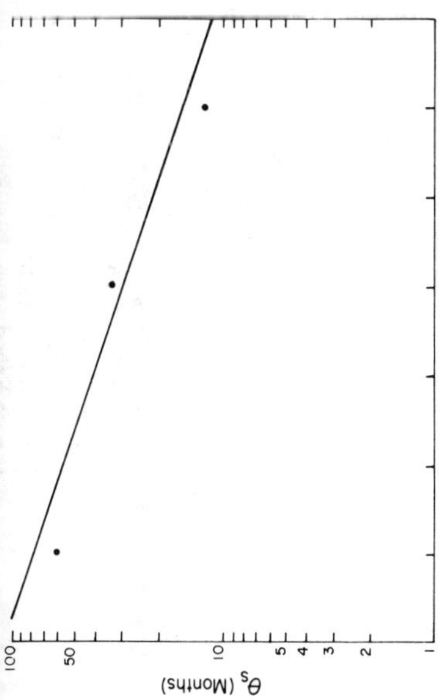

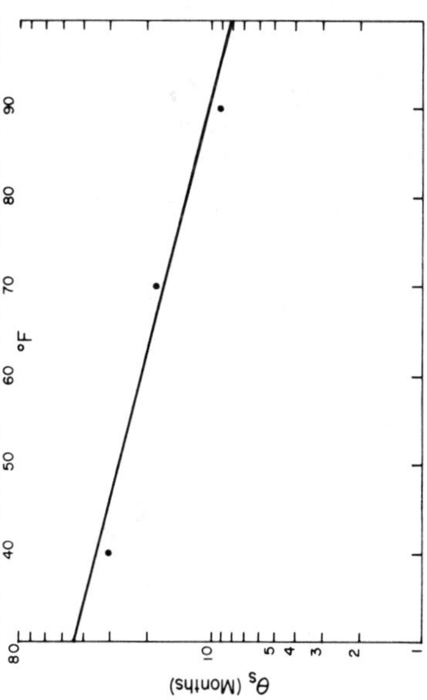

FIG. 13.9.(Top). APRICOTS (REGULAR PACK, CAN)—TIME TO LOSS OF OVERALL QUALITY
(From Congressional Record 1969).
FIG. 13.10.(Bottom). APRICOTS (BABY FOOD STRAINED, JAR)—TIME TO LOSS OF OVERALL QUALITY

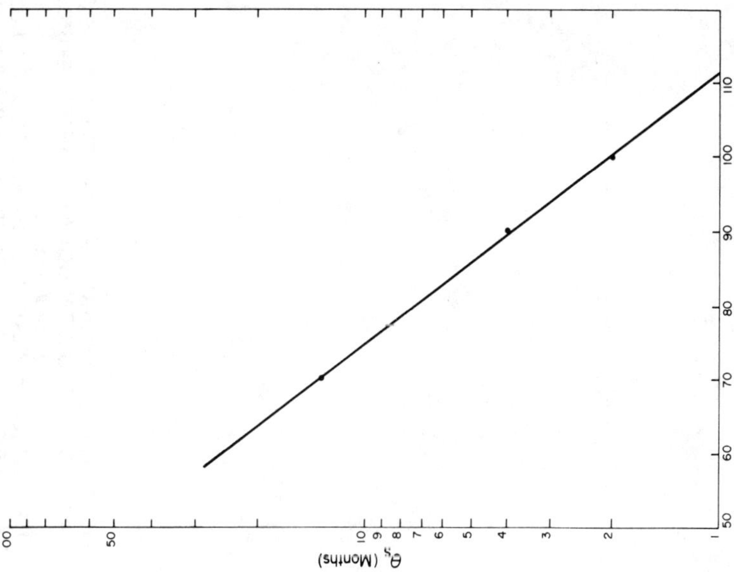

FIG. 13.11. APRICOTS—TIME TO 20% LOSS VITAMIN C
(From Freed *et al.* 1949).

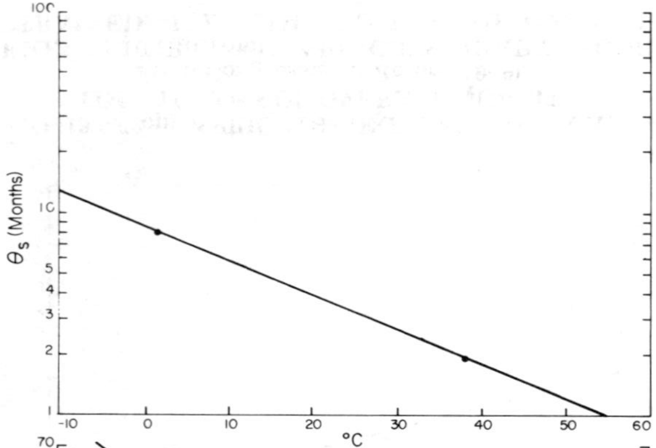

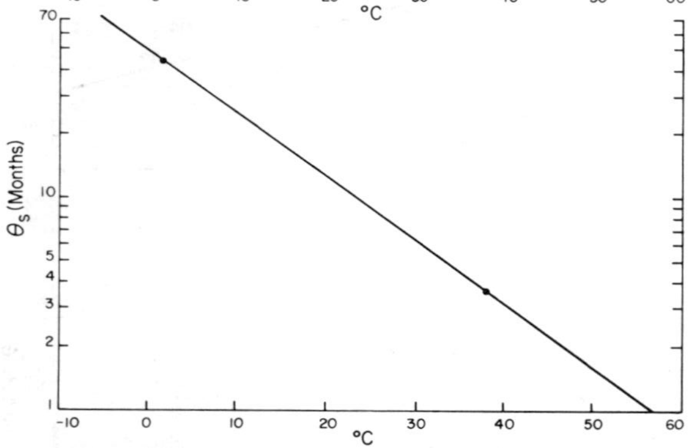

FIG. 13.12.(Top). APRICOTS—TIME TO 20% LOSS THIAMIN
(From Freed *et al.* 1949).

FIG. 13.13.(Bottom). LIMA BEANS—TIME TO 20% LOSS THIAMIN
(From Freed *et al.* 1949).

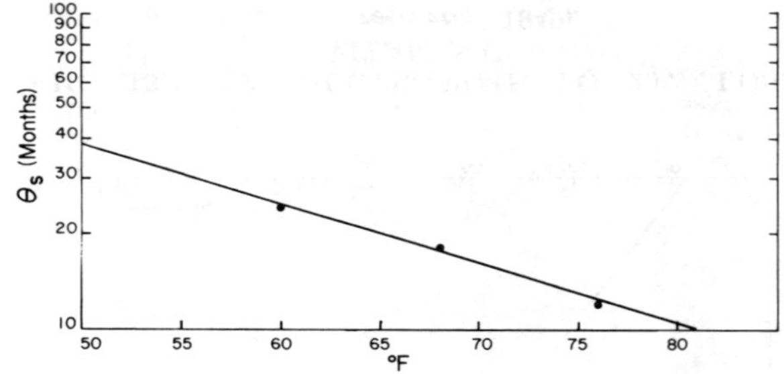

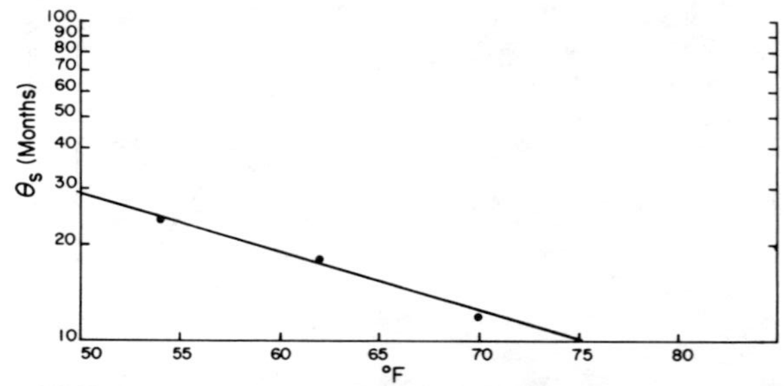

FIG. 13.14.(Top). APRICOTS—TIME TO 10% LOSS OF ASCORBIC ACID AT VARIOUS TEMPERATURES
(From Kramer 1974).

FIG. 13.15.(Bottom). APRICOTS—TIME TO 10% LOSS OF CAROTENE AT VARIOUS TEMPERATURES
(From Kramer 1974).

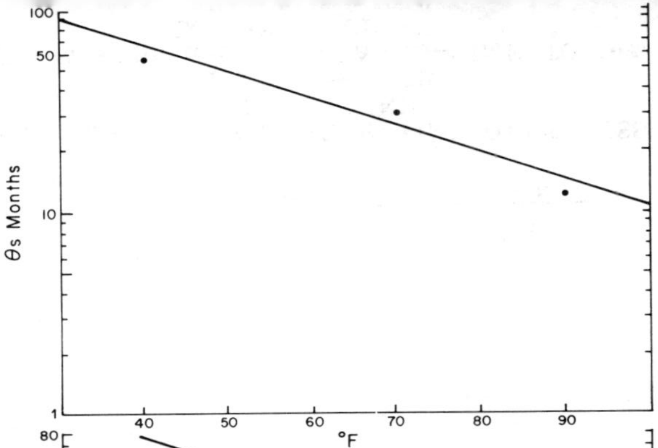

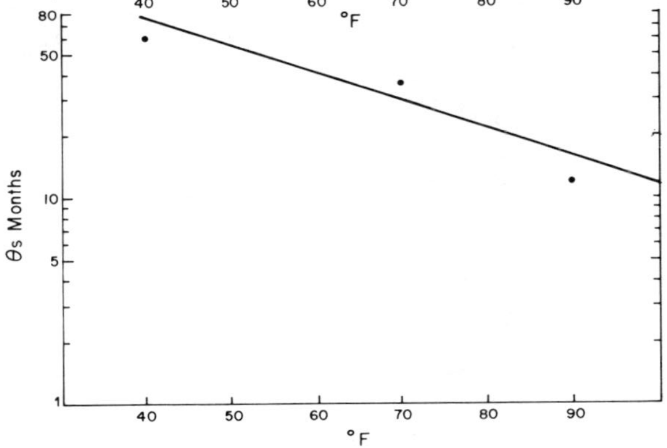

FIG. 13.16.(Top). APRICOTS (DIETARY PACK, CAN)—TIME TO LOSS OF OVERALL QUALITY (From Congressional Record 1969).

FIG. 13.17.(Bottom). ASPARAGUS (CAN)—TIME TO LOSS OF OVERALL QUALITY (From Congressional Record 1969).

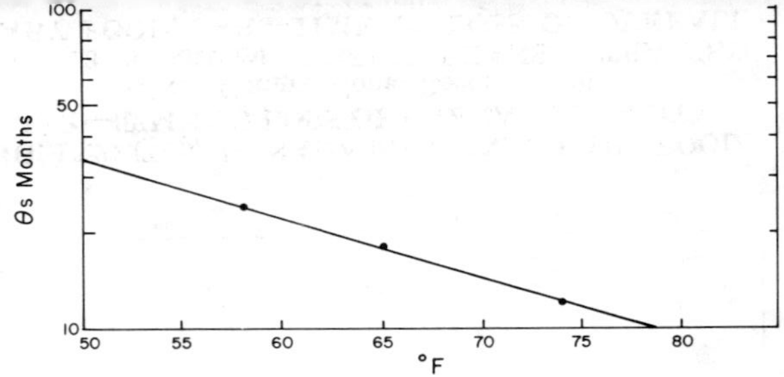

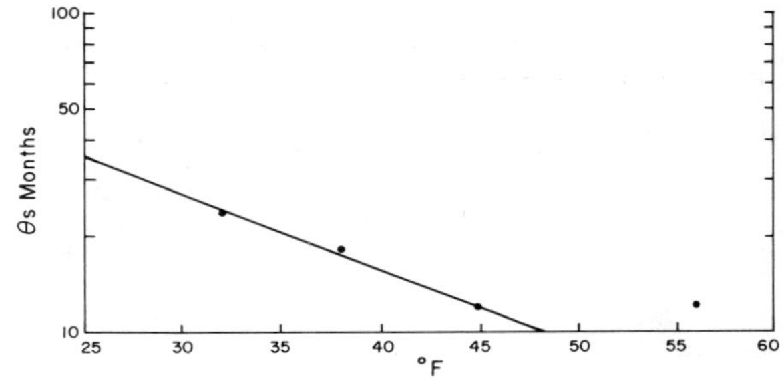

FIG. 13.18.(Top). ASPARAGUS—TIME TO 10% LOSS OF ASCORBIC ACID (From Kramer 1974).

FIG. 13.19.(Bottom). ASPARAGUS—TIME TO 10% LOSS OF THIAMINE (From Kramer 1974).

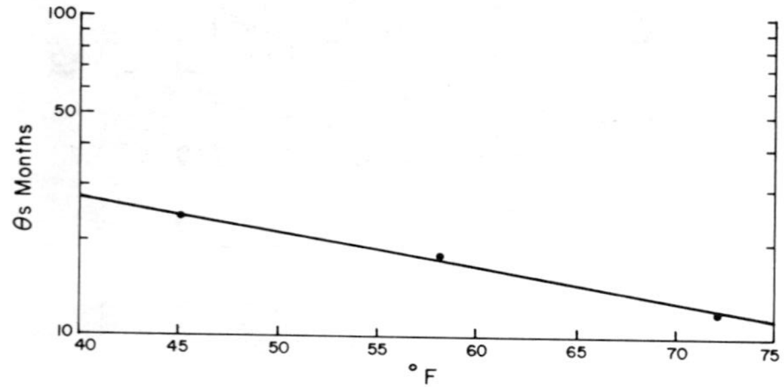

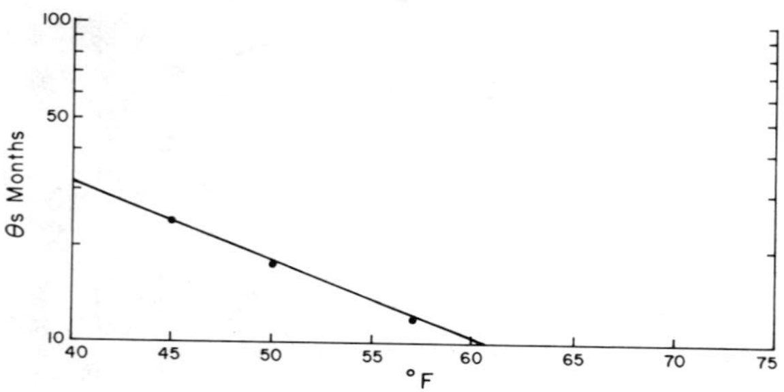

FIG. 13.20.(TOP). ASPARAGUS—TIME TO 10% LOSS OF CAROTENE
(From Kramer 1974).

FIG. 13.21.(Bottom). ASPARAGUS—TIME TO 10% LOSS OF RIBOFLAVIN

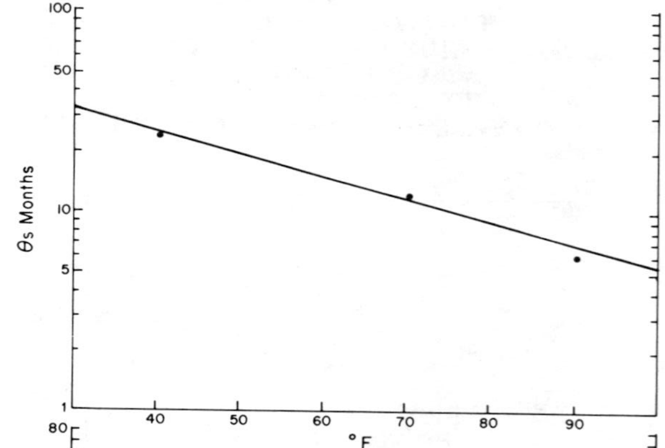

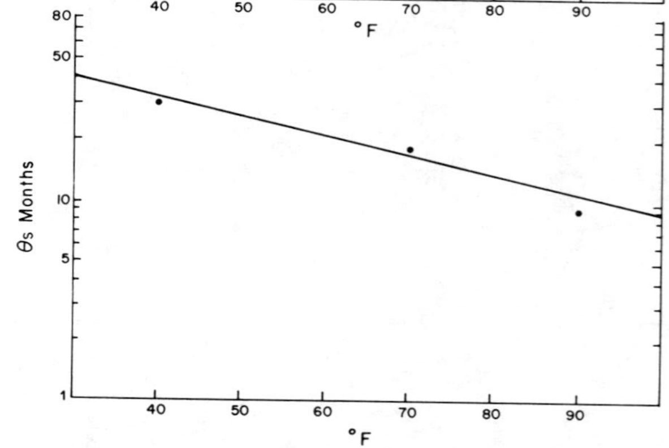

FIG. 13.22.(Top). BANANA (STRAINED BABY FOOD, JAR)—TIME TO LOSS OF OVERALL QUALITY
(From Congressional Record 1969).

FIG. 13.23.(Bottom). GREEN BEANS (STRAINED BABY FOOD, JAR)—TIME TO LOSS OF OVERALL

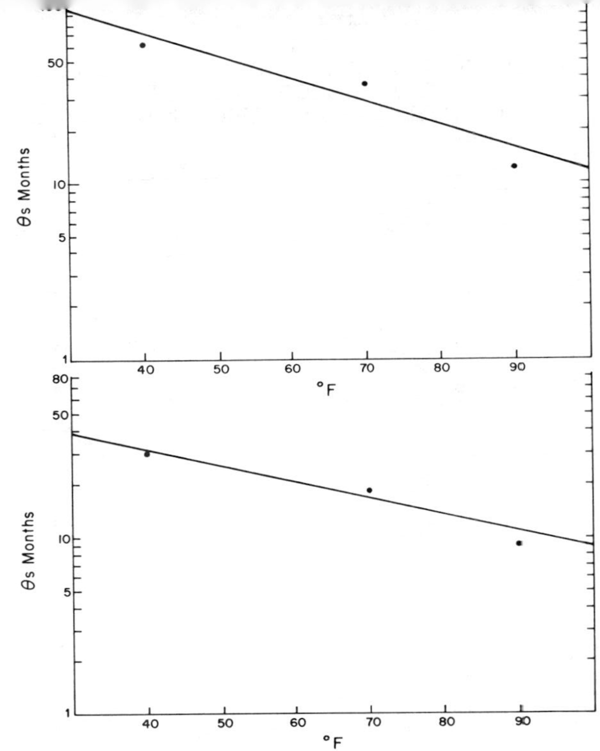

FIG. 13.24.(Top). GREEN BEANS (REGULAR, CAN)—TIME TO LOSS OF OVERALL QUALITY
FIG. 13.25.(Bottom). GREEN BEANS (JUNIOR BABY FOOD, JAR)—TIME TO LOSS OF OVERALL QUALITY
(From Congressional Record 1969).

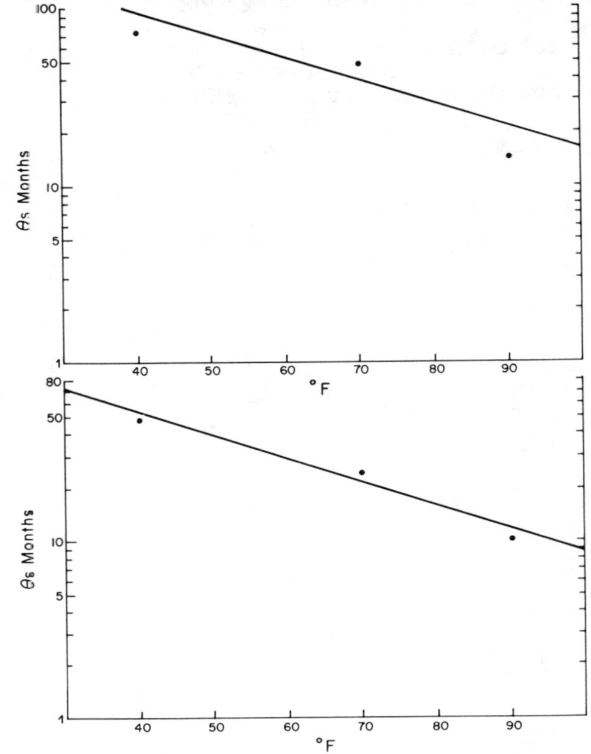

FIG. 13.26.(Top). KIDNEY BEANS (CAN)—TIME TO LOSS OF OVERALL QUALITY
FIG. 13.27.(Bottom). BEAN SPROUTS (CAN)—TIME TO LOSS OF OVERALL QUALITY
(From Congressional Record 1969).

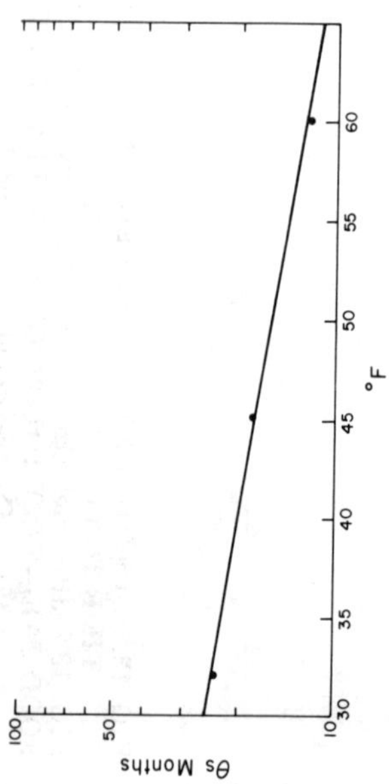

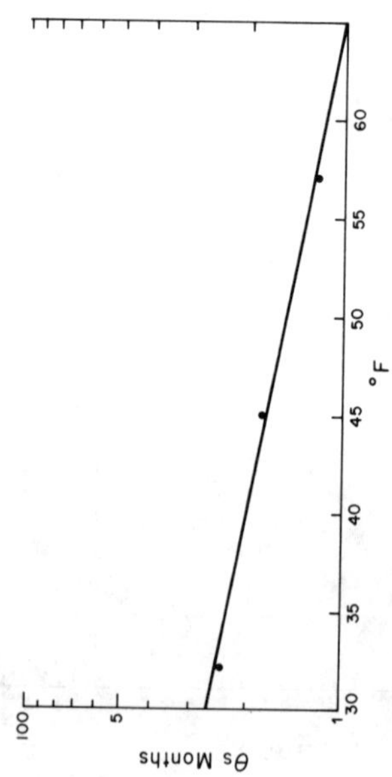

FIG. 13.28.(Top). GREEN BEANS—TIME TO 10% LOSS OF ASCORBIC ACID
FIG. 13.29.(Bottom). GREEN BEANS—TIME TO 10% LOSS OF THIAMIN
(From Kramer 1974).

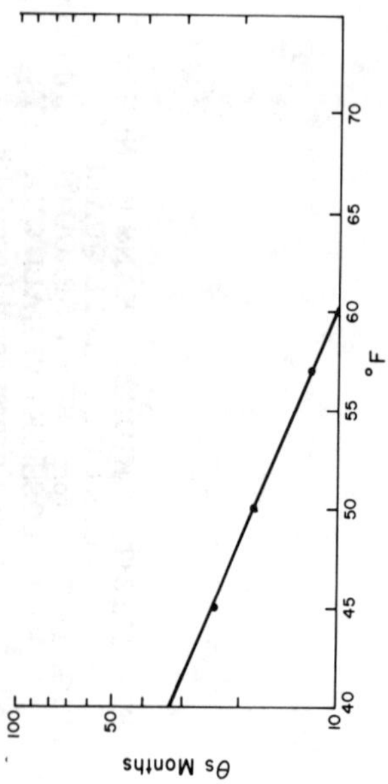

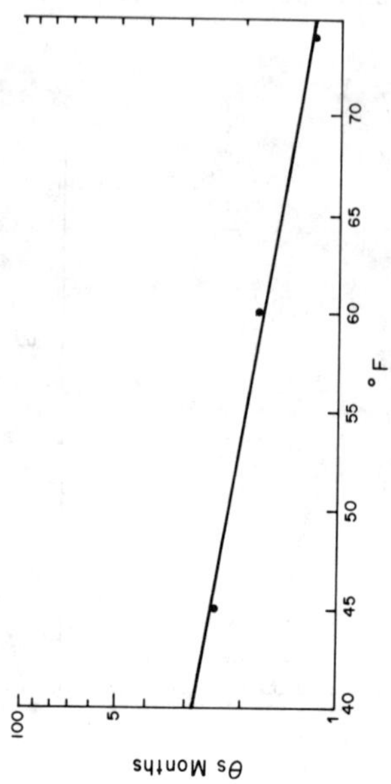

FIG. 13.30.(Top). GREEN BEANS—TIME TO 10% LOSS OF RIBOFLAVIN
FIG. 13.31.(Bottom). LIMA BEANS—TIME TO 10% LOSS OF ASCORBIC ACID
(From Kramer 1974).

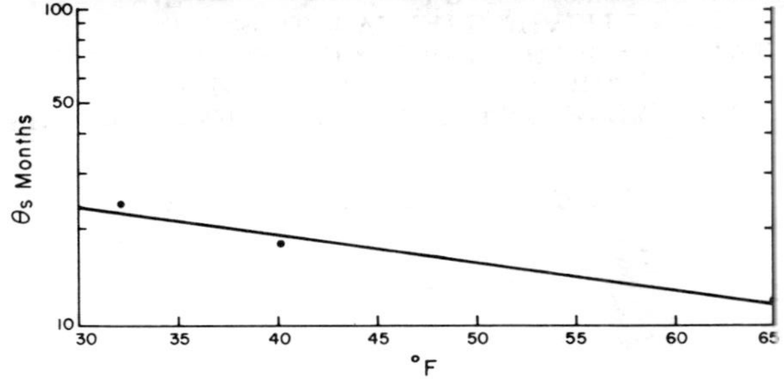

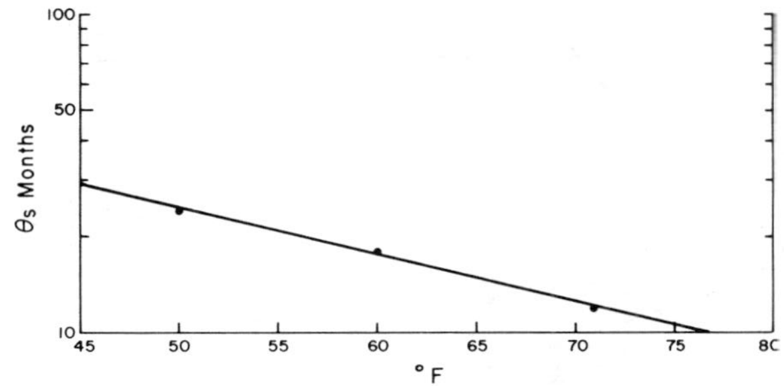

FIG. 13.32.(Top). LIMA BEANS—TIME TO 10% LOSS OF RIBOFLAVIN
FIG. 13.33.(Bottom). SWEET CORN—TIME TO 10% LOSS OF ASCORBIC ACID
(From Kramer 1974).

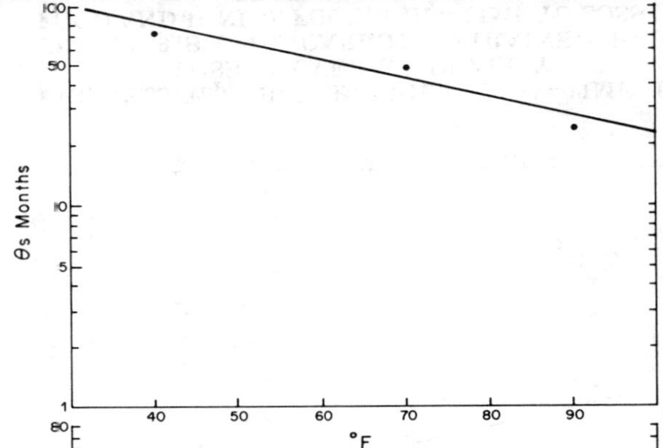

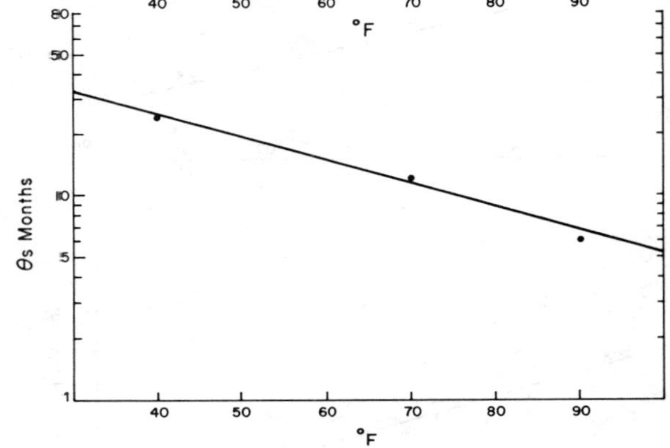

FIG. 13.34.(Top). LIMA BEANS (CAN)—TIME TO LOSS OF OVERALL QUALITY
FIG. 13.35.(Bottom). BEETS BABY FOOD STRAINED—TIME TO LOSS OF OVERALL QUALITY
(From Congressional Record 1969).

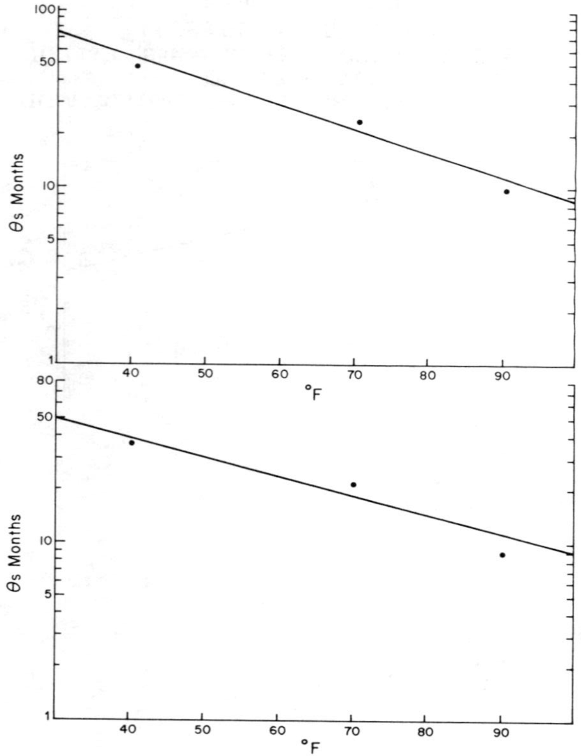

FIG. 13.36.(Top). BEETS (REGULAR PACK, CAN)—TIME TO LOSS OF OVERALL QUALITY

FIG. 13.37.(Bottom). BLACKBERRIES (CAN)—TIME TO LOSS OF OVERALL QUALITY

(From Congressional Record 1969)

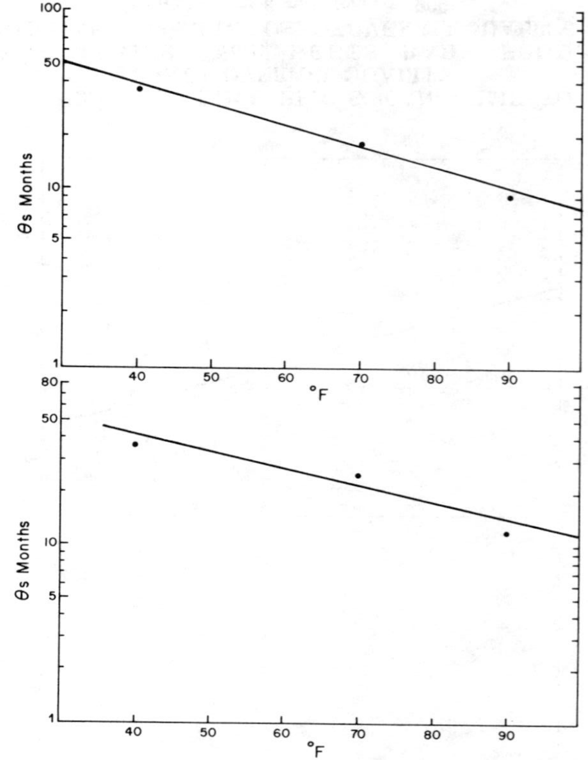

FIG. 13.38.(Top). BLUEBERRIES (CAN)—TIME TO LOSS OF OVERALL QUALITY

FIG. 13.39.(Bottom). CARROTS (STRAINED BABY FOOD AND JUNIOR FOOD, JAR)—TIME TO LOSS OF OVERALL QUALITY

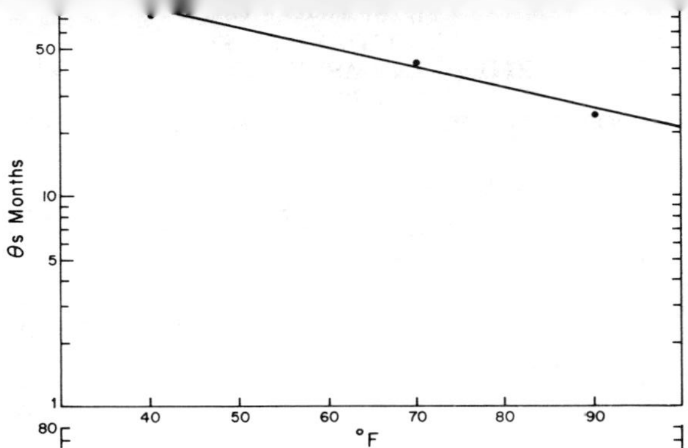

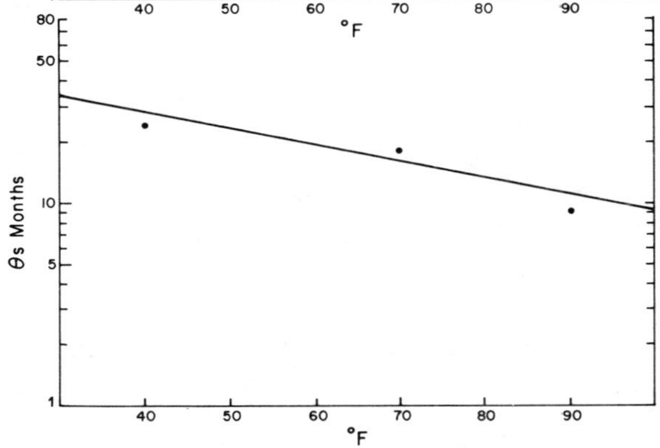

FIG. 13.40.(Top). CARROTS (PUREE AND REGULAR PACKS, CAN)—TIME TO LOSS OF OVERALL QUALITY

FIG. 13.41.(Bottom). CHERRIES DIETETIC AND RED SOUR PITTED)—TIME TO LOSS OF OVERALL QUALITY

(From Congressional Record 1969).

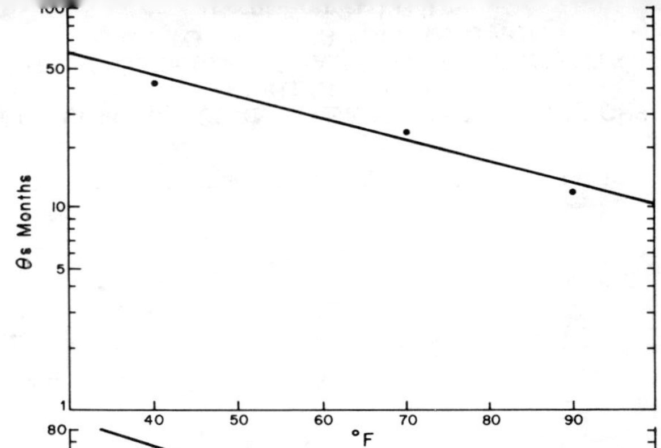

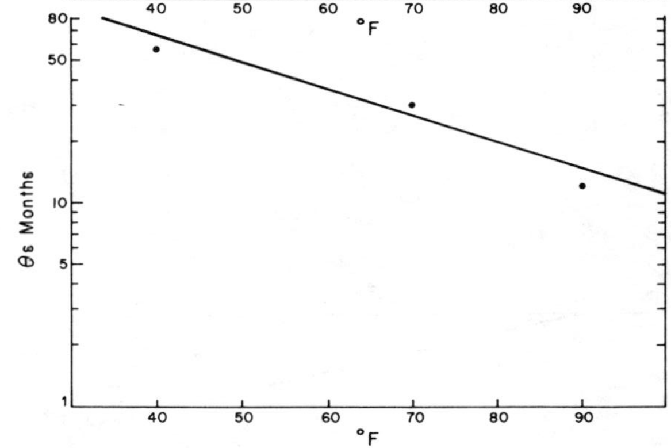

FIG. 13.42.(Top). CHERRIES (SWEET, DARK, CAN)—TIME TO LOSS OF OVERALL QUALITY

FIG. 13.43.(Bottom). CHERRIES (SWEET, LIGHT, CAN)—TIME TO LOSS OF OVERALL QUALITY

(From Congressional Record 1969).

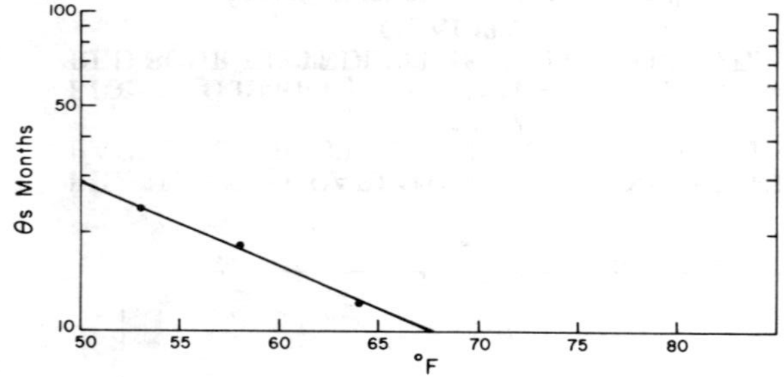

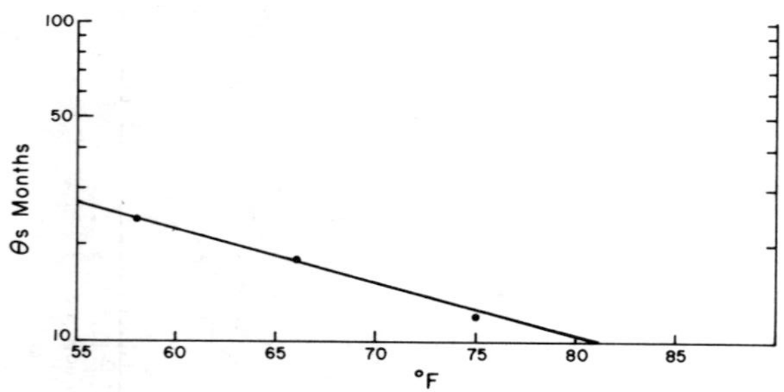

FIG. 13.44.(Top). CORN (SWEET)—TIME TO 10% LOSS OF THIAMIN
FIG. 13.45.(Bottom). CORN (SWEET)—TIME TO 10% LOSS OF CAROTENE
(From Kramer 1974)

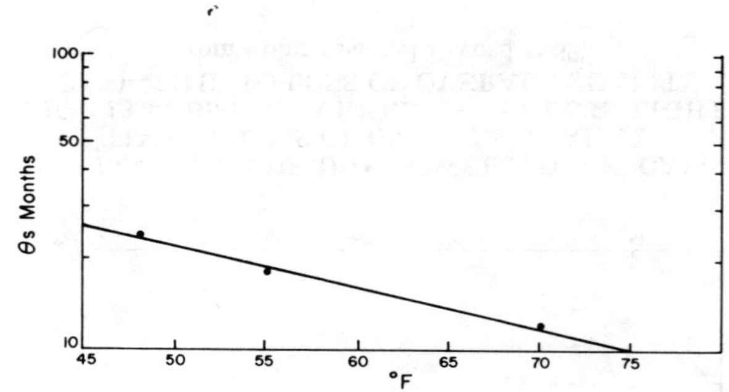

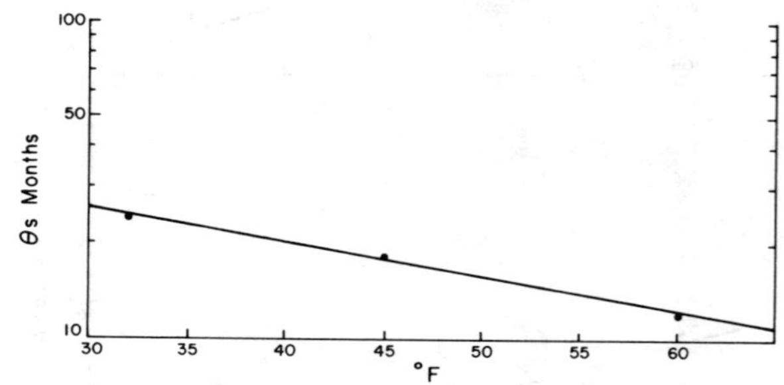

FIG. 13.46.(Top). CORN (SWEET)—TIME TO 10% LOSS OF RIBOFLAVIN
FIG. 13.47.(Bottom). GRAPEFRUIT SEGMENTS—TIME TO 10% LOSS ASCORBIC ACID
(From Kramer 1974)

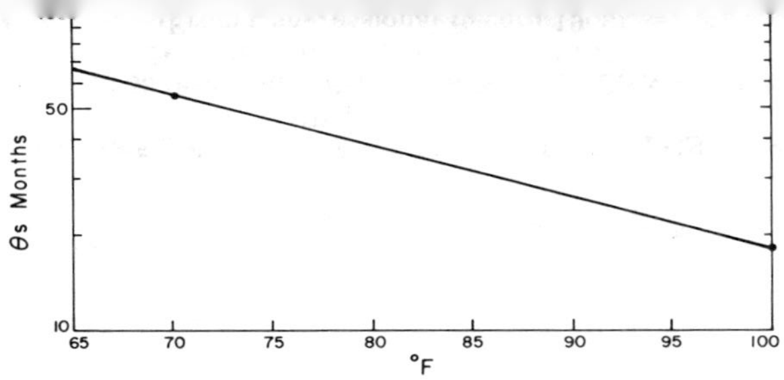

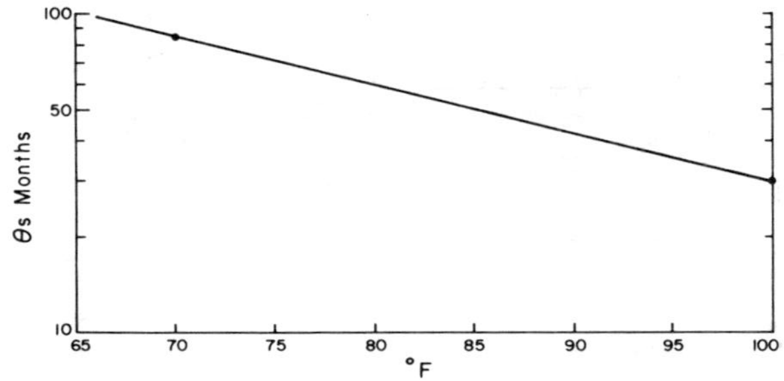

FIG. 13.48.(Top). CORN (WHOLE GRAIN)—TIME TO 50% DEGRADATION OF FLAVOR BASED ON ORGANOLEPTIC RATINGS

FIG. 13.49.(Bottom). TOMATOES—TIME TO 50% DEGRADATION OF FLAVOR BASED ON ORGANOLEPTIC RATINGS

(From Cecil and Woodroof 1963).

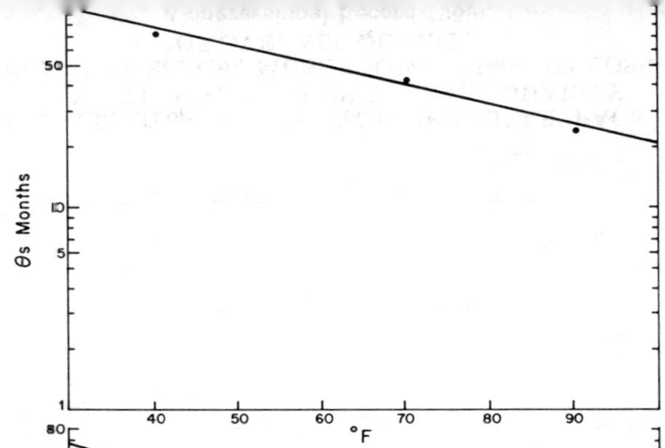

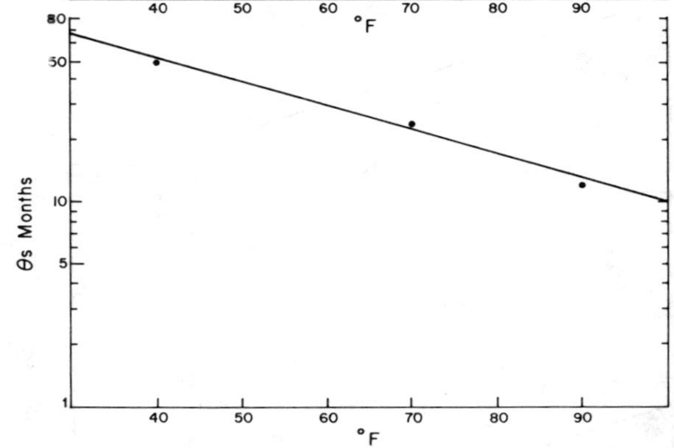

FIG. 13.50.(Top). CORN (CREAM AND WHOLE GRAIN STYLES, CAN)— TIME TO LOSS OF OVERALL QUALITY

FIG. 13.51.(Bottom). CRANBERRY SAUCE—TIME TO LOSS OF OVERALL QUALITY

(From Congressional Record 1969).

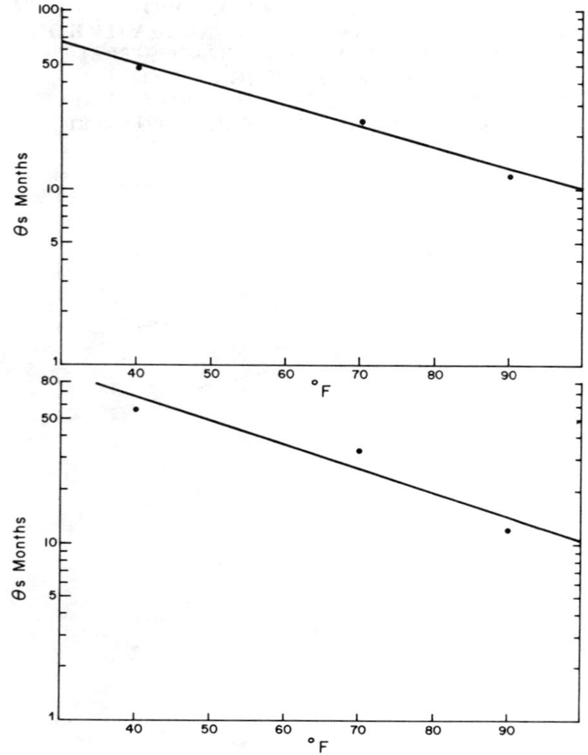

FIG. 13.52.(Top). FIGS (CAN)—TIME TO LOSS OF OVERALL QUALITY
FIG. 13.53.(Bottom). FRUIT COCKTAIL (CAN)—TIME TO LOSS OF OVERALL QUALITY
(From Congressional Record 1969).

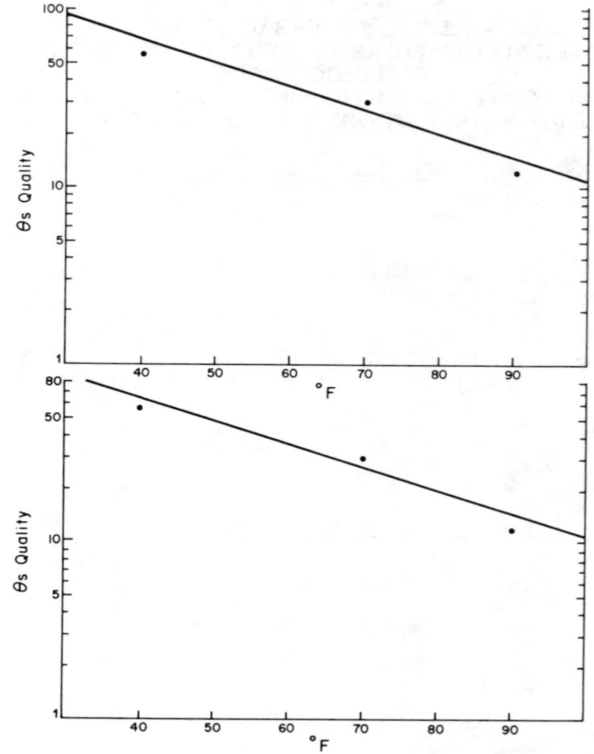

FIG. 13.54.(Top). GRAPEFRUIT (REGULAR PACK, CAN)—TIME TO LOSS OF OVERALL QUALITY
FIG. 13.55.(Bottom). MUSHROOMS—TIME TO LOSS OF OVERALL QUALITY
(Congressional Record 1969).

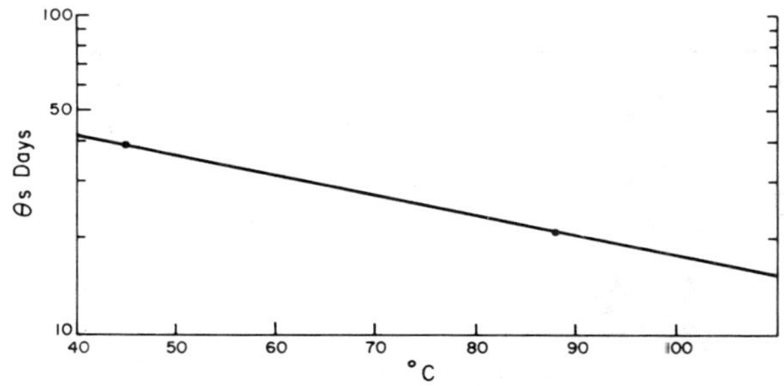

FIG. 13.56. MANGO SQUASH—TIME TO 10% LOSS OF ASCORBIC ACID
(From Sneed and Muvarek 1971).

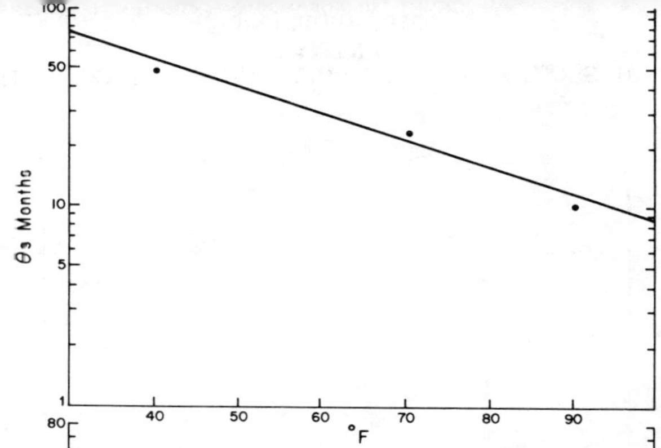

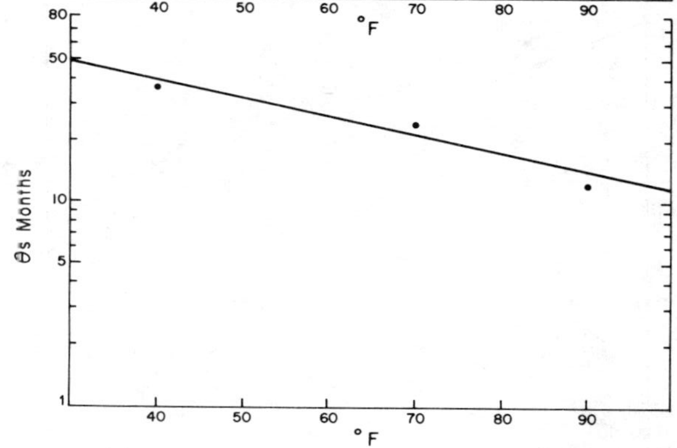

FIG. 13.57.(Top). OKRA (CAN)—TIME TO LOSS OF OVERALL QUALITY
FIG. 13.58.(Bottom). OLIVES (GREEN AND RIPE, CAN)—TIME TO LOSS OF OVERALL QUALITY
(From Congressional Record 1969).

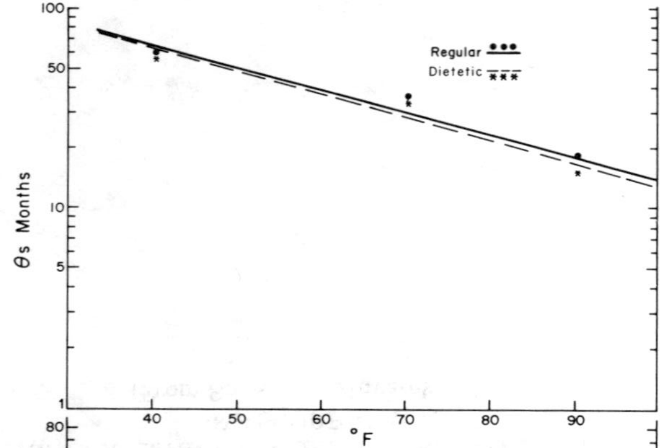

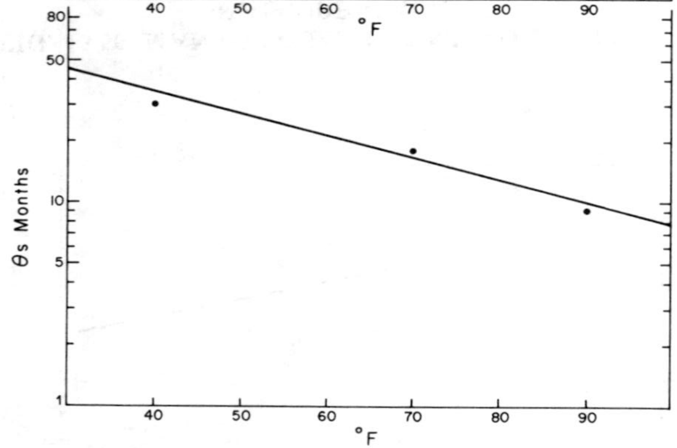

FIG. 13.59.(Top). PEACHES (REGULAR AND DIETETIC PACKS, CAN)—TIME TO LOSS OF OVERALL QUALITY

FIG. 13.60.(Bottom). PEACHES (BABY FOOD STRAINED, JAR)—TIME TO LOSS OF OVERALL

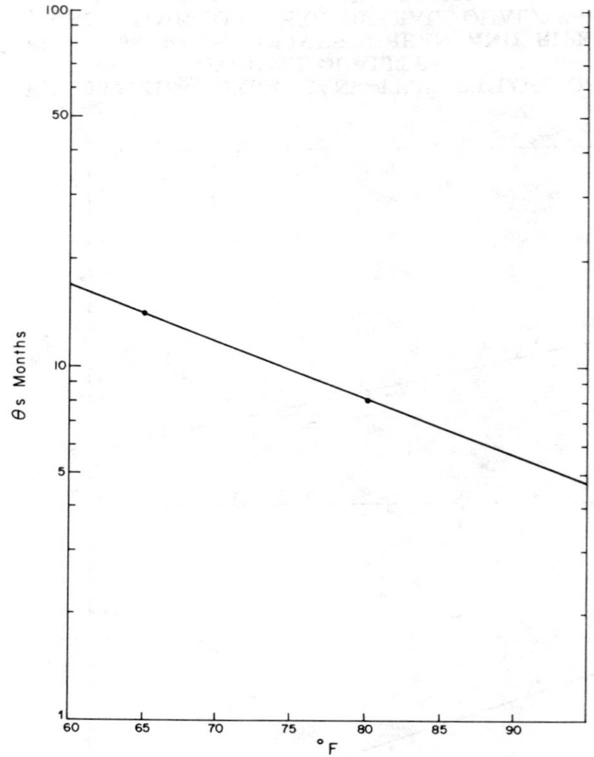

FIG. 13.61. PEACHES (CAN)—TIME TO 20% LOSS OF VITAMIN C
(From Clifcorn 1948).

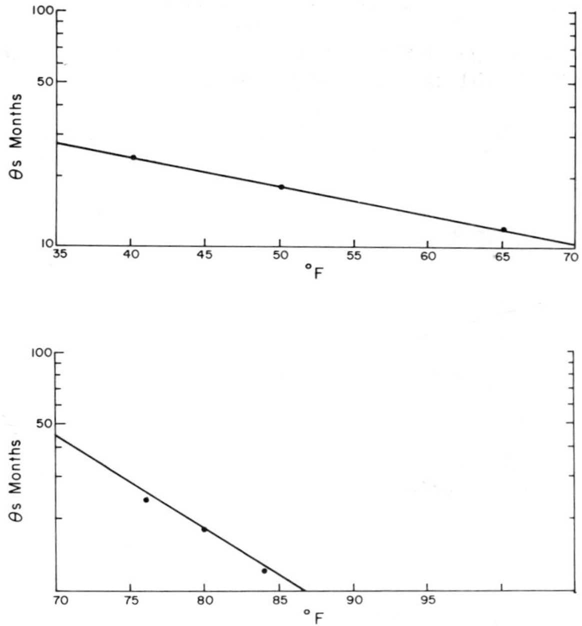

FIG. 13.62.(Top). PEACHES—TIME TO 10% LOSS OF ASCORBIC ACID
FIG. 13.63.(Bottom). PEACHES—TIME TO 10% LOSS OF THIAMIN
(From Kramer 1974).

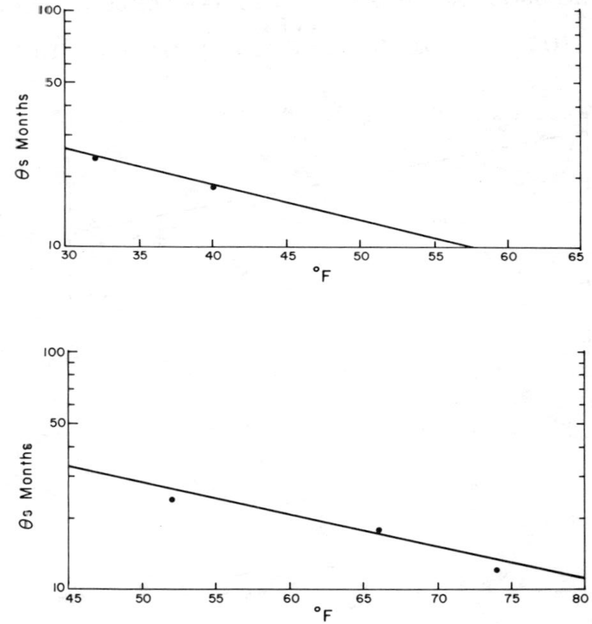

FIG. 13.64.(Top). PEACHES—TIME TO 10% LOSS CAROTENE
FIG. 13.65.(Bottom). PEAS—TIME TO 10% LOSS OF ASCORBIC ACID
(From Kramer 1974).

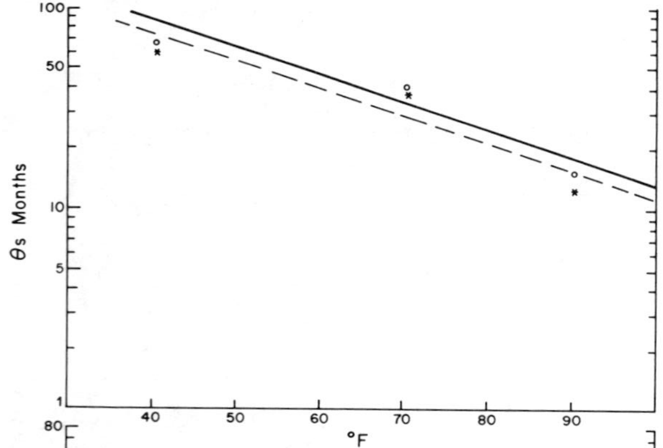

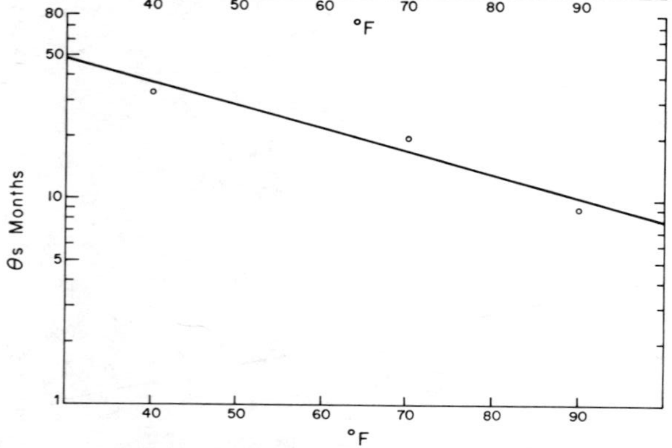

FIG. 13.66.(Top). PEARS (REGULAR AND DIETETIC PACKS, CAN)—TIME TO LOSS OF OVERALL QUALITY

Regular . . . Dietetic* * *

(From Congressional Record 1969).

FIG. 13.67.(Bottom). PEAS AND PEARS (BABY FOOD,

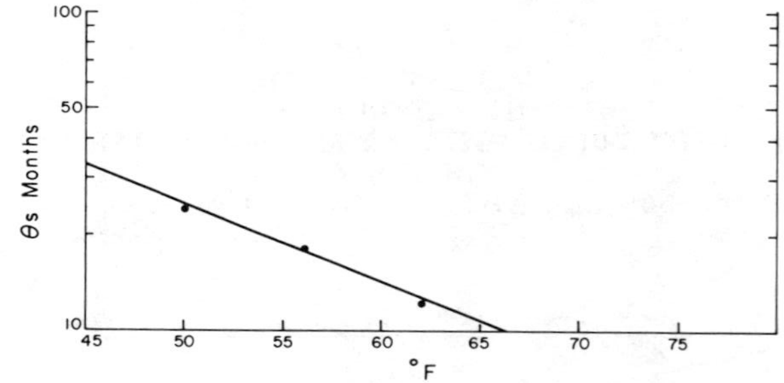

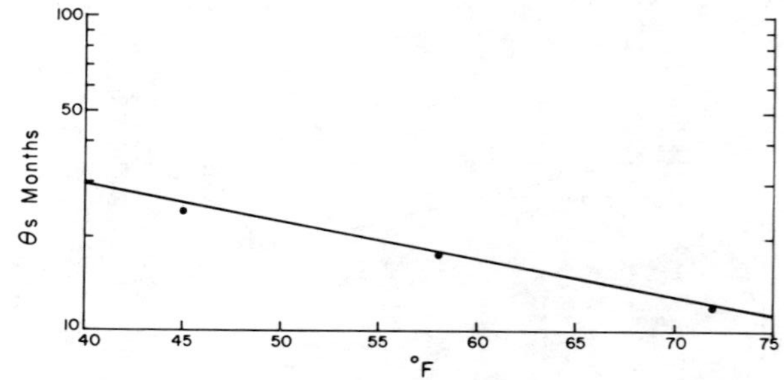

FIG. 13.68.(Top). PEAS—TIME TO 10% LOSS THIAMIN

FIG. 13.69.(Bottom). PEAS—TIME TO 10% LOSS OF CAROTENE

(From Kramer, 1974).

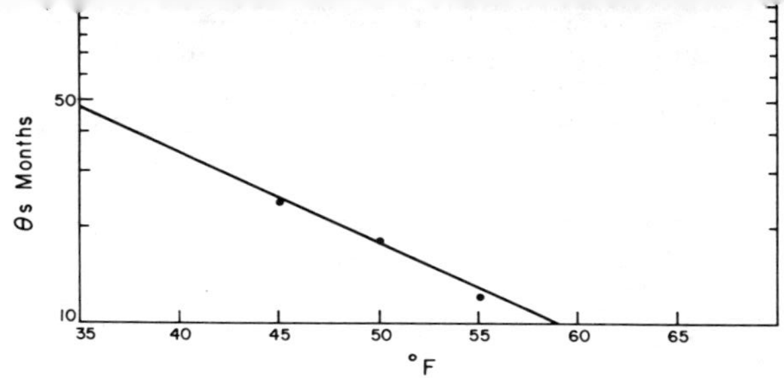

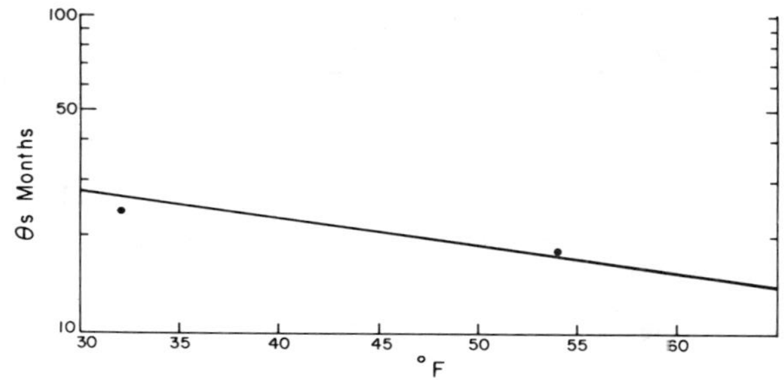

FIG. 13.70.(Top). PEAS—TIME TO 10% LOSS OF RIBOFLAVIN

FIG. 13.71.(Bottom). PINEAPPLE SLICES—TIME TO 10% LOSS OF ASCORBIC ACID.

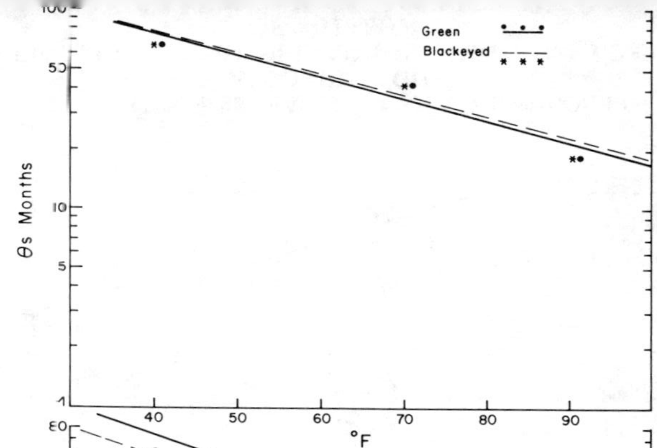

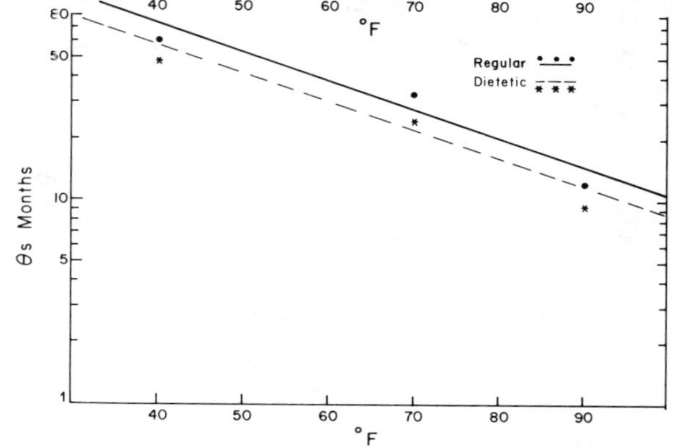

FIG. 13.72.(Top). PEAS (GREEN AND BLACKEYED, CAN)—TIME TO LOSS OF OVERALL QUALITY

FIG. 13.73.(Bottom). PINEAPPLE (REGULAR AND DIETETIC)—TIME TO LOSS OF OVERALL QUALITY

(From Congressional Record 1969).

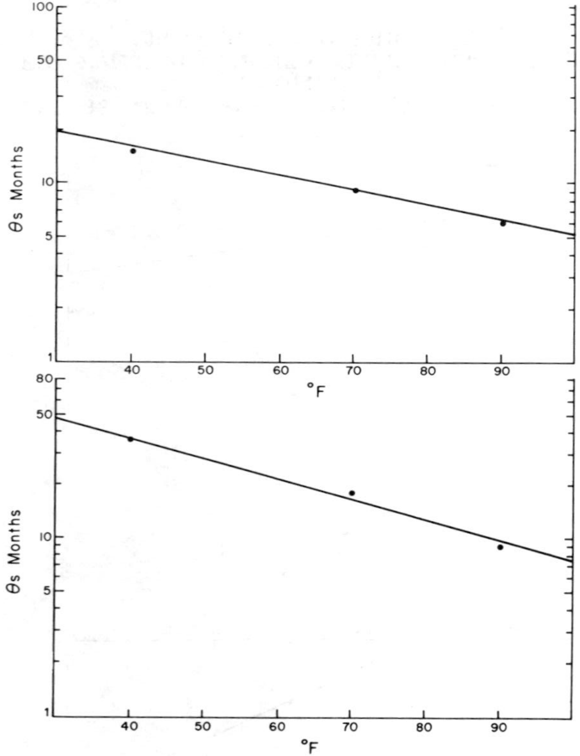

FIG. 13.74.(Top). PRUNES (BABY FOOD, JAR)—TIME TO LOSS OF OVERALL QUALITY
FIG. 13.75.(Bottom). SAUERKRAUT (CAN)—TIME TO LOSS OF TOTAL QUALITY

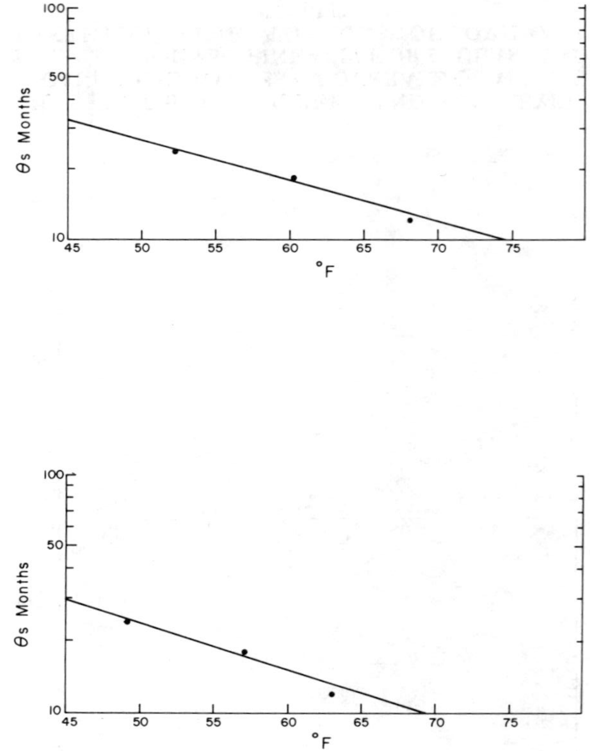

FIG. 13.76.(Top). SPINACH—TIME TO 10% LOSS OF ASCORBIC ACID
FIG. 13.77.(Bottom). SPINACH—TIME TO 10% LOSS OF THIAMIN

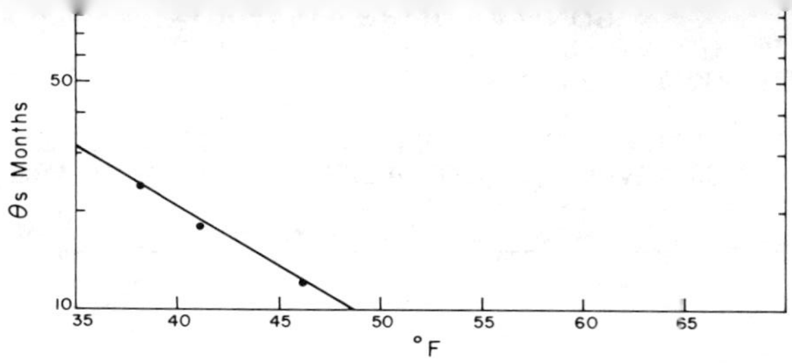

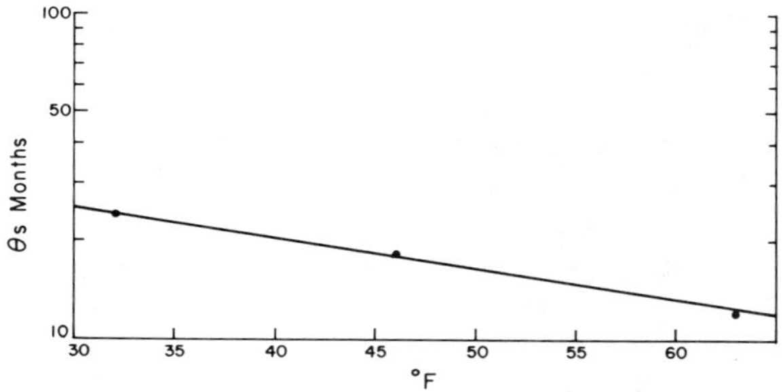

FIG. 13.78.(Top). SPINACH—TIME TO 10% LOSS CAROTENE

FIG. 13.79.(Bottom). SPINACH—TIME TO 10% LOSS RIBOFLAVIN

(From Kramer 1974).

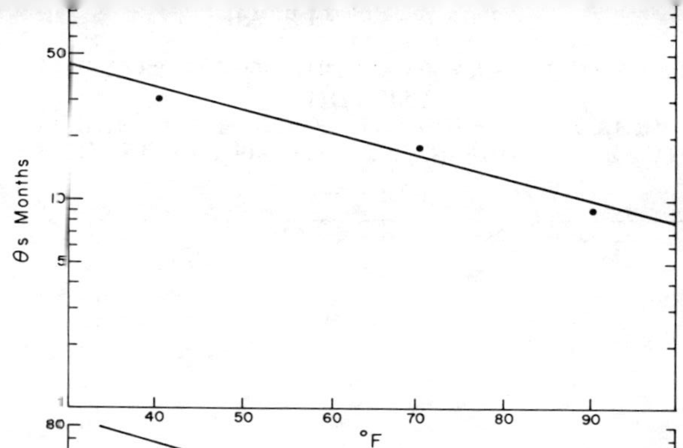

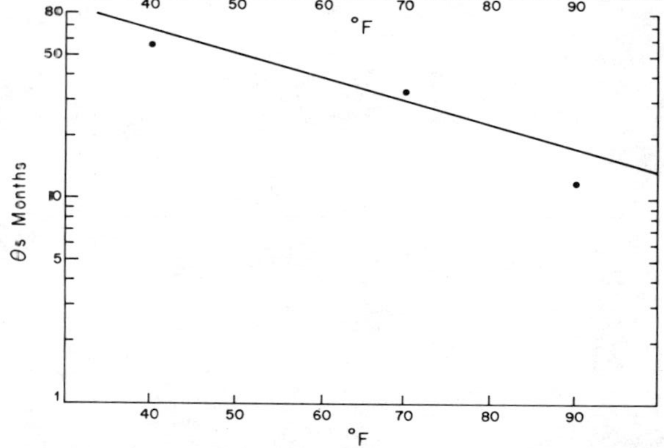

FIG. 13.80.(Top). SPINACH (STRAINED AND JUNIOR BABY FOODS, JAR)—TIME TO LOSS OF OVERALL QUALITY

FIG. 13.81.(Bottom). SPINACH (REGULAR AND PUREE, JAR)— TIME TO LOSS OF OVERALL QUALITY

(From Congressional Record 1969).

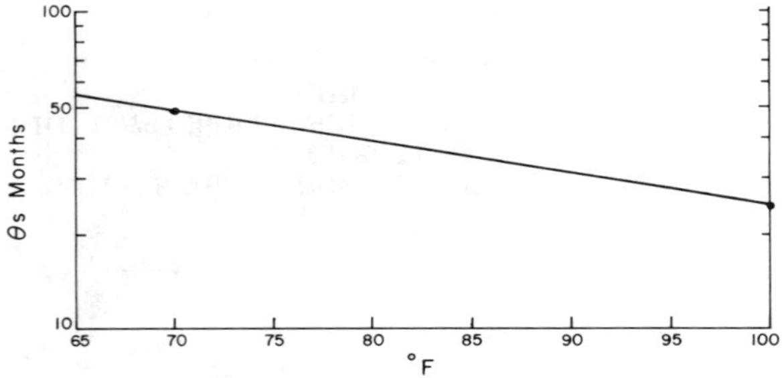

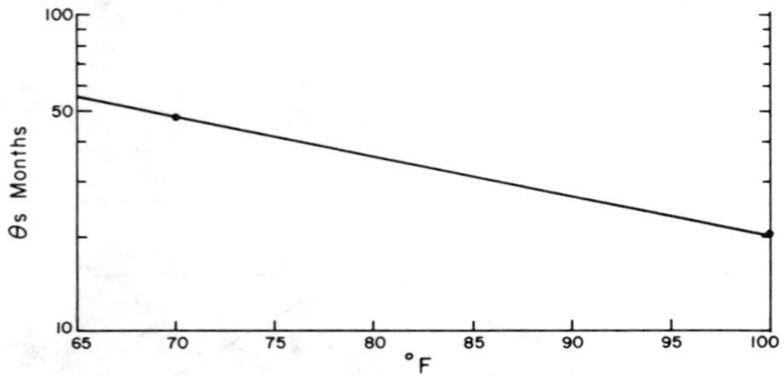

FIG. 13.82.(Top). SUMMER SQUASH—TIME TO 50% DEGRADATION OF TEXTURE BASED ON ORGANOLEPTIC RATINGS

FIG. 13.83.(Bottom). SUMMER SQUASH—TIME TO 50% DEGRADATION OF FLAVOR BASED ON ORGANOLEPTIC RATINGS

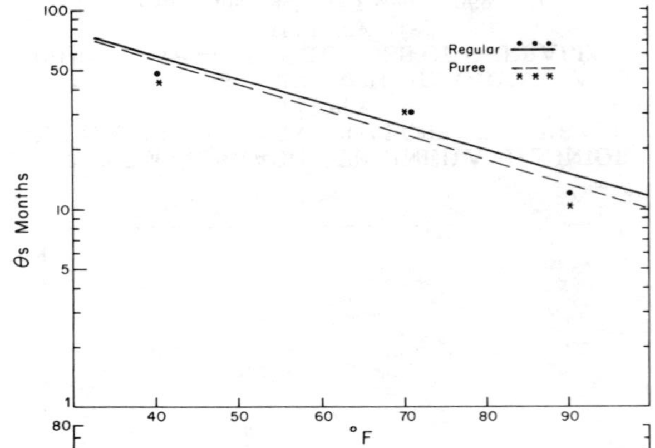

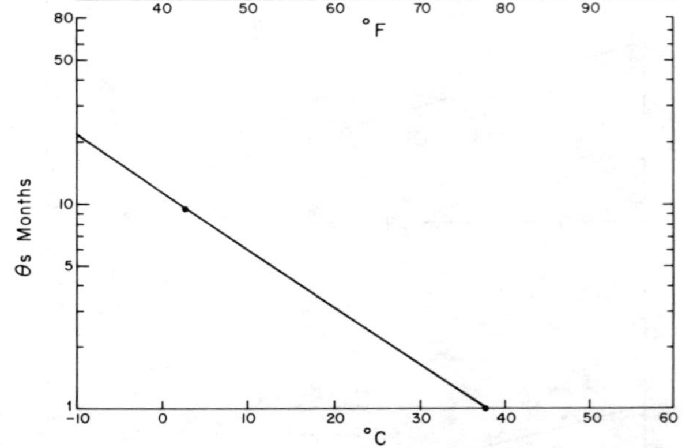

FIG. 13.84.(Top). TOMATOES (REGULAR AND PUREE, CAN)—TIME TO LOSS OF OVERALL QUALITY

FIG. 13.85.(Bottom). GREEN BEANS—TIME TO 20% LOSS THIAMIN

(From Freed *et al.* 1949).

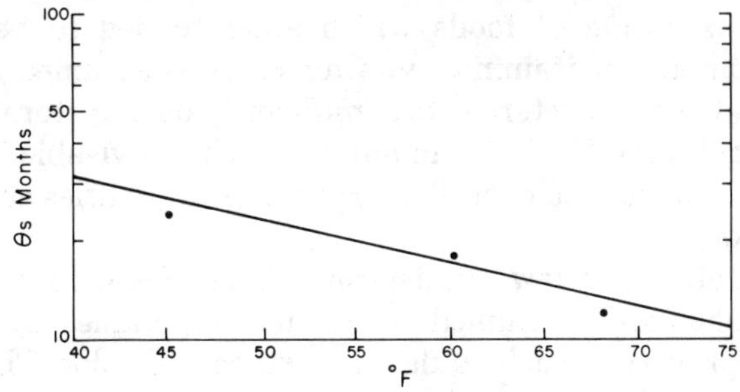

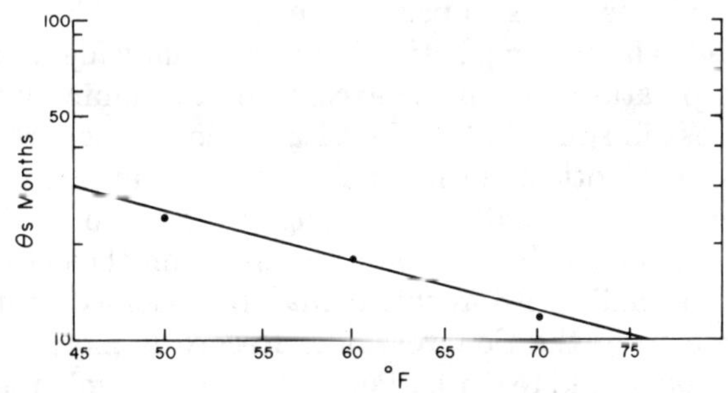

FIG. 13.86.(Top). TOMATOES—TIME TO 10% LOSS OF ASCORBIC ACID
FIG. 13.87.(Bottom). TOMATOES—TIME TO 10% LOSS OF THIAMINE
(From Kramer 1974).

Containers used for canned fruits and vegetables also deteriorate during storage. Corrosive products such as fruits tend to have shorter lives than bland vegetables, due to a more rapid deterioration of tin containers (cans).

Slight imperfections in the double seams of cans can also lead to a loss of vacuum during long term storage. Extremely low temperature storage can also lead to damage of can seams and subsequent loss of vacuum.

It must be remembered that changes in color, flavor and texture may differ in nature depending upon storage temperature, so some changes will occur at a higher temperature and not occur at all at a lower one.

With the exception of foods which are intended to be significant sources of thiamin or vitamin C, vitamins can be assumed to be among the last components to deteriorate significantly during storage of canned fruits and vegetables. With this in mind, it seems advisable to base shelf-life of canned products on overall or organoleptic qualities such as flavor, taste and color.

Unfortunately, very few studies have been found in the literature, which base shelf-life of canned fruits and vegetables specifically on organoleptic properties such as flavor, texture and color. The only other shelf-life data which correspond to this sort of evaluation have been based on overall quality, a rather ill defined term.

The data in Tables 13.3 and 13.4 and Figs. 13.1 to 13.87 summarize data for a number of fruits and vegetables. In considering the data furnished by the Congressional Record, it must be remembered that this information is not based on experimental or actual findings, but upon estimations. This becomes apparent when the shelf-lives of products which differ radically in composition have essentially identical shelf-lives at various temperatures. With the exception of thiamin loss in peaches, and carotene loss in spinach, Q_{10}s for vitamin loss range from 1.3 to 3.1. The Q_{10}s for organoleptic qualities such as flavor and texture range from 1.5 to 1.7. The Q_{10}s for overall quality range from 1.4 to 1.8. Q_{10}s for color and vitamin loss tend to be somewhat higher than those for flavor, texture and overall quality. From this it may be assumed that the overall quality referred to in the Congressional Record is more likely to have been based on flavor and texture than on color or vitamin retention. This may not always be the case, however, as some of the Q_{10}s for vitamin loss fall in the same range as for overall quality.

Products which have a higher Q_{10} for a particular condition, i.e., vitamin loss, color loss or overall quality, will be more temperature sensitive.

Again, it must be remembered that the data for vitamin loss and color, flavor, and texture degradation are based on actual experimental results, while those for overall quality are not.

In some products, vitamin loss seems to occur more rapidly than color, flavor or texture degradation and in other products, it occurs at the same time. This is consistent with the findings of Cecil and Woodroof (1963).

The dependence of the retention of vitamin C, thiamin, and riboflavin in canned fruits and vegetables on the type of container has received the attention of various workers. Andrae (1974) has gone so far as to state that the shelf-life of many canned fruits should be based on the degree of container corrosion in cans.

From Figs 13.1 to 13.87, it is apparent that the shelf-lives for various fruits and vegetables are substantially longer in cans than in jars. Unfortunately, since these results are based on overall quality, it is impossible to state which component is deteriorating more rapidly in the jars. As was stated earlier, color changes and loss of riboflavin tend to occur more rapidly in the presence of light. Browning reactions could also lead to flavor changes.

OPEN DATING BENEFITS VS NONBENEFITS

The National Canners' Association (NCA), which represents the canning industry as a whole, has proposed a system of voluntary open dating for canned foods which would be uniform throughout the United States.

According to the NCA, the date of pack would be the easiest to implement, but would not tell the consumer anything about the shelf-life of the product. Canners who have seasonal packs would be in a difficult position because the date of the cans would seem old when actually the product was still well within the shelf-life for the product. This would be especially true in years when an over-abundant crop would force the canner to sell some product the following year. Since the canning industry usually figures that a three year shelf-life for most fruits and vegetables is the norm, a one year delay would still result in a more than adequate shelf-life for a given product. However, the consumer would have to be convinced of this fact. This would take much time, effort and money. There is also some chance for confusion among consumers who could mistake the "pack date" for a "use by date".

The "sell by date" is not really applicable to canned foods which are often stored in the home for a long period of time after being sold. However, if some system which indicates shelf-life beyond the selling date were indicated, this could be the best system. It would not, however, account for abuse.

The "best if used by" date could be useful to consumers because it would give an idea of the shelf-life of the product if conditions of storage were known or uniform. This would also be useful for rotation of stock at the grocery level. However, with all such dating, the actual end of shelf-life would vary with processing, distribution and home storage conditions. Another useful way to present this information would be to give label information of shelf-life at several temperatures of storage. It is doubtful at the present time if there are sufficient good data for this format, or room on the label. However, since there are data for products at ambient conditions (single temperature), single "date of best quality if used by" could be embossed on the can with or without an explanation of the temperature of storage on which it is based. The canning industry could, however, collect data on each product for each mode of deterioration, estimate time-temperature distributions and then estimate shelf-life left at several home storage conditions. If this is not done, then at least a "pack date" would be useful.

REFERENCES

ADAMS, H.W. and YAWGER, E.S. 1961. Enzyme inactivation and color of processed peas. Food Technol. *15*, 314-317.

ANDRAE, W. 1974. Effect of can materials on the shelf life and storage of stability of canned foods. III. Verpackung. 15(1), 14-16.

BENDIX, G.H., HEBERLEIN, D.G., PTAK, L.R. and CLIFCORN, L.E. 1951. Thiamin destruction in peas, corn, lima beans, and tomato juice from 104.5°C to 132°C. J. Food Sci. *16*, 494-503.

BRENNER, S., WODICKA, B.O. and DUNLOP, S.G. 1948. Effect of high temperature storage on the retention of nutrients in canned foods. Food Technol. *2*, 207-222.

CAIN, R.F. 1967. Water soluble vitamins. Changes during processing and storage of fruits and vegetables. Food Technol. *21*(2), 998-1007.

CAMERON, E.J. 1955. Retention of Nutrients During Canning. Research Laboratories, National Canners' Association, Washington, DC.

CECIL, S.R. and WOODROOF, J.G. 1963. The stability of canned foods in long term storage. Food Technol. *17*, 131-138.

CLIFCORN, L.E. 1948. Factors influencing the vitamin content of canned foods. Advan. Food Res. *1*, 39-104.

CLIFCORN, L.E. and HEBERLEIN, D.G. 1944. Thiamin content of vegetables. Effect of commercial canning. Ind. Eng. Chem. *36*, 168.

CONGRESSIONAL RECORD. 1977. Based on data supplied by the Army, Navy, Marines, Air Force manuals and publications. Depository publication. US-GPO-D-295.

EVERSON, G.J., CHANG, J., LEONARD, S., LUH, B.S. and SIMONE, M. 1964. Aseptic canning of foods. II. Thiamin retention as influenced by processing method, storage time and temperature and type of container. Food Technol. *18*, 84-86.

FARRER, R.T.H. 1955. The thermal destruction of vitamin B_1 in foods. Advan. Food Res. *6*, 257-311.

FEASTER, J.F., TOMPKINS, M.D., and IVES, M. 1948. Retention of vitamins in low acid canned foods. Food Ind. *20*, 14.

FELICIOTTI, E. and ESSELEN, W.B. 1957. Thermal destruction rates of thiamin in pureed meats and vegetables. Food Technol. *11*, 77-84.

FELLERS, C.R., ESSELEN, W.B. and FITZGERALD, G.A. 1940. Vitamin B_1 and Vitamin B_2 content of vegetables as influenced by quick freezing and canning. Food Res. *5*, 495.

FREED, M., BRENNER, S. and WODICKA, V.O. 1949. Prediction of thiamin and ascorbic acid stability in canned foods. Food Technol. *3*, 148.

GOLD, H.J. and WECKEL, K.G. 1959. Degradation of chlorophyll to pheophytin during sterilization of green peas by heat. Food Technol. *13*, 281-286.

GUERRANT, N.B., VAVICH, M.G., FARDIG, O.B., DUTCHER, R.A. and STERN, R.M. 1946. The nutritive value of canned foods. Changes in the vitamin content of foods during canning. J. Nutr. *32*, 435.

GUERRANT, N.B. and O'HARA, M.B. 1953. Vitamin retention in peas after processing in tin and glass. Food Technol. *7*, 473.

GUPTE, S.M., EL-BISI, H.M. and FRANCIS, F.J. 1964. Kinetics of thermal degradation of chlorophyll in spinach puree. J. Food Sci. *29*, 379-382.

HEBERLEIN, D.G., PTAK, L.R., MEDOFF, S. and CLIFCORN, L.E. 1950. Quality and nutritive value of peas as affected by blanching. Food Technol. *4*, 109.

HERRMANN, J. 1970. Calculation of the chemical and sensory alterations in food during heating and storage processes. Ernaehrungsforschung *15*, 279-299.

KRAMER, A. 1974. Storage retention of nutrients. Food Technol. *28*, 50-60.

LENZ, M.K. and LUND, D.B. 1977. The lethality fourier method: Experimental verification of a model for calculating average quality factor retention in conduction heating canned foods. J. Food Sci. *42*(4) 997-1001.

LIVINGSTON, G.E., ESSELEN, W.B. and FELLERS, C.R. 1954. Storage changes in processed applesauce. Food Technol. *8*, 116-120.

LUDIN, A. 1969. Studies on the quality characteristics of canned grapefruit segments. J. Food Technol. *4*(2), 171-177.

LUH, B.S. and WOODROOF, J.G., 1975a, Commercial Vegetable Processing. AVI Publishing Co., Westport, Conn.

LUH, B.S. and WOODROOF, J.G. 1975b. Commercial Fruit Processing. AVI Publishing Co., Westport, Conn.

LUND, D.B. 1975. Effects of blanching, pasteurization, and sterilization on nutrients. In Nutritional Evaluation of Food Processing. R.S. Harris and E. Karmas (Editors). AVI Publishing Co., Westport, Conn.

LUNDE, G., KRINGSTAD, H. and OLSEN, A. 1940. Verhalten des vitamins B_1 beim kochen und konservieren von gemusen. Angew. Chem. *53*, 123 (German).

MULLEY, E.A., STUMBO, L.R. and HUNTING, W.M. 1975. Kinetics of thiamin degradation by heat: A new method for studying reaction rates in model systems and food products. J. Food Sci. *40*, 985-988.

RUTGERS UNIVERSITY. 1971. Food Stability Survey. Rutgers University.

SNEED, A.R. and EL MUVARAK, A. 1971. Technical studies on mango squash. II. Effects of food storage on the shelf life of canned mango squash. Sudan J. Food Technol. *3*, 38-55.

VON ELBE, J., MAING, I.Y. and AMUNDSON, C.H. 1974. J. Food Sci. *39*, 334.

WILLIAMS, M.P. and NELSON, P.E. 1974. Kinetics of the thermal degradation of methyl methionine sulfonium ions in citrate buffers and in sweet corn and tomato serum. J. Food Sci. *39*, 457-460.

WODSAK, W. 1969. Stability of vitamins in vitamin enriched baby foods during storage and preparation. Ernaehr. Umsch. *17*(6) 234-236.

ZHUK, Yu. T. and ROD'KINA, N.A. 1975. Preservation of vitamins during the production of canned mushrooms. Konservn. Ovoshchesush. Prom. No. 12, 21-22.

CHAPTER 14

SHELF-LIFE OF FROZEN FRUITS AND VEGETABLES

INTRODUCTION

Preservation of fruits and vegetables by freezing maintains the most garden-fresh quality of any of the economically feasible approaches. Typically, frozen fruits and vegetables (FFV) are processed through a series of operations: harvesting, post-harvesting handling and/or storage, transport, cleaning, trimming, sizing, sorting, blanching, cooling, freezing and packaging. The initial product quality can be affected by the various processing steps as much as by the quality of the raw material. However, the final product quality is affected by postprocessing handling, storage, and distribution temperatures as well as by thawing and cooking (if it is a vegetable). Quality deterioration of FFV through chemical and physical changes in this distribution can eventually reach the point where the product is no longer acceptable. Proper dating of FFV would give the consumer more information about the expected quality of the FFV at the time of sale or purchase. Dating could also facilitate stock rotation in distribution channels, retail stores, as well as at home. It is the purpose of this chapter to report scientific data regarding the shelf-life of FFV and the problems that may be encountered in open dating of FFV.

FACTORS AFFECTING QUALITY OF FFV

Raw Material

The premium quality of FFV primarily depends on raw material quality. Color, flavor, texture and nutritive value can be genetically controlled to varying degrees and thus certain varieties of a given species are usually more adaptable to freezing. These qualities attributes can be manipulated through plant breeding practices. The quality of fruits and vegetables is also influenced by the type of soil on which they are grown, soil fertility, soil moisture, soil microflora, sunlight, day length, temperature, pollination and cultural practices. This aspect has been described by Olson and Dietrich (1968) and Ponting *et al.* (1968).

Maturity is another factor which drastically affects FFV quality. The ever-increasing trend toward mechanization of fruit and vegetable harvesting has introduced many problems in preparing raw products for freezing. These problems must be considered if uniform quality is to be maintained.

Cooling to remove field heat and proper storage for the short time between harvesting and processing is extremely important. The temperature during this holding period can affect chemical reaction rates and can be extremely detrimental to FFV quality.

Cleaning, sizing, trimming, reducing microbial load, and removing foreign material and minimizing product variation are all essential steps in producing clean and wholesome FFV products.

Processing

Most vegetables are blanched (a short heat treatment) to inactivate some enzymes, affect color, soften texture, and reduce microbial population. Time-temperature control in blanching is critical to provide sufficient protection against enzymatic deterioration for prolonged subsequent storage at subfreezing temperature. However, the heat treatment must be kept to a minimum to reduce quality loss. The adequacy of blanching is judged with the peroxidase test (Masure and Campbell 1944). Underblanching will result in undesirable enzymatic changes, drastically shortening the shelf-life of FFV products. Over-blanching, on the other hand, can result in leaching of soluble nutrients, destruction of heat labile vitamins, poor color and poor texture. Immediate cooling following blanching also minimizes further quality loss. Loss of nutrients during blanching and cooling is reviewed by Fennema (1975). Summarized data are shown in Table 14.1.

The flavor and color of most frozen concentrated fruit juices is adversely affected by heat during concentration. Modern technology permits better flavor retention through low temperature evaporation and through techniques such as "cut-back" and "stripping". Color can be controlled by blending. Color loss in juice concentration during heating was investigated by Ponting *et al.* (1960).

The freezing rate is the major processing factor influencing the extent of textural damage. Rapid freezing results in less damage to texture than slow freezing. However, the final texture of FFV is not solely a function of freezing rate but also depends on the storage condition, packaging and thawing method. The loss of vitamins during freezing per se is negligible. The holding time between the end of blanching and freezing, used in the commercial situation for grading, packaging and handling of the products before freezing, is much more damaging to the product quality than the actual freezing.

TABLE 14.1
LOSS OF VITAMINS C AND B_1 FROM VEGETABLES DURING BLANCHING AND COOLING

Product	Mean % (Range) Loss of Vitamin C	Loss of Vitamin B_1
Asparagus	10 (6—15)	
Beans, green	23 (12—42)	9 (0—14)
Beans, lima	24 (19—40)	36 (20—76)
Broccoli	36 (12—50)	
Brussels sprouts	22 (21—25)	
Cauliflower	20 (18—25)	
Peas, green	21 (1—35)	11 (3—23)
Spinach	50 (40—76)	60 (41—80)

From Fennema (1975).

Postprocessing Distribution and Storage

The rate of quality deterioration during frozen storage depends primarily on the temperature and the type of product. The mode of failure or type of change may include loss of palatability and nutritive value. Microbiological spoilage is not likely to be a problem in FFV if the product is stored at -18°C or below. In fact, the microbial population will gradually decline, especially that of gram-negative bacteria during subfreezing storage. People eat fruits and vegetables for pleasure and as a source of vitamin C and minerals. Therefore, the loss of palatability (color, flavor and texture) and vitamin C degradation are the two main concerns in determining the shelf-life of FFV. Other changes, such as protein degradation, which is of concern in meats and dairy products, are not of interest to the consumer of FFV.

The types of changes that may affect FFV quality are chlorophyll degradation, ascorbic acid oxidation, off-flavor development, lipid autoxidation, loss of characteristic volatile flavor compounds, gellation in concentrated juice product, loss of cloud in juice, crystallization of solute, volume change, recrystallization (or package ice formation), freezer burn (or surface dehydration), separation of meta-cryotic liquid, and cellular structure breakdown (or loss of crispiness). The effects of desiccation can cause a loss of as much as one-fifth of the weight of frozen green beans, corn, spinach and peas during a storage period of one year at —18°C. This will result in evident changes in appearance but has little or no effect on palatability (including surface appearance) or nutritive value (ascorbic acid and carotene) of the cooked product (Volz *et al.* 1949). Surface dehydration of FFV without adequate packaging protection may advance to a stage where objectionable color, textural changes as well as a dry appearance are developed.

In today's market many FFV are packed in lightweight waxed boxes which are over-wrapped with heavier weight waxed paper. Other popular retail packages are the poly-bag and the boil-in-pouch made of plastic material which prevent most moisture loss. Retail packages are then packed in corrugated cartons for easy handling. Bulk storage of individual quick frozen (IQF) FFV items is commonly done in plastic film-lined tote bins that hold up to a ton.

FFV are usually stored in the producer's warehouse at a temperature of −18 °C or below and a relative humidity of about 90%. Poor sanitation and odor control in the freezer could cause quality failures of stored FFV. Excess air circulation is avoided by stacking in solid piles to reduce moisture loss and possible oxidation. FFV are mainly transported with trailers, piggyback rail trucks and mechanical refrigerator rail cars. Loading and unloading are usually carried out with the aid of a fork-lift and should be done as fast as possible to reduce quality loss. Thawing due to mishandling is extremely detrimental to quality, and furthermore, may lead to growth of pathogens. Automatic temperature controls, air circulation systems, a self-contained power supply and efficient heat insulation are necessary for both the stationary freezer warehouse and the mobile shipping vehicle.

When FFV reach the marketplace, they are often further kept in a wholesale freezer warehouse and then shipped to the retail supermarket in trucks. In the retail store, FFV are displayed in a frozen cabinet for sale. For maximum convenience an air-screened, fully displayed, automatic defrosting frozen cabinet is commonly used and inevitable temperature fluctuations occur. Mishandling at the retail stage is quite common, especially on the loading dock and in over-filled cabinets.

Home Handling and Consumption

Fully processed FFV have an initial nutrient concentration or quality level which is predetermined by the raw material and by the various processing variables and distribution conditions to which they have been subjected. The quality loss following freezing is a function of time and temperature. For FFV, temperature is the most important factor due to the large Q_{10}, as will be evident in later discussion. In addition, textural change in FFV is influenced by temperature fluctuations rather than by temperature per se. Most quality losses in FFV follow a pattern predictable by zero order kinetics. The rate of these changes is independent of the initial value, but varies with different temperatures. Transporting FFV from the retail frozen cabinet to home freezer often elevates product temperature and can result in a great amount of quality loss. Thawing and cooking methods (for vegetables) used by the consumer can also be one of the most serious factors affecting FFV quality.

SHELF-LIFE OF FFV

Shelf-life is a rather ill-defined term that frequently confuses the consumer, as well as the food researcher. Some investigators assume that shelf-life ends when it is possible to detect a "just noticeable difference" (JND) in the quality of the food product, as compared to a control product. Others may define shelf-life in terms of the time that the product will remain acceptable, which could be substantially longer than the JND shelf-life. Another term used is "practical storage life" (PSL) or the length of time the product will remain acceptable to the consumer. High quality life (HQL) is also used. HQL is defined as the storage time at which 70% of taste testers in a triangle test correctly indicate a quality difference(s) between a control and stored FFV samples. PSL of FFV is about 3.1 to 3.5 times longer than HQL, as has been determined by the Refrigeration Research Foundation (Information Bulletin No. 73-1, 1971). This ratio varies for different foods and storage temperatures.

Nutritional value can also be used as an index of the end of shelf-life. Ascorbic acid, an unstable vitamin, is commonly used for this purpose. Other vitamins are generally stable at low temperatures.

Literature data regarding FFV shelf-life may, therefore, vary considerably, not only because different definitions of shelf-life are used, but also as the result of initial varietal differences of products, preparation method (e.g., thawing method is poorly specified), type (e.g., whole vs sliced) of product, size of package (bulk vs retail), and poor experimental control, which can even given contradictory data. Such questionable data were excluded from this report to avoid confusion.

Another problem is that a good deal of the data on the shelf-life of FFV have been generated only at a single storage temperature (Table 14.2). These data have little use in shelf-life prediction or open dating of FFV. Other over-simplified or generalized data (Table 14.3) may only have very limited value.

Vegetables

Asparagus: Van Arsdel *et al.* (1969) reported the approximate storage life in months of frozen asparagus: 4—6 (at —12 °C), 8—12 (at —18 °C) and 16—18 (at —23 °C); See Fig. 14.1. Kramer (1974) summarized the shelf-life data based on Shepherd (1960), Davis (1958), DuBois and Kew (1951), and Huggart *et al.* (1954), and indicated:

(1) The shelf-life in months (sensory quality) was 6 (at 0 °F), 12 (at —5 °F), 18 (at —8 °F) and 24 (at —12 °F); see Fig. 14.2.

(2) The shelf-life in months (10% ascorbic acid loss) was 12 (at 0 °F), 18 (15 —2 °F), 24 (at —2 °F); see Fig. 14.3.

TABLE 14.2
STORAGE LIFE OF FFV AT −18°C OR BELOW[1]

Product	Approximate Storage Life (Months)
Apples	18
Apple juice, concentrated	30
Asparagus	10
Blackberries	18
Blueberries	18
Boysenberries	18
Broccoli	14
Brussels sprouts	11
Carrots	24
Cauliflower	14
Cherries	24
Corn	24
Corn on the cob	9
Dates	12
Grape juice, concentrated	24
Grapefruit juice, concentrated	24
Grapefruit/orange juice, concentrated	24
Grapefruit sections	12
Greens, leafy	14
Lemon juice, concentrated	18
Lime juice, concentrated	18
Lime juice, single strength	18
Okra	12
Orange juice, concentrated	24
Peaches	18
Peas, black eyed	12
Peas, green	14
Peas and carrots	14
Pineapple	12
Pineapple juice, concentrated	24
Potatoes, white, French fried	12
Spinach	14
Squash, summer	24
Strawberries	18
Succotash	12
Vegetables, mixed	10

[1]From the Technical Manual for Storage and Material Handling for Department of the Army — A Congressional Record.

TABLE 14.3
TIME-TEMPERATURE COMBINATIONS WHICH CAUSE EQUIVALENT QUALITY CHANGES IN SOME FROZEN VEGETABLES AND FRUITS[1]

Temperature (°F)	Sensitive Type	Other Type
0	1 year	1 year
5	5 months	5 months
10	6 weeks	2 months
15	3 weeks	1 month
20	1 week	2 weeks
25	2 days	1 week
30	1 day	3 days

[1]Guadagni (1968)

(3) The shelf-life in months (25% ascorbic acid loss) was 6 (at 7 °F), 12 (at 3 °F), 18 (at 0 °F) and 24 (at —1 °F); see Fig. 14.4.

(4) The shelf-life in months (50% ascorbic acid loss) was 6 (at 8 °F), 12 (at 4 °F), 18 (at 2 °F), and 24 (at 0 °F); see Fig. 14.5.

Jenkins *et al.* (1940) reported shelf-life in months based on 10% loss of ascorbic acid: 5.4 (at —20 °F), 3.2 (at 0 °F), 2.1 (at 10 °F) and 1.7 (at 16 °F); see Fig. 14.6.

Beans, Lima: — Van Arsdel *et al.* (1969) reported the approximate storage life in months: 6—8 (at —12 °C), 14—16 (at —18 °C) and 24 (at —23 °C); see Fig. 14.7. Kramer (1974) indicated:

(1) The shelf-life in months (sensory quality): 6 (at 4 °F), 12 (at —3 °F), 18 (at —6 °F) and 24 (at —8 °F); see Fig. 14.8.

(2) The shelf-life in months (10% ascorbic acid loss): 6 (at 5 °F), 12 (at 5 °F), 18 (at 2 °F) and 24 (at 0 °F); see Fig. 14.9.

(3) The shelf-life in months (25% ascorbic acid loss): 12 (at 5 °F), 18 (at 2 °F) and 24 (at 0 °F); see Fig. 14.10.

(4) The shelf-life in months (50% ascorbic acid loss): 6 (at 20 °F), 12 (at 9 °F), 18 (at 5 °F) and 234 (at 2 °F); see Fig. 14.11.

Beans, Snap: — Van Arsdel *et al.* (1969) reported the approximate storage life in months: 4—6 (at —12 °C), 8—12 (at —18 °C) and 16—18 (at —23 °C); See Fig. 14.12. Derse and Tepley (1958) studied French cut green beans and found:

(1) The shelf-life in months (25% ascorbic acid loss): 2.1(—18 °C) and 1.2 (at 7 °C); see Fig. 14.13.

(2) The shelf-life in months (25% carotene loss): 3.7 (at —18 °C) and 2.2 (at —7 °C); see Fig. 14.14.

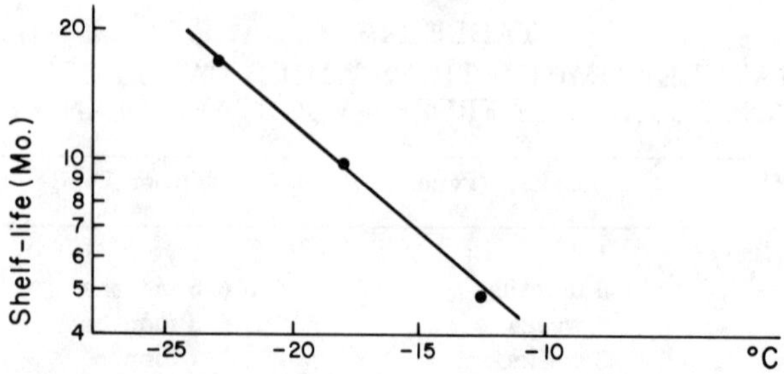

14.1

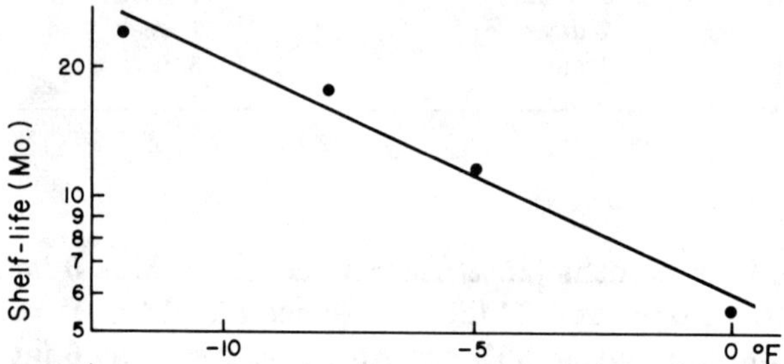

14.2

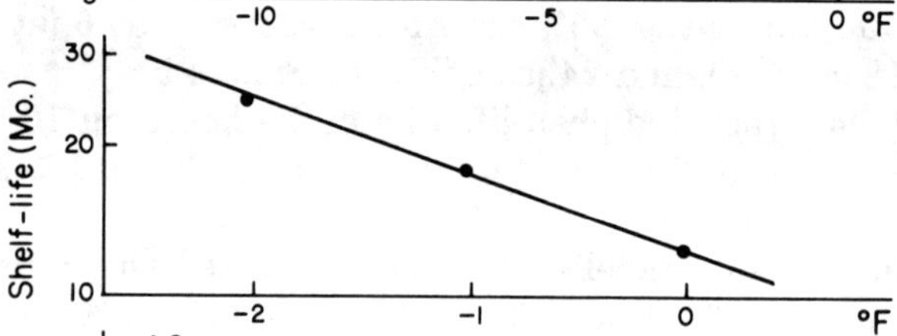

14.3

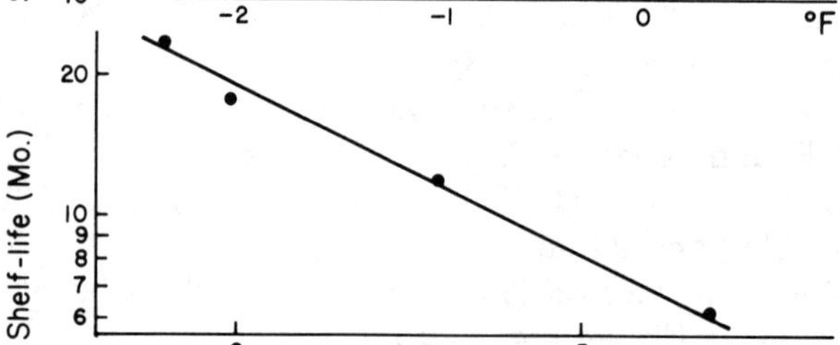

14.4

FIG. 14.1. APPROXIMATE STORAGE LIFE OF FROZEN ASPARAGUS
(From Van Arsdel *et al.* 1969).

FIG. 14.2. SENSORY QUALITY OF FROZEN ASPARAGUS
(From Kramer 1974).

FIG. 14.3. 10% ASCORBIC ACID LOSS IN FROZEN ASPARAGUS
(From Kramer 1974).

FIG. 14.4. 25% ASCORBIC ACID LOSS IN FROZEN ASPARAGUS
(From Kramer 1974).

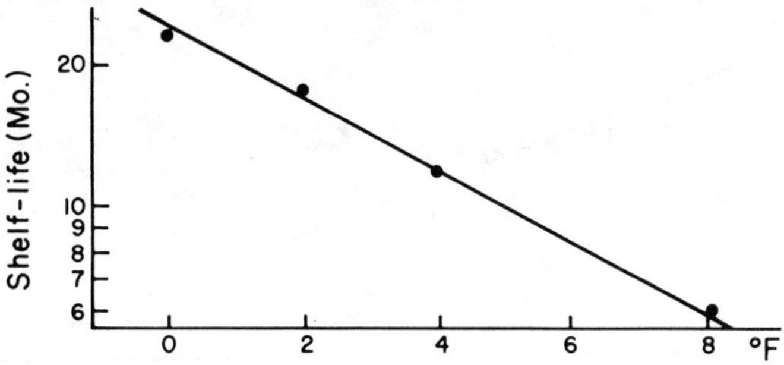

14.5

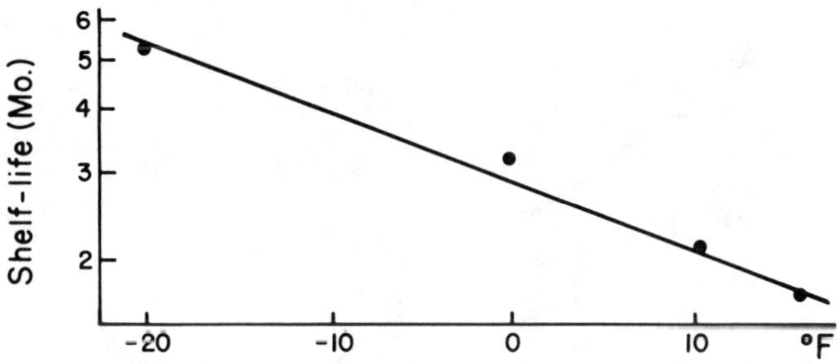

14.6

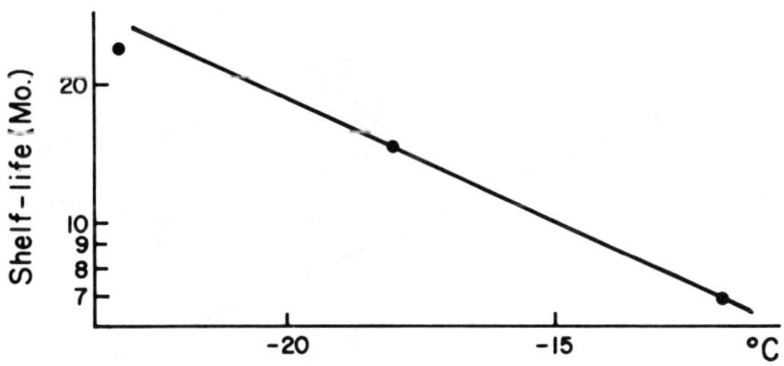

14.7

FIG. 14.5. 50% ASCORBIC ACID LOSS IN FROZEN ASPARAGUS (From Kramer 1974).

FIG. 14.6. 10% ASCORBIC ACID LOSS IN FROZEN ASPARAGUS (From Jenkins *et al.* 1940).

FIG. 14.7. APPROXIMATE STORAGE LIFE OF FROZEN LIMA BEANS (From Van Arsdel *et al.* 1969).

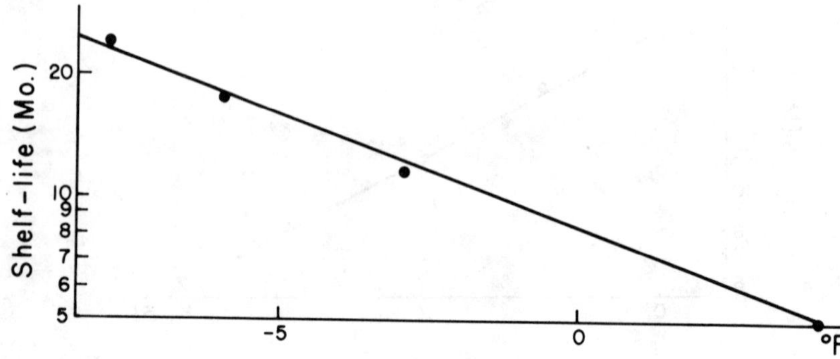

14.8

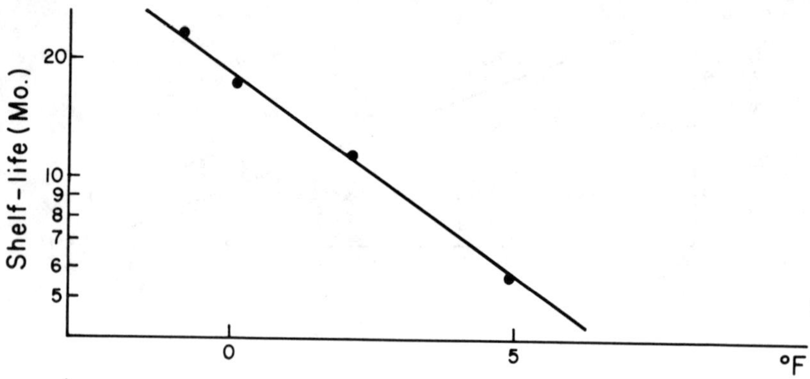

14.9

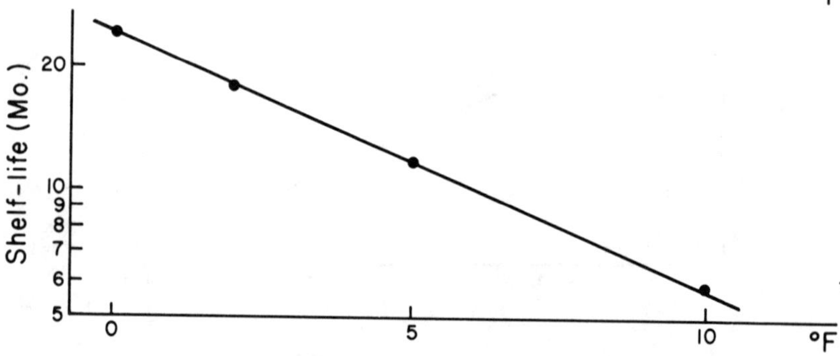

14.10

FIG. 14.8. SENSORY QUALITY OF FROZEN LIMA BEANS (From Kramer 1974).

FIG. 14.9. 10% ASCORBIC ACID LOSS IN FROZEN LIMA BEANS (From Kramer 1974).

FIG. 14.10. 25% ASCORBIC ACID LOSS IN FROZEN LIMA BEANS (From Kramer 1974).

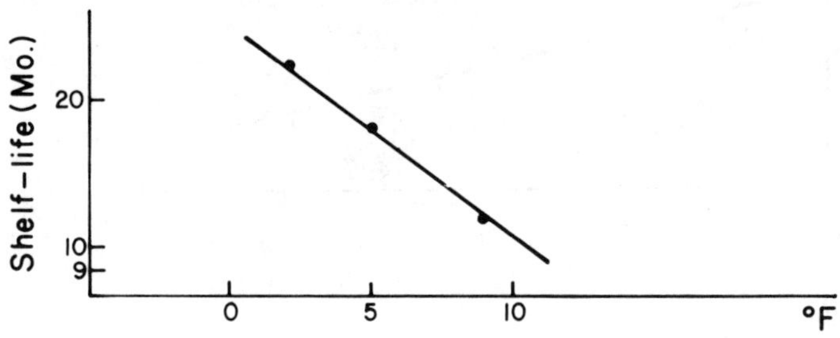

14.11

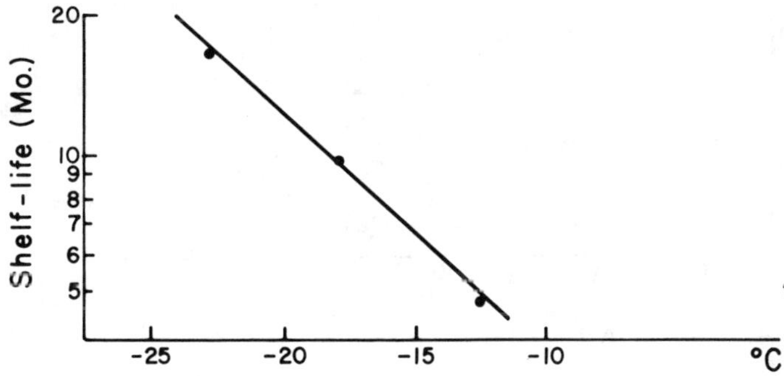

14.12

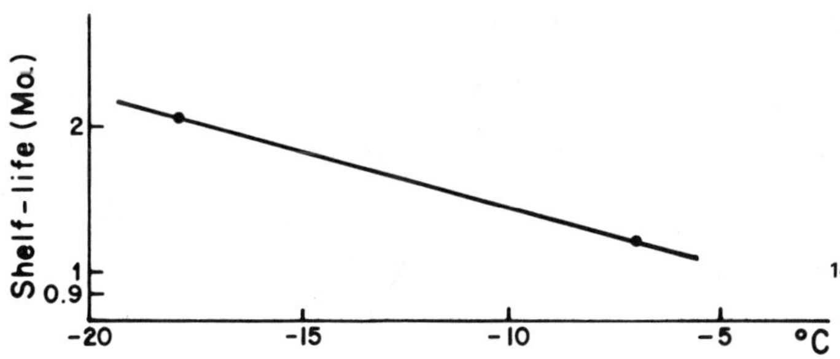

14.13

FIG. 14.11. 50% ASCORBIC ACID LOSS IN FROZEN LIMA BEANS
(From Kramer 1974).

FIG. 14.12. APPROXIMATE STORAGE LIFE OF FROZEN SNAP BEANS
(From Van Arsdel *et al.* 1969).

FIG. 14.13. 25% ASCORBIC ACID LOSS IN FROZEN SNAP BEANS
(From Derse and Teply 1958).

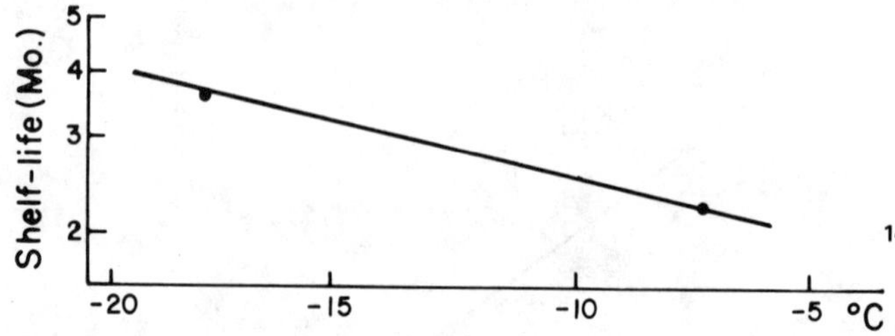

14.14

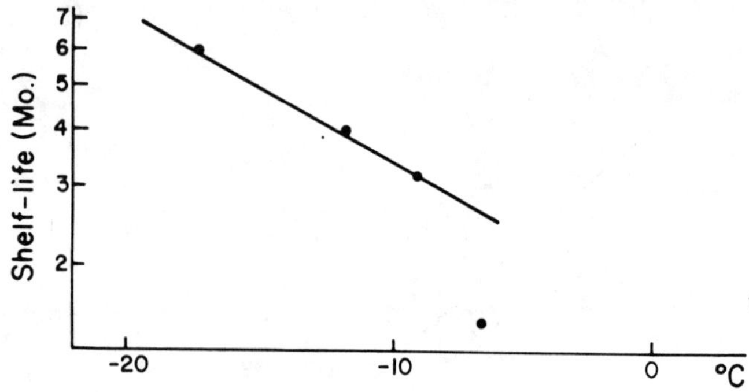

14.15

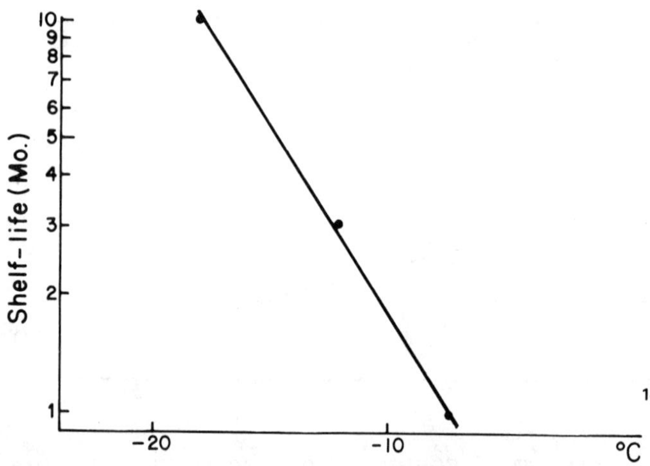

14.16

FIG. 14.14. 25% CAROTENE LOSS IN FROZEN SNAP BEANS (From Derse and Topley 1958).

FIG. 14.15. VITAMIN C DEGRADATION IN FROZEN SNAP BEANS (From Jurics 1970).

FIG. 14.16. FLAVOR DIFFERENCE SHELF-LIFE IN FROZEN SNAP BEANS (From Dietrich *et al.* 1959).

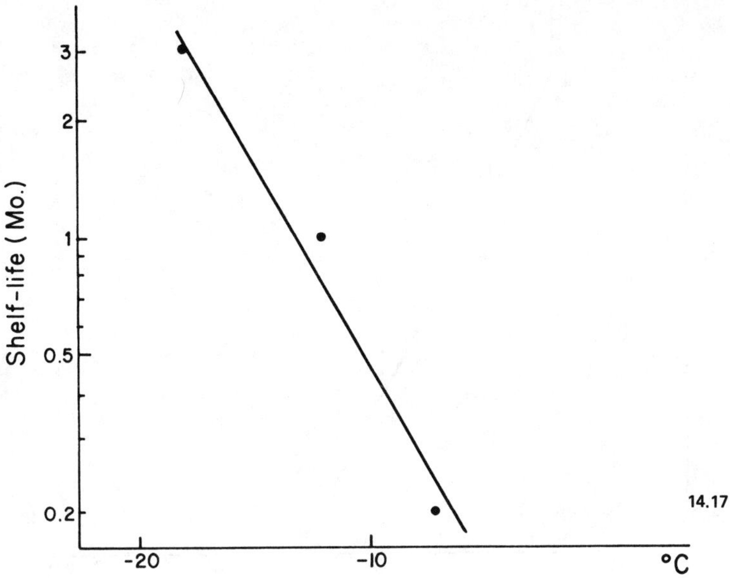

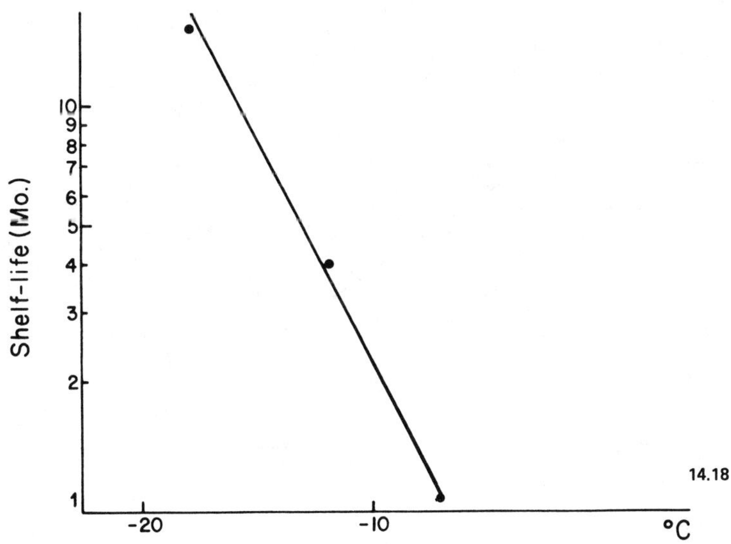

FIG. 14.17. COLOR DIFFERENCE SHELF-LIFE IN FROZEN SNAP BEANS (From Dietrich *et al.* 1959).

FIG. 14.18. 50% ASCORBIC ACID LOSS IN FROZEN SNAP BEANS (From Dietrich *et al.* 1959).

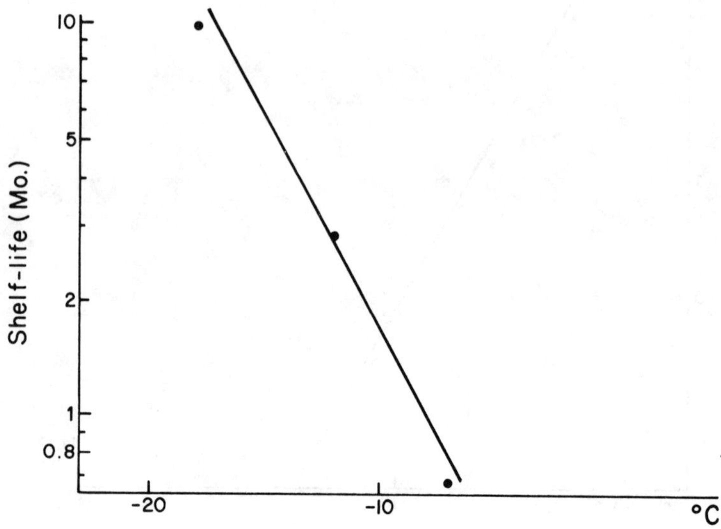

14.19

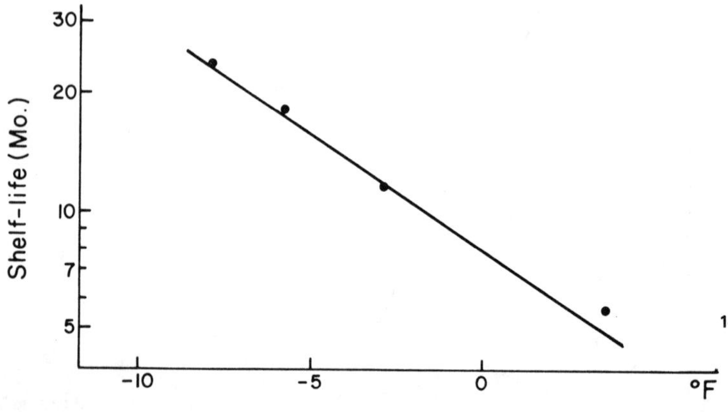

14.20

FIG. 14.19. 10% CHLOROPHYLL LOSS IN FROZEN SNAP BEANS
(From Dietrich *et al.* 1959).

FIG. 14.20. 10% ASCORBIC ACID LOSS IN FROZEN SNAP BEANS
(From Kramer 1974).

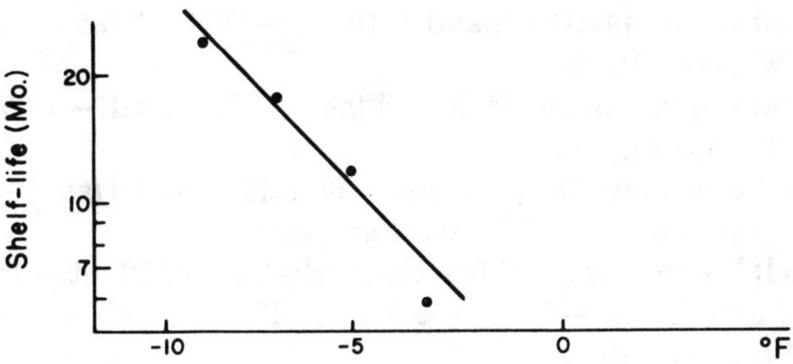

14.21

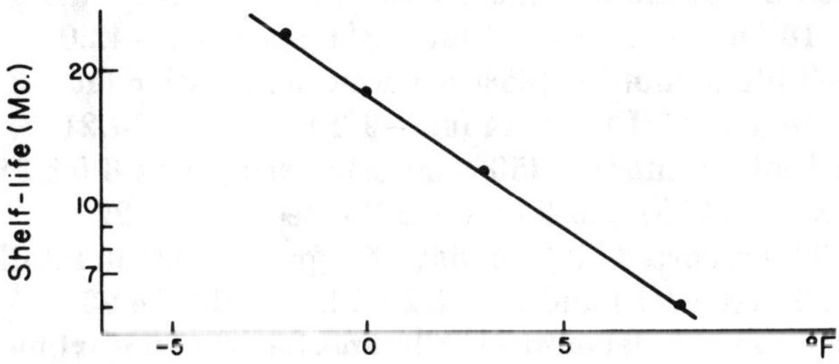

14.22

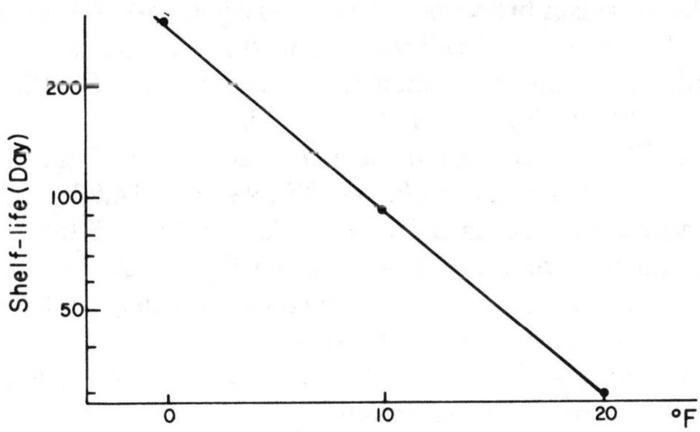

14.23

FIG. 14.21. 25% ASCORBIC ACID LOSS IN FROZEN SNAP BEANS
(From Kramer 1974).

FIG. 14.22. 50% ASCORBIC ACID LOSS IN FROZEN SNAP BEANS
(From Kramer 1974).

FIG 14.23. HIGH QUALITY LIFE OF FROZEN BEANS
(From Guadagni 1968).

Jurics (1970) showed shelf-life in months (vitamin C degradation): 3 (at −9 °C), 4 (at −12 °C) and 6 (at −18 °C); see Fig. 14.15. Dietrich *et al.* (1959) reported:

(1) The shelf-life in months (flavor): 10 (at −18 °C), 3 (at −12 °C) and 1 (at −7 °C); see Fig. 14.16.
(2) The shelf-life in months (color): 3 (at −18 °C), 1 (at −12 °C) and 0.2 (at −7 °C); see Fig. 14.17.
(3) The shelf-life in months (50% ascorbic acid loss); 16 (at −18 °C), 4 (at −12 °C) and 1.0 (at −7 °C); see Fig. 14.18.
(4) The shelf-life in months (10% chlorophyll loss): 10 (at −18 °C), 3 (at −12 °C) and 0.7 (at −7 °C); see Fig. 14.19.

Kramer (1974) reported:

(1) The shelf-life in months (10% ascorbic acid loss): 6 (at 4 °F), 12 (at −3 °F), 18 (at −6 °F) and 24 (at −8 °F); see Fig. 14.20.
(2) The shelf-life in months (25% ascorbic acid loss); 6 (at −3 °F), 12 (at −5 °F), 18 (at −7 °F) and 24 (at −9 °F); see Fig. 14.21.
(3) The shelf-life in months (50% ascorbic acid loss): 6 (at 3 °F), 12 (at 0 °F), 18 (at −7 °F) and 24 (at −9 °F); see Fig. 14.22.

Guadagni (1968) reported HQL in days for green beans in retail package: 296 (at 0 °F), 94 (at 10 °F) and 30 (at 20 °F); see Fig. 14.23.

Broccoli: — Van Arsdel *et al.* (1969) reported the approximate storage life in months of frozen broccoli: 6—8 (at −12 °C), 14—16 (at −18 °C) and 24 (at −23 °C); see Fig. 14.24. Kramer (1974) indicated:

(1) The shelf-life in months (sensory quality): 6 (at 0 °F), 12 (at −5 °F), 18 (at −8 °F) and 24 (at −12 °F); see Fig. 14.25.
(2) The shelf-life in months (10% ascorbic acid loss); 6 (at 6 °F), 12 (at 0 °F), 18 (at −1 °F), and 24 (at −2 °F); see Fig. 14.26.
(3) The shelf-life in months (25% ascorbic acid loss); 6 (at 7 °F), 12 (at 3 °F), 18 (at 0 °F) and 24 (at −1 °F); see Fig. 14.27.
(4) The shelf-life in months (50% ascorbic acid loss); 6 (at 9 °F), 12 (at 7 °F), 18 (at 4 °F) and 24 (0 °F); see Fig. 14.28.

Brussels sprouts: — Van Arsdel *et al.* (1969) reported approximate storage life in months of frozen brussels sprouts: 4—6 (at −12 °C), 8—12 (at −18 °C) and 16—18 (at −23 °C); see Fig. 14.29.

Carrots: Van Arsdel *et al.* (1969) reported approximate storage life in months of frozen carrots: 12 (at −12 °C), 24 (at −18 °C) and 236 (at −23 °C); see Fig. 14.30.

Cauliflower: Van Arsdel *et al.* (1969) reported approximate storage life in months: 6—8 (at −12 °C), 14—16 (at −18 °C) and 24 (at 23 °C); see Fig. 14.31. Bennet *et al.* (1954), Dietrich *et al.* (1957) and Jenkins *et al.* (1940) studied vitamin C degradation in frozen cauliflower and reported shelf-life in months: 2 (at −7 °C), 3 (at −9 °C), 4 (at −12 °C) and 6 (at −18 °C); see Fig. 14.32. Dietrich *et al.* (1962) reported months required to reach a

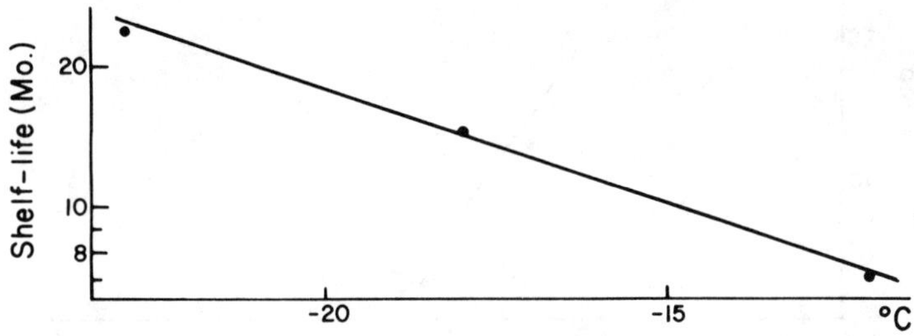

14.24

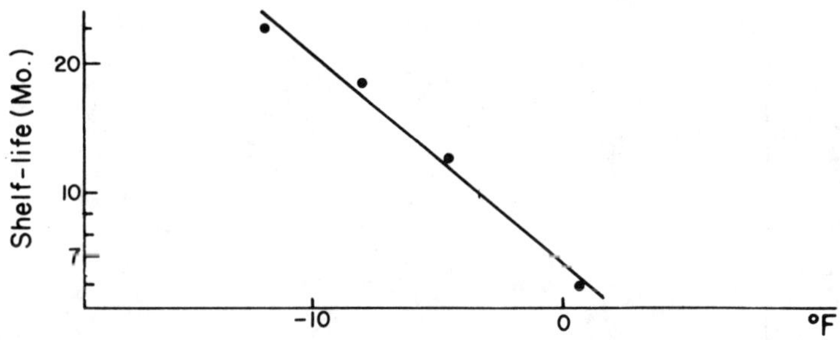

14.25

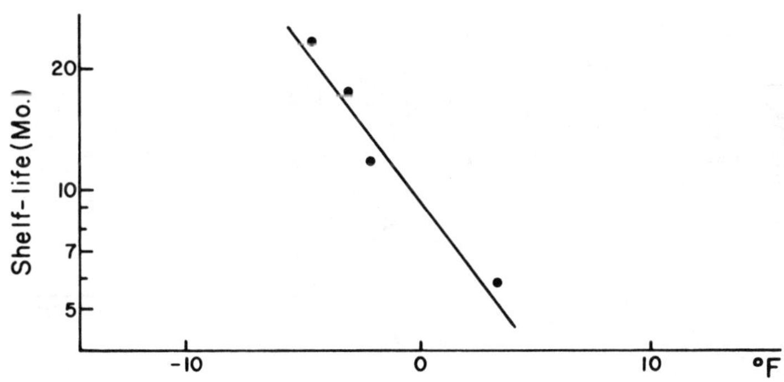

14.26

FIG. 14.24. APPROXIMATE STORAGE LIFE OF FROZEN BROCCOLI (From Van Arsdel *et al.* 1969).

FIG. 14.25. SENSORY QUALITY OF FROZEN BROCCOLI (From Kramer 1974).

FIG. 14.26. 10% ASCORBIC ACID LOSS IN FROZEN BROCCOLI (From Kramer 1974).

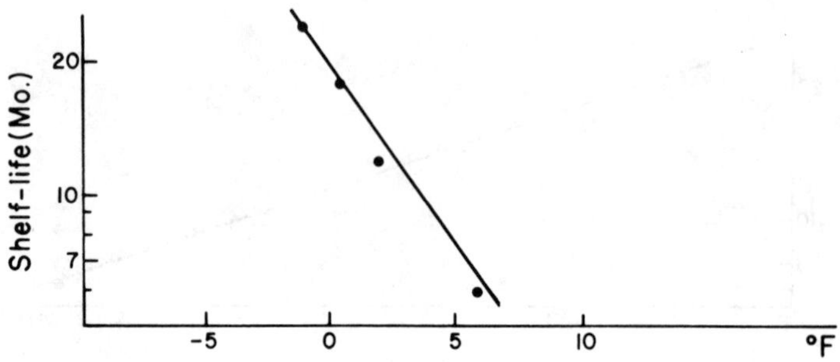

14.27

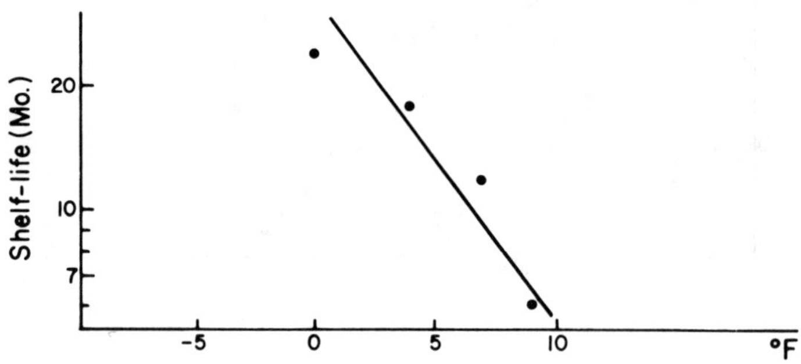

14.28

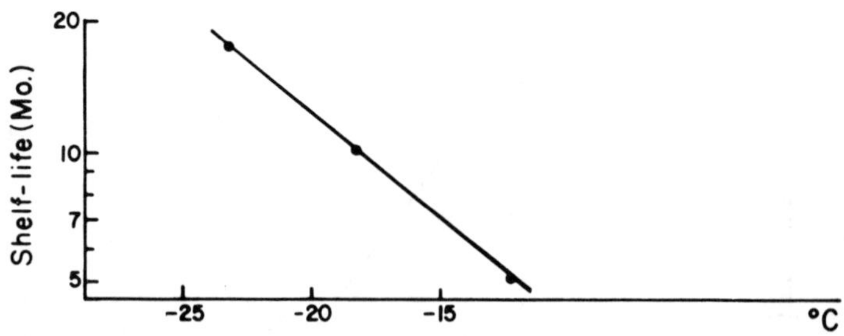

14.29

FIG. 14.27. 25% ASCORBIC ACID LOSS IN FROZEN BROCCOLI (From Kramer 1974).

FIG. 14.28. 50% ASCORBIC ACID LOSS IN FROZEN BROCCOLI (From Kramer 1974).

FIG. 14.29. APPROXIMATE STORAGE LIFE OF FROZEN BRUSSEL SPROUTS (From Van Arsdel *et al.* 1969).

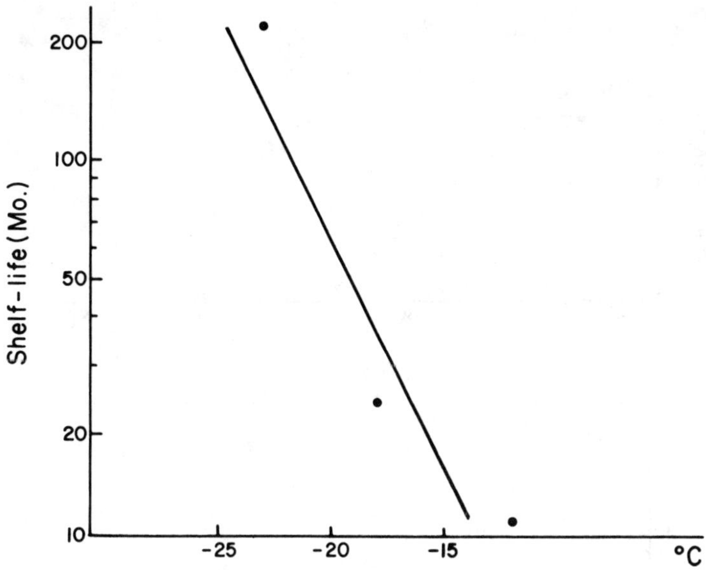

14.30

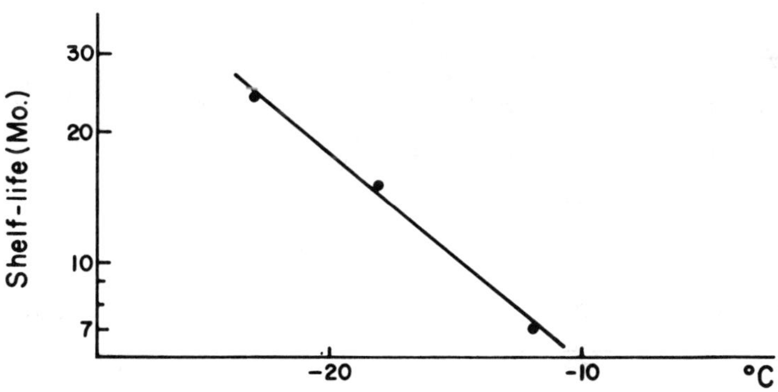

14.31

FIG. 14.30. APPROXIMATE STORAGE LIFE OF FROZEN CARROTS
(From Van Arsdel *et al.* 1969).

FIG. 14.31. APPROXIMATE STORAGE LIFE OF FROZEN CAULIFLOWER
(From Van Arsdel *et al.* 1969).

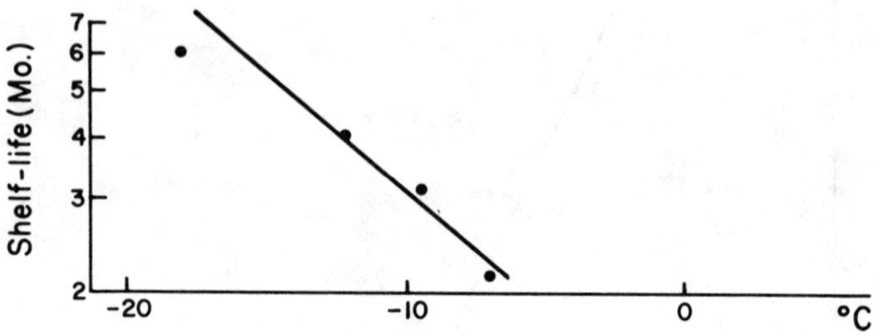

14.32

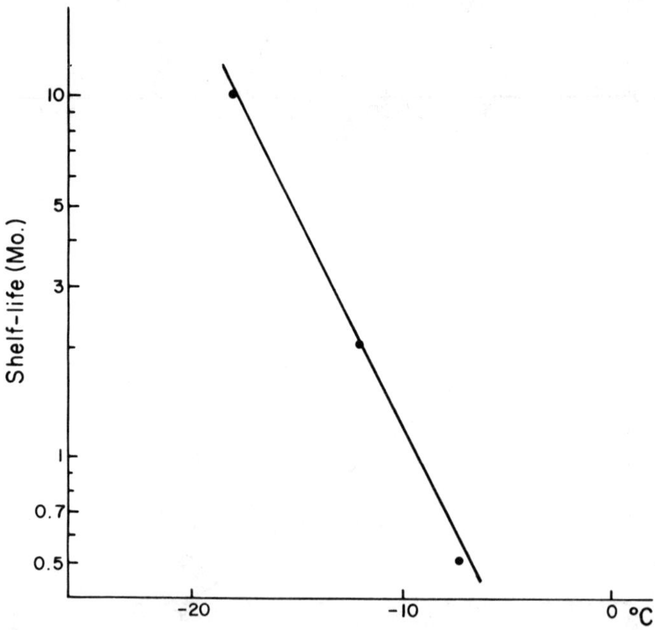

14.33

FIG. 14.32. VITAMIN C DEGRADATION IN FROZEN CAULIFLOWER
(From Bennet *et al.* 1954; Dietrich *et al.* 1957; and Jenkins *et al.* 1940).

FIG. 14.33. PERCEPTIBLE FLAVOR DIFFERENCE IN FROZEN CAULIFLOWER
(From Dietrich *et al.* 1962).

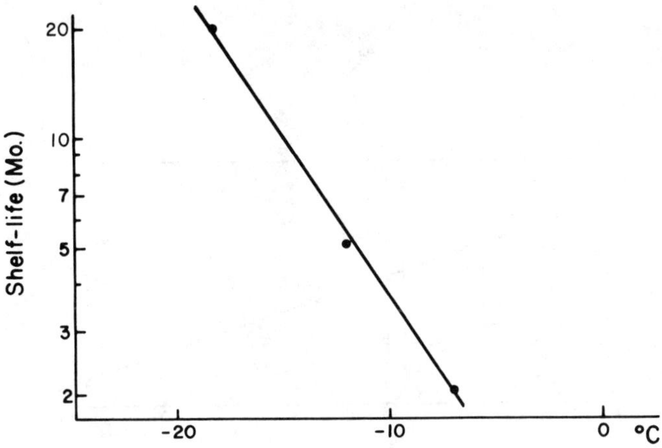

14.34

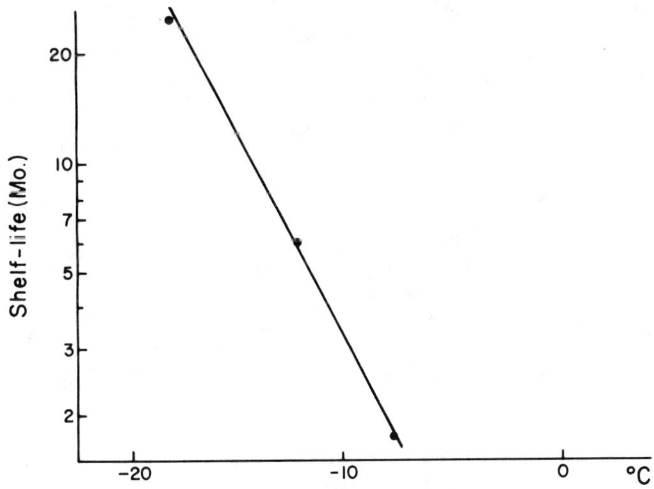

14.35

FIG. 14.34. PERCEPTIVE COLOR DIFFERENCE IN FROZEN CAULIFLOWER
(From Dietrich *et al.* 1962).

FIG. 14.35. 50% VITAMIN C LOSS IN FROZEN CAULIFLOWER
(From Dietrich *et al.* 1962).

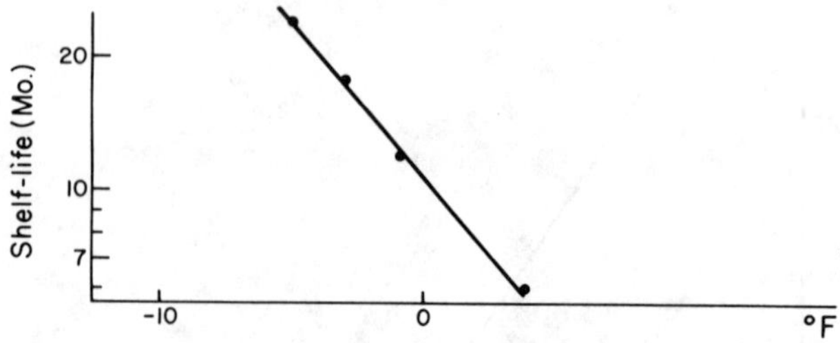

14.36

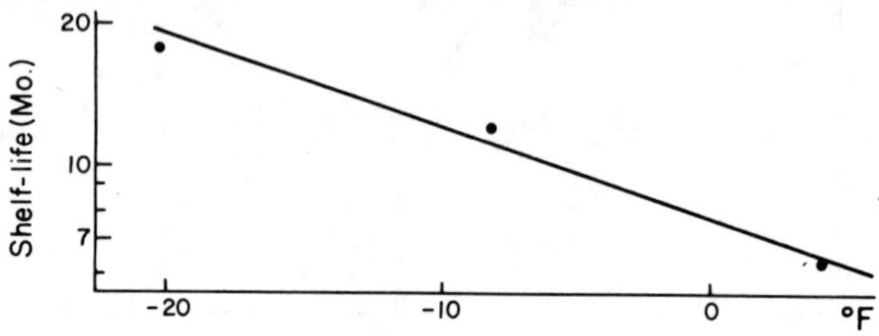

14.37

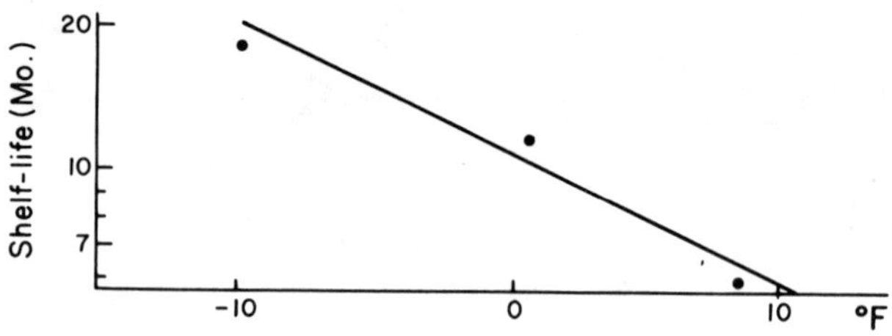

14.38

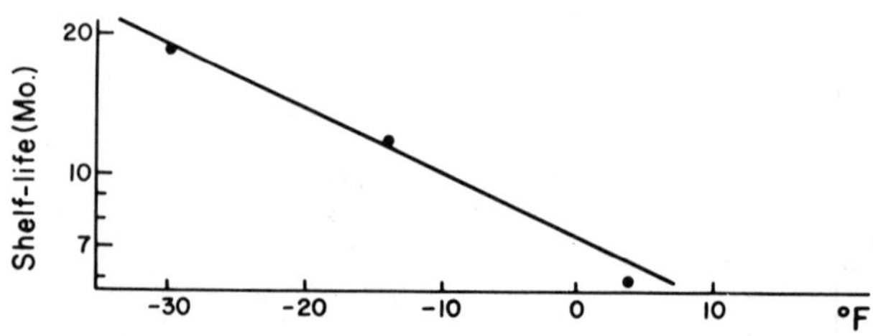

14.39

FIG. 14.36. SENSORY QUALITY IN FROZEN CAULIFLOWER (From Kramer 1974).

FIG. 14.37. 10% ASCORBIC ACID LOSS IN FROZEN CAULIFLOWER (From Kramer 1974).

FIG. 14.38. 25% ASCORBIC ACID LOSS IN FROZEN CAULIFLOWER (From Kramer 1974).

FIG. 14.39. 50% ASCORBIC ACID LOSS IN FROZEN CAULIFLOWER (From Kramer 1974).

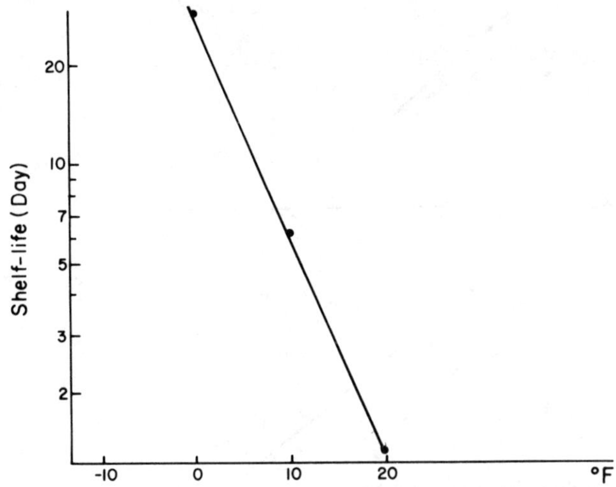

14.40

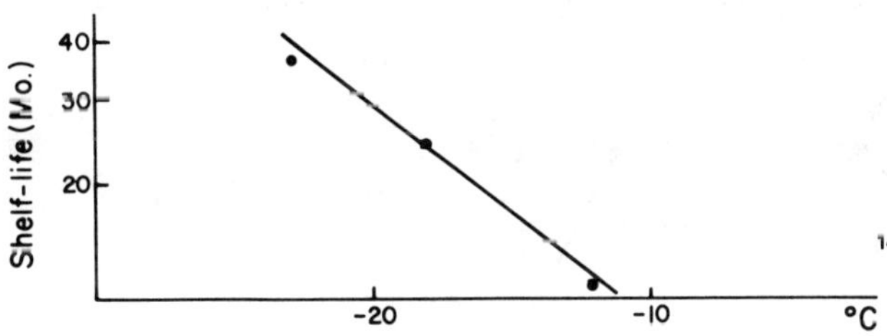

14.41

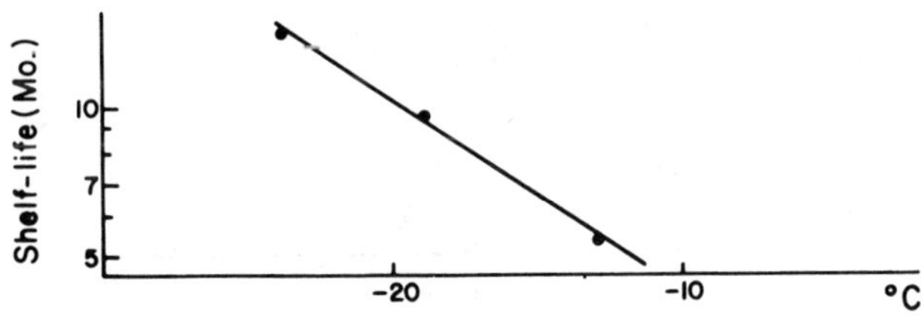

14.42

FIG. 14.40. HIGH QUALITY LIFE OF FROZEN CAULIFLOWER
(From Guadagni 1968).

FIG. 14.41. APPROXIMATE STORAGE LIFE OF FROZEN CUT CORN
(From Van Arsdel *et al.* 1969).

FIG. 14.42. APPROXIMATE STORAGE LIFE OF FROZEN CORN ON THE COB
(From Van Arsdel *et al.* 1969).

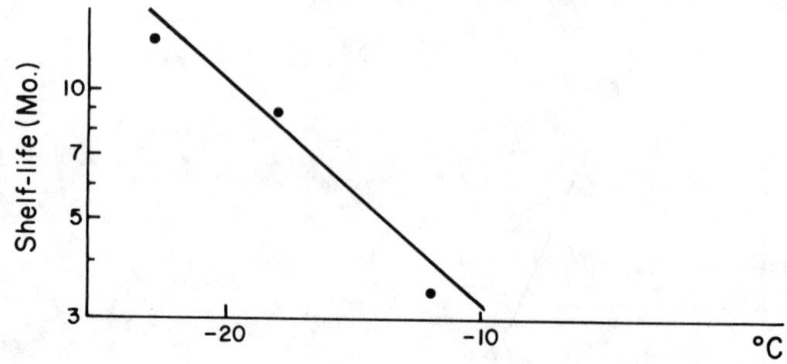

14.43

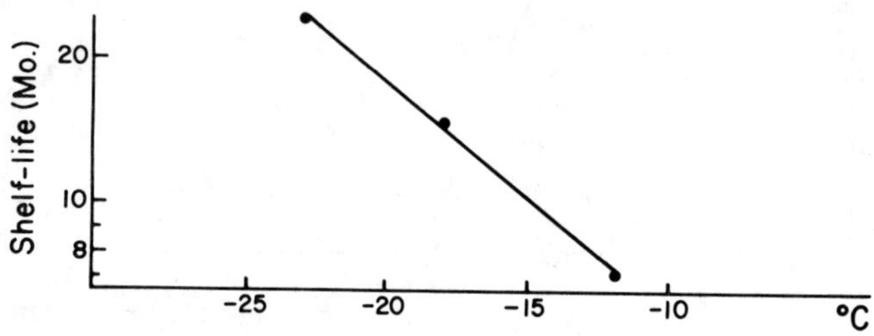

14.44

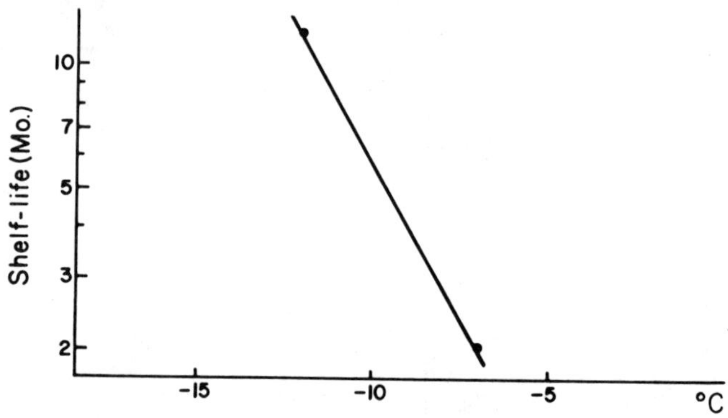

14.45

FIG. 14.43. APPROXIMATE STORAGE LIFE OF FROZEN MUSHROOMS
(From Van Arsdel *et al.* 1969).

FIG. 14.44. APPROXIMATE STORAGE LIFE OF FROZEN PEAS
(From Van Arsdel *et al.* 1969).

FIG. 14.45. VITAMIN C DEGRADATION IN FROZEN PEAS
(From Guerrant *et al.* 1947 and Lindquist *et al.* 1950).

perceptible flavor difference: 10 (at −18 °C), 2 (at −12 °C) and 0.5 (at −7 °C); see Fig. 14.33; a perceptible color difference: 2 (at −18 °C), 0.5 (at −12 °C), and 0.2 (at −7 °C); see Fig. 14.34, and 50% loss of vitamin C: 25 (at −18 °C), 6 (at −12 °C) and 1.7 (at −7 °C); see Fig. 14.35. Kramer (1974) also reported:

(1) The shelf-life in months (sensory quality): 6 (at 4 °F), 12 (at −1 °F), 18 (at −3 °F), and 24 (at −5 °F); see Fig. 14.36.
(2) The shelf-life in months (10% ascorbic acid loss); 6 (at 2 °F), 12 (at −12 °F), 18 (at −30 °F); see Fig. 14.37.
(3) The shelf-life in months (25% ascorbic acid loss); 6 (at 4 °F), 12 (at −8 °F), 18 (at −20 °F); see Fig. 14.38.
(4) The shelf-life in months (50% ascorbic acid loss); 6 (at 8 °F), 12 (at 0 °F) and 18 (at −10 °F); see Fig. 14.39.

Guadagni (1968) showed HQL in days: 291 (0 °F), 61 (10 °F) and 13 (20 °F); see Fig. 14.40.

Corn: Van Arsdel *et al.* (1969) reported approximate storage life in months for cut corn and corn on the cob. They are 12 (at −12 °C), 24 (at −18 °C) and 36 (at −23 °C) for cut corn; see Fig. 14.41; and 4—6 (at −12 °C), 8—10 (at −18 °C) and 12—14 (at −23 °C) for corn on the cob; see Fig. 14.42.

Mushroom: — Van Arsdel *et al.* (1969) also reported approximate storage life in months for frozen mushrooms: 3—4 (at −12 °C), 8—10 (at −18 °C) and 12—14 (at −23 °C); see Fig. 14.43.

Peas: Van Arsdel *et al.* (1969) gave approximate storage life in months for frozen peas: 6—8 (at −12 °C), 14—16 (at −18 °C) and 24 (at −23 °C); see Fig. 14.44. Lindquist *et al.* (1950) reported shelf-life in months based on vitamin C degradation: 2 (at −7 °C), 12 (at −12 °C) and >12 (at −18 °C); see Fig. 14.45. Boggs *et al.* (1960) reported the months to reach a perceptible flavor difference: 10 (at −18 °C(, 3 (at −12 °C) and 1 (at −7 °C) and 0.3 (at −7 °C); see Fig. 14.46; a perceptible color difference: 7 (at—18 °C), 1.5 (at −12 °C) and 0.3 (at −7 °C); see Fig. 14.47; 50% ascorbic acid loss: 48 (at −18 °C), 10 (at −12 °C) and 1.8 (at 7 °C); see Fig. 14.48; and 10% chlorophyll loss: 43 (at −18 °C), 12 (at −12 °C); see Fig. 14.46; a perceptible color difference: 7(at −18 °C), 1.5 (at −12 °C) and 0.3 (at −7 °C); see Fig. 14.47; 50% ascorbic acid loss: 48 (at −18 °C), 10 (at −12 °C) and 1.8 (at 7 °C); see Fig. 14.48; and 10% chlorophyll loss: 43 (at −18 °C), 12 (at −12 °C) and 2.5 (at −7 °C); see Fig. 14.49 Kramer (1974) reported:

(1) The shelf-life in months (sensory quality); 6 (at 4 °F), 12 (at −3 °F), 18 (at −6 °F) and 24 (at −8 °F); see Fig. 14.50.
(2) The shelf-life in months (10% ascorbic acid loss; 6 (at 4 °F), 12 (at −1 °F), 18 (at −3 °F) and 24 (at −8 °F); see Fig. 14.51.
(3) The shelf-life in months (25% ascorbic acid loss); 6 (at 9 °F), 12 (at 5 °F), 18 (at 2 °F) and 24 (at 0 °F); see Fig. 14.52.

(4) The shelf-life in months (50% ascorbic acid loss); 6 (at 11 °F), 12 (at 8 °F), 18 (at 7 °F) and 24 (at 5 °F); see Fig. 14.53.

HQL in days was reported by Guadagni (1968): 305 (at 10 °F), and 27 (at 20 °F); see Fig. 14.54.

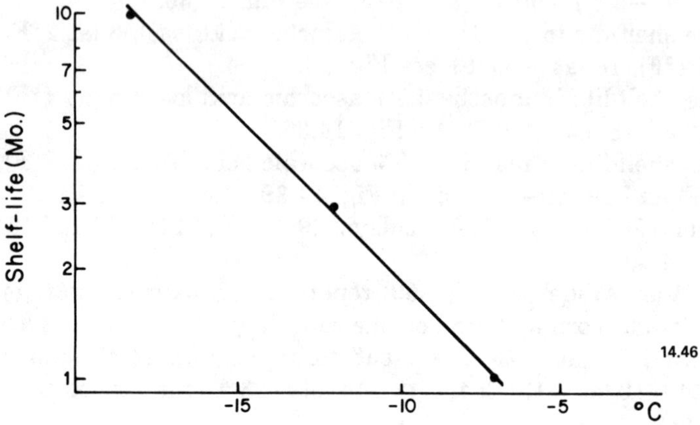

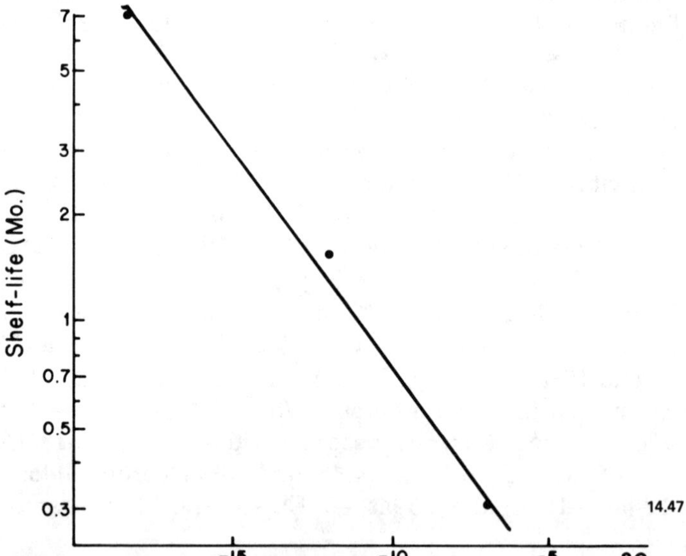

FIG. 14.46. PERCEPTIBLE FLAVOR DIFFERENCE IN FROZEN PEAS
(From Boggs *et al.* 1960).

FIG. 14.47. PERCEPTIBLE COLOR DIFFERENCE IN FROZEN PEAS
(From Boggs *et al.* 1960).

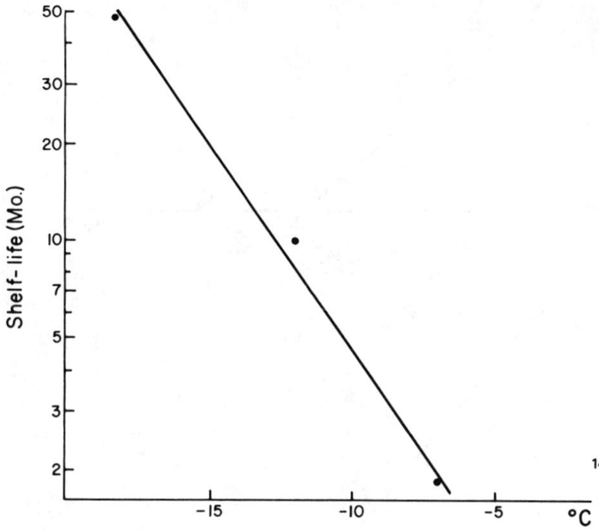

14.48

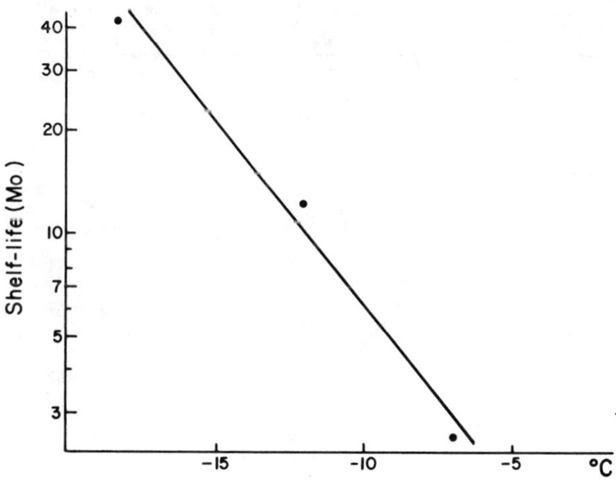

14.49

FIG. 14.48. 50% ASCORBIC ACID LOSS IN FROZEN PEAS (From Boggs *et al.* 1960).

FIG. 14.49. 10% CHLOROPHYLL LOSS IN FROZEN PEAS (From Boggs *et al.* 1960).

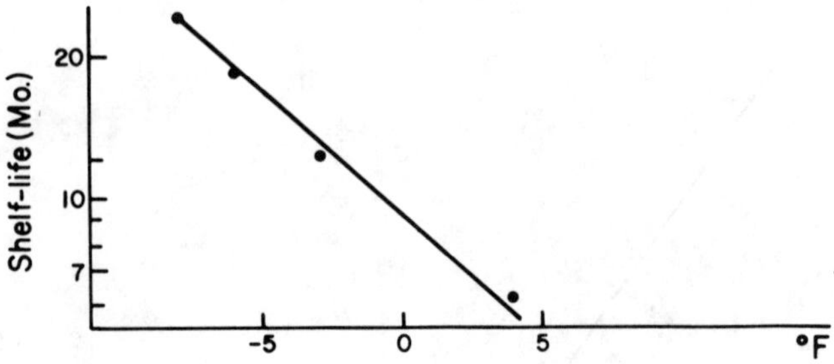

14.50

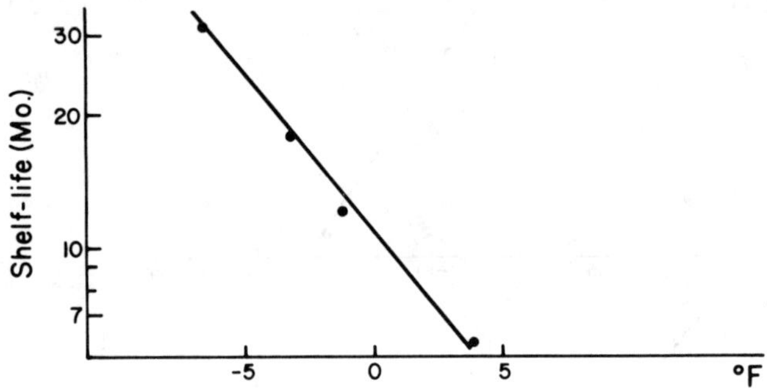

14.51

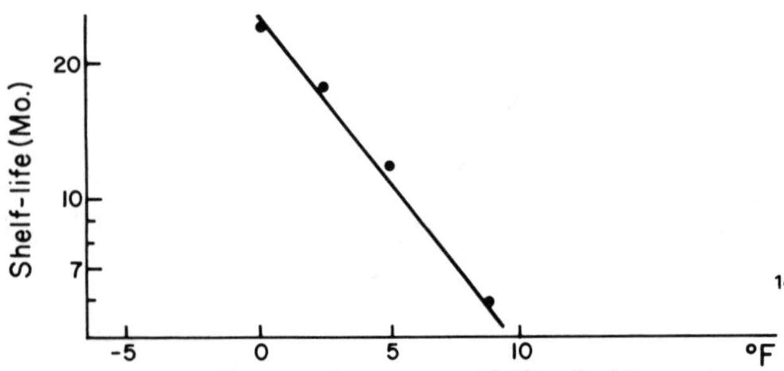

14.52

FIG. 14.50. SENSORY QUALITY LOSS IN FROZEN PEAS (From Kramer 1974).

FIG. 14.51. 10% ASCORBIC ACID LOSS IN FROZEN PEAS (From Kramer 1974).

FIG. 14.52. 25% ASCORBIC ACID LOSS IN FROZEN PEAS (From Kramer 1974).

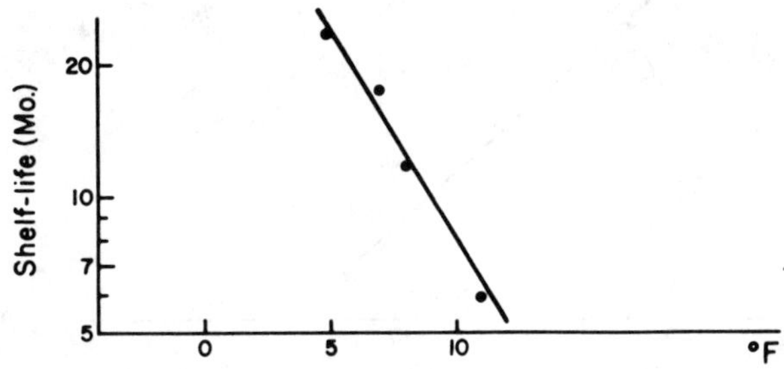

14.53

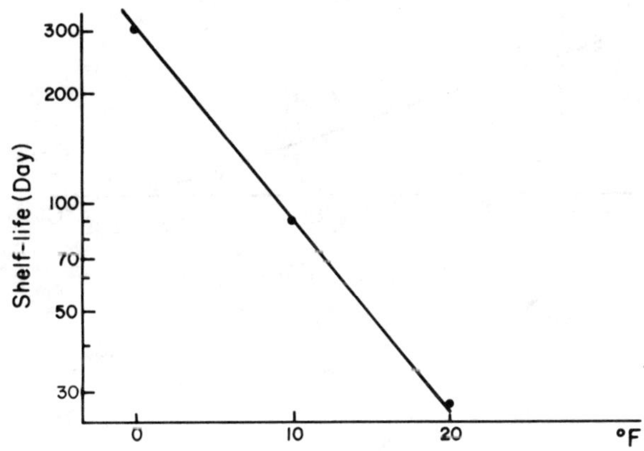

14.54

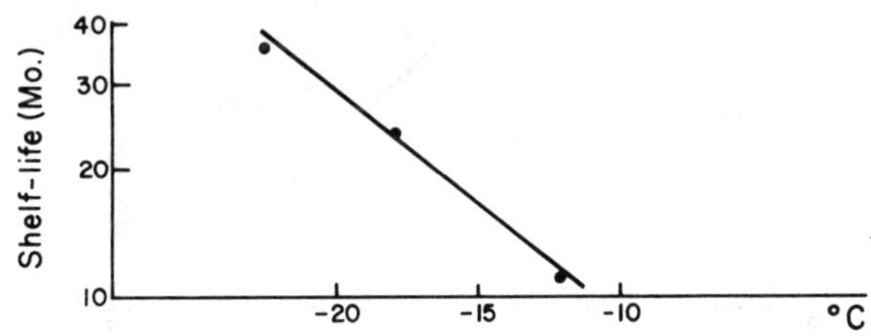

14.55

FIG. 14.53. 50% ASCORBIC ACID LOSS IN FROZEN PEAS (From Kramer 1974).

FIG. 14.54. HIGH QUALITY LIFE OF FROZEN PEAS (From Guadagni 1968).

FIG. 14.55. APPROXIMATE STORAGE LIFE OF FROZEN PUMPKIN (From Van Arsdel *et al.* 1969).

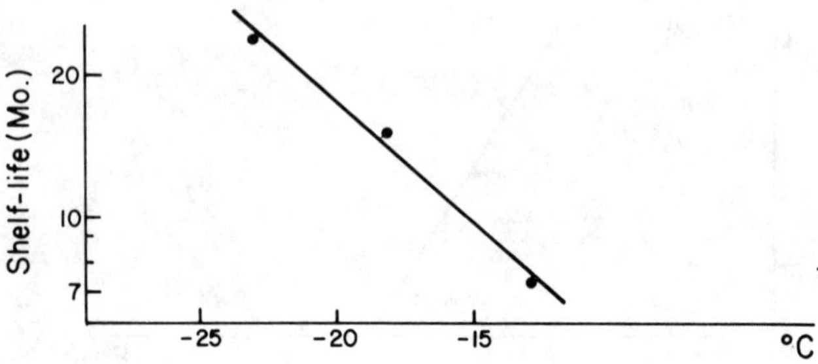

14.56

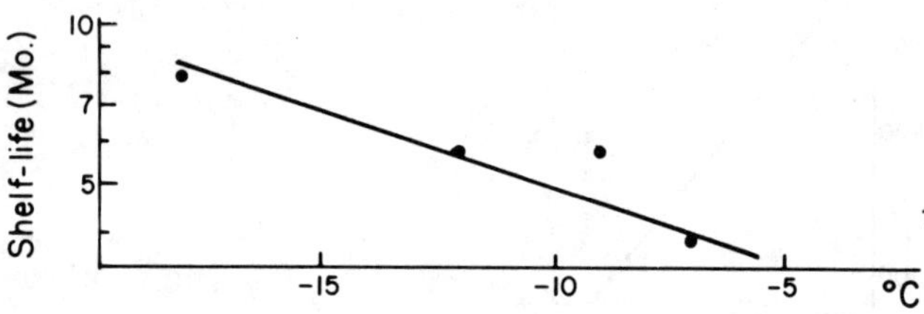

14.57

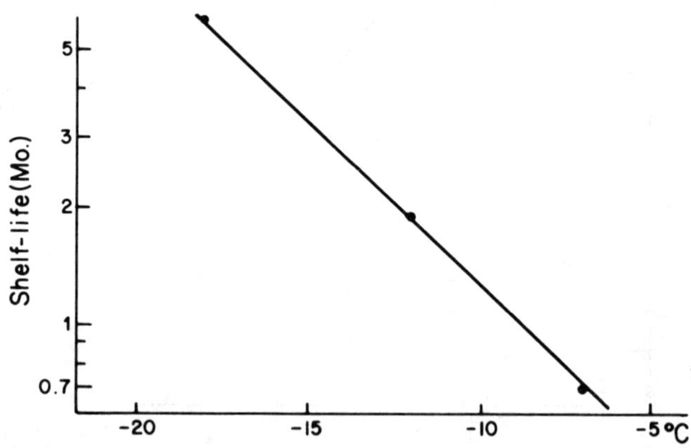

14.58

FIG. 14.56. APPROXIMATE STORAGE LIFE OF FROZEN SPINACH
(From Van Arsdel *et al.* 1969).

FIG. 14.57. VITAMIN C LOSS IN FROZEN SPINACH
(From Jurics 1970).

FIG. 14.58. PERCEPTIBLE COLOR OF FLAVOR DIFFERENCE IN FROZEN SPINACH
(From Dietrich *et al.* 1960).

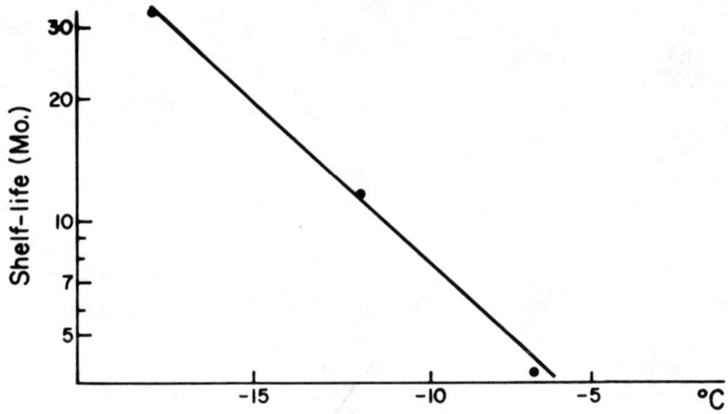

14.59

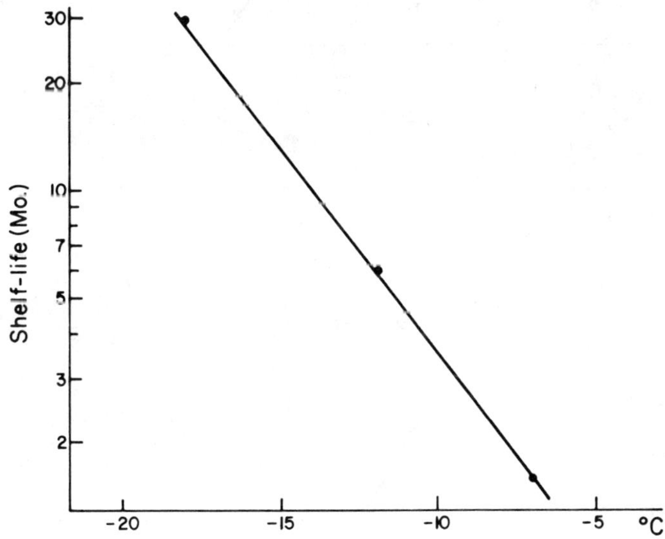

14.60

FIG. 14.59. 50% ASCORBIC ACID LOSS IN FROZEN SPINACH (From Dietrich *et al.* 1960).

FIG. 14.60. 10% CHLOROPHYLL LOSS IN FROZEN LEAF SPINACH (From Dietrich *et al.* 1960).

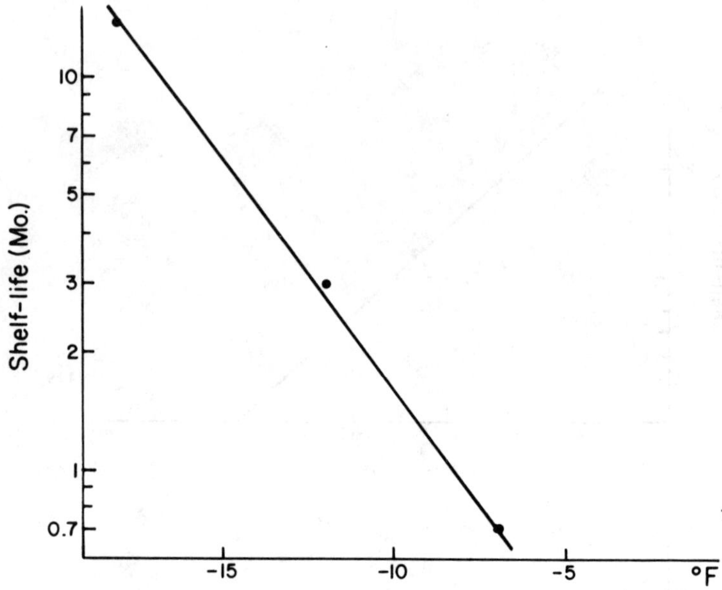

14.61

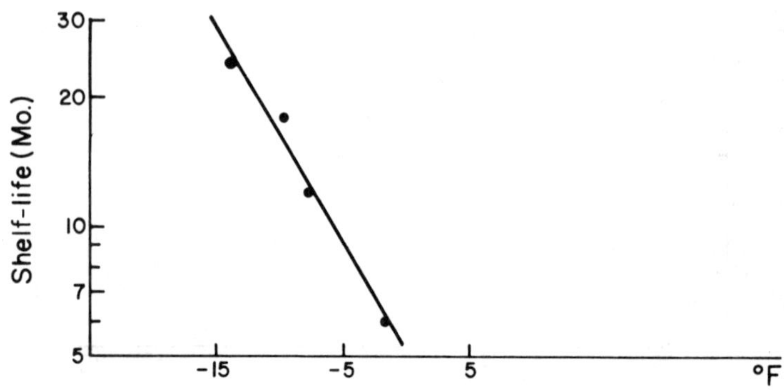

14.62

FIG. 14.61. 10% CHLOROPHYLL LOSS IN FROZEN AND CHOPPED SPINACH
(From Dietrich *et al.* 1960).

FIG. 14.62. SENSORY QUALITY LOSS IN FROZEN SPINACH
(From Kramer 1974).

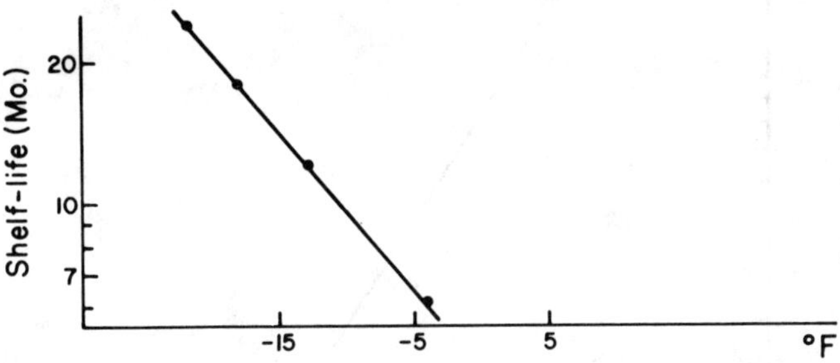

14.63

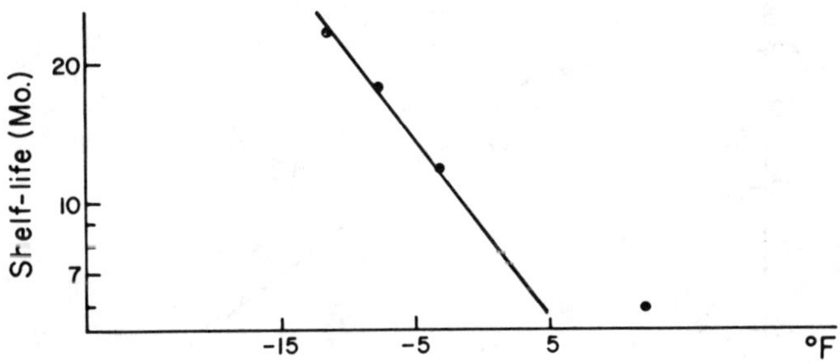

14.64

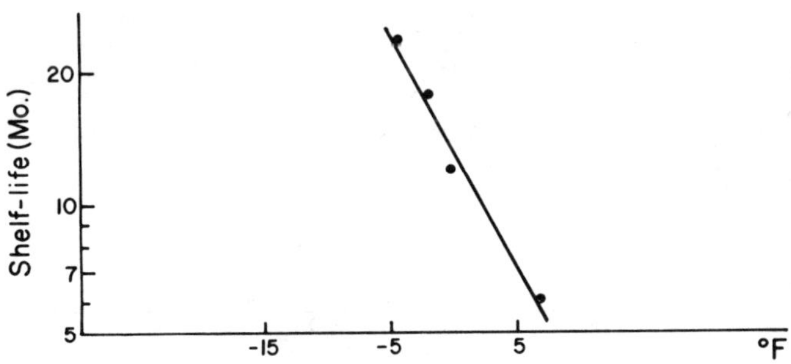

14.65

FIG. 14.63. 10% ASCORBIC ACID LOSS IN FROZEN SPINACH (From Kramer 1974).

FIG. 14.64. 25% ASCORBIC ACID LOSS IN FROZEN SPINACH (From Kramer 1974).

FIG. 14.65. 50% ASCORBIC ACID LOSS IN FROZEN SPINACH (From Kramer 1974).

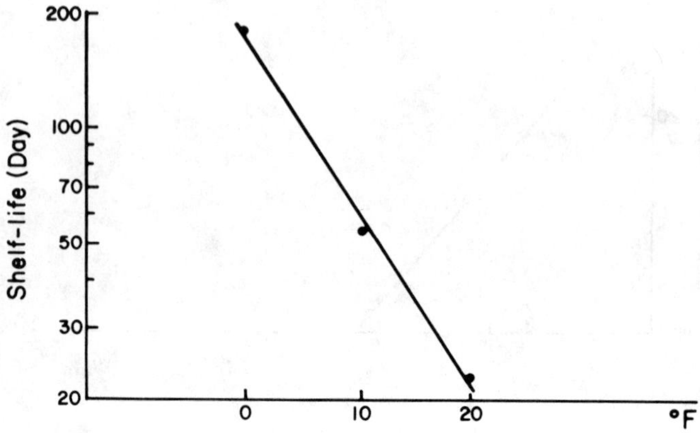

14.66

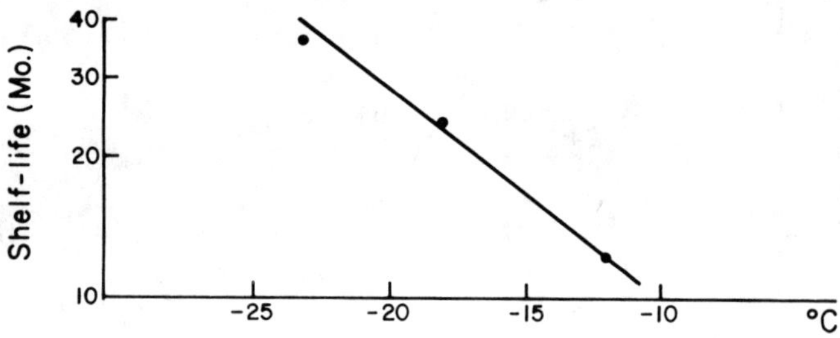

14.67

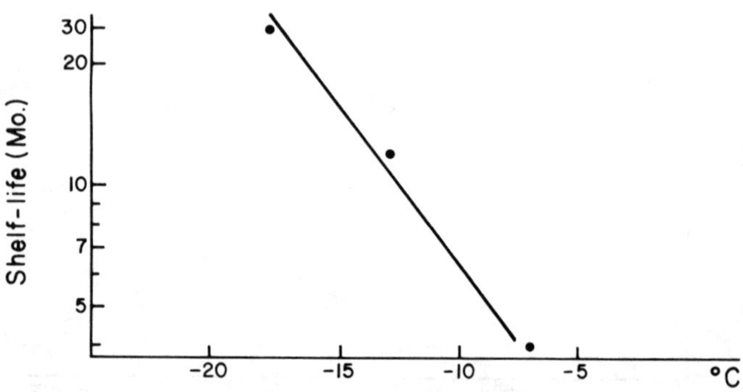

14.68

FIG. 14.66. HIGH QUALITY LIFE OF FROZEN SPINACH (From Guadagni 1968).

FIG. 14.67. APPROXIMATE STORAGE LIFE OF FROZEN SQUASH (From Van Arsdel *et al.* 1969).

FIG. 14.68. FLAVOR STABILITY OF FROZEN APPLE JUICE (From Guadagni and Harris 1967).

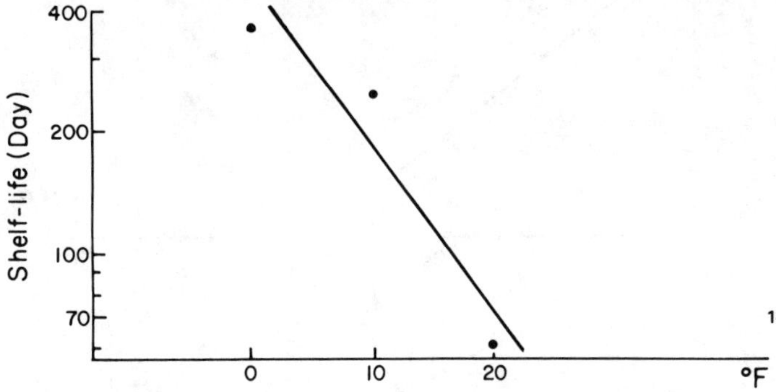

14.69

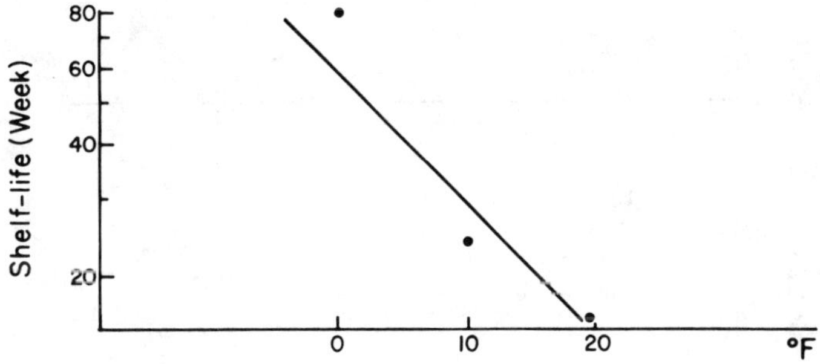

14.70

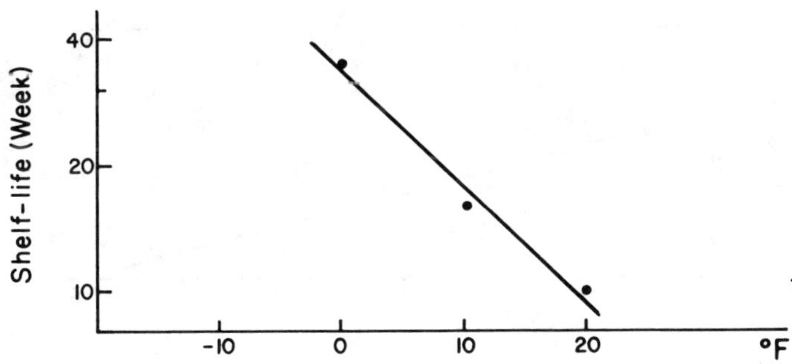

14.71

FIG. 14.69. HIGH QUALITY LIFE OF FROZEN APPLE PIE FILLING
(From Guadagni 1968).

FIG. 14.70. TASTE STABILITY OF FROZEN CONCENTRATED ORANGE JUICE
(From Guadagni *et al.* 1970).

FIG. 14.71. AROMA STABILITY IN CONCENTRATED FROZEN ORANGE JUICE
(From Guadagni *et al.* 1970).

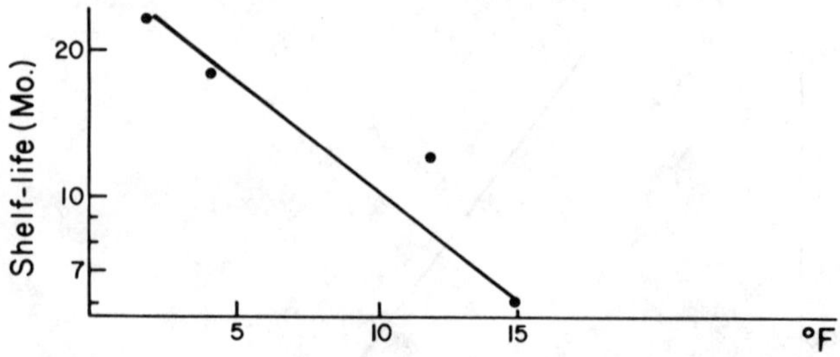

14.72

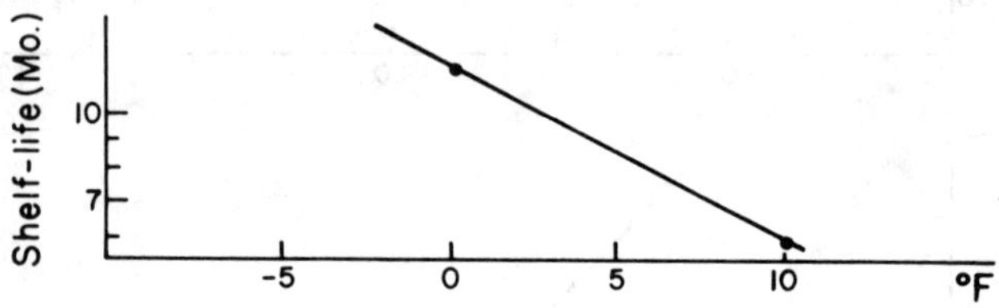

14.73

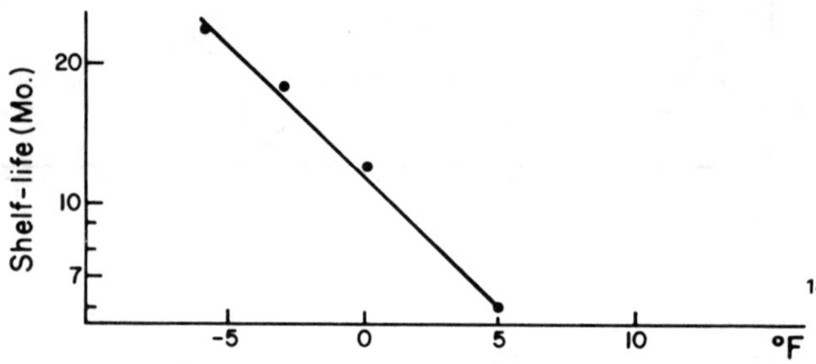

14.74

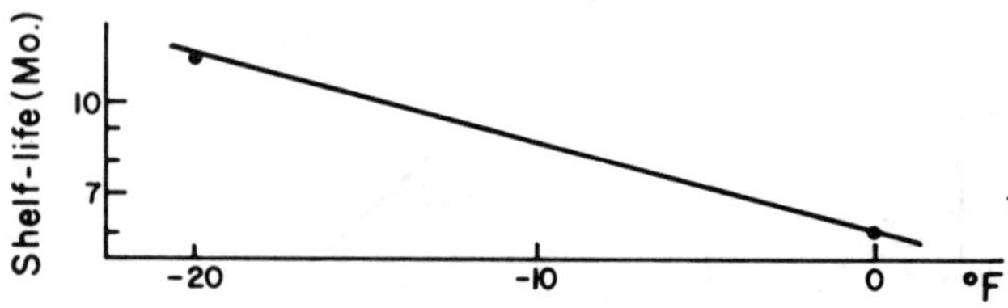

14.75

FIG. 14.72. SENSORY QUALITY IN FROZEN CONCENTRATED ORANGE/GRAPEFRUIT JUICE (From Kramer 1974).

FIG. 14.73. SENSORY QUALITY STABILITY IN FROZEN PEACHES (From Kramer 1974).

FIG. 14.74. 25% ASCORBIC ACID LOSS IN FROZEN PEACHES (From Kramer 1974).

FIG. 14.75. 50% ASCORBIC ACID LOSS IN FROZEN PEACHES (From Kramer 1974).

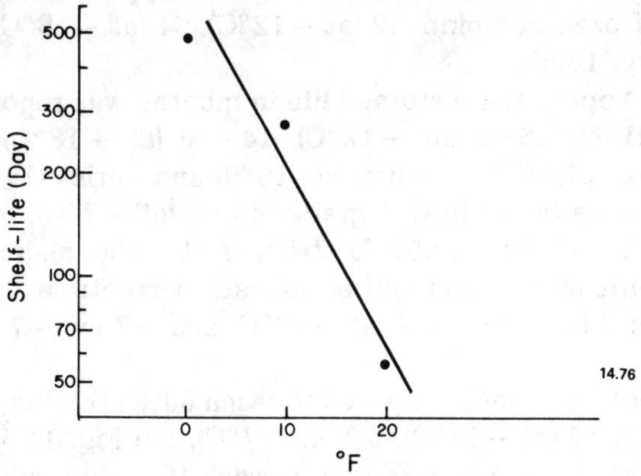

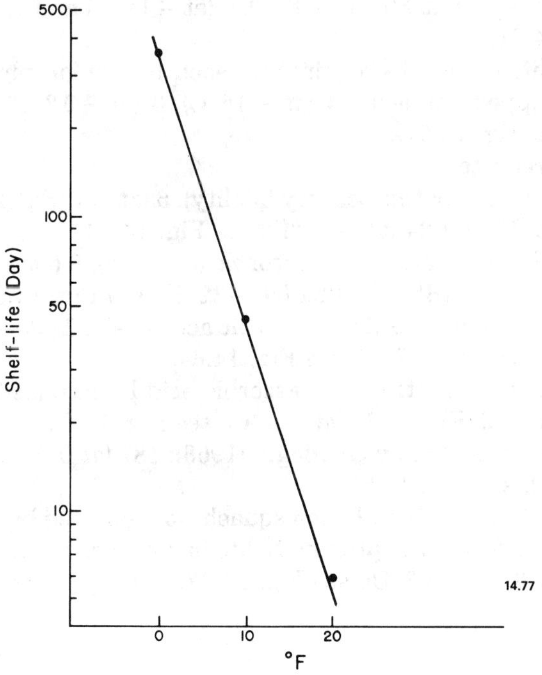

FIG. 14.76. HIGH QUALITY LIFE OF FROZEN PEACH PIE FILLING
(From Guadagni 1968 and 1957).

FIG. 14.77. HIGH QUALITY LIFE OF FROZEN RETAIL PEACHES IN SYRUP
(From Guadagni 1957 and 1968).

Pumpkin: — Van Arsdel *et al.* (1969) reported approximate storage life in months for frozen pumpkin: 12 (at −12 °C), 24 (at −18 °C), and 36 (at −23 °C); see Fig. 14.55.

Spinach: — Approximate storage life in months was reported by Van Arsdel *et al.* (1969): 6—8 (at −12 °C), 14—16 (at −18 °C) and 24 (at −23 °C); see Fig. 14.56. Dietrich *et al.* (1960) and Jurics (1970) reported shelf-life in months (vitamin C degradation): 4 (at −7 °C), 6 (at −12 °C) and 8 (at −18 °C); see Fig. 14.57. Dietrich *et al.* (1960) also reported:

(1) The shelf-life in months required to reach perceptible flavor or color difference: 6 (at −18 °C), 2 (at −12 °C) and 0.7 (at −7 °C); see Fig. 14.58.
(2) The shelf-life in months required to reach 50% ascorbic acid loss: 33 (at −18 °C), 12 (at −12 °C), 4.2 (at −7 °C); see Fig. 14.59.
(3) The shelf-life in months required to reach 10% chlorophyll degradation for leaf spinach: 30 (at −18 °C), 6 (at −12 °C) and 1.6 (at −7 °C); see Fig. 14.61.
(4) The shelf-life in months required to reach 10% chlorophyll degradation of chopped spinach: 14 (at −18 °C), 3 (at −12 °C) and 0.7 (at −7 °C); see Fig. 14.61.

Kramer (1974) reported:

(1) The shelf-life in months (sensory quality): 6 (at −1 °F), 12 (at −8 °F), 18 (at −10 °F) and 24 (at −14 °F); see Fig. 14.62.
(2) The shelf-life in months (10% ascorbic acid loss); 6 (at −4 °F), 12 (at −13 °F), 18 (at −18 °F) and 24 (at −22 °F); see Fig. 14.63.
(3) The shelf-life in months (25% ascorbic acid loss): 12 (at −4 °F), 18 (at −8 °F) and 24 (at −12 °F); see Fig. 14.64.
(4) The shelf-life in months (50% ascorbic acid loss): 6 (at 7 °F), 12 (at 0 °F), 18 (at −2 °F) and 24 (at −4 °F); see Fig. 14.65.

HQL in days was reported by Guadagni (1968): 187 (at 0 °F), 57 (at 10 °F) and 23 (at 20 °F); see Fig. 14.66.

Squash: — Only data about frozen squash was reported by Van Arsdel *et al.* (1969) in the form of approximate life in months: 12 (at −12 °C), 24 (at −18 °C) and 36 (at −23 °C); see Fig. 14.67.

Fruits

Apple: — Guadagni and Harris (1967) studied the stability of frozen concentrated apple juice and found its shelf-life to be: 2 years (at −18 °C) 1 year (at −12 °C) and 2—4 months (at −1 to −7 °C); see Fig. 14.68. Guadagni (1968) reported HQL in days of apple pie filling; 360 (at 0 °F), 250 (at 10 °F) and 60 (at 20 °F); see Fig. 14.69.

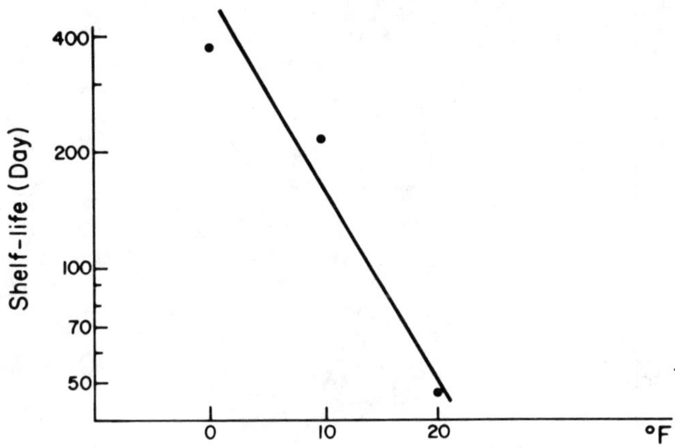

14.78

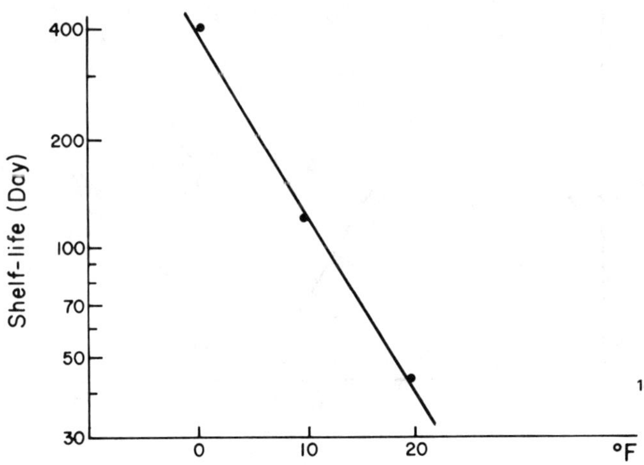

14.79

FIG. 14.78. HIGH QUALITY LIFE IN FROZEN BOYSENBERRY PIE FILLING
(From Guadagni 1960 and 1968).

FIG. 14.79. HIGH QUALITY LIFE OF FROZEN BULK BOYSENBERRIES WITH NO SUGAR
(From Guadagni 1960 and 1968).

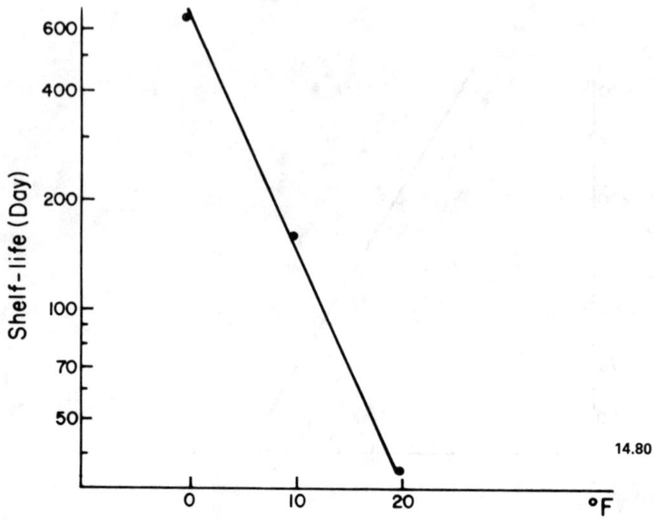

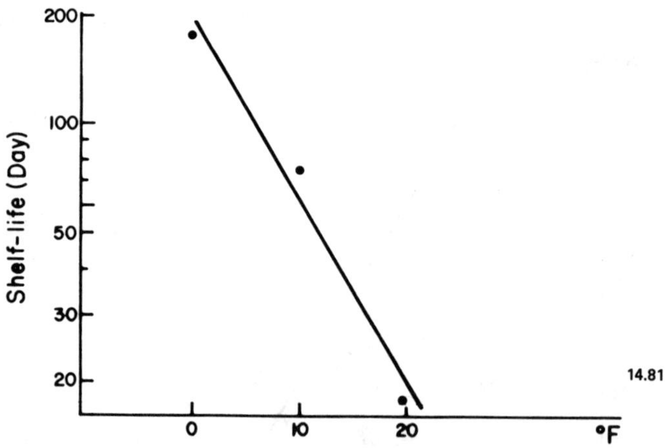

FIG. 14.80. HIGH QUALITY LIFE OF FROZEN RETAIL BOYSENBERRIES IN SYRUP
(From Guadagni 1960 and 1968).

FIG. 14.81. HIGH QUALITY LIFE OF FROZEN BLUEBERRY PIE FILLING
(From Guadagni 1968).

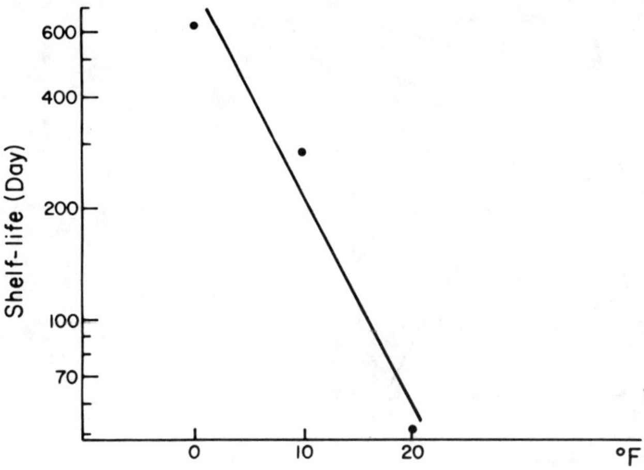

14.82

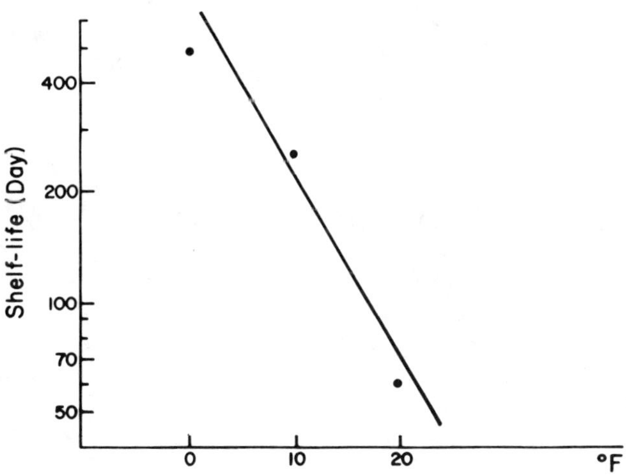

14.83

FIG. 14.82. HIGH QUALITY LIFE OF FROZEN BULK BLACKBERRIES WITH NO SUGAR
(From Guadagni *et al.* 1961 and 1968).

FIG. 14.83. HIGH QUALITY LIFE OF FROZEN CHERRY PIE FILLING
(From Guadagni 1968).

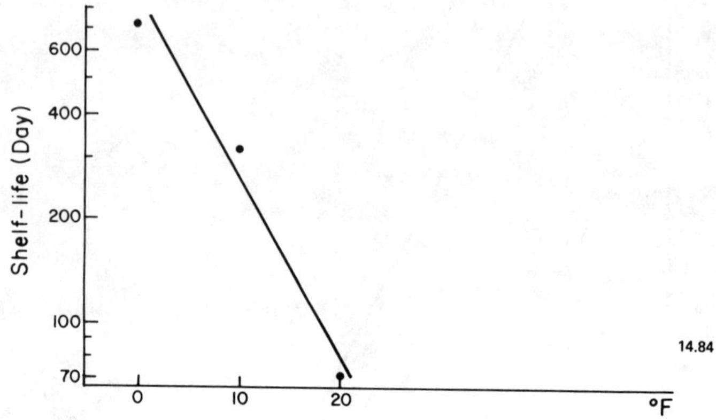

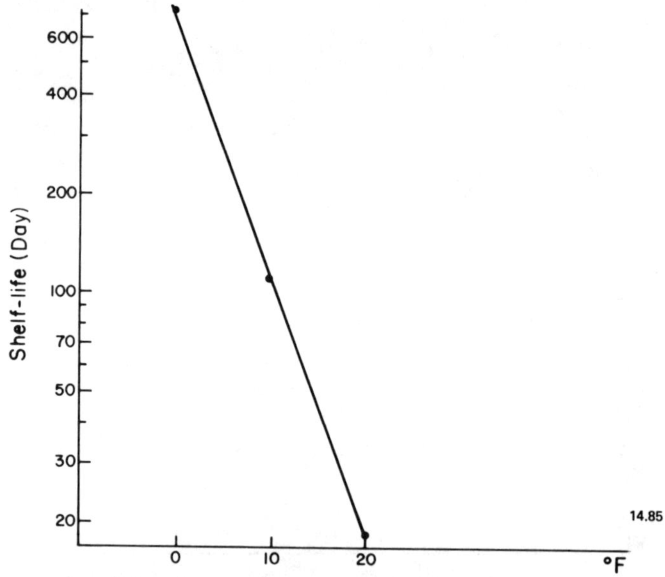

FIG. 14.84. HIGH QUALITY LIFE OF FROZEN BULK RASPBERRIES WITH NO SUGAR
(From Guadagni *et al.* 1957a, 1957c, 1958 and 1961).

FIG. 14.85. HIGH QUALITY LIFE OF FROZEN RETAIL RASPBERRIES IN SYRUP
(From Guadagni *et al.* 1957a, 1957c, 1968 and 1961).

Orange: — Guadagni *et al.*(1970) studied frozen orange concentrate and reported the shelf-life in weeks (taste stability): 80 (at 0 °F), 24 (at 10 °F) and 16 (at 20 °F); see Fig. 14.70; and the shelf-life in weeks (aroma stability): 36 (at 0 °F), 16 (at 10 °F) and 10 (at 20 °F); see Fig. 14.71. Kramer (1974) reported shelf-life in months for frozen orange/grapefruit concentrate: 6 (at 15 °F), 12 (at 8 °F), 18 (at 4 °F) and 24 (at 2 °F); see Fig. 14.72.

Peach: — Kramer (1974) reported:

(1) The shelf-life in months (sensory quality): 6 (at 5 °F), 12 (at 0 °F), 18 (at —3 °F) and 24 (at —6 °F); see Fig. 14.73.

(2) The shelf-life in months (25% ascorbic acid loss): 6 (at 0 °F) and 12 (at —20 °F); see Fig. 14.74.

(3) The shelf-life in months (50% ascorbic acid loss): 6 (at 10 °F) and 12 (at 0 °F); see Fig. 14.75.

Guadagni (1957; 1968) reported HQL in days for frozen peach pie filling: 490 (at 0 °F), 280 (at 10 °F) and 56 (at 20 °F); see Fig. 14.76; and HQL in days for frozen retail peach (in syrup): 360 (at 0 °F), 45 (at 10 °F) and 6 (at 20 °F); see Fig. 14.77.

Boysenberries — Guadagni *et al.* (1960) and Guadagni (1968) reported HQL in days for frozen boysenberries (pie filling): 375 (at 0 °F), 210 (at 10 °F) and 45 (at 20 °F); see Fig. 14.78; for frozen boysenberries in bulk without sugar added: 405 (at 0 °F), 125 (at 10 °F) and 45 (at 20 °F); see Fig. 14.79; and for retail frozen boysenberries in syrup: 650 (at 0 °F), 160 (at 10 °F) and 35 (at 20 °F); see Fig. 14.80.

Blueberries: — Guadagni (1968) reported HQL in days for blueberry pie filling: 175 (at 0 °F), 77 (at 10 °F) and 18 (at 20 °F); see Fig. 14.81.

Blackberries: — Guadagni *et al.* (1961) and Guadagni (1968) reported HQL in days for frozen blackberries in bulk without sugar added: 630 (at 0 °F), 280 (at 10 °F) and 50 (at 20 °F); see Fig. 14.82.

Cherries: — Guadagni (1968) reported HQL in days for frozen cherry pie filling: 490 (at 0 °F), 260 (at 10 °F) and 60 (at 20 °F); see Fig. 14.83.

Raspberries: — Guadagni (1957); Guadagni *et al.* (1957a); Guadagni and Nimmo (1958) studied raspberries and reported HQL in days for frozen raspberries in bulk without sugar added: 720 (at 0 °F), 315 (at 10 °F) and 70 (at 20 °F); see Fig. 14.84; and for retail frozen raspberries in syrup: 720 (at 0 °F), 110 (at 10 °F) and 18 (at 20 °F); see Fig. 14.85.

Strawberries: — Guadagni (1957), Guadagni *et al.* (1957a), and Guadagni and Nimmo (1958) studied frozen strawberry products and reported:

(1) The HQL in days of strawberries (in bulk, no sugar): 630 (at 0 °F), 90 (at 10 °F) and 18 (at 20 °F); see Fig. 14.86.

(2) HQL in days of strawberries (retail): 360 (at 0 °F), 60 (at 10 °F) and 10 (at 20 °F); see Fig. 14.87.

(3) The shelf-life (30% ascorbic acid loss) in days: 225 (at 10 °F), 50 (at 20 °F) and 12 (at 30 °F); see Fig. 14.88.

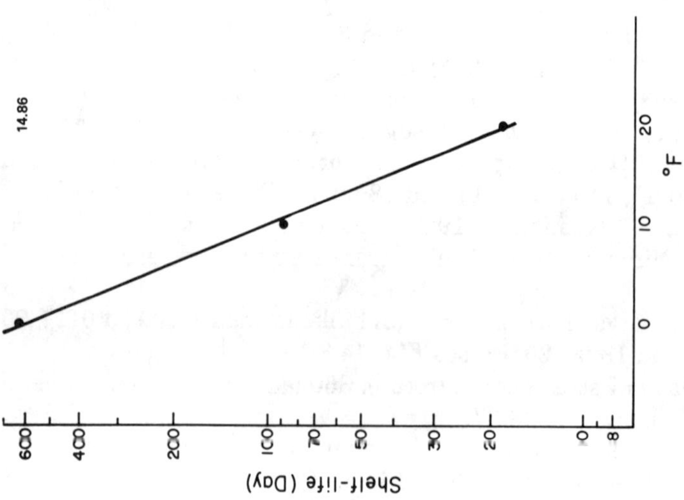

Fig. 14.86. HIGH QUALITY LIFE OF FROZEN BULK STRAWBERRIES WITH NO SYRUP
(From Guadagni *et al.* 1957a, 1957b, 1958 and 1961).

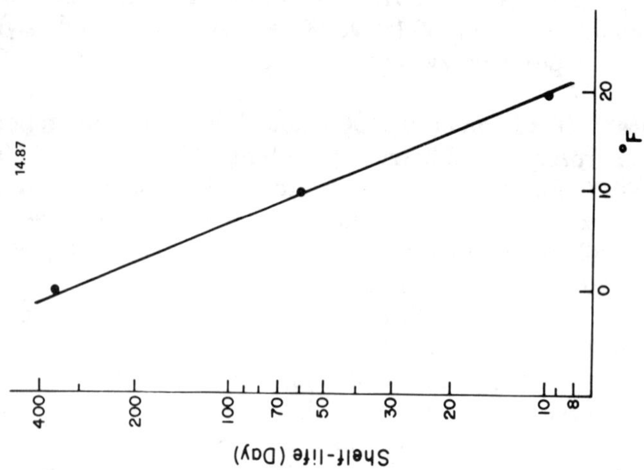

FIG. 14.87. HIGH QUALITY LIFE IN FROZEN RETAIL STRAWBERRIES
(From Guadagni 1957a, 1957b, 1958 and 1961).

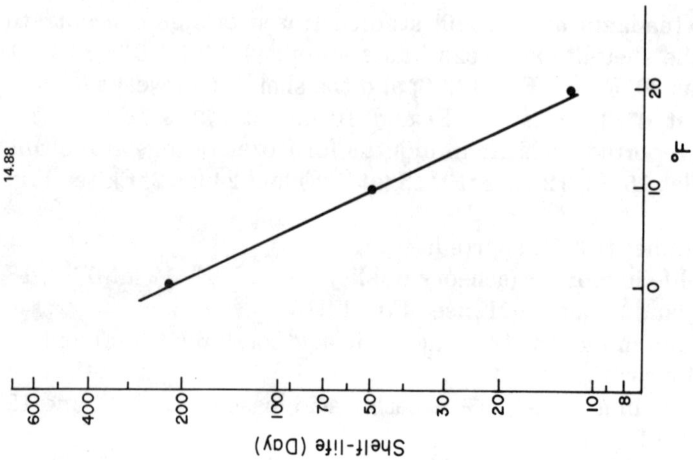

FIG. 14.88. 30% ASCORBIC ACID LOSS IN STRAWBERRIES
(From Guadagni 1957a, 1957b, 1958 and 1961).

In order to make a visual comparison of shelf-life data of FFV, Table 14.4 was made by converting the previously mentioned shelf-life data into months at $-10\,°C$ and $-20\,°C$ storage temperature. Linearity between variables (i.e., shelf-life and temperature) in shelf-life plots can be justified in most cases. This indicates that the activation energy (E_a) for the specific deteriorative reaction remains constant. However, in a very few cases the E_a does show a significant change, especially at relatively higher temperature (i.e., just below freezing). Increase of water activity (a_w), change of phase, release of enzymes and many other factors may cause considerable changes in the mechanism of deterioration at higher temperatures and thus change the E_a. The data (shelf-lives, E_a and Q_{10}) in Table 14.4 are computed from the original data presented in this report using simple linear regression.

SHELF-LIFE PREDICTION OF FFV

The stability of FFV is dependent on variety: growing conditions; methods of harvesting, preparation and freezing; and packaging method and material. However, as soon as the product is frozen, the initial quality (A_o) is fixed. The rate of quality loss for a given FFV product thereafter is dependent on the time and temperature of storage and distribution. It is found that most reactions which lower the quality of FFV follow a zero order reaction (i.e., reaction rate is independent of A_o). If shelf-life of FFV can be accurately defined in terms of degree of quality loss, shelf-life prediction can be fairly precise and reproducible using the equations developed in Chapter 3.

Guadagni (1961) evaluated the time-temperature effect of various commercial practices. The percentage loss in HQL was computed for each individual handling or storage stage and when these percentages were summed, total loss was found to be close to actual values.

OPEN DATING OF FFV

Ninety percent of the 1400 respondents to the USDA's survey felt open dating on food labels was extremely useful. However, some felt open dating could be misleading, confusing and even deceiving. Many problems regarding open dating still remain unsolved, such as listed below:

(1) Definition of "the end of shelf-life". — In order to preserve the fair competition among processors of FFV, the end of shelf-life must be defined as a uniform quality level, rather than a uniform length of time-temperature conditions. Thus, a better product will take longer to reach the quality level which is the end of shelf-life.

TABLE 14.4
SUMMARIZED SHELF-LIFE DATA OF FFV

Product	Fig.	Basis of Shelf-life	Shelf-life (months) −10°C	Shelf-life (months) −20°C	E_a Kcal/mole	Q_{10}	Reference
Asparagus green	14.1	approximate storage life	4.08	12.05	14.33	2.95	Van Arsdel *et al.* (1969)
Asparagus, green	14.2	sensory quality	1.33	9.82	26.52	7.40	Kramer (1974)
Asparagus, green	14.3	10% vitamin C loss	0.18	34.81	69.55	190.00	Kramer (1974)
Asparagus, green	14.4	25% vitamin C loss	1.89	35.85	38.95	18.90	Kramer (1974)
Asparagus, green	14.5	50% vitamin C loss	2.08	47.93	41.53	22.96	Kramer (1974)
Asparagus, green	14.6	10% vitamin C loss	1.97	3.32	6.90	1.68	Jenkins *et al.* (1940)
Beans, lima	14.7	approximate storage life	5.40	18.97	16.64	3.51	Van Arsdel *et al.* (1969)
Beans, lima	14.8	sensory quality	1.93	13.88	26.10	7.17	Kramer (1974)
Beans, lima	14.9	10% vitamin C loss	0.81	43.52	52.79	53.66	Kramer (1974)
Beans, lima	14.10	25% vitamin C loss	3.47	40.09	32.40	11.53	Kramer (1974)
Beans, lima	14.11	50% vitamin C loss	8.81	35.69	18.53	4.05	Kramer (1974)
Beans, snap	14.12	approximate storage life	4.04	11.98	14.41	2.97	Van Arsdel *et al.* (1965)
Beans, (French cut)	14.13	25% vitamin C loss	1.38	2.31	6.82	1.67	Derse and Tepley (1958)
Beans, (French cut)	14.14	25% Carotene loss	2.51	4.05	6.34	1.61	Derse and Tepley (1958)
Beans, snap	14.15	vitamin C degradation	3.28	7.01	10.05	2.13	Jurics (1970)
Beans, snap	14.16	flavor difference	1.84	15.19	27.99	2.11	Dietrich *et al.* (1959)
Beans, snap	14.17	color difference	0.51	18.94	47.80	36.84	Dietrich *et al.* (1959)
Beans, snap	14.18	50% vitamin C loss	2.13	26.95	33.65	2.54	Dietrich *et al.* (1959)
Beans, snap	14.19	10% chlorophyll loss	1.51	17.08	32.15	2.43	Dietrich *et al.* (1959)
Beans, snap	14.20	10% vitamin C loss	1.92	13.65	25.97	7.10	Kramer (1974)
Beans, snap	14.21	25% vitamin C loss	0.18	8.06	50.34	44.60	Kramer (1974)
Beans, snap	14.22	50% vitamin C loss	2.60	30.46	32.58	11.69	Kramer (1974)
Beans, (retail)	14.23	HQL	1.89	15.56	27.91	8.21	Gaudagni (1968)
Broccoli	14.24	approximate storage life	5.40	18.97	16.64	3.51	Van Arsdel *et al.* (1969)
Broccoli	14.25	sensory quality	1.33	9.82	26.52	2.00	Kramer (1974)

continued

TABLE 14.4 (continued)

Product	Fig.	Basis of Shelf-life	Shelf-life (months) −10°C	Shelf-life (months) −20°C	E_a Kcal/mole	Q_{10}	Reference
Broccoli	14.26	10% vitamin C loss	1.54	27.49	38.15	17.79	Kramer (1974)
Broccoli	14.27	25% vitamin C loss	1.89	35.85	38.95	18.90	Kramer (1974)
Broccoli	14.28	50% vitamin C loss	3.61	47.06	34.02	13.03	Kramer (1974)
Brussels sprouts	14.29	approximate storage life	4.04	11.98	14.41	2.97	Van Arsdel *et al.* (1969)
Carrots	14.30	approximate storage life	5.30	71.52	34.48	3.51	Van Arsdel *et al.* (1969)
Cauliflower	14.31	approximate storage life	5.40	18.97	16.64	3.51	Van Arsdel *et al.* (1969)
Cauliflower	14.32	vitamin C degradation	2.96	7.63	12.54	2.58	Jenkins *et al.* (1940) Bennett *et al.* (1954) Dietrich *et al.* (1957)
Cauliflower	14.33	flavor difference	1.09	17.03	36.46	15.66	Dietrich *et al.* (1962)
Cauliflower	14.34	color difference	.35	2.89	28.16	8.37	Dietrich *et al.* (1962)
Cauliflower	14.35	50% vitamin C loss	3.43	40.50	32.70	11.79	Dietrich *et al.* (1962)
Cauliflower	14.36	sensory quality	1.29	19.37	35.88	14.99	Kramer (1974)
Cauliflower	14.37	10% vitamin C loss	5.06	8.39	6.71	1.66	Kramer (1974)
Cauliflower	14.38	25% vitamin C loss	4.11	8.93	10.28	2.17	Kramer (1974)
Cauliflower	14.39	50% vitamin C loss	4.55	13.02	13.94	2.86	Kramer (1974)
Cauliflower (retail)	14.40	HQL	1.02	18.01	37.98	3.13	Guadagni (1968)
Corn, cut	14.41	approximate storage life	9.43	29.71	15.14	3.13	Van Arsdel *et al.* (1969)
Corn, on the cob	14.42	approximate storage life	4.29	10.05	11.27	2.34	Van Arsdel *et al.* (1969)
Mushroom	14.43	approximate storage life	2.95	9.57	15.57	3.24	Van Arsdel *et al.* (1969)
Peas	14.44	approximate storage life	5.40	18.97	16.64	3.51	Van Arsdel *et al.* (1969)
Peas	14.45	vitamin C degradation	5.55	231.9	49.45	41.72	Guerrant and O'Hara (1953) Lindquist *et al.* (1950)
Peas	14.46	flavor difference	1.84	15.19	27.99	8.26	Boggs *et al.* (1960)
Peas	14.47	color difference	0.72	12.78	38.19	17.84	Boggs *et al.* (1960)
Peas	14.48	50% vitamin C loss	4.51	90.85	39.78	20.11	Boggs *et al.* (1960)

continued

TABLE 14.4 (continued)

Product	Fig.	Basis of Shelf-life	Shelf-life (months) −10°C	Shelf-life (months) −20°C	E_a Kcal/mole	Q_{10}	Reference
Peas	14.49	10% chlorophyll loss	5.71	76.49	34.39	13.39	Boggs *et al.* (1960)
Peas	14.50	sensory quality	0.28	9.60	46.66	33.81	Kramer (1974)
Peas	14.51	10% vitamin C loss	2.12	16.07	26.84	7.58	Kramer (1974)
Peas	14.52	25% vitamin C loss	2.82	43.99	36.39	15.58	Kramer (1974)
Peas	14.53	50% vitamin C loss	5.58	42.67	26.94	7.63	Kramer (1974)
Peas	14.54	HQL	1.77	16.44	29.56	9.30	Guadagni (1968)
Pumpkin	14.55	approximate storage life	9.48	29.71	15.14	3.13	Van Arsdel *et al.* (1969)
Spinach	14.56	approximate storage life	5.40	18.97	16.64	3.51	Van Arsdel *et al.* (1969)
Spinach	14.57	vitamin C degradation	4.93	9.27	8.36	1.88	Jurics (1970) Dietrich *et al.* (1960)
Spinach	14.58	flavor or color difference	1.24	8.93	26.10	7.16	Dietrich *et al.* (1960)
Spinach	14.59	50% vitamin C loss	7.41	48.89	25.00	6.59	Dietrich *et al.* (1960)
Spinach (leaf)	14.60	10% chlorophyll loss	3.38	50.01	35.71	14.79	Dietrich *et al.* (1960)
Spinach (chopped)	14.61	10% chlorophyll loss	1.56	24.30	36.39	15.58	Dietrich *et al.* (1960)
Spinach	14.62	sensory quality	1.24	8.03	24.72	6.46	Kramer (1974)
Spinach	14.63	10% vitamin C loss	1.63	5.90	17.01	3.61	Kramer (1974)
Spinach	14.64	25% vitamin C loss	3.36	12.24	17.04	3.62	Kramer (1974)
Spinach	14.65	50% vitamin C loss	2.44	21.65	28.90	8.85	Kramer (1974)
Spinach	14.66	HQL	1.32	9.02	25.51	6.85	Guadagni (1968)
Squash	14.67	approximate storage life	9.48	29.71	15.14	3.13	Van Arsdel *et al.* (1969)
Apple, concentrated juice	14.68	flavor stability	6.99	35.58	21.55	5.08	Guadagni and Harris (1967)
Apple, pie filling	14.69	HQL	3.94	20.35	21.76	5.17	Guadagni (1968)
Orange, concentrated juice	14.70	taste stability	5.09	22.71	19.81	4.46	Guadagni *et al.* (1970)
Orange , concentrated juice	14.71	aroma stability	3.13	10.66	16.24	3.41	Guadagni *et al.* (1970)
Orange/grapefruit (concentrated juice)	14.72	sensory quality	6.93	42.83	25.20	6.69	Kramer (1974)
Peach	14.73	sensory quality	2.00	18.66	29.56	9.30	Kramer (1974)
Peach	14.74	25% vitamin C loss	3.79	6.80	7.74	1.79	Kramer (1974)

continued

TABLE 14.4 (concluded)

Product	Fig.	Basis of Shelf-life	Shelf-life (months) −10°C	Shelf-life (months) −20°C	E_a Kcal/mole	Q_{10}	Reference
Peach	14.75	50% vitamin C loss	4.48	15.68	16.59	3.50	Kramer (1974)
Peach (pie filling)	14.76	HQL	4.08	29.73	26.31	7.28	Guadagni (1968) Guadagni (1957)
Peach (retail/syrup)	14.77	HQL	0.62	26.85	49.91	43.19	Guadagni (1968) Guadagni (1957)
Boysenberries (pie filling)	14.78	HQL	3.19	22.29	25.77	6.99	Guadagni (1968) Guadagni *et al.* (1960)
Boysenberries (bulk, no sugar)	14.79	HQL	2.70	20.41	26.79	7.55	Guadagni (1968) Guadagni *et al.* (1960)
Boysenberries (retail/syrup)	14.80	HQL	2.69	39.49	35.57	14.88	Guadagni (1968) Guadagni *et al.* (1960)
Blueberries (pie filling)	14.81	HQL	1.23	10.17	27.67	8.06	Guadagni (1968)
Blackberries (bulk, no sugar)	14.82	HQL	3.94	40.31	30.79	10.23	Guadagni (1968) Guadagni *et al.* (1961)
Cherries (pie filling)	14.83	HQL	4.13	28.36	25.51	6.85	Guadagni (1968)
Raspberries (bulk, no sugar)	14.84	HQL	4.84	41.29	28.39	2.14	Guadagni (1957) Guadagni *et al.* (1961) Guadagni *et al.* (1957b) Guadagni and Nimmo (1958)
Raspberries (retail/syrup)	14.85	HQL	1.66	49.52	44.97	29.75	Guadagni and Nimmo (1958)
Strawberries (bulk, no sugar)	14.86	HQL	1.53	40.39	43.36	26.35	Guadagni (1957) Guadagni *et al.* (1961) Guadagni *et al.* (1957a) Guadagni and Kelly (1958)
Strawberries (retail/syrup)	14.87	HQL	0.90	24.60	43.80	27.74	Guadagni and Kelly (1958)
Strawberries	14.88	30% vitamin C loss	3.89	64.02	37.10	16.53	Guadagni and Kelly (1958)

(2) How are the quality levels measured? — Are there available objective measurements to do this? If these problems cannot be solved, the enforcement of proposed open dating regulations may cause a great deal of argument. In addition, because the variations expected are large, a sound statistical sampling procedure must be developed for judging the compliance or adulteration. Who should be held responsible for failure in meeting specified shelf-life?

(3) Temperature vs time. FFV quality is more seriously affected by temperature than by time. A single mishandling could destroy FFV quality in a relatively short time period. Therefore a question is raised whether open dating is actually useful. The answer could be positive if a maximum storage temperature at any point in the distribution channel can be specified and regulated by law. Mishandling of FFV may not be a source of significant health problems, but the possibility exists.

(4) Type of dating for FFV. A "pack date" would be inappropriate for FFV since exposure to high or fluctuating temperatures can be more critical than length of storage. The use of a "pull date" or "sell by date" would be meaningless unless it is accompanied by storage and handling instructions. In addition, the length of time that the product can be kept after the "sell by date" under various practical conditions should be specified. A nationwide uniform dating system backed by a strong educational program is preferred in order to enable the general consumer to properly handle the FFV product and to interpret the open dating formation. A "use by date" would be impractical for FFV, since surveys have shown that a major portion of degradation of FFV occurs while in the hands of the housewife or end-user (Guadagni 1961). Probably the best date would be a "best if used by date" since it is most appropriate for a food with long shelf-life under controlled conditions.

REFERENCES

BENNET, G. *et al.* 1954. Some factors affecting the quality of frozen foods. II. Bull. 580, Penn. State University, State College, Penn.

BOGGS, M.M., *et al.* 1960. Time-temperature tolerance of frozen foods. XXI. Frozen peas. Food Technol. *14,* 181-185.

DAVIS, L.G. 1958. Food Can. *16,* 4.

DERSE, P.H. and TEPLEY, L.J. 1958. Effect of storage conditions on nutrients in frozen green beans, peas, orange juice and strawberries. J. Agric. Food Chem. *6,* 309-312.

DIETRICH, W.C., LINDQUIST, F.E., MIERS, J.C., BOHART, G.S., NEUMANN, N.J. and TALBURT, W.F. 1957. The time-temperature tolerance of frozen foods. IV. Objective tests to measure adverse changes in frozen vegetables. Food Technol. *11,* 109-113.

DIETRICH, W.C. *et al.* 1959. Time-temperature tolerance of frozen foods. XVI. Quality retention of frozen green snap beans in retail packages. Food Technol. *13,* 136-145.

DIETRICH, W.C., BOGGS, M.M., NUTTING, M.D. and WEINSTEIN, N.E., 1960. Time-temperature tolerance of frozen foods. XXIII. Quality changes in frozen spinach. Food Technol. *14,* 522-527.

DIETRICH, W.C., NUTTING, M.D., BOGGS, M.M. and WEINSTEIN, N.E. 1962. Time-temperature tolerance in frozen foods. XXIV. Quality changes in cauliflower. Food Technol. *16* (10), 123-128.

DuBOIS, C.W. and KEW, T.S. 1951. Storage temperature effects on frozen citrus concentrates. Refrig. Eng. *59,* 772.

FENNEMA, O. 1975. In Nutritional Evaluation of Food Processing, 2nd Ed, R.S. Harris and E. Karmas (Editors). AVI Publishing Co., Westport, Conn.

GUADAGNI, D.G. 1957. Time-temperature tolerance of frozen foods. VII. Organoleptic evaluation of frozen strawberries, raspberries and peaches. Food Technol. *11,* 471.

GUADAGNI, D.G. 1968. Cold storage life of frozen fruits and vegetables as a function of time and temperature. *In* Low Temperature Biology of Foodstuffs. J. Hawthorn (Editor). Pergamon Press, New York.

GUADAGNI, D.G., NIMMO C.C. and E.F. JANSEN. 1957a. Time-temperature tolerance of frozen foods, VI. Retail packages of frozen strawberries. Food Technol. *11,* 389-397.

GUADAGNI, D.G. and KELLY, S.H. 1958. Time-temperature tolerance of frozen foods. XIV. Ascorbic acid and its oxidation products as a measure of temperature history in frozen strawberries. Food Technol. *12,* 645-647.

GUADAGNI, D.G. and NIMMO, C.C. 1958. Time-temperature tolerance of frozen foods. XIII. Effect of regularly fluctuating temperature in retail packages of frozen strawberries and raspberries. Food Technol. *12,* 306-310.

GUADAGNI, D.G., EREMIA, K.M., KELLY, S.H. and HARRIS, J. 1960. Time-temperature tolerance of frozen foods. XX. Boysenberries. Food Technol. *14,* 148-150.

GUADAGNI, D.G., DOWNES, N.J., SANSHUCK, D.W. and SHINODA, S. 1961. Effect of temperature on stability of commercially frozen bulk pack fruits — strawberries, raspberries and blackberries Food Technol. *15,* 207-209.

GUADAGNI, D.C. 1961. Time-temperature experience of food quality. ASHRAE J. 3(4), 66-69, 83.

GUADAGNI, D.C. and HARRIS, J. 1967. Stability of frozen concentrated apple juice with and without added essence. Food Technol. *21,* 454.

GUADAGNI, D.C., BOMBEN, J.L. and MANNHEIM, H.C. 1970. Storage stability of frozen orange juice concentrate made with aroma solution of cutback juice. Food Technol. *24,* 1012-1016.

GUERRANT, N.B. and O'HARA, M.B. 1953. Vitamin retention in peas and lima beans after blanching, freezing, processing in tin and in glass, after storage and after cooking. Food Technol. *7,* 473.

HUGGART, R.L., HARMAN, D.A. and MOORE, E.L. 1954. Ascorbic acid retention in frozen concentrated citrus fruits. J. Am. Diet. Assoc. *39,* 682.

JENKINS, R.R., TRESSLER, D.K., MOYER, A. and McINTOSH, J. 1940. Storage of frozen vegetables. Vitamin C experiments. Refrig. Eng. *39,* 381.

JURICS, E.W. 1970. Vergleichende Untersuchungen uber den vitamin — C — Gehalt von tiefekuhltem und frischem Gemuse im rohen und gekochten Zustand. Nahrung. *14*(2) 104-114. (German).

KRAMER, A. 1974. Storage retention of nutrients. Food Technol. *28*(1), 50-60.

LINDQUIST, F.E., DIETRICH, W.C. and BOGGS, M.M. 1950. Effect of storage temperature on quality of frozen peas. Food Technol. *4,* 5.

MASURE, M.P. and CAMPBELL, H. 1944. Rapid estimation of peroxidase in vegetable extracts — An index of blanching adequacy for frozen vegetables. Fruit Prod. J. Am. Food Manufac. *23,* 369-74.

OLSON, R.L., DIETRICH, W.C. 1968. *In* The Freezing Preservation of Foods, Vol. 2, D.K. Tressler, W.B. Van Arsdel and M.J. Copley (Editors). AVI Publishing Co. Westport, Conn.

PONTING, J.D., SANSHUCK, D.W. and BREKKE, J.E. 1960. Color measurement and deterioration in grape and berry juices and concentrates. Food Res. *25,* 471-478.

PONTING, J.D., FEINBERG, B. and BOYLE, F.P. 1968. *In* The Freezing Preservation of Foods. AVI Publishing Co., Westport, Conn.

SHEPHERD, A.D. 1960. Relative stabilities of various frozen foods. *In* Conference on Frozen Food Quality. USDA Western Regional Research Laboratory, Albany, CA.

USDA. Food Dating: Shoppers' Reaction and Impact on Retail Food Stores. Market Research Report 984.

VAN ARSDEL, W.B., COPLEY, M.J. and OLSON, R.J. 1969. Quality and Stability of Frozen Foods. John Wiley & Sons, New York.

VOLZ, F.E., GORTNER, W.A. and DELWICK, C.V. 1949. Effect of desiccation in frozen vegetables. Food Technol. *3,* 307.

CHAPTER 15

SHELF-LIFE OF CONCENTRATED JUICES

INITIAL PROCESSING AND PACKAGING

The general processing steps for concentrated juices start with cleaning, grading, peeling, cutting, and juicing of the fruit, followed by concentrating. In most cases, concentrates are made by concentrating fresh juice to slightly less than one quarter of the original volume. Usually a small amount of unconcentrated juice is added to the concentrated juice to restore fresh flavor. This process is called "add back". The juice is now a four-fold concentrate and is diluted with three volumes of water to prepare it for consumption. Small amounts of orange peel oil or volatile flavoring constituents may be added to give a full flavor concentrate and to compensate for flavor lost during the concentrating process. This is referred to as "stripping". At some stage, commercial citrus processors generally inactivate the enzyme pectin-methylesterase (PME) with high temperature — short time (HTST) pasteurization to improve the retention of natural cloudiness in the original juice (Stevens 1940). This treatment is kept to a minimum due to the fact that high temperatures tend to impart a "cooked" off-flavor to juices.

Packaging of concentrated juices is usually done in laminated containers which are hermetically sealed. These containers may be foil covered paper bodies with metal ends, aluminum bodies with aluminum or tin plate ends, or enameled tin plate.

Freezing is accomplished in air blast freezers or by liquid immersion freezing to achieve a temperature of lower than 0 °F (—18 °C) as soon as possible after processing. The major advantage of liquid immersion freezing is that it results in moderately rapid freezing, as indicated by the fact that 6 oz cans of orange juice concentrate are cooled from 4° to —18 °C (40° to 0 °F) in 10—15 min using commercially available equipment (Fennema 1975).

PRESERVATION

Freezing is unquestionably the most satisfactory method currently available for long term preservation of foods. Preservation by freezing provides the closest approach to maintaining fresh quality of foods. Frozen foods can be considered extremely stable products if they are prepared under sanitary conditions and kept below 0 °F in the interval from production to consumption. The preservative benefits of freezing are: arresting growth of microorganisms; preserving nutritional values by reduction of chemical reaction rates; controlling rodents, insects and parasites due to their inability to live at low temperatures; retarding chemical activity; and retarding or arresting enzyme activity (Rutgers University 1971).

An excellent example of the quality of frozen foods is citrus fruit juice, particularly orange juice concentrate, which will retain its quality for over two years at 0 °F, and will lose less than 10% of vitamin C even at temperatures as high as 40 °F (Kramer 1974). In addition, when frozen concentrated orange juice was subjected to improper conditions, it required at least three days at room temperature (70 °F) and at least 5 weeks at 40 °F to cause cans to swell or burst. During these periods of time, only yeast organisms grew (Rutgers University 1971).

Superior packaging also has an important role in preservation of concentrated juices. Proper packaging prevents recontamination by microorganisms because the cans are hermetically sealed. Care must be taken to utilize the proper enamels to prevent iron and other trace metal accumulations in the product. In addition, cans are deaerated to prevent oxidation of ascorbic acid. Packaging of concentrated juices also prohibits the potential destruction of ascorbic acid by light.

Cloudiness or turbidity is a physical characteristic indicative of good quality in frozen concentrated juices. High temperature—short time pasteurization is employed in concentrates in order to inactivate pectinmethylesterase (PME) so cloudiness will be maintained in the concentrated juice. High temperture—short time pasteurization also significantly reduces the number of microorganisms.

In addition, sorbic acid and sodium benzoate may be added to orange juice and orange juice concentrates prepared for further manufacture (Federal Register 1961, 1963). Sorbic acid and sodium benzoate are used to inhibit the growth of molds and yeast associated with food spoilage.

DISTRIBUTION

The maintenance of low temperatures and the use of good handling practices and stock rotation throughout transportation, warehousing, and retailing are important to frozen food quality. In the United States, −18 °C (0 °F) is generally accepted as a satisfactory storage temperature for frozen foods (lower temperatures are more common in Europe). The length of time that frozen foods such as concentrated juices can be maintained in good condition depends on the quality of the fresh fruit, the maintenance of sanitary conditions, the methods of processing and packaging and the control of storage temperatures.

In spite of the fact that frozen foods should be maintained at −18 °C or lower during storage and marketing, sizable quantities are routinely exposed to higher temperatures. Frozen foods may be kept for up to one year in warehouses due to marketing considerations, yet it appears that most mishandling occurs at locations other than storage warehouses, especially in assembly rooms, delivery trucks and retail cabinets (Fennema 1975). The nonuniformity of temperatures that can occur even in properly operated retail cabinets was demonstrated by Bodyfelt and Davidson (1975).

Nonrotational handling by the distribution trade and consumer errors in home storage and preparation can lead to quality losses. Although citrus fruit concentrates will retain quality for over two years at 0 °F, and will lose less than 10% ascorbic acid at temperatures as high as 40 °F, other frozen foods are more vulnerable. Kramer (1974) stated that −5 °F is adequate to maintain sensory quality of broccoli, cauliflower, spinach, and peaches for 12 months or longer, yet these products may lose 20 to 50% of their vitamin C concent under these storage conditions. Thus, due to the differences in products and product losses (i.e., sensory vs nutritional) it is important to maintain 0 °F (−18 °C) or lower in the interval from production to consumption to ensure the maintenance of proper quality.

MODES OF DETERIORATION

Nutrient Retention

As stated earlier, the sensory quality of citrus fruit juices may deteriorate more rapidly than the vitamin content. Numerous articles report that nutrient retention during storage, especially that of ascorbic acid in frozen and canned citrus fruits, is good. Huggart *et al.* (1954) reported that no appreciable decrease in ascorbic acid occurred in packs of Florida frozen orange, tangerine, and grapefruit concentrates stored for twelve months at −8 °, 10 °, 20 °, 32 ° and 40 °F. In addition, Huggart *et al.* (1954) cited evidence that ascorbic acid losses in Florida frozen citrus concentrate were exceedingly low at temperatures as high as 75 °F for periods up to 11 months. The figures for percent retention of ascorbic acid in six citrus juices are given in Table 15.1.

Kramer (1974) stated that canned citrus juices intended for storage of up to two years should be kept at not higher than 45 °F if 90% of their vitamin C is to be retained. Canned pineapple and tomato juice must be stored at less than 70 °F and 60 °F respectively, while carrot juice may be

TABLE 15.1
RETENTION OF ASCORBIC ACID IN 42° BRIX-CONCENTRATED CITRUS JUICES STORED FOR 12 MONTHS[1]

Storage Temperature (°F)	% Retention Hamlin Orange	Pineapple Orange	Valencia Orange	Dancy Tangerine	Duncan Grapefruit	Marsh Grapefruit
−8	100	98.7	99.2	94.0	98.4	98.8
10	99.9	98.0	97.9	93.5	97.9	98.8
20	98.7	96.7	96.7	90.7	98.1	98.3
32	97.6	96.0	96.2	90.9	97.7	98.6
40	97.1	94.7	95.9	89.7	97.1	97.1

[1]Adapted from Huggart *et al.* (1954)

stored at ambient temperatures (21 °C) with no appreciable loss in vitamin A, due to the fact that vitamin A or its precursor carotene is more stable than vitamin C.

Microbial

In normal situations, the public health hazards of frozen foods are negligible. If the product is maintained at low temperatures, no possible public health hazards arise. As was stated earlier, even when frozen concentrated juice was subjected to improper storage conditions, it required three days at 70 °F for cans to burst or swell, and then only yeast organisms grew.

Canned concentrated juices should not present a public health hazard if proper sanitary conditions and retort conditions are met.

Color and Flavor

The frozen food industry acknowledges the main basis for consumer quality judgments to be color and flavor (Rutgers University 1971). Early studies by Kew and Veldhius (1962) showed that a combination of heat with high yield reaming appeared to reduce stability of flavor. Recently, new methods for aroma recovery have led to the production of aroma concentrates which possess many of the characteristics of fresh orange aroma (Guadagni 1970a). Guadagni studied the stability of aroma and taste in frozen orange juice concentrate (FOJC). Basically he found FOJC made with aroma solutions stored at 0 °F were stable for periods of up to a year. In addition, taste was stable for these storage conditions. Saldana *et al.* (1976) prepared canned beverages from combinations of carrot juices, carrot puree, whole orange puree, grapefruit and pineapple juices and lemon juice concentrate. The beverages were stored at 20 °C for 9 months. Flavor and aroma in these beverages did not change significantly with storage. Ponting *et al.* (1960) stated that the flavor and color of the concentrates can be protected from heat damage by confining heat treatment to a minimum.

Guadagni (1970b) has suggested that concentrates with aroma solutions be stored at 55 ° Brix instead of the standard 42 ° Brix. Gaudagni feels that concentrates stored at 55 ° Brix will provide important savings in containers, storage space and transportation costs. There has been some question as to how this concentrate would reconstitute.

Cloud Stability

Cloud or turbidity in reconstituted juice is a physical characteristic indicative of good quality in frozen concentrated orange juices. Concentrates which retain desirable cloud after being subject to short term elevated temperature are accepted as stable products by the citrus industry (Rouse *et al.* 1957). Studies in the early 1950s on stability of orange juice concentrate indicated cloud loss as the first serious quality defect upon storage (Guadagni 1970b). These juices were not pasteurized. Today commercial processors have alleviated this problem by HTST pasteurization which inactivates pectin-methylesterase and prevents cloud loss or gelatin. Rouse in 1957 stated that the storage life of frozen concentrates with respect to cloud stability can be increased by keeping the product at 0 °F or below, concentrating the product to 57 ° Brix to 75 ° Brix, and by controlling heat treatment. Today, with the common practice of HTST pasteurization, cloud stability has been significantly improved.

SHELF-LIFE DATA

The kinetic data presented in Table 15.2 were obtained from the lines corresponding to the references given in the figures. In many cases, data were found for various storage times but only one temperature. These data may not represent true shelf-life data. More information on true storage stability studies carried out at three different temperatures for various lengths of time is necessary.

With respect to orange juice concentrate, Figs. 15.1 to 15.4 give data on shelf-life as measured organoleptically. The Q_{10}s reported for the frozen concentrate vary from 5.5 to 12, while the Q_{10} for the refrigerated product is around 2. At 5 °F the reported shelf-life for the frozen product

TABLE 15.2

KINETIC PARAMETERS FOR STORAGE OF JUICE CONCENTRATES

Figure No.	Product	Criteria	Comments	E_a (Kcal/mole)	Q_{10}	Reference
15.1	orange juice (concentrate)	sensory	—	10.3	2.0	Kramer 1974
15.2	orange and grapefruit (concentrate)	sensory	—	26.0	6.8	Kramer 1974
15.3	orange juice (frozen)	relative stability	—	24.2	5.49	Shephard 1960
15.4	orange aroma (solution)	aroma	θ_s based on 50% correct responses	26.8	7.7	Guadagni 1970b
15.5	orange juice (COJ — chilled)	time to reach fermentation (yeast growth)	COJ inoculated with 1 organism/ml	40.5	8.0	Murdock and Hatcher 1975
15.6	apple juice (concentrate)	organoleptic	—	12.3	2.05	Czapski 1976
15.7	Strawberry, boysenberry grape juice	10% loss in color intensity just noticeable to the eye	color loss at high evaporation temperatures	15.1 17.5 24.2	2.0 2.1 2.8	Ponting 1960 Ponting 1960 Ponting 1960

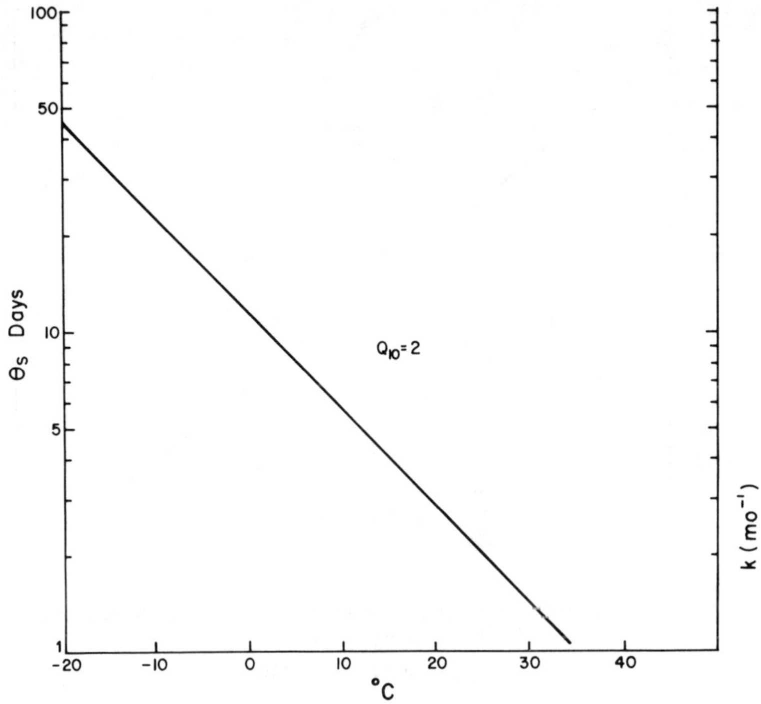

FIG. 15.1. PACKAGED ORANGE JUICE CONCENTRATE SHELF-LIFE (From Amman 1976).

ranges from 4 weeks to 20 months. The refrigerated concentrate (unfrozen) lasts only a few days above 0 °C. Obviously, the systems studied varied greatly in their actual composition but the data show the definite need for freezing.

Murdock and Hatcher (1975) reported the times for yeast fermentation of chilled orange juice in Fig. 15.5. The Q_{10} is around 8 to 26 depending on the inoculum, and above 45 °F the product is fermented in two days to one week. Yeast can easily contaminate orange juice in preparation from concentrate, so it should be used rapidly. It is interesting to note that the shelf-life data for flavor show only a Q_{10} of 2 for a similar product. Recently (Kopelman and Effroni 1977) did an excellent kinetic shelf-life study on chilled reconstituted juice. They found that mild pasteurization trebles the shelf-life under refrigeration based on microbial growth. In addition, below 8 °C the Q_{10} was 7.5, but above it the mechanism changed to give a Q_{10} of 36. Similarly, above 8 °C the Q_{10} for flavor deterioration increased from 3 to a value of 10. What is most interesting is that they used first

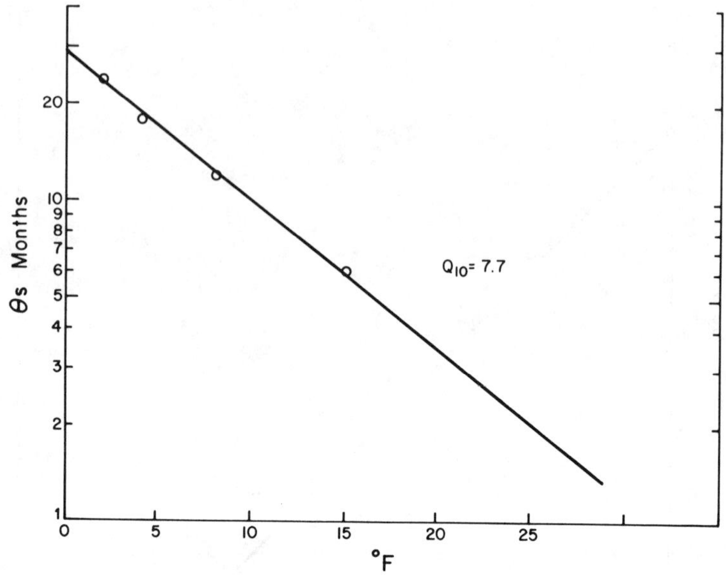

FIG. 15.2. FROZEN ORANGE AND GRAPEFRUIT CONCENTRATE SHELF-LIFE
(From Kramer 1974).

order kinetics to predict the yeast population in two variable temperature situations (e.g., 40 h at 5 °C, 10 hr at 11 °C, 20 hr at 6.5 °C and 125 hr at 8.0 °C) and got very close results as compared to actual growth levels. This verifies the use of the equations for a first order reaction developed in Chapter 3 with respect to microbial growth.

Figure 15.6 shows data for heat processed canned apple juice concentrate. These data are similar to those for the low Q_{10} in refrigerated orange juice but do not fit a very good straight line. A low Q_{10} is expected for a nonfrozen product.

Figure 15.7 gives results for the time to loss of 10% color for various juices undergoing the thermal process during evaporation as well as storage. As seen, at 40—45 °C, significant losses could take place. The study points out the need for rapid evaporation to achieve good color.

Table 15.3 shows data on nutrient losses during storage. The data of Huggart *et al.* (1954) showed very little change for vitamin C loss over the period of one year storage at —10 to 36 °F and for storage of the reconstituted product for two days at 50 °F. Thus, the Q_{10}s are very small. In most cases the loss was less than 5%.

TABLE 15.3
EFFECT OF VARIETY ON KINETIC PARAMETERS FOR FROZEN JUICE STORAGE

Product	Criteria	Comments	E_a (Kcal/mole)	Q_{10}	Reference
Concentrated citrus juices	Ascorbic acid retention after 12 months storage at −10 to 36°F				Huggart *et al.* 1954
(a) Duncan and Marsh grapefruit			—	1.01	Huggart *et al.* 1954
(b) Hamline			—	1.01	Huggart *et al.* 1954
(c) Valencia orange and pineapple			—	1.02	Huggart *et al.* 1954
(d) Dancy			—	1.04	Huggart *et al.* 1954
Average			13.31	1.013	
(a) Duncan and Marsh	Ascorbic acid retention after 2 days at 50°F		—	1.01	Huggart *et al.* 1954
(b) Hamline			—	1.02	Huggart *et al.* 1954
(c) Pineapple			—	1.02	Huggart *et al.* 1954
(d) Valencia			—	1.03	Huggart *et al.* 1954
(e) Dancy			—	1.04	Huggart *et al.* 1954
Blueberry juice	Pantothenic acid	nutrient loss	23.4	4.4	Eitenmiller *et al.* 1977
	Riboflavin		25.6	4.79	Eitenmiller *et al.* 1977
	Thiamin		2.7	1.18	Eitenmiller *et al.* 1977
	Niacin Ascorbic Acid	amount retention increased at 21°C as compared to 40°C			
	B_6		12.3	4.78	Eitenmiller *et al.* 1977
	Biotin		1.9	1.12	Eitenmiller *et al.* 1977
	Folacin		1.2	1.08	Eitenmiller *et al.* 1977

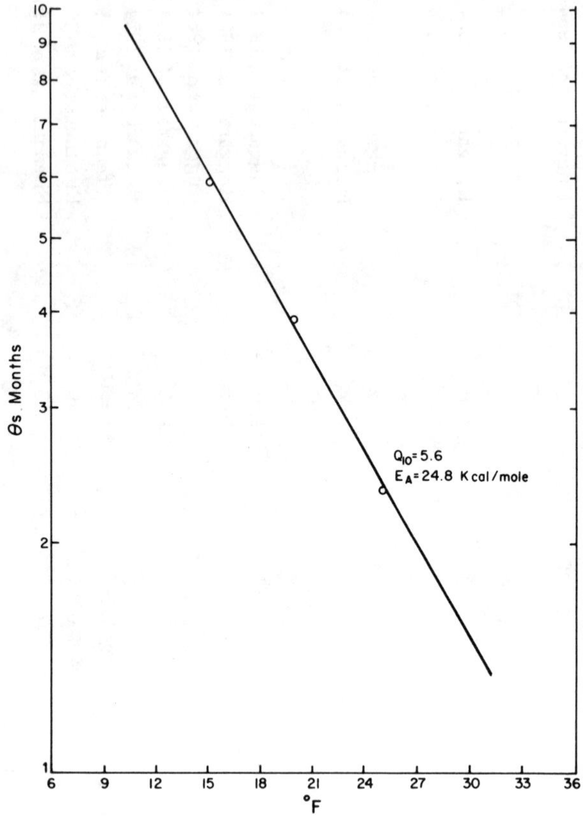

FIG. 15.3. RELATIVE STABILITY OF FROZEN ORANGE JUICE

(From Shepherd 1960)

TABLE 15.4
APPROXIMATE STORAGE LIFE OF FROZEN JUICES AT 0°F OR BELOW[1]

Product (Concentrated)	Months
Apple juice	30
Grape juice	24
Grapefruit juice	24
Grapefruit-orange juice	24
Lemon juice	18
Lime juice	18
Orange juice	24
Pineapple juice	24

[1]Department of the Army (1971).

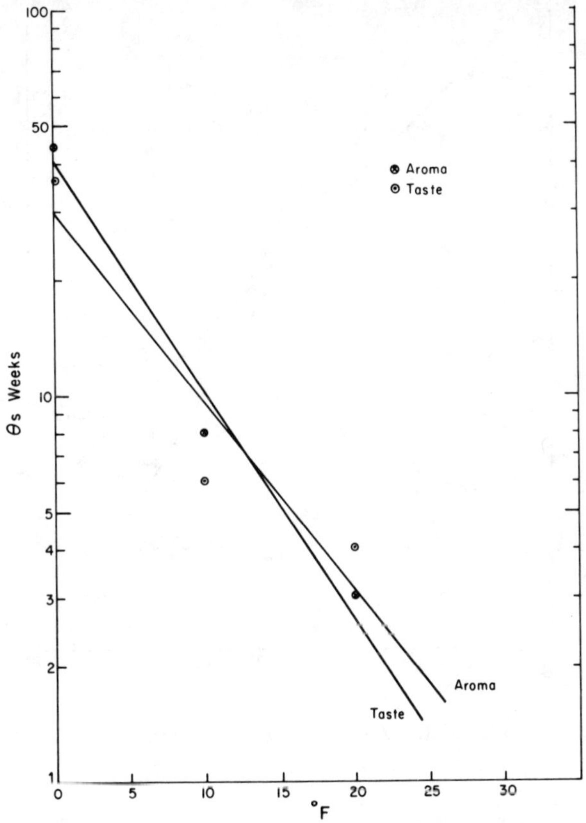

FIG. 15.4. FROZEN ORANGE JUICE — θ_s BASED ON 50% CORRECT RESPONSES (From Guadagni *et al.* 1970).

TABLE 15.5
LOSS OF VITAMIN C FROM FRUITS DURING THE ENTIRE FREEZING PROCESS

Product	Loss of Vitamin C (mean %)	Storage Time at −18°C (months)
Citrus products:		
orange juice concentrate, 42° Brix	1	9
Orange juice, unconcentrated	32	6
Grapefruit juice concentrate, 42° Brix	5	9

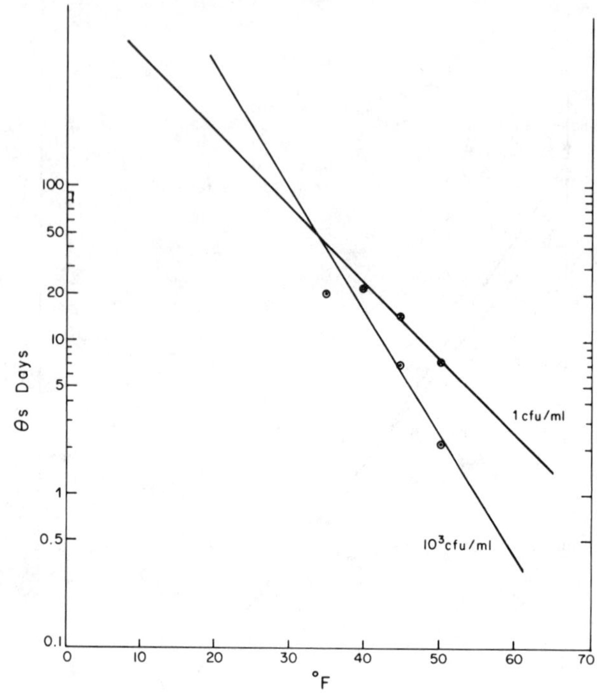

FIG. 15.5. YEAST GROWTH IN CHILLED ORANGE JUICE (From Murdock and Hatcher 1975).

Figures 15.8 and 15.9 show nutrient losses in blueberry juice during storage at 4 and 21 °C. The Q_{10}s vary with the different vitamins as is shown in Table 15.3. For vitamin C and niacin, the retention increases at the higher temperature, which is not expected.

Table 15.4 shows the Army shelf-life data for various juices. Only one temperature is reported, so no Q_{10} could be calculated. Table 15.5 lists values for loss of vitamin C from fruits during the entire freezing process.

OPEN DATING

Quality retention is based on surveillance of the product at every stage in its life cycle, including maintenance of low storage temperatures (0 °F or below) as well as good manufacturing practices in selection of raw materials and sanitation and speed in handling and processing. Frozen food companies generally practice industrial coding on packages by openly placing the date of final packaging on the exterior of the individual packages of frozen food. Date of final packaging or "pack date" is used because it permits and encourages first-in, first-out stock rotation in distribution and retail store operations. The stamping of individual food packages with date of shelf display is proposed to assure stock rotation at the retail store operations. The stamping of individual food packages with date of shelf display is proposed to assure stock rotation at the retail store level but is useless for frozen concentrates unless locally reconstituted. The adoption and enforcement of storage and transportation regulations that would require frozen foods to be held at or below 0 °F is recommended as a better method of quality assurance. Time-temperature recording devices with warning devices (alarms, bells) for temperatures greater than 0 °F in warehouses, transportation equipment, and retail cabinets would also help insure better quality of frozen food products such as concentrated juices.

Due to the nonuniformity of temperatures that occur even in properly operating retail cabinets, retail units should be vertical, door-closing freezer cabinets fitted with air-curtains to reduce mishandling of foods by retailers and consumers. These units should be maintained at 0 °F or preferably −5 °F.

Use of a "pack date" is not recommended for open dating of these foods since exposure to high temperature for relatively short times is more critical than longer times at low temperatures and a "pack date" tells the consumer nothing about the storage conditions.

The use of a "sell by date" is not meaningful unless combined with storage information. In the United Kingdom, for example, frozen food industry trade associations and refrigerated freezer manufacturers cooperated in developing a unique system that provides consumers with knowledge of recommended home storage life. This system, known as the Three-Star System, defines time and temperature allowances for home storage protection for each type of refrigerator-freezer or freezer unit. If a freezer can maintain a temperature of 21 °F, food should be used within one week; if 10 °F, within one month; and if 0 °F, within 3 months. The refrigerator-freezer or freezer units receive one (*), two (**), or three-star (***) ratings based on their ability to achieve such temperatures. It should be noted that the Three-Star System correlates rather well with the times of storage commonly found in randomly chosen households in the United States (Rutgers University 1971). Product packages would then be labeled, for example:

"If your frozen food compartment has the new 'star' rating, here are the recommended storage times: * 10 days; ** 1 month; *** 6 months."

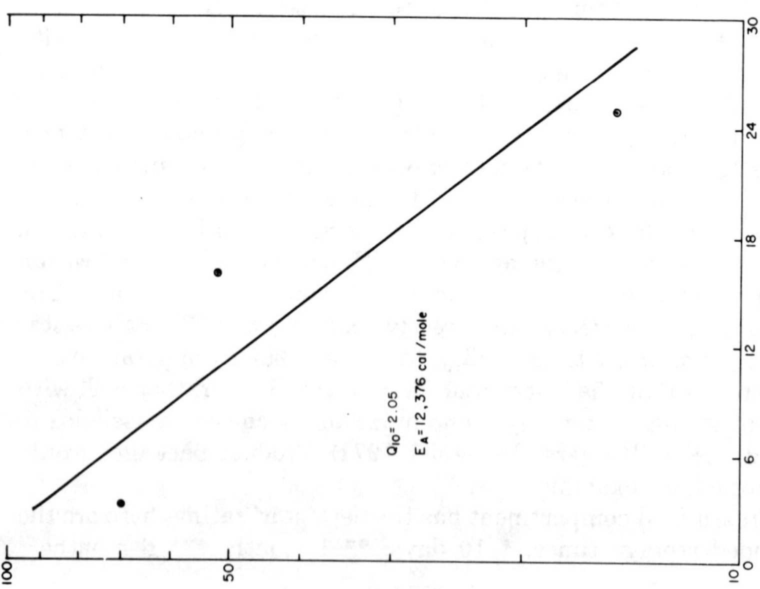

FIG. 15.6. APPLE JUICE (CONCENTRATED) — θ_s ORGANOLEPTICALLY BASED
(From Czapski 1976).

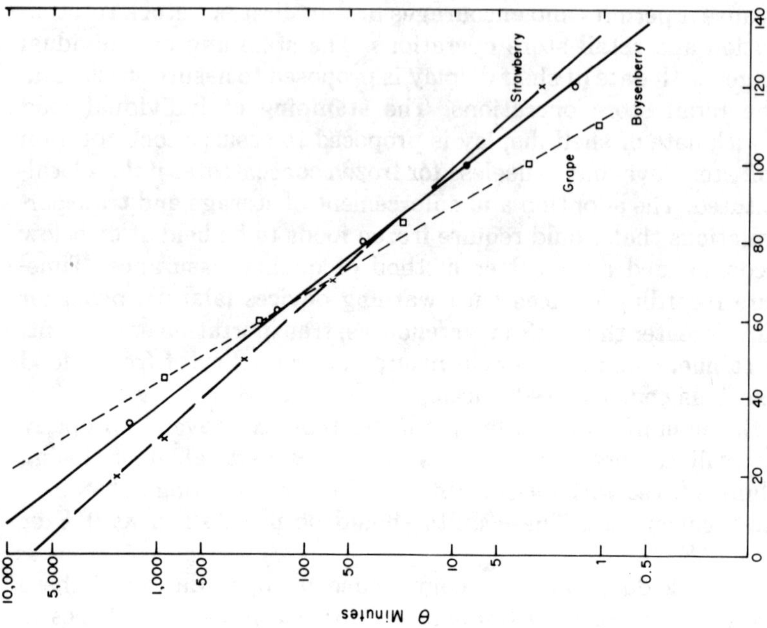

FIG. 15.7. TIME FOR 10% LOSS OF COLOR IN JUICES AT VARIOUS TEMPERATURES

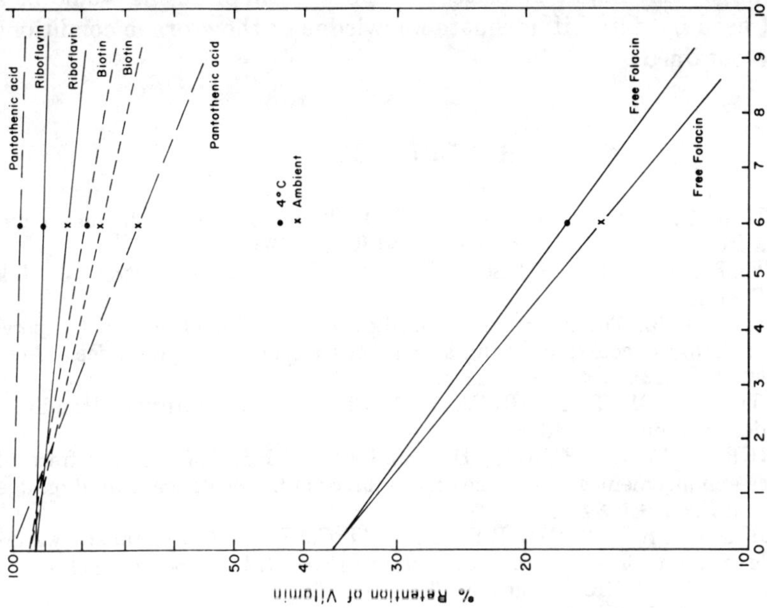

FIG. 15.9. BLUEBERRY JUICE
(From Eitenmiller *et al.* 1977).

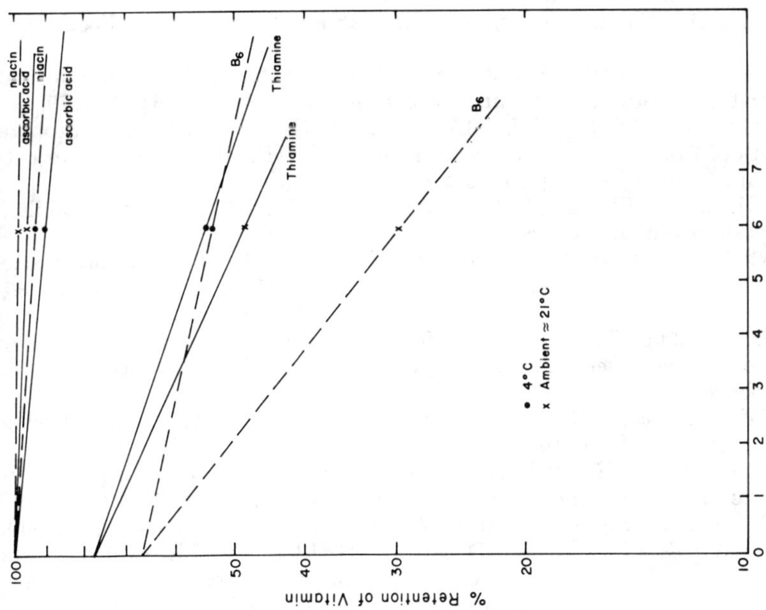

FIG. 15.8. BLUEBERRY JUICE
(From Eitenmiller *et al.* 1977).

However, most households would have a freezer that would have a three-star rating so this might be useless. The best form of dating would be a "best if used by date" if adequate knowledge of the storage conditions could be obtained.

REFERENCES

BEATTIE, H.G., WHEELER, K.A. and PEDERSON, C.S. 1943. Changes occurring in fruit juices during storage. Food Res. *8,* 395.

BODYFELT, F.W. and DAVIDSON, W.D. 1975. Temperature control. J. Milk Food Technol. *38,* 12.

CZAPSKI, J. 1976. The influence of clarification, concentration and temperature on changes occurring during storage of concentrated apple juice. Acta Aliment. Polonica. *2,* 4.

DEPARTMENT OF THE ARMY. 1971. Storage and Materials Handling. Technical Manual TM 743-200.

DOUGHERTY, M.H., PETRUS, D.R. and FELLERS, P.J. 1974. Effect of essence enhancement and storage on the flavor of frozen concentrated orange juice. J. Food Sci. *39,* 855.

EITENMILLER, R.R., KUHL, R.F. and SMIT, C.J.B. 1977. Mineral and water-soluble vitamin content of rabbiteye blueberries. J. Food Sci. *42,* 311.

FEDERAL REGISTER. January 31, 1961. Vol. 26.

FEDERAL REGISTER. October 11, 1963. Vol. 28.

FENNEMA, O. 1975. Freezing preservation. *In* Principles of Food Science, Part II. O. Fennema (Editor) Marcel Dekker, New York.

FENNEMA, O. 1977. Loss of vitamins in fresh and frozen foods. Food Technol. *31,* 12.

GUADAGNI, D.G., BOMBEN, J.L. and MANNHEIM, H.C. 1970a. Effect of temperature on stability of orange aroma solution. J. Food Sci. *35,* 279.

GUADAGNI, D.G., BOMBEN, J.L. and MANNHEIM, H.C. 1970b. Storage stability of frozen orange juice concentrate made with aroma solution or cutback juice. Food Technol. *24,* 1012.

HOLLAND, R.R., REEDER, S.K. and PRITCHETT, D.E. 1976. Cloud stability test for pasteurized citrus juices. J. Food Sci. *41,* 813.

HUGGART, R.L., HARMAN, D.A. and MOORE, E.L. 1954. Ascorbic acid retention in frozen concentrated citrus juices. J. Am. Diet. Assoc. *30,* 682.

JOHNSON, R.L. and TOLEDO, R.T. 1975. Storage stability of 55° brix orange juice concentrate aseptically packaged in plastic and glass containers. J. Food Sci. *40,* 433.

KEW, T.J. and VELDHIUS, M.K. 1962. Stability of citrus juices following adverse storage. Food Technol. *16*(10), 119.

KOPELMAN, I. and EFFRONI, D. 1977. Shelf life and microbial growth of chilled reconstituted orange juice. Lebensm. Wiss. Technol. *10,* 131.

KRAMER, A. 1974. Storage retention of nutrients. Food Technol. *28*(1), 50-60.

LEE, Y.C., KIRK, J.R., BEDFORD, C.L. and HELDMAN, D.R. 1977. Kinetics and computer simulation of ascorbic acid stability of tomato juice as functions of temperature, pH and metal catalysts. J. Food Sci. *42,* 640.

McCOLLOCH, R.J., RICE, R.G., BANDURSKI, M.B. and GENTILI, B. 1957. Time-temperature tolerance of frozen foods. VII. Frozen concentrated orange juice. Food Technol. *11,* 444.

MURDOCK, D.I. and HATCHER, W.S. 1975. Growth of microorganisms in chilled orange juice. J. Milk Food Technol. *38,* 7.

NIMMO, C.C., WALKER, L.H. AND SEAMANS, V.S. 1952. Influence of storage conditions on frozen and canned apple juice concentrates. Food Technol. *6,* 31.

PETERSON, A.C. 1961. *In* Proceedings of the Low Temperature Microbiology Symposium, Campbell Soup Co., Camden, NJ.

PONTING, J.D., SANSHUCK, D.W. and BREKKEE, J.E. 1960. Color measurement and determination in grape and berry juices and concentrates. Food Res. *25,* 471-478.

ROUSE, A.H., ATKINS, C.D. and MOORE, E.L. 1957. Factors contributing to the storage life of frozen concentrated orange juice. Food Technol. *11,* 218.

RUTGERS UNIVERSITY. 1971. Food Stability Survey. Rutgers University Department of Food Science for the State of New Jersey Department of Health. In cooperation with the U.S. Department of Agriculture/Economic Research Service.

SALDANA, G., STEPHENS, T.S. and LIME, B.J. 1976. Carrot beverages. J. Food Sci. *41,* 1243.

SHEPHARD, A.D. 1960. Frozen juice concentrates. *In* Conference on Food Quality. USDA-WRRL, Albany, California. ARS 74-21, Nov. 4.

STEVENS, J.W. 1940. Method of conserving fruit juices. U.S. Patent 2,216,261.

TRINGLEFF, A.J. and MILLER, E.V. 1959. Studies on ascorbic acid retention in frozen juice, segments and whole oranges. Food Res. *25,* 145.

CHAPTER 16

SHELF-LIFE OF COFFEE AND TEA

COFFEE PROCESSING

In the United States coffee is produced as roasted and ground coffee which is extracted with water prior to consumption by percolation or by the "drip-through" method; or it is produced as soluble (instant) coffee which is dissolved in water before it is consumed. Roasted and ground coffee is made by roasting the dried green coffee beans, grinding the roasted beans, and packaging the ground beans for sale. Soluble coffee is made by extracting the roasted ground coffee with very hot water and then either spray-drying or freeze-drying the extract.

When coffee is roasted, the green beans are quickly heated in order to drive off all of the moisture. The beans are then heated to a temperature greater than 360°F (180°C), where pyrolysis occurs and exothermic chemical reactions produce the roasted coffee aroma. At this point the temperature in the beans rises to between 392° and 410°F (200—210°C) (Sivetz and Foote 1963). During this time, a large amount of carbon dioxide is evolved, mainly from the decomposition of carbohydrates and acids (Rutgers University 1971). This carbon dioxide plays an important role in the preservation of the roasted coffee after packaging, as will be shown below. Because of the high temperatures used in processing both roasted and instant coffee, and because of the low moisture content of the coffee, there are no known hazards to roasted and ground or instant coffee from microorganisms (Rutgers University 1971).

MODE OF DETERIORATION OF COFFEE

The mode of deterioration in coffee is staling, especially in roasted and ground coffee. However, most consumers have become so used to drinking stale coffee that they have developed a taste for it (Lee 1975). Instant coffee is not so susceptible to staling as roasted and ground coffee since it has already lost a considerable amount of aroma during extraction and drying (Rutgers University 1971). However, in order to recover some of the aroma lost in extraction and drying, coffee producers add natural coffee aroma as coffee oil to the dried powder. When more volatile and unstable flavor compounds are added to soluble coffee, the coffee becomes more susceptible to staling (Harris *et al.* 1974).

Staling was previously thought to be due to rancidity of the coffee oil but Elder (1940) showed that coffee oil stabilized from oxidation with an antioxidant still did not taste fresh compared to vacuum packed coffee. Staling is now thought to be due to loss of flavor volatiles or to chemical changes in the volatile components caused by moisture and oxygen absorption (Lee 1975; Rutgers University 1971). Staling in roasted and ground coffee can occur to a moderate extent after one week and to a considerable extent after three weeks (Rutgers University 1971). Sivetz and Foote (1963) described the aroma degeneration during staling as changing from flat to old to sharply rancid, after which cocoa odor appears in the advanced stage. The taste of the coffee concurrently changes from flat to bitter, old, and rancid. At this point the coffee should no longer be sold. If the coffee is unprotected, the coffee borders on unsalability in seven to fourteen days depending on the storage conditions and the sensitivity of the taste buds.

SHELF-LIFE OF GROUND COFFEE

Moisture is a critical factor in staling in both roasted and ground coffee and soluble coffee. In fact, moisture seems to be more important to the stability of coffee aroma in soluble coffee than oxygen (Harris *et al.* 1974; Sivetz and Foote 1963). When unpackaged roast coffee is exposed to air at various relative humidities, the rate of staling increases as the humidity increases. At 100% RH, an old taste develops after 3—4 days, at 50% RH an old taste develops after 7—8 days and at 0% RH an old taste does not develop until 3—4 weeks. Moist oxygen is more harmful than moist nitrogen or dry oxygen. A relative humidity of only 25% will cause the moisture content of unprotected coffee to increase to 5% (Sivetz and Foote 1963). As reported by Lee in Harris *et al.* (1974), moisture in air on a fairly dry day can cause hydrolysis of the esters, acetals, and ketals in coffee aroma to other compounds which do not have as pleasing an aroma.

SHELF-LIFE OF INSTANT COFFE

Harris *et al.* (1974), in a study on soluble coffee shelf-life, found very few differences in color, odor, flavor, or appearance in both spray-dried and freeze-dried coffee stored in zero oxygen, 2% oxygen and air at storage times up to one year. In spray-dried soluble coffee, the odor after one week and after two months in zero oxygen was judged to be significantly better than the odor of 2% oxygen or airpack coffee. After nine months the flavor of airpack spray-dried coffee was judged significantly worse than that in 2% oxygen or zero oxygen. In freeze-dried coffee, no significant differences in odor, color, flavor, or appearance were noted for storage times up to one year except after three months. At this time, the coffee stored in zero oxygen was judged to be better than that stored in 2% oxygen or in air. The researchers also served spray-dried and freeze-dried coffee stored for one year in air, 2% oxygen and zero oxygen to a consumer panel. The panel found no difference in the various coffees after zero storage time but after one year storage time, the spray-dried coffee packed in air was judged to be significantly worse than the coffee packed in 2% oxygen or zero oxygen. The researchers then served the panel a new sample to see if they could tell a difference between it and the coffee aged for one year. The panel could not detect any differences in any of the freeze-dried samples and judged that only the air-packed sample was significantly worse than the other three. The researchers concluded that the freeze-dried coffee had a longer shelf-life than the spray-dried coffee and that this extended shelf-life was probably due to the difference in the moisture contents of the two coffees. The freeze-dried coffee had an initial moisture value of 2.0% while that of the spray-dried coffee was 4.5%. They also concluded that moisture content had a greater effect on shelf-life than headspace gas treatment.

PACKAGING OF COFFEE

In order to protect coffee from staling, roasted and ground coffee is usually packaged in a metal can under vacuum with a resealable plastic lid. It may also be packed with an inert gas.

When coffee is roasted, a large amount of carbon dioxide is emitted both from the pyrolysis of the beans and the heating gases. The beans absorb a large amount of this CO_2 and a large part of this is lost during grinding of the beans. The coffee is stored from 2—8 hr after grinding to allow more CO_2 to escape. When the coffee is packaged, a vacuum of 29 in. of mercury is drawn to remove oxygen from the cans. The can is then sealed and CO_2 begins to evolve from the coffee. The evolution of CO_2 continues until the interior pressure of the can is greater than the outside pressure. In order to insure the greatest product stability, it is necessary to have no residual oxygen in the can. If the can is evacuated at 27 in. of mercury instead of 29 in., a very small amount of oxygen, 2% or less, will remain, which is sufficient to oxidize the flavor compounds in the coffee (Rutgers University 1971).

Coffee may also be sold in paper bags laminated with plastic, but this type of packaging is becoming scarce. This fold-top bag is more common when the beans are ground at the grocery store and sold under a chain supermarket private label. Since coffee sold in this way undergoes staling at a much faster rate, the stores arrange for frequent delivery and rely on a fast turnover rate (Rutgers University 1971; Sivetz and Foote 1963).

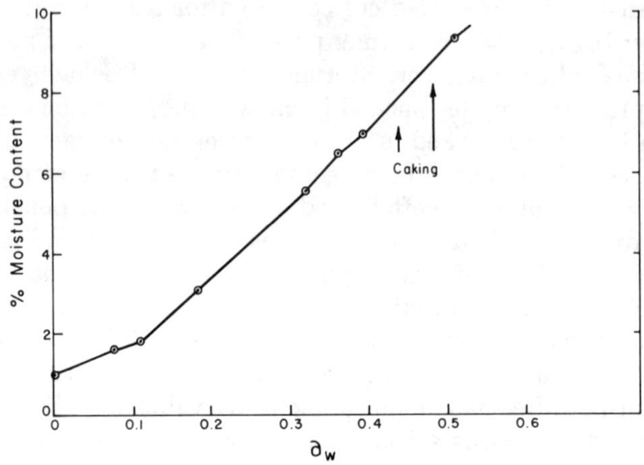

FIG. 16.1. SOLUBLE COFFEE ISOTHERM (23 °C)
(From Pintauro 1969).

In addition to loss of flavor, aromatized instant coffee has the problem of moisture pickup and caking when it is exposed to the atmosphere. To prevent these problems, soluble coffee is usually packaged in a glass jar with a paper seal under an inert gas. As the isotherms of soluble coffee show, (Figs. 16.1 and 16.2), the moisture content rises rapidly when the coffee is exposed to increasing relative humidities (Pintauro 1969; Quast and Neto 1976). Upon exposure to the atmosphere, the product will begin to cake, and if exposed to high humidities for an extended period of time, will turn into a tarry mass (Pintauro 1969). As can be seen from the isotherm, soluble coffee will begin to agglomerate at around 50% relative humidty. Above 75% RH soluble coffee will turn into a liquid. Because of the hygroscopic nature of coffee, it must be packaged in humidity-controlled areas. The equations developed in Chapter 3 can be used to predict moisture gain for semi-permeable pouches.

Coffee extract that is lyophilized is usually dried to below 1.7% moisture. Above this level the coffee will absorb too much moisture during further processing and will deteriorate rapidly upon storage. Drying to levels below 1%, however, will cause excess loss of aroma volatiles. Therefore, coffee should be dried to a level of moisture between 1.0 and

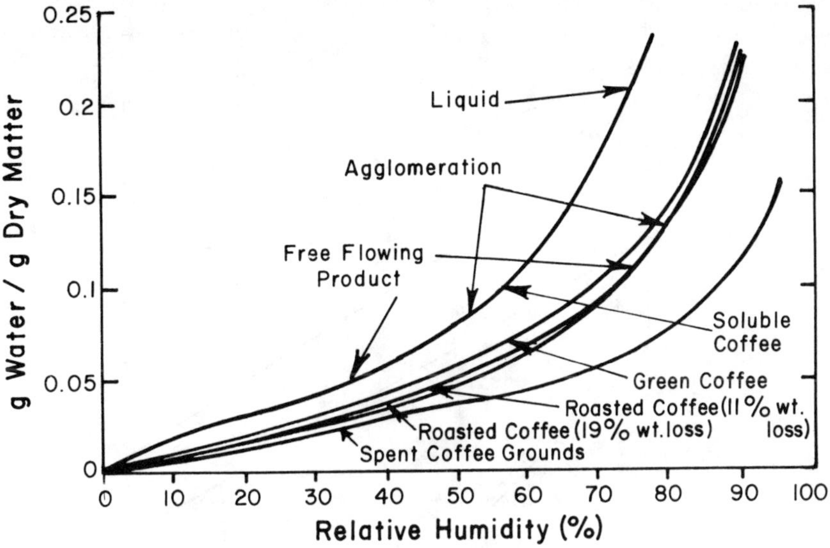

FIG. 16.2. COFFEE MOISTURE SORPTION ISOTHERMS AT 28°C, AS DETERMINED BY THE DESICCATOR METHOD
(From Quast and Teixeira Neeto 1976).

TABLE 16.1
SHELF-LIFE OF COFFEE

Type of Coffee	Shelf-Life (months) 40°F	70°F	90°F	Q_{10}	E_a (Kcal/mole)
Roasted and ground —					
can	18	12	5	1.57	7.40
pouch	9	2	1	2.24	13.30
Instant — jar	60	36	24	1.39	5.46
envelope	36	18	9	1.63	8.03

1.7%. In order to prevent the moisture level from exceeding 2.5% and the oxygen level from exceeding 2% and preferably 1% in the packaged product, the vacuum in the freeze-drier should be "broken" with an inert gas such as carbon dioxide, nitrogen or argon and the product should be shielded as much as possible from atmospheric oxygen and moisture. The inert gas used to break the vacuum will permeate the product and form a

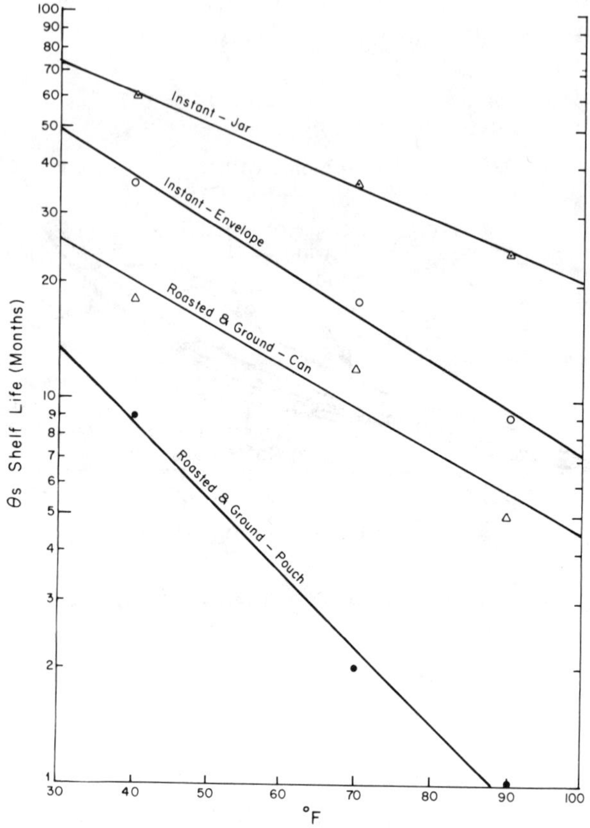

FIG. 16.3. SHELF-LIFE PLOTS OF COFFEE

protective layer around the particles, especially when the frozen extract has been ground into particles prior to freeze-drying. Exposure of the coffee to ambient conditions after this step should be kept at a minimum to insure that the moisture level remains below 2.5% and that the coffee does not cake during storage. The rapid pickup of moisture in the dried coffee can be seen in the following example. When the extract has been dried to below 1.7% moisture, coated with nitrogen and then exposed for 5 min to 80°F and 70% RH, the coffee will absorb about 0.5 to 0.8% moisture. Another 0.2% of moisture will be gained during packaging, and additional 0.2% moisture will dvelop during storage due to organic reactions (Pintauro 1969).

After coffee has been packaged, it is distributed from the factory according to normal distribution paths and conditions for semi-perishable foods. The coffee is transported from the factory and stored in warehouses under ambient conditions which may vary widely throughout the country. The distance the coffee must travel from the factory to the store depends both on the number of plants in the country and whether or not the company distributes their product nationally. One of the largest national manufacturers of coffee in the country, General Foods, has four plants in the country. They are located in Hoboken, New Jersey Houston, Texas, Jacksonville, Florida, and San Leandro, California. Therefore, coffee may have to travel over 1000 miles before it reaches the grocery shelf. Major coffee brands have a turnover rate from packaging to sales of two months (Rutgers University 1971).

Values for the actual shelf-life of coffee vary widely. In roasted and ground coffee packed in cans, the shelf-life depends on the efficiency with which the oxygen is removed during vacuum packaging. Nine months is usually considered to be the maximum shelf-life of unopened cans (Rutgers University 1971). Table 16.1 and Fig. 16.3 show shelf-lives for coffee, which are given in the Technical Manual for Storage and Materials Handling for the Department of the Army (1971). The Q_{10}s were calculated from the E_a at 50 to 68 °F.

It can be seen that the product with the longest shelf-life is instant coffee packed in a jar and that with the shortest is roasted and ground coffee packaged in a pouch. Other food industry sources give a shelf-life of one year for instant coffee and a shelf-life of 21 days for unground roasted coffee in double wall bags. Coffee ground in the home is expected to be used within one week after purchase (Rutgers University 1971).

TEA PROCESSING

Tea, like coffee, is made in both soluble and insoluble forms. The insoluble tea leaves are extracted with hot water, either loose or through a cloth bag. Soluble "instant" tea is made by extracting the tea in hot water and then either spray-drying or, less commonly, freeze-drying the extract. Tea may also be sold in cans or bottles in ready-to-drink form with added sugar and lemon, or as a dry mix with lemon flavoring and sweetener.

Three different types of tea can be made, depending on the degree of fermentation: black, oolong, and green teas.

Black tea goes through four processes: withering, rolling, fermentation, and firing. After the tea leaves have been picked, they are placed on trays to wither, or dry, for about 18 hr. Heat may be applied to reduce the withering time to 6 to 8 hr. During this time the moisture content of the leaves drops from 75—80% moisture to 58—68%, depending on the area of production (Lee 1975).

After withering, the tea leaves are rolled, which distorts the shape and crushes the cell walls. Oxidizing enzymes are released and allowed to mix with the flavonols to start the fermentation process (Lee 1975).

Fermentation follows the rolling step. The leaves are spread out and placed in a room at ambient temperature with a relative humidity near 100%. The leaves are allowed to ferment for about three hours, during which the leaves change from green to copper-red and the flavor is further developed (Lee 1975).

Following fermentation, the leaves are fired by heating them to 82—93 °C (180—200 °C). This heating denatures the enzymes and stops fermentation. During the heating, the moisture content is reduced to about 3% (Lee 1975).

Oolong tea is a semi-fermented tea. After the leaves are picked, they are spread in bamboo baskets which are held in the shade for 5—6 hr at a temperature of 28.3 to 29.4 °C (83—85 °F). This period allows for a small amount of fermentation. At the end of this time the leaves have changed in color and give off an odor similar to apples. Fermentation is then stopped by drying the leaves with agitation in a pan at about 204 °C (400 °F). The first firing lasts for about 3 hr; the second firing lasts from 5—12 hr (Lee 1975).

Green tea is not withered or fermented. After the leaves have been picked, they are steamed or heated to denature the enzymes. They are then rolled until they are dried. Further drying decreases the moisture content to about 2% (Lee 1975).

Tea is preserved generally by its low moisture content which inhibits the growth of microorganisms. Tea is a very stable food and even if stored for a long period of time does not result in any health hazard, either in leaf or instant form (Rutgers University 1971).

PACKAGING AND DISTRIBUTION

Tea is usually packaged so as to exclude moisture and sometimes light (Rutgers University 1971b). Loose tea is usually placed in metal cans but is not sealed under vacuum. Tea bags are individually wrapped in paper and then placed in a cardboard box with a plastic overwrap. Instant teas and tea mixes are usually packaged in glass jars with a sealed paper liner or in envelopes. The glass jars may be made of grown glass to exclude light. Ready-to-drink tea is packed in cans or bottles.

Tea follows normal distribution paths after leaving the factory and is stored in warehouses in which the temperatures may vary but in which extremes of temperature are avoided. Tea mixes are usually stored in areas in which the relative humidity does not exceed 50% (Rutgers University 1971).

MODES OF DETERIORATION

During storage, tea may undergo staling or may lose some of its aroma. Sometimes foreign or incompatible odors may be absorbed. Staling and mustiness can occur from oxidation and moisture adsorption. Moisture adsorption can also result in caking of instant tea (Rutgers University 1971). Freshly made black tea has a raw or green taste which mellows when stored for a few weeks. Longer storage, especially when the tea is exposed to light and moisture, will result in the tea having a "flat" taste and lacking in briskness. Tea in this condition is said to be "soft" (Wickremasinghe and Perera 1972). One study showed that when tea was exposed to moist air but not light the tea gained moisture at a rate of 0.227% per week. Of course, this would depend on the % RH, which was not given. When the tea is protected from moisture, it will gain moisture at a rate of only 0.0425% per week as seen in Fig. 16.4. The researchers

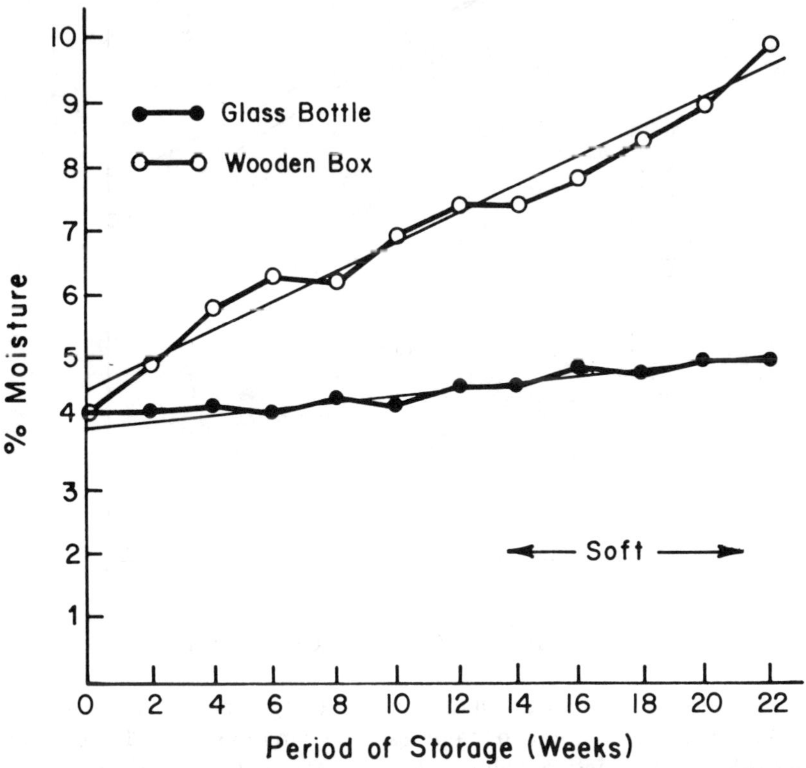

FIG. 16.4. CHANGES IN MOISTURE CONTENT OF BLACK TEA SAMPLES STORED IN GLASS BOTTLE AND WOODEN BOX

(From Wickremasinghe and Perera 1972).

TABLE 16.2
SHELF-LIFE OF TEA

Form of Tea	Shelf-Life (months) 40°F	70°F	90°F	Q_{10}	E_a (Kcal/mole)
Black, bags or loose in can/carton	36	18	12	1.49	6.53
Instant — envelope	36	18	9	1.63	8.03

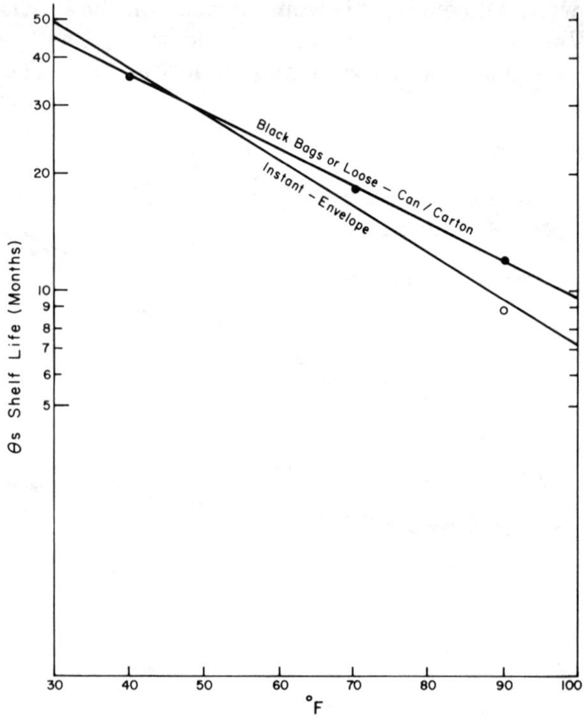

FIG. 16.5. SHELF-LIFE PLOTS OF TEA

found that, even when the tea had gained a large amount of moisture, the market value was similar to tea protected from moisture. The researchers concluded that moisture value alone does not lead to deterioration of tea. Studies on the levels of various chemical substances in the stored tea led to the suggestion that a reduced level of epicatechen gallate contributed to the "softness" of tea and that catechins were more photolabile than theaflavins (Wickremasinghe and Perera 1972).

According to the Technical Manual for Storage and Materials Handling for the Department of the Army (1971), the different forms of tea have the shelf-lives shown in Table 16.2 and Fig. 16.5.

According to the data plotted in Fig. 16.5, above 55 °F, loose tea in cans or tea bags in cartons has a slightly longer shelf-life than instant tea.

Other sources give canned or bottled tea a shelf-life of one year (Pintauro 1977), packaged tea a shelf-life of 24 months and tea bags a shelf life of 18 months (Rutgers University 1971). The following list gives the shelf-lives of tea in various forms as reported by various industry sources (Rutgers University 1971).

Form of Tea	*Shelf-Life (years)*
Tea	5
bags	1.5
bags	1
instant	indefinite
instant	1
loose/carton	1
mix	2
mix, iced	3
mix, iced	1
packaged/carton	2

ANALYSIS OF OPEN DATING

Consumer groups suggest that consumers have the right to know the age of foods they purchase in grocery stores (Rutgers University 1971), and how long foods can be expected to last before they should not be used. Open dating gives consumers psychological assurance that the food manufacturer is taking them into consideration and implies that the consumer could make more intelligent choices at the supermarket. The principle of open dating is commendable, but due to the lack of understanding of food deterioration, the practices of open dating may have no beneficial effect for certain foods. A few of the disadvantages of open dating for three of the different types of open dating are discussed below.

Pack Date

Open dating of the "pack date" would not be advantageous to the consumer for tea or coffee because it would not provide any information about the shelf-life of the product. An open date of manufacture might result in considerable wastage of the product since the consumer might conclude that an older product is not as good as a newer one, and would buy the product with the latest date on it. The conclusion would be particularly erroneous in the case of roasted and ground coffee since the greatest consumption of shelf-life occurs after the product is opened. The date of manufacture also does not give any indication of the true age of the coffee or tea since the green coffee beans or tea leaves could vary in age considerably from the time they were harvested until they were processed and packaged. The date of manufacture would also not reflect any differences in shelf-life due to different processing procedures among manufacturers. For example, two manufacturers of roasted and ground coffee may package on the same day and have the same date of manufacture. One manufacturer, however, evacuates the cans to 29 in. of mercury and thereby rids the cans of essentially all of the oxygen, while a second manufacturer evacuates the cans to 27 in. of mercury and leaves a residual amount of oxygen (Rutgers University 1971). The coffee produced by the first manufacturer would be expected to have a longer shelf-life than that of the second, yet this fact would not be reflected on the "pack date". The "pack date" placed on a product with no explanation of what kind of date it was would also tend to confuse the consumer who might interpret it as an expiration date and assume that it was already beyond its predicted shelf-life.

"Sell by Date"

The practice of placing a "sell by or pull date" on coffee or tea products would be almost meaningless and would cause an unnecessary expense to the manufacturer since the shelf-life of these products is long. The only product for which a "pull or sell by date" would be applicable would be roasted and ground coffee packaged in bags since the shelf-life of this product is much shorter than that of coffee packaged in vacuum cans. Some manufacturers already place an open "pull date" on this product for the benefit of the consumer and as an aid in stock rotation, but the practice of selling roasted and ground coffee in fold-top bags is usually localized and is becoming rather scarce (Rutgers University 1971).

"Best If Used By", or "Use By Date"

The practice of placing an open expiration "use by date" on coffee or tea should not be initiated. The shelf-life of coffee or tea depends not only on the age of the product, but on other storage conditions such as temperature and relative humidity, especially after the product has been opened (Rutgers University 1971). Storage of instant coffee or tea mix, for example, with the lids open or loosely screwed on would result in moisture pickup and caking of the product. Storage of roasted and ground coffee in an unsealed container would result in faster staling. An expiration date would also result in wastage of the product not only because the consumer might reject the food in the grocery store because of the date but because an expiration date would give the impression that the product should not be consumed for health reasons after a certain period of time when in fact, no health hazard exists when aged coffee or tea is consumed (Rutgers University 1971). Food deterioration is also a gradual process and rarely is a product good one day, and bad the next (Rutgers University 1971). Shelf-life predictions for the same product can differ from one manufacturer to the next, since the end of shelf-life is often a subjective decision, and a consumer may unjustly reject a product with a conservative shelf-life in favor of the same product produced by a different manufacturer with a more liberal shelf-life prediction (Rutgers University 1971). Inclusion of an expiration date would be costly to the manufacturer and ultimately to the consumer (Rutgers University 1971). On the other hand, the same storage information collected by the manufacturer can be used to implement a "best if used by date" based on minimal changes in flavor/odor during storage. This could be used to a marketing advantage.

In summary, open dating through a "best if used by date" for tea and coffee can be implemented to the consumers' advantage except that a "sell by date" for roasted and ground coffee packaged in bags should be used. The manufacturers should label each package with the proper storage instructions as well. Roasted and ground coffee, for example, should be labeled, "for maximum freshness reseal after use and refrigerate after opening" (Rutgers University 1971). In this way the consumer will realize that refrigeration is recommended not to prevent a health hazard but to retard staling. Instant coffee and tea should be labeled "close cap tightly after use" so that caking may be prevented.

REFERENCES

COOK, L. 1977. Product dating discussed. St. Paul Dispatch. Dec. 20, p. 11.

DEPARTMENT OF THE ARMY. 1971. Storage and Materials Handling. Technical Manual TM 743-200.

ELDER, L.W. 1940. Staling vs rancidity in roasted coffee. Ind. Eng. Chem. *32,* 798.

HARRIS, N.E., BISHOV, S.J., RAHMAN, A.R., ROBERTSON, M.M., and MABROUK, A.F. 1974. Soluble coffee: Shelf-life studies. J. Food Sci. *39,* 192.

LEE, F.A. 1975. Basic Food Chemistry. AVI Publishing Co., Westport, Conn.
PINTAURO, N. 1969. Soluble Coffee Manufacturing Processes. Noyes Development Corp., Park Ridge, N.J.
PINTAURO, N. 1977. Tea and Soluble Tea Products Manufacture. Noyes Development Corp., Park Ridge, N.J.
QUAST, D.G., and TEIXEIRA NETO, R.O. 1976. Moisture problems of foods in tropical climates. Food Technol. *30* (5) 98.
RUTGERS UNIVERSITY, 1971. Food Stability Survey, Rutgers University
Department of Food Science, for the State of New Jersey Department of Health. In cooperation with the U.S. Department of Agriculture/Economic Research Service.
SIVETZ, M., and FOOTE, H. 1963. Coffee Processing Technology, Vol. 1. AVI Publishing Co., Westport, Conn.
WICKREMASINGHE, P.L., and PERERA, K.P.W.C. 1972. Chemical changes during storage of black tea. Tea Q. *43* (4) 147.

CHAPTER 17

SHELF-LIFE OF SPICES, SUGAR AND SALT

INTRODUCTION

Spices are dried plant products added to foods in small quantities for flavor and/or color. In most spicees the aromatic and pungent principles are components of the volatile (or essential) oil fraction. Notable exceptions are ginger and pepper, in which the principles are in the resin.

Various parts of the spice plant may be used, depending on the localization of the oil sacs containing the essential oils. Table 17.1 lists the most commonly used spices along with botanic source, portion of the plant used and major active principle. As can be seen, seeds, leaves, flowers, fruits, bark, rhizomes or bulb are used.

PRESERVATION AND PACKAGING

Spices are preserved by drying, often at or near the point of harvest. Since many spices are grown in Africa, India and South and Central America, they are frequently dried by the sun. Spices are usually imported whole, processed domestically, then packaged for industrial or retail market. The major forms used by food processors are spice oils, oleo resins or extract. At the retail level whole, ground, powdered, crushed, dehydrated and flaked and tincture products are available, depending on the spice. These products are sold in metal tins, glass jars (clear or amber) and cardboard boxes.

FACTORS LIMITING ACCEPTABILITY

Spices are susceptible to two major factors which limit acceptability of the products: contamination and deterioration. Contamination may be particulate, insect or rodent infestation, or microbial. Deterioration concerns loss of color or flavor — or both — by chemical or physical means. Each of these factors will be discussed separately. Another mode of deterioration is excessive moisture gain through the package, leading to caking.

TABLE 17.1
COMMON SPICES, BOTANICAL SOURCES AND PRINCIPAL COMPONENTS[1]

Spice	Plant Sourcd	Portion of Plant Used	Major Component(s) of Volatile Oil
Allspice	*Pimenta officinalis* Lindl.	fruit	eugenol
Anise	*Pimpinella anisum* L.	seed	anethole
Basil	*Ocimum basilicum* L.	leaves	methyl chavicol, d-linalool cineole, eugenol
Capsicum spices			
Paprika	*Capsicum annum* L.	fruit	capsorubin, capsanthin (color) capsaicin (flavor)
Cayenne pepper (Red pepper)	*C. frutescens* L. *C. boccatum* L.	fruit	as above
Caraway	*Carum carvi* L.	seed	d-carvone, d-limonene
Cardamon	*Elettaria cardamomum* Maton	fruit	cineole, α-terpinyl acetate
Celery	*Apium graveoleus* L.	seed	d-limonene, selinene, sedanolide, sedanonic acid anhydride
Cinnamon	*Cinnamomum zeylanicum* Nees *C. cassia* L. *C. burmanni* Blume *C. loureirii* N.	bark	cinnamic aldehyde
Clove	*Carophyllus aromaticus* L.	flower buds[1]	eugenol
Coriander	*Coriandrum sativum* L.	fruit	coriandrol (d-linalool)
Cumin	*Cumin cyminum* L.	fruit	cumaldehyde
Dill seed	*Anethum graveoleus* L.	fruit	carvone, d-limonene, α-phellandrene
Dill weed	*Anethum graveoleus* L.	plant	as above

continued . . .

TABLE 17.1. *continued*

Spice	Plant Source	Portion of Plant Used	Major Component(s) of Volatile Oil
Fennel	*Foeniculum vulgare* Miller	fruit	anethole, fenchone
Garlic	*Allium sativum* L.	bulb	diallyl disulfide, diallyl trisulfide, allyl propyl disulfide
Ginger	*Zingiber officinale* Roscoe	rhizome	λ-zingiberene, zingerone
Laurel leaves	*Laurus nobilis* L.	leaves	cineole
Mace	*Myristica fragans* Houttyn	arillus	d-camphene, α-, β-pinene, limonene, 4-terpineol, α-terpineol
Marjoram	*Marjorana hortensis* M.	leaves	terpinene, d-α-terpineol 4-terpineol
Mint			
Peppermint	*Mentha piperita* L.	leaves and flower tops	λ-mentol, λ-menthone, λ-carvone
Spearmint	*M. spicata* L.		
Mustard			
Black	*Brassica nigra* (L.) Koch	seed	allylisothiocyanate (enzymatic hydrolysis product of glucoside potassium myronate)
White	*Sinapsis alba* L.	seed	p-hydroxybenzyl isothiocyanate (enzymatic hydrolysis product of glucoside sinalbin)
Nutmeg	*Myristica fragrans* Houttyn	seed	(same as mace)
Onion	*Allium cepa* L.	bulb	disulfide
Oregano	*Origanum vulgare* L.	leaves and flowering tops	thymol, carvacol
Parsley	*Petroselinum sativum* Hoffm.	leaves	apiol
Pepper			
blackpepper peppercorn	*Piper nigrum* L.	immature berry	α-, β-pinene, λ-phellandrene piperine, chavicine, piperidine

continued . . .

TABLE 17.1 *concluded*

Spice	Plant Source	Portion of Plant Used	Major Component(s) of Volatile Oil
white pepper		mature berry	piperine
Rosemary	*Rosmarinus officinalis* L.	leaves	borneol, pinene, cineole, camphene, camphor
Saffron	*Crocus sativus* L.	stigmas	safranal (hydrolysis product of picrocrocin) crocetin (hydrolysis product of crocin)
Sage	*Salvia officinalis* L.	leaves	thujone, borneol
Savory	*Satureia hortensis* L.	leaves and flowering tops	carvacol
Sesame	*Sesamum indicum* L.	seed	sesamin, sesamolin
Tarragon	*Artemisia dracunulus* L.	leaves	methyl chavicol
Thyme	*Thymus vulgaris* L.	leaves and flowering tops	thymol, carvacrol
Turmeric	*Curcuma longa* L.	rhizome	turmerone, curcumin
Vanilla	*Vanilla planifolia* Andr. *V. tahiteusis* (J.F. Moor) F. and B. *V. pompona* Schiede F.	bean	vanillin

[1]Merory 1968; Parry 1969.

Contamination

Particulate contamination is usually the result of inclusion of extraneous plant material such as stems, leaves or other parts not containing the pungent and flavor principles. United States government standards limit the amount of foreign material allowed as well as limit the total ash and ash insoluble in hydrochloric acid.

Contamination of spices via rodent or insect infestation is usually a warehouse problem of bulk spices although Christensen *et al.* (1967) found evidence of rodent excreta in whole peppercorns purchased at the retail level. Neither particulate nor rodent or insect contamination affect shelf-life of a spice although it may have an adverse effect on consumer acceptability.

Spices are frequently imported from areas which do not have facilities for sanitary handling, drying or storing spice. As a result, many spices have a high load of microorganisms. Pepper has been one of the highly contaminated products. Christensen *et al.* (1967) examined ground black pepper, whole peppercorns and red pepper for microflora. Black pepper and peppercorns showed high counts of *E. coli, Serratia* sp., *Klebsiella* sp., *Bacillus* sp., *Staphylococcus* sp., *Streptococcus* sp., along with numerous fungi. Among the *Aspergillus* species present were *A. flavus* and *A. ochracens,* termed "storage" fungi and also aflatoxin producers. Suzuki *et al.* (1973) was able to detect aflatoxin at levels of 0.75 to 5.5 ppb in samples of black pepper and nutmeg. Julseth and Diebel (1974), however, in work supported in part by American Spice Trade Association, examined documented samples of spices and herbs (import and domestic) and found no bacteria of public health significance. Black pepper and paprika were found to have high levels of aerobic spore-formers, with celery and ginger somewhat lower. Mold counts varied from very high to very low in both cassia and black pepper. More recently Powers *et al.* (1975, 1976) detected *Clostridium perfringens* in 15% of selected spices examined and *Bacillus cereus* in 53% of the samples. Both organisms pose a potential for food poisoning. No coliforms or coagulase positive *S. aureus* were found and only low levels of yeasts and molds were present.

In order to decrease the levels of microorganisms many spices are now gassed with ethylene oxide to achieve a 90% or greater reduction in microbial population. This method has drawbacks as residual ethylene oxide must be eliminated to levels below those set by the Food and Drug Administration. Also, ethylene oxide treatment has undesirable effects on the oil content, flavor and color of some spices, notably paprika (Vajdi and Pereira 1973). Gamma irradiation has been studied as an alternative method for sterilizing species (Vajdi and Pereira 1973; Bachman and

Gresczynska 1973; Farkas 1975). Results indicate that irradiation is more effective than ethylene oxide in reducing the population of microbes and has minimal effects on the quality of the spices. Microwave treatment was found to be ineffective as local heating only is achieved due to low moisture content of most spices (Vajdi and Pereira 1973).

It is interesting to note that some spices or spice extracts possess antimicrobial properties (Johnson and Vaughn 1969; Bullerman 1974; Farbood *et al.* 1976).

Microbial contamination *per se* does not limit shelf-life of spices because most spices are too dry to permit growth. Growth can occur however, if spices are held at a relative humidity greater than 75%. However, contaminated spices could be sources of inoculum for foods or may contain aflatoxins as shown by Suzuki *et al.* (1973).

Loss of Flavor, Pungency and Color

Flavor, pungency and color may be lost from spices by either physical or chemical routes. As mentioned earlier, the active principles of most spices are organic compounds in the volatile oil fraction. As would be expected, loss of these volatiles by evaporation can be a problem, especially in ground spices (Parry 1969). Georgiev and Khadzhiiski (1970) studied the effect of storage temperature on loss of essential oils and cumaldehyde from cumin seeds. As can be seen from the plot of the data (Fig. 17.1), the shelf-life at room temperature (20 °C) is about 5 years. If the data are representative of loss of volatile oils from other whole spices, temperature would not be a major factor in limiting shelf-life.

In contrast to the limited work done on loss of volatiles, much work has been done in the past 30 years with factors affecting loss of color from capsicum spices, paprika and various spices of red peppers. This area is of importance to both growers and processors as price is directly related to color intensity of the product. The major pigments of capsicums have been identified as capsanthin, capsorubin and β-carotene (Curl 1962).

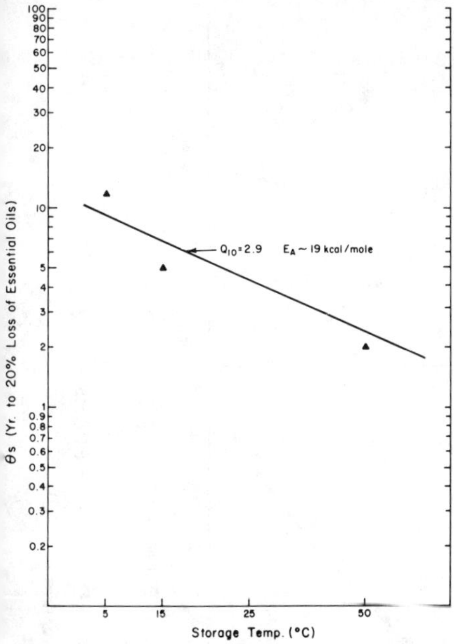

FIG. 17.1. EFFECT OF STORAGE TEMPERATURE ON SHELF-LIFE OF CUMIN SEEDS

Shelf-Life is time to 20% loss of essential oils. (From data of Georgiev and Khadzhiiski 1970).

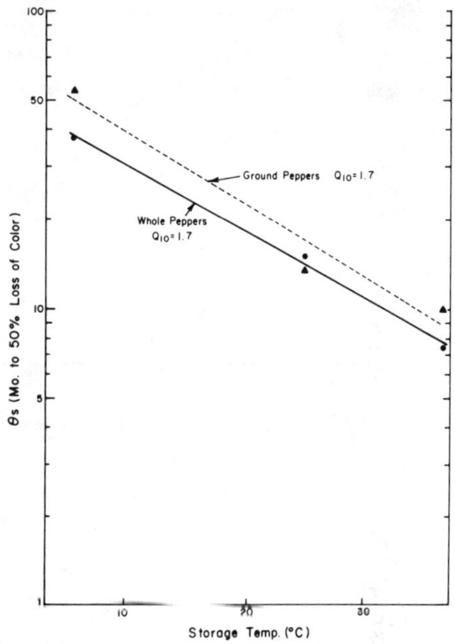

FIG. 17.2. EFFECT OF STORAGE TEMPERATURE ON SHELF-LIFE (50% COLOR LOSS) OF WHOLE AND GROUND CAYENNE PEPPERS

(Adapted from Lease & Lease, 1956a).

Extensively conjugated molecules such as the carotene types are liable to oxidation which may be induced by light, prooxidants or coupled with other oxidations (Kanner *et al.* 1977).

Early efforts to study color retention in capsicums were not concerned with mechanisms or kinetics but rather were designed to help the grower find ways to improve storage of his red pepper crop. Lease and Lease 1956a,b) found that color retention is a function of the variety of pepper, harvest condition, drying method, drying temperature and, most importantly, storage temperature. The color loss observed appears to follow zero order rate kinetics. Using 50% color loss as end of shelf-life (arbitrary choice) and zero order kinetics, shelf-life plots for whole and ground peppers yield identical Q_{10}s of 1.7 (Fig. 17.2). This indicates an E_a on the order of a little less than 10 Kcal/mole. This appears to be somewhat low for the activation energy for an oxidation reaction if that

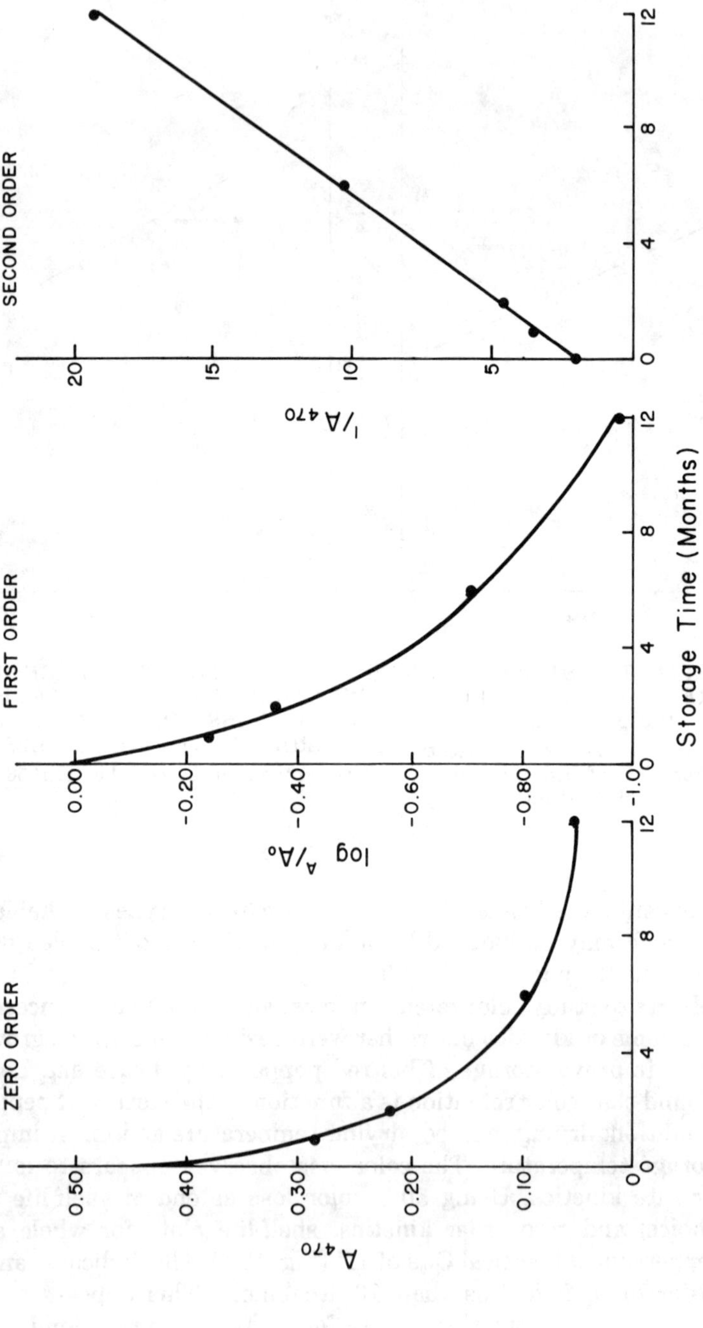

FIG. 17.3. LOSS OF COLOR FROM GROUND CHILI PEPPERS (*C. annum L.*)
(From Chen and Gutmanis 1968).

in fact is the mechanism. However, presence of prooxidants may act to lower the E_a. Then again, the data may not be too accurate.

de la Mar and Francis (1969) studied the pigments of paprika that had undergone severe bleaching (3 months in direct sunlight). They found the presence of ketonic and epoxide derivatives of the normal pigments of unbleached paprika correlated with the loss of red color. No kinetics were done.

Chen and Gutmanis (1968) found that second order kinetics (Fig. 17.3) best describe the oxidation of extractable color pigments from chili pepper. The effect of water activity on reaction rates was also determined. Recently Kanner *et al.* (1977) also observed the influence of moisture for color retention in sweet red paprika (*Capsicum annum* L.). The isotherms (Fig. 17.4) show that paprika powder is very sensitive to moisture gain at an a_w above 0.6. As can be seen from Fig. 17.5, the color is most stable at a_w 0.65. However, at this a_w, caking and browning occur. The pepper fruit is abundant in linoleic acid. Philip *et al.* (1971) proposed that the degradation of carotenoids is coupled with the oxidation of unsaturated fatty acids.

In efforts to retard color loss in capsicum spices, numerous antioxidants have been tested. BHA, hydroquinones, propyl gallate, citric acid and ethoxyquin have proven to be effective in retarding color losses to varying degrees (Van Blaricom and Martin 1951; Lease and Lease 1956a; Chen and Gutmanis 1968).

Very limited studies on other species have shown that temperatures during and immediately after grinding were important in retention of essential oils (Lichey and Genchev 1972; Georgiev and Van Khong 1973; Koller 1976).

OPEN DATING CONSIDERATIONS

Quality (aroma, pungency, taste, color) is the determining factor for shelf-life of spices. Although some spices, notably paprika, are rich in vitamins (de la Mar and Francis 1969) they are not consumed for their nutritive value.

As was evident from the preceeding section, very little published data are available on deterioration of spices, especially kinetic data. However, since wholesalers sell oleoresin, oils and extracts to industrial users at certain specification, e.g., color in paprika, it would seem surprising if these wholesalers do not have data on stability of spice products in storage.

Even with such data available, the critical question remains: at what point does a spice product become acceptable? Furthermore, who

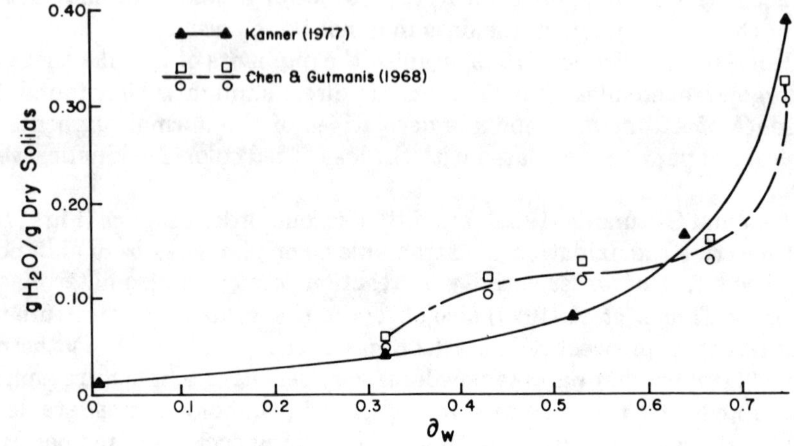

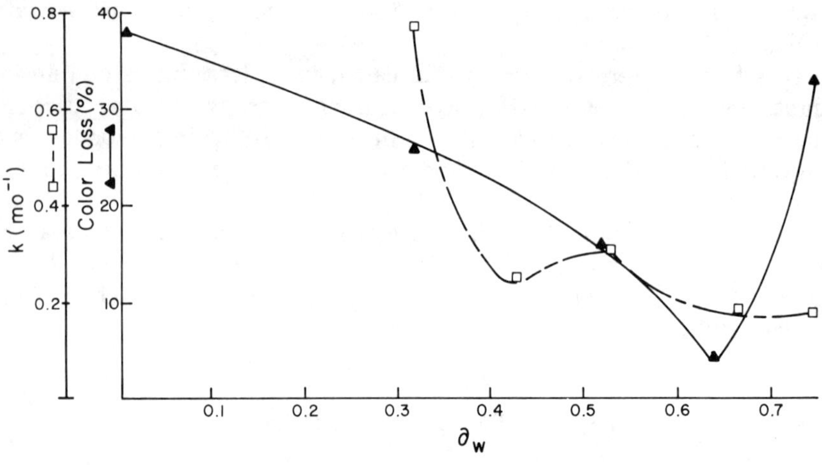

FIG. 17.4. ISOTHERM OF PAPRIKA (*C. annum* L.) POWDER (TOP)

FIG. 17.5. EFFECT OF a_w ON LOSS OF COLOR IN PAPRIKA POWDER IN AIR (BOTTOM)

determines this limit? At present, U.S. government standards are concerned with truth in labeling (botanic source, and portion of plant used) and extraneous material. It is interesting to speculate whether or not the majority of consumers with no standard for comparison have any idea as to the strength of spices in terms of taste, pungency or color.

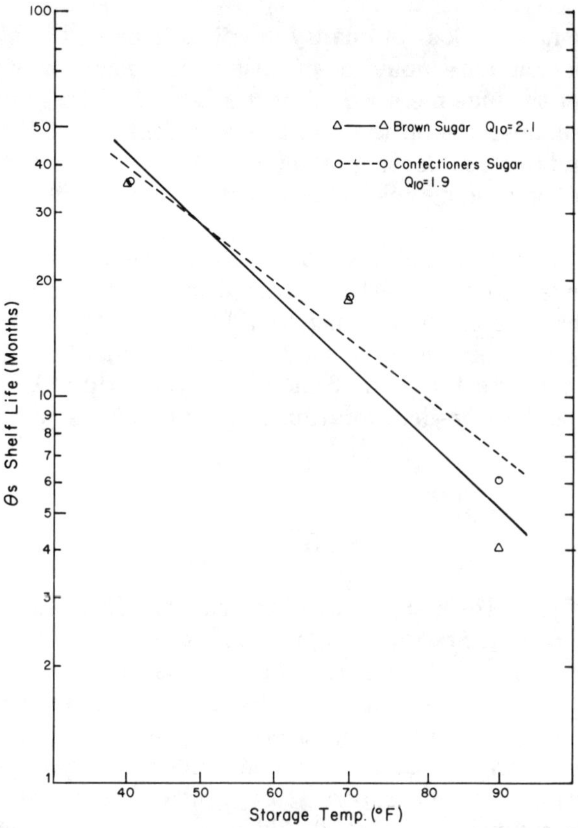

FIG. 17.6. SHELF-LIFE PLOTS OF BROWN AND CONFECTIONERS SUGAR

(Data from *Tech. Manual for Storage and Material Handling for the Dept. of Army*).

Currently spices for retail sale are stamped with a coded number probably indicating pack date and location. Crown Colony (Safeway Stores, Inc., Oakland, CA) on the side of cans of ground spices advises purchasers "for best flavor results use all ground spices within one year of purchase". Furthermore, Crown Colony spices are dated, e.g., 7-1-78. It is unclear as to whether this is a sell-by date or expiration date.

CONCLUSIONS

(1) Accurate data on loss of quality in spices is needed.

(2) A legible pack date would be of little value to consumers.

(3) Beneficial to consumers would be a sell-by date on ground spices with printed suggestions on the box to use within a specified time for best results, and to store closed, protected from direct light and excessive heat. On the other hand a "best if used by date" would give the same information.

(4) A sell-by date on whole spices is of questionable value. If the stability of cumin seeds, discussed earlier, is representative of stability of whole spices, then the date on the product would be several years beyond the time of packaging. Surveys have shown that consumers are doubtful of dates on products greater than 18 months in the future. As mentioned before, accurate data on deterioration of products is required to make such decisions.

SUGAR

Table sugar and brown sugar are obtained from different cuts during the processing of sugar beets or sugar cane. Powdered, or confectioner's sugar is made from table sugar. Pure sucrose is not susceptible to microbial or chemical deterioration. Sugar can become unacceptable to the consumer if contamination by insects or rodents occurs. Excessive moisture gain leading to caking can also render the package unacceptable. These are indications of poor storage or packaging failure. Under proper storage conditions, sugar should be definitely shelf stable. The Technical Manual for Storage and Material Handling for the Department of the Army lists sugar stored in a bag, can or envelope as indefinitely stable at 40°, 70°, and 90°F.

Brown sugar is susceptible to moisture loss resulting in an extremely hard mass. Retail packages are either sealed in plastic bags or in waxed bags enclosed within boxes. Confectioner's sugar has a problem with moisture gain leading to caking. To combat this, anticaking agents such as cornstarch are included. Confectioner's sugar is packaged for retail sale in the same way as brown sugar. Using the Department of Army data, a shelf-life plot (Fig. 17.6) shows approximately the same response over normal temperature range.

Open dating on granulated sugar would be of little value since sugar is indefinitely shelf stable. Open dating on brown sugar and confectioner's sugar might be beneficial. However, of more value would be instructions on the package advising steps to take if brown sugar loses moisture or confectioner's sugar gains moisture.

SALT

Table salt (NaCl) is not susceptible to microbial or chemical degradation. However, pure salt is very hygroscopic and will absorb moisture from the surroundings when the relative humidity is about 75%. For this reason, anticaking agents are added to salt to insure its free flowing property. Stored in moisture-proof containers, salt will remain indefinitely stable, as stated by the Department of the Army Technical Manual for Storage and Material Handling, and needs no open dating.

REFERENCES

BACHMAN, S. and GRESZCZYNSKA, J. 1973. Studies on some microbiological and chemical aspects of irradiated spices. *In* Aspects of the Introduction of Food Irradiation in Developing Countries. Conference Proceedings. Vienna, Austria. Abstracted in FSTA *7* (1975) No. 04 4T173.

BULLERMAN, L.B. 1974. Inhibition of aflatoxin production by cinnamon. J. Food Sci. *39,* 1163-1165.

CHEN, SL.L and GUTMANIS, F. 1968. Auto-oxidation of extractable color pigments in chili pepper with special reference to ethoxyquin treatment. J. Food Sci. *33,* 274-280.

CHRISTENSEN, C.M., FANSE, H.A., NELSON, G.H., BATES, F. and MIROCHA, C.J. 1967. Microflora of black and red papper. Appl. Microbiol. *15,* 622-626.

CURL, A.L., 1962. The carotenoids of red bell peppers. J. Agric. Food Chem. *12,* 522-524.

de la MAR, R.R., and FRANCIS, F.J. 1969. Carotenoid degradation in bleached paprika. J. Food Sci. *34,* 287-290.

DEPARTMENT OF THE ARMY. 1971. Storage and Materials Handling. Technical Manual TM 743-200.

FARBOOD, M.I., MACNEIL, J.H., and OSTOVAR, K. 1976. Effect of rosemary spice extractive on growth of microorganisms in meats. J. Milk Food Techol. *39,* 675-679.

FARKAS, J. 1973. Radurization and radicidation of spices. *In* Aspects of the Introduction of Food Irradiation in Developing Countries. Conference Proceedings. Vienna, Austria. Abstracted in FSTA *7* (1975) No. 04 4T172.

GEORGIEV, E.V. and KHADZHIISKI, TsT. 1970. Changes in essential oils and glycerides during storage of raw materials: Oil changes during storage of cumin (*Cumin cyminum*) seed. Nauchni Tr. Vissh Inst. Krhanit. Vkusova Prom. *17*(2) 97-106. Abstract FSTA *5* (1973) 4T194.

GEORGIEV, E.V. and VAN KHONG, T.M. 1973. Changes in the essential oils and glycerides during storage of raw materials. Changes in the essential oils of ground cumin fruits during short term storage. Nauchni Tr. Vissh Inst. Khranit. Vkusova Prom. *20* (1) 99-106. Abstract FSTA *6* (1974) 9T510.

JOHNSON, M.G. and VAUGHN, R.H. 1969. Death of *Salmonella typimurium* and *Escherichia coli* in the presence of freshly reconstituted dehydrated garlic and onion. Appl. Microbiol. *17,* 903-905.

JULSETH, R.M. and DIEBEL, R.H. 1974. Microbial profile of selected spices and herbs at import. J. Milk Food Technol. *37,* 414-419.

KANNER, J.S. HAREL, PAEVETCH, D. and BEN-GERA, I. 1977. Colour retention in sweet red paprika (*Capsicum annum* L.) powder as affected by moisture contents and ripening stage. J. Food Technol. *12,* 59-64.

KOLLER, W.D. 1976. Temperature — an important factor in the storage of ground natural spices. Lebensm. Unters. Forsch. *160,* 143-147. Abstract FSTA *8* (1976) 8T372.

LEASE, J.G. and LEASE, E.J., 1956a. Factors affecting the retention of red color in peppers. Food Technol. *10,* 368-373.

LEASE, J.G. and LEASE, E.J. 1956b. Effect of fat-soluble antioxidants on the stability of the red color of peppers. Food Technol. *10,* 403-405.

LEASE, J.G. and LEASE, E.J. 1962. Effect of drying conditions on initial color, color retention and pungency of red peppers. Food Technol. *17,* 104-106.

LICHEV, I.V. and GENCHEV, L.N. 1972. Effect of initial product temperature on the colour stability of packaged ground paprika during storage. Nauchni Tr. Vissh Inst. Khranit. Vkusova Prom. *19,* 117-123. Abstract FSTA *6* (1974) 9T513.

MACLEOD, A.J. 1974. Spices. Chem. Ind. 778-780, Oct. 5.

MERORY, J. 1968. Food Flavorings: Composition, Manufacture and Use, 2nd Ed. AVI Publishing Co., Westport, Conn.

PARRY, J.W. 1969. Spices. Vol. I, II. Chemical Publishing Co., New York.

PHILIP, T., NAWAR, W.W. and FRANCIS, F.J. 1971. The nature of fatty acids and capsanthin esters in paprika. J. Food Sci. *36,* 98-102.

POWERS, E.M., LAWYER, R. and MASOUKA, Y. 1975. Microbiology of processed spices. J. Milk Food Technol. *38,* 683-687.

POWERS, E.M., LATT, T.G. and BROWN, T. 1976. Incidence and levels of *Bacillus cereus* in processed spices. J. Milk Food Technol. *39,* 668-670.

SUZUKI, J.I., DAINIUS, B. and KILBACK, J.H. 1973. A modified method for aflatoxin determination in spices. J. Food Sci. *38,* 949-950.

TASSAN, C.G. and RUSSELL, G.F. 1975. Chemical and sensory studies on cumin. J. Food Sci. *40,* 1185-1188.

VAJDI, M. and PEREIRA, R.R. 1973. Comparative effects of ethylene oxide, gamma irradiation and microwave treatment on selected spices. J. Food Sci. *38,* 893-895.

VAN BLARICOM, L.O. and MARTIN, J.A. 1951. Retarding the loss of red color in cayenne pepper with oil-antioxidants. Food Technol. *5,* 337-339.

CHAPTER 18

SHELF-LIFE OF DEHYDRATED FOODS

INTRODUCTION

Dehydrated foods comprise a significant part of food consumption if all forms of dehydration are considered. The shelf-life data for cereals, pasta, fried snacks, baked goods, dry milk, tea and coffee, all of which are dehydrated by some means, have been presented in other parts of this book. This chapter covers the drying of particulate foods such as vegetables, fruits and meats. Consumer use of these products is usually limited to dry meal and soup mixes and some vegetable spices such as powdered garlic.

PROCESSING

Processing of particulate foods requires the normal preprocessing steps such as washing, cutting, peeling and blanching. Fruits may not be blanched if they develop an undesirable cooked flavor. Garlic and onion are not blanched since the characteristic flavor is the result of enzyme activity. Meats may be precooked. In most cases drying is done on trays in an air tunnel. Temperature control is necessary to prevent scorching. Some fruits such as raisins are still sun dried, but this is being done less because of the problems of microbial and filth contamination. The dry products usually are packaged in fairly impermeable pouches except for fruits which are only dried to an a_w of about 0.6.

The major modes of deterioration will be considered separately for each type of dry food. In summary, they include: (1) loss of nutrients; (2) nonenzymatic browning; (3) lipid oxidation; (4) color loss; and (5) moisture gain to a critical level. To insure against these, drying is done close to the BET (Brunauer-Emmet-Teller) monolayer value, a good water impermeable pouch is used, the package is vacuum sealed or gas flushed, and the package should be opaque.

VEGETABLES

Dehydrated vegetables deteriorate primarily through: (1) lipid oxidation reactions, causing rancid or "hay-like" off-flavors; (2) nonenzymatic browning reactions, causing darkening, hardness and loss of available protein; (3) oxidation, causing loss of vitamins such as vitamin C and thiamin; and (4) oxidation of pigments such as chlorophyll and carotene, causing unacceptable colors.

For dehydrated vegetables, as in all dehydrated foods, the moisture content has a great effect on the rate of each of these reactions and on how much the rate increases with increased temperature.

The first three of these modes of degradation are illustrated by the reactions occurring in dehydrated potato products. Pigment degradation has been studied in spinach, carrots, and freeze-dried peas, among others. Rates of vitamin loss at different temperatures have been studied in several different vegetables.

Potatoes

Work done by Sapers *et al.* (1973, 1974) and Sapers (1975) at the USDA Eastern Regional Laboratory indicates that lipid oxidation is the limiting factor in the shelf-life of dehydrated potato products. In 1973 they found that the rate of lipid oxidation at 23 °C in air is increased by the presence of peel, use of defective raw materials, over-drying, and large amounts of process water. Earlier workers (cited by Copley and Van Arsdel 1964) found that the rate of lipid oxidation in stored dried potato products decreased with decreasing a_w down to the monolayer and increased at a_w levels below the monolayer. The data of Sapers (1975) is shown in Figure 18.1. The initial level of oxidation is higher with a more

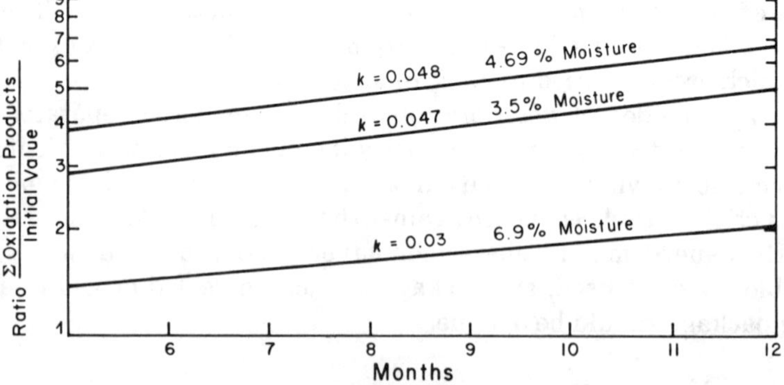

FIG. 18.1. RATE OF LIPID OXIDATION IN STORED DRIED POTATO PRODUCTS

(From Sapers 1975).

strenuous drying process as indicated for the 3.5 and 4% moisture systems, but the rate itself is not significantly changed, as indicated by the rate constants shown in the figure. The Q_{10} of the rate of lipid oxidation in potatoes was found by Burton (1949, as cited in Copley and Van Arsdel 1964) to be 1.2 to 1.4, so higher temperature has only a slight effect. This value is less than expected and may be a Q_{10} °F rather than a Q_{10} °C. It is not indicated. The presence of oxygen accelerates lipid oxidation; however, the cost of packing in N_2 makes the use of BHA and BHT (allowed by FDA standards to a level of 10 ppm) preferable.

Dried potato products also deteriorate by nonenzymatic browning (NEB). Copley and Van Arsdel give a Q_{10} of 5 to 7 for NEB in potatoes. The Q_{10} decreases with higher moisture content and lower temperature ranges. Burton (1945) as cited in Copley and Van Arsdel (1964) found a high correlation between reducing sugar content of the potato and the rate of NEB during storage at high temperatures of the dry product. Sulfite or sulfur dioxide increases the shelf-life (with a given degree of NEB as the end-point) by 1.9 to 5.1 times (Legault *et al.* 1951). However, this protection is lowered by a higher content of reducing sugars in the potatoes (Ross 1948). The reducing sugar content in potatoes is increased by a long holding time prior to drying at lower temperatures (~50 °F) to prevent sprouting. Hendel (1959) found that less than 1% reducing sugar content is best for the manufacture and the storage of dried potato, but potatoes held at 50 °F to retard sprouting, can have up to 4% reducing sugars. Therefore, the use of sprout inhibitors (i.e., irradiation) and higher storage temperatures of raw potatoes is recommended as a control measure for NEB in dehydrated potato products.

Sulfite or sulfur dioxide was found by Legault *et al.* (1951) to increase the time to a given amount of browning by a factor of 1.9 to 5.1. Ross in 1948 found similar results and also that the protection factor was less with greater reducing sugar content.

The difference in the Q_{10}s for NEB (5 to 7) and for lipid oxidation (about 1.3 to 2) in dehydrated potato products can be used to show why at normal storage temperatures lipid oxidation determines the end of shelf-life. Sullivan *et al.* (1974) found a noticeable difference in flavor due to NEB at the end of two months in N_2 packed, explosion puffed potatoes stored at 38 °C. Using a Q_{10} of 6, the end of shelf-life due to NEB shown in Fig. 18.2 could be obtained. Sapers *et al.* (1974) found a noticeable difference in the concentration of oxidation volatile products after 6 months. Using a Q_{10} of 1.3 the end of shelf-life also plotted due to rancidity is in Fig. 18.2. Using these data it can be seen that end of shelf-life due to lipid oxidation occurs sooner at temperatures below 33 °C to 36 °C, while browning becomes the major mode above this temperature range. Thus, accelerated shelf-life studies done at 40—45 °C would give incorrect results if only browning were used as the end-point.

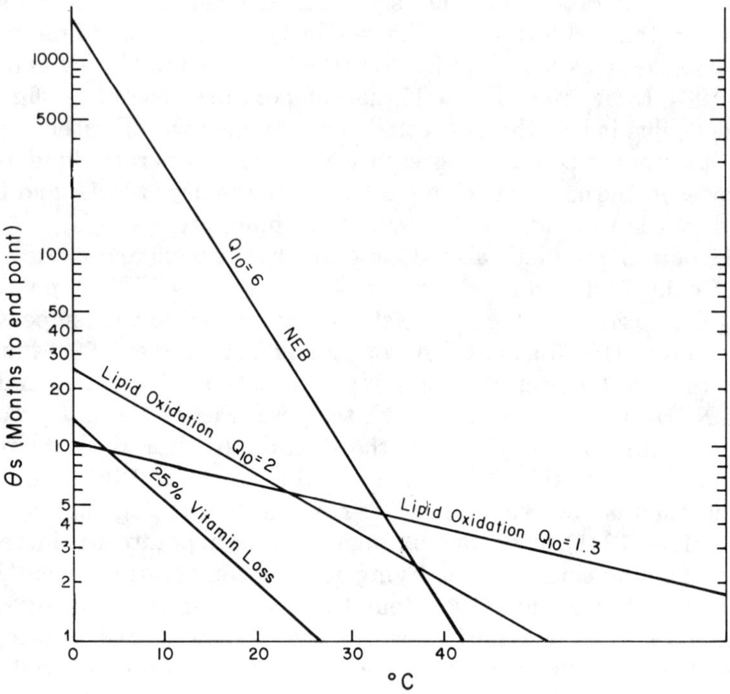

FIG. 18.2. DEHYDRATED POTATOES (FLAKES)
(From Sapers 1975).

The Q_{10} for the loss of vitamin C in dehydrated white potatoes as extrapolated by Kramer (1974) is also shown in Fig. 18.2. At 70 °F it takes only one month or less to lose 10% of the vitamin C in dried white potatoes (Kramer 1974). Using these data to produce a 25% vitamin C loss line, it is evident that loss of shelf-life due to this parameter would predominate at all temperatures above 4 °C. However, these data say nothing about the processing method or moisture content of the potatoes, which could be a significant factor in vitamin C loss.

Spinach

The effect of moisture content, as expressed in water activity, on the rate of chlorophyll pigment loss can be seen in Fig. 18.3 (LaJolla *et al.* 1971) for freeze-dried spinach. Table 18.1 shows the first order rate constants, the activation energies, and the Q_{10}s for chlorophyll degradation

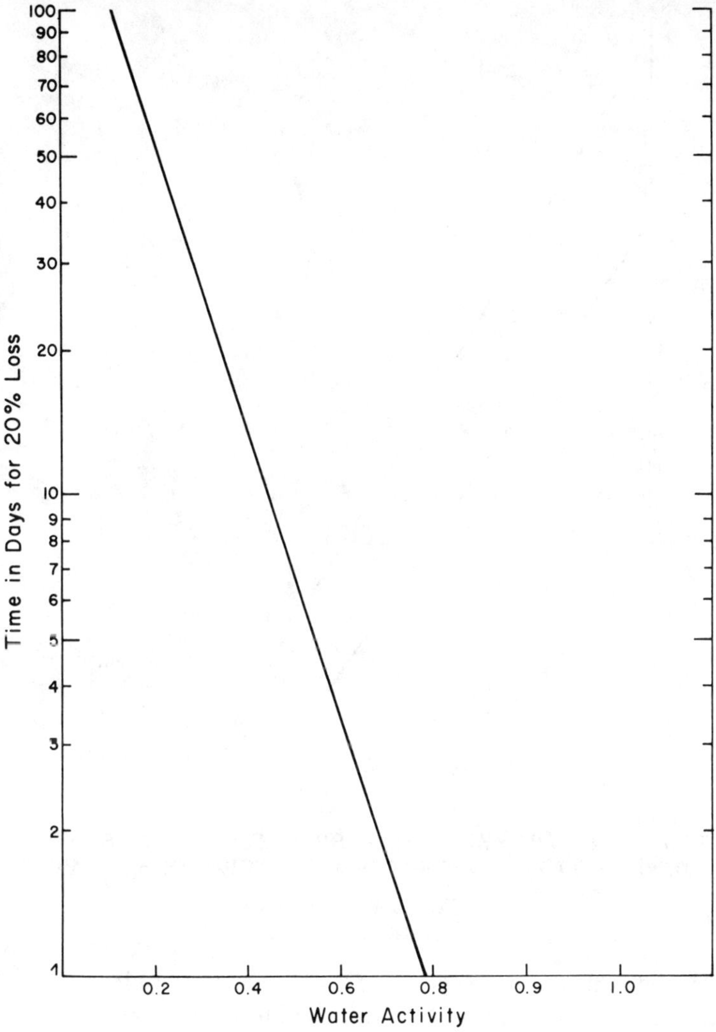

FIG. 18.3. FREEZE-DRIED SPINACH — DAYS AT 37°C TO 20% LOSS OF CHLOROPHYLL VERSUS WATER ACTIVITY
(From LaJolla *et al.* 1974).

TABLE 18.1
CHLOROPHYLL LOSS IN SPINACH[1]; KINETIC DATA

	Rate constant $\times 10^{-2}$ (hr^{-1})							
	Chlorophyll a		Chlorophyll b		Chlorophyll a		Chlorophyll b	
a_w	37 °C	55 °C	37 °C	55 °C	E_a (Kcal/mole)	Q_{10}	E_a (Kcal/mole)	Q_{10}
0.75	2.74	14.7	0.92	5.4	19	2.6	20	2.7
0.62	1.12	7.2	0.42	3.3	21	2.8	23	3.2

[1]From LaJolla *et al.* 1971.

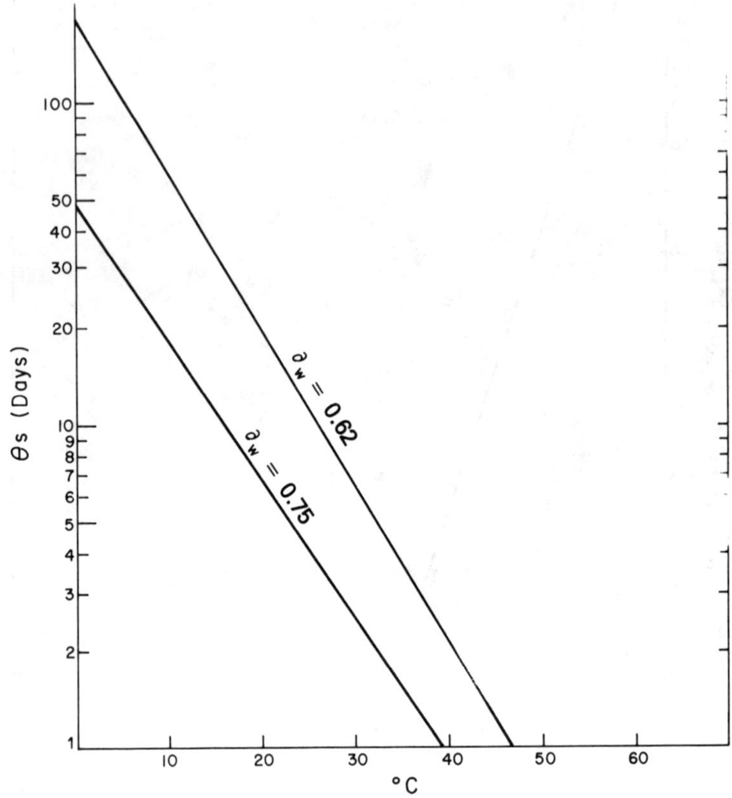

FIG. 18.4. FREEZE-DRIED SPINACH — DAYS TO 20%. CHLROPHYLL LOSS VERSUS TEMPERATURE FOR a_w .62 AND a_w .75

(From LaJolla *et al.* 1977).

at 0.75 and 0.62 water activities. This is shown graphically for 20% loss of chlorophyll in Fig. 18.4. As seen, the lines are nearly parallel and the loss rate is high at high a_w. This means good protection is needed against moisture gain. They showed that at a_w 0.11 no loss of chlorophyll occurred during the two month storage study.

Freeze-dried Peas

Kapsalis *et al.* (1967) at the U.S. Army Natick Food Laboratories studied the effect of a_w and temperature on the storage of freeze-dried peas with respect to thiamin and carotene retention, chlorophyll stability, and O_2 uptake (a measure of lipid oxidation resulting in hay-like

TABLE 18.2
FREEZE-DRIED PEAS[1]; RATE CONSTANTS (DAY^{-1})

% RH	Thiamine Loss 21.1 °C	Thiamine Loss 43.3 °C	Q_{10}	Carotene Loss 21.1 °C	Carotene Loss 43.3 °C	Q_{10}	O_2 Uptake 43.3 °C
0	3.6×10^{-4}	—	—	.012	.012	—	.0058
5	1.2×10^{-4}	—	—	.010	.011	—	—
11	4.9×10^{-4}	4.9×10^{-4}	—	.005	.009	1.3	.0154
23	1.1×10^{-4}	7.4×10^{-4}	2.4	.004	.008	1.35	—
33	1.4×10^{-3}	2.5×10^{-3}	3.6	.002	.008	1.85	.0327
50	1.3×10^{-3}	8.3×10^{-3}	6.5	.003	.009	—	—

[1]From Kapsalis 1973.

off-flavors). Table 18.2 gives the rate constants and Q_{10}s of the reactions at each moisture level (% RH) and temperature (°C).

Thiamin loss is more temperature sensitive, but carotene loss occurs more quickly until temperatures above 40 °C are reached at the higher humidities, as seen in Fig. 18.5. Chlorophyll retention was stable at 21.1 °C at all % RHs and at 43.3 °C at low a_w. However, at 43.3 °C and a_ws above 0.23, progressively greater amounts of chlorophyll were lost in 84 days of storage. The rate of oxygen uptake also increased with the a_w of the product and was greater than the rates of thiamin and carotene loss. Which parameter would determine the end of shelf-life of freeze-dried peas would depend on the degree of loss that would be unacceptable.

Tomato Flakes

Moisture content and exposure to oxygen in air both have an effect on the rate of oxidative loss of vitamin C in dried tomato flakes. In vacuum at an unspecified moisture content as seen in Fig. 18.6, the Q_{10} of vitamin C loss is 1.4 (Kramer 1974). The results for storage in air at 1% and 5% moisture are in Table 18.3 and Fig. 18.6. In air at 1% moisture the Q_{10} is 2.1 and at 5% moisture the Q_{10} is 2.5, only slightly higher (Tressler 1956). Exposure to oxygen in air seems to have a greater effect on temperature sensitivity than does moisture content. If we assume that the Q_{10} in vacuum remains at 1.4 regardless of moisture content (further study would be needed to show this) a storage temperature below 38 °F (3.3 °C) would be needed at 5% moisture to give the same or better protection as vacuum packing, and below 83 °F (28 °C) for 1% moisture. Therefore, the importance of complete drying for vitamin C retention is obvious. However, faster degradation through carotene loss and development of rancid off-flavors at lower moisture contents could offset this advantage if dried tomato flakes follow the same pattern as other dried vegetables.

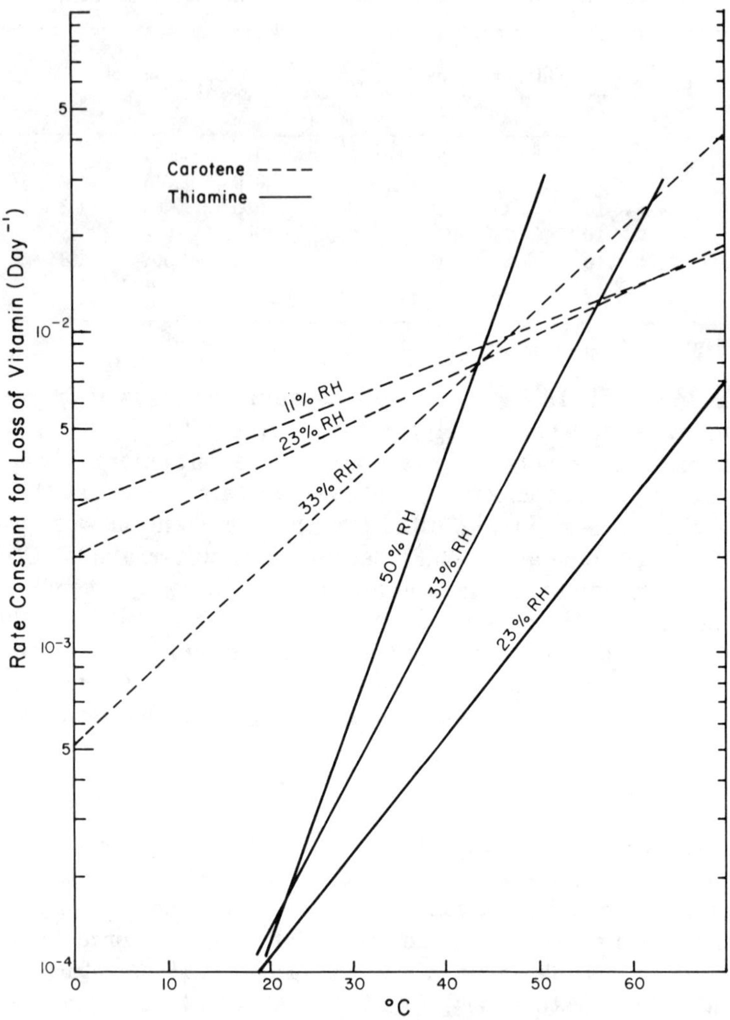

FIG. 18.5. VITAMIN LOSS AS A FUNCTION OF TEMPERATURE IN FREEZE-DRIED PEAS
(From Kapsalis 1967).

Bell Peppers

Daoud and Luh (1967, as cited in Kramer 1974) have studied the stability of protein and vitamins A and C in bell peppers at different temperatures during storage.

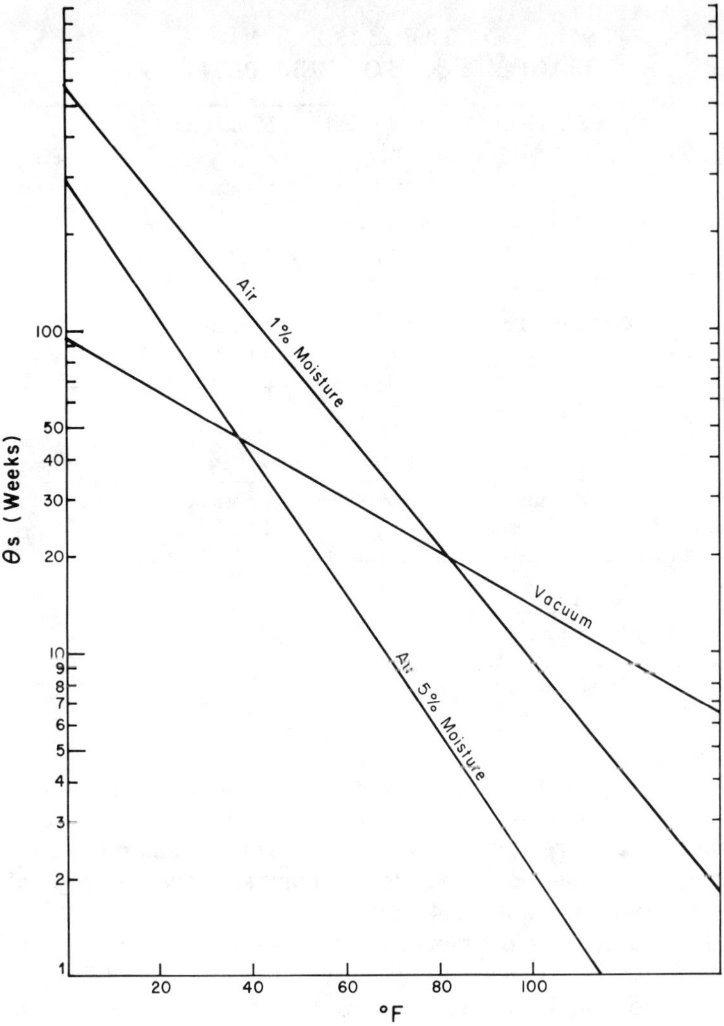

FIG. 18.6. TOMATO FLAKES — 10% VITAMIN C LOSS (From Kramer 1974; Tressler 1956).

TABLE 18.3

VITAMIN C LOSS IN TOMATO FLAKES AFTER 32 WEEKS IN AIR[1]

Temperature	% Moisture	% Vitamin C Lost	$k(wk)^{-1}$	Weeks to 10% Loss
40	1%	none	—	—
70	1%	10%	0.0033	32
100	1%	30%	0.0111	9.5
40	5%	none	—	—
70	5%	30%	0.0111	9.5
100	5%	80%	0.0503	2.1

[1]Adapted from Tressler (1956). Q_{10} = 2.1 at 1% moisture; Q_{10} = 2.5 at 5% moisture

TABLE 18.4
STORAGE EFFECTS ON BELL PEPPERS[1]

Temperature °F	% Lysine Loss in 12 Months	Rate Constant $(mo)^{-1}$	Months to 10% Loss	Q_{10}
32	0	—	—	
68	10	8.78×10^{-3}	12.0	
86	87	0.17	0.62	20

Temperature °F	% Methionine Loss in 12 Months	Rate Constant $(mo)^{-1}$	Months to 10% Loss	Q_{10}
32	0	—	—	
68	12	0.011	9.9	
86	75	0.116	0.91	12

Temperature °F	% Vitamin A and C Loss		Months to 10% Loss	Q_{10}
32	10 in 12 months		12.0	
58	5 in 6 months		0.9	
86	50 in 3.5 months		0.52	3.1

[1]Daoud and Luh 1967 (cited in Kramer 1974).

Lysine and methionine are both amino acids that are degradated through nonenzymatic browning reactions with the normal reducing sugars such as glucose and fructose. Lysine is more susceptible to this type of loss than is methionine and is also more sensitive to temperature, as the Q_{10}s derived in Table 18.4 show.

Vitamins A and C are lost more quickly than the two amino acids, but are less sensitive to changes in temperature, as seen in Fig. 18.7. It is obvious that, below 65 °F, protein losses occurring during normal storage are negligible, especially since peppers are not considered to be a source of obtaining protein in the diet. However, the vitamin losses are significant.

Vitamin C Loss in General

Vitamin C loss has been studied in several dried vegetables. Kramer (1974) gives data on several of these. The Q_{10}, activation energy and loss rate constant, assuming a first order reaction, derived from this data are shown in Table 18.5. These data are shown graphically in Figures 18.8 to 18.12. As seen, the Q_{10}s run from about 1.5 to 4 depending on the product.

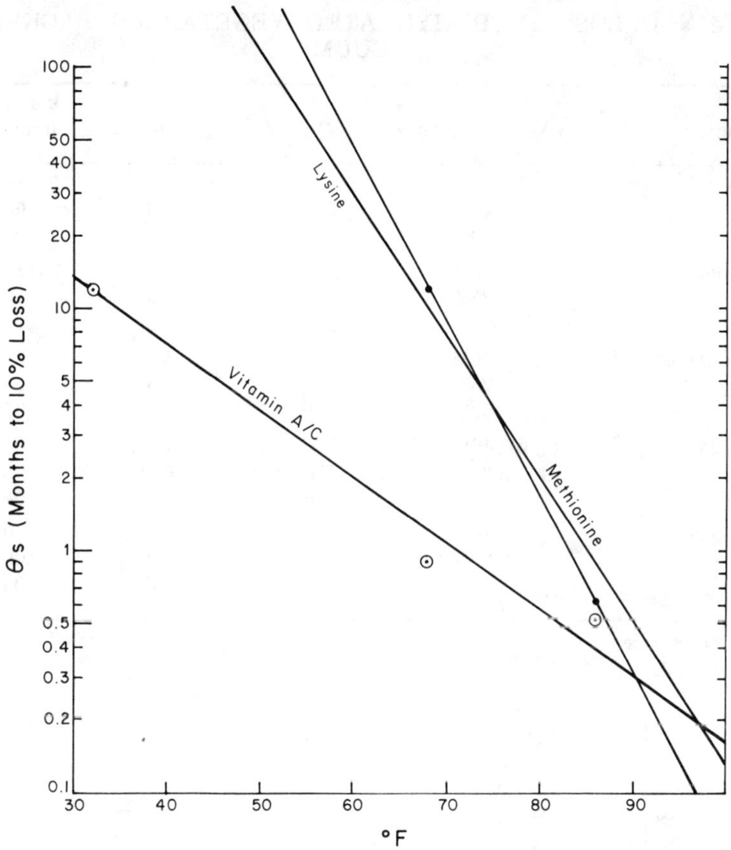

FIG. 18.7. DEHYDRATED BELL PEPPERS
(From Daoud and Luh 1967 as cited in Kramer 1974).

Unfortunately the moisture contents were not indicated. Examining the figures, it can be seen that there are significant losses at 80—100 °F.

Other Data

Data on shelf-life and quality of vegetables from earlier studies and some data from which rates and Q_{10}s cannot be derived are summarized in Table 18.6.

TABLE 18.5
VITAMIN C LOSS IN DEHYDRATED VEGETABLES PACKED IN VACUUM[1]

Vegetable	Vitamin C Loss	Q_{10}	E_a Kcal/mole	k at 70°F ($month^{-1}$)
Onions	10%	3.9	22.5	.105
	25%	3.3	20.0	.058
	50%	3.0	18.0	.035
White potatoes	10%	2.3	13.8	.105
	25%	2.7	16.5	.169
	50%	2.9	17.6	.099
Tomato flakes	10%	1.4	5.6	.018
	25%	1.4	5.6	.033
	50%	1.4	5.6	.053
Cabbage	10%	1.61	7.9	.013
	25%	1.49	6.6	.064
	50%	1.46	6.3	.043
Rutabagas	10%	3.7	21.7	.105
	25%	3.2	19.3	.064
	50%	2.9	17.6	.036

[1]From Kramer (1974).

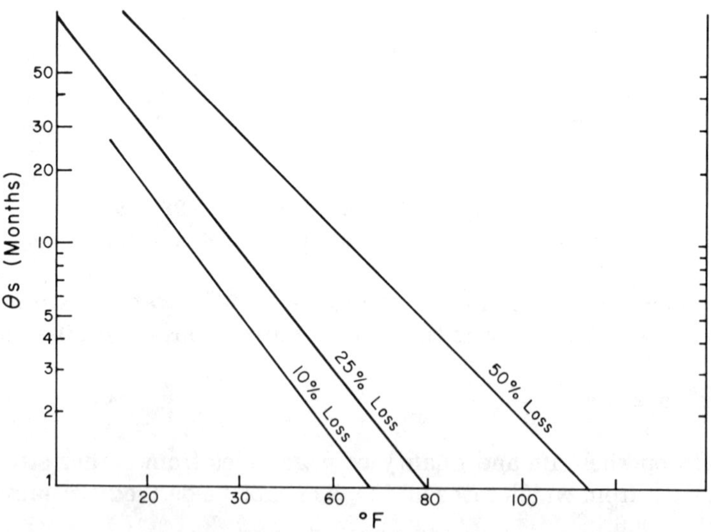

FIG. 18.8. WHITE POTATOES – VITAMIN C LOSS (From Kramer 1974).

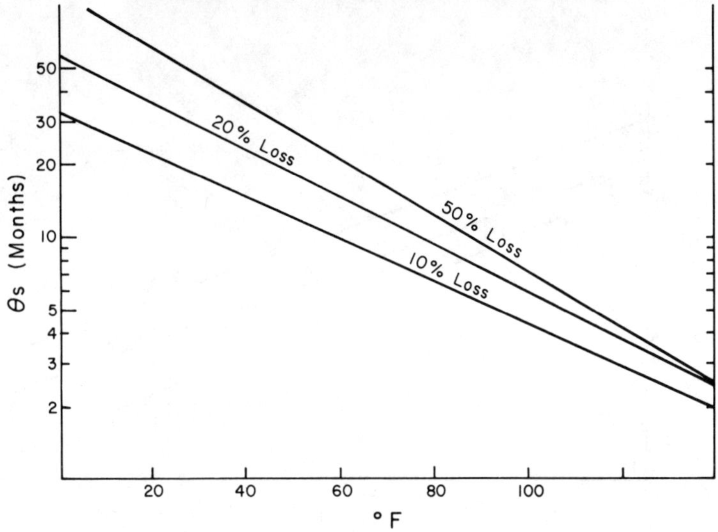

FIG. 18.9. CABBAGE — VITAMIN C LOSS
(From Kramer 1974).

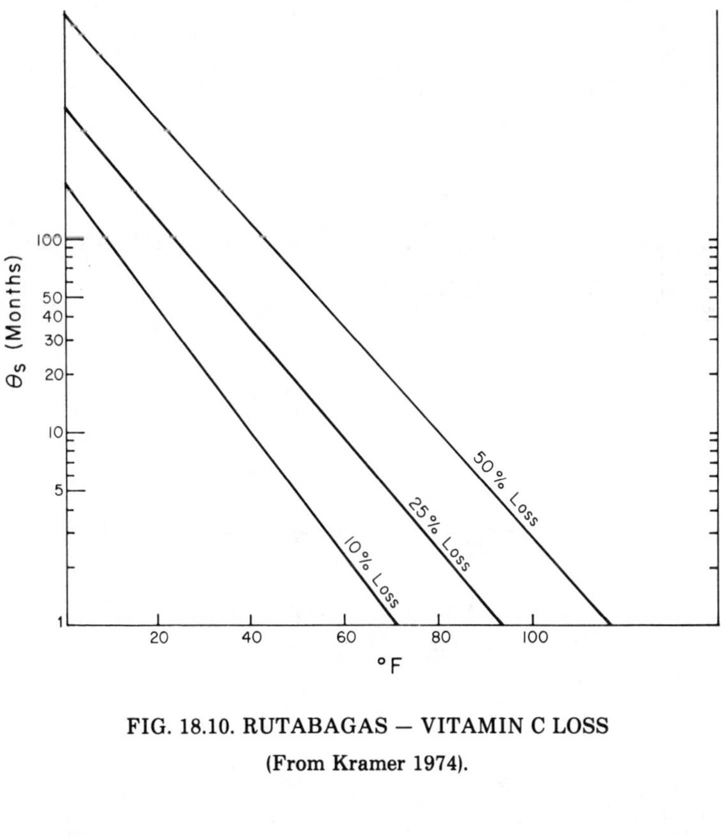

FIG. 18.10. RUTABAGAS — VITAMIN C LOSS
(From Kramer 1974).

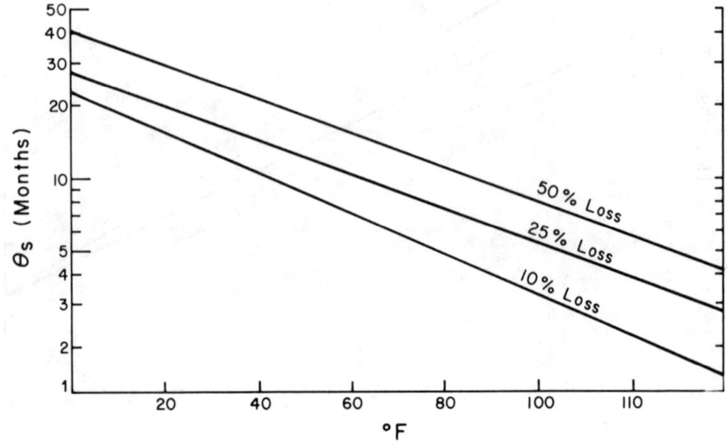

FIG. 18.11. TOMATO FLAKES — VITAMIN C LOSS
(From Kramer 1974).

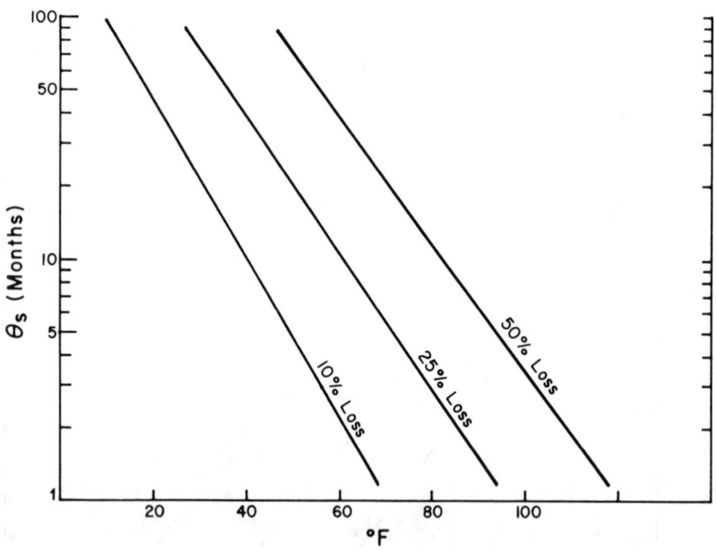

FIG. 18.12. ONIONS — VITAMIN C LOSS
(From Kramer 1974).

TABLE 18.6
QUALITY EFFECTS DURING STORAGE OF VEGETABLES

Product Vegetable	Quality Measured	Retention	Temperature (°F)	Length of Storage
(Copley and Van Arsdel 1972)				
Green snap beans	color and flavor	good	100	6 months
Beets (2.4% moisture)	general quality	good	100	48 weeks
Beets (2.4% moisture)	general quality	good	—30	48 weeks
Beets (7% moisture)	general quality	inedible	100	48 weeks
Cabbage (7% moisture)	color and flavor	inedible	100	2-3 months
Cabbage (5% moisture)	color and flavor	inedible	100	5-6 months
Cabbage (3% moisture)	color and flavor	inedible	100	10-12 months
(Kramer 1974)				
Carrot flakes	vitamin C	80%	ambient	2 months
Carrot flakes	carotene	30%	ambient	2 months
(Copley and Van Arsdel 1972)				
Carrots in air				
Unblanched	carotene	8.2%	84	6 months
Blanched	carotene	29.8%	84	6 months
Blanched and sulfited	carotene	25.5%	84	6 months
blanched and starched	carotene	63.6%	84	6 months
Control in N_2	carotene	97.3%	—30	6 months
(Tally et al. *1966)*				
Pumpkin	noticeable difference from			
N_2	hidden standard		73	>12 months
In air with antioxidant			73	12 months
In air with no antioxidant			73	5 months

DEHYDRATED MEATS, POULTRY AND SEAFOOD

Dried meats, poultry and seafood, like the other dry foods, deteriorate by nonenzymatic browning, oxidation, and enzymatic reactions. Raw products also are subject to continued protein denaturation during storage. Combinations of these four modes of deterioration lead to pigment changes, loss of texture, loss of original flavor with development of burned, rancid flavors and loss of rehydration.

NEB is the most important deterioration reaction and is slower with low pH, temperature and moisture content. It leads to color, texture and flavor change and loss of rehydration.

Oxidation of lipids by oxygen leads to development of rancid, burned flavors, loss of change of pigments and loss of vitamins. Exclusion of oxygen, very low temperatures and/or use of antioxidants are necessary to control oxidation. Oxidation is extremely dependent also on moisture content, being lowest at the monolayer, but increasing above and below this level. Precooked beef seems more susceptible to oxidation than raw beef (Watts 1962, as cited in Copley and Van Arsdel 1964), although the reverse is true for most meats. Enzyme and protein degradation are much more important in raw than in precooked dried meats.

Beef

Karel and Labuza (1969) found that 200 μl of O_2 absorbed per gram of reconstituted beef was the cutoff point for acceptability. Tuomy and Hinnergardt (1968) studied the effect of the amount of vacuum on oxidation of freeze-dried raw beef patties. Using Karel's cutoff point with Tuomy's data in Fig. 18.13 shows the effect of vacuum packing on the shelf-life of freeze dried raw beef.

Results shown in Table 18.7 from a study done by Whirlpool Corporation (1965, cited in Brockman 1966) on precooked beef, freeze-dried to 2% moisture content also show the importance of the level of oxygen on oxidation. They found that the product stored in 2% oxygen was significantly more acceptable to taste panels than that stored in 20% oxygen even at the end of one month.

Thompson *et al.* (1962) studied the effect of moisture content and temperature on the quality of freeze-dried raw beef. They found that moisture contents from 1.7 to 5.1% had only a slight effect on rehydration rate after storage for five months. Temperature of storage however, had a greater effect, with decreased rehydration at higher temperatures, as is shown in Table 18.8.

TABLE 18.7
COOKED BEEF FREEZE-DRIED TO 2% MOISTURE

% Oxygen Concentration in Headspace at 100°F		
Initial	1 Month	6 Months
2	0.11	0.11
4	0.22	0.22
20	0.57	1.29

Whirlpool Corporation (U.S. Army Contract, 1965).

TABLE 18.8
EFFECT OF STORAGE TEMPERATURE ON REHYDRATION OF FREEZE-DRIED BEEF[1]

Temperature (°F)	Time	% Rehydration 30 Sec	Final
0	5 months	79.2 ± 2.3	81.2 ± 2.3
68	5 months	61.2 ± 6.6	74.5 ± 1.7
98	5 months	44.2 ± 6.6	60.2 ± 5.8

[1]From Thompson *et al.* (1962).

TABLE 18.9
THIAMIN LOSS OF DEHYDRATED PORK[1]

% Loss of Thiamin	Q_{10}	E_a	Temperature Range (°F)
10	137	77.7	46—55
25	35	60.1	56—68
50	8.6	38.9	68—88

[1]Rice and Robinson 1944, cited in Kramer, 1974.

Pork

Antioxidants can be applied to ground products to control oxidation. Sharp and Rolfe (1958, as cited in Copley and Van Arsdel 1964) found that 0.1 percent of Tenox II or Tenox IV per weight of fat extended the shelf-life of ground cooked dehydrated pork when stored in air at 100°F from one month to four months.

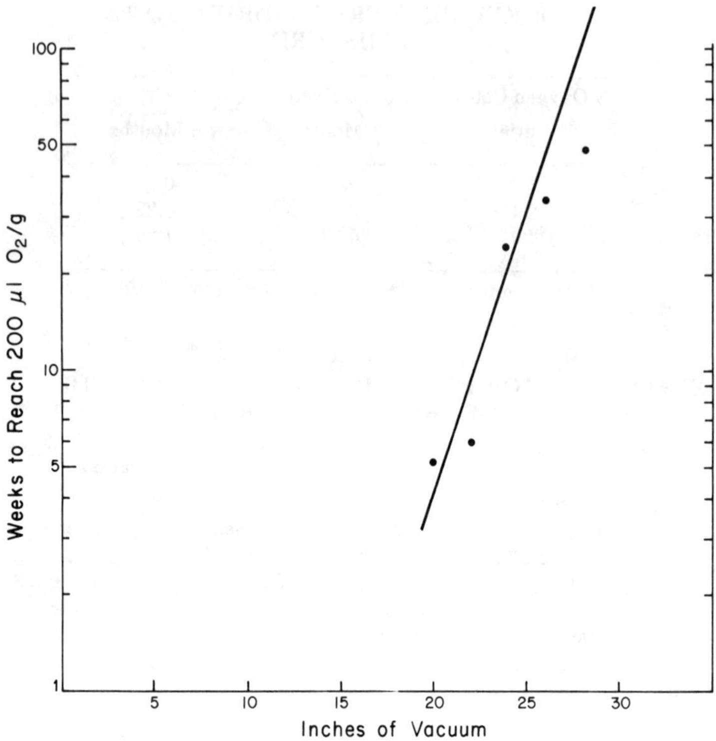

FIG. 18.13. FREEZE-DRIED RAW BEEF — EFFECT OF VACUUM ON TIME TO REACH UNACCEPTABLE RANCIDITY

(From Toumy *et al.* 1968).

Moisture content or water activity has been found by Sharp (1962) to be important to the rate of nonenzymatic browning in pork, as seen in Fig. 18.14.

Rice and Robinson (1944, cited in Kramer 1974) studied the loss of thiamin in pork dried to an unspecified water activity. A summary of Q_{10}s derived from their data is given in Table 18.9 and the shelf-life is plotted in Fig. 18.15. The lines are not parallel and the Q_{10}s are extremely high. Labuza (1972) found an overall activation energy of 22 Kcal/mole and a Q_{10} of 3.22 for the same data. How Kramer calculated his data for Fig. 18.15 is not known, but it is very suspect. The half lives reported should be 63 days at 23 °C, 17 days at 37 °C and 3 days at 49 °C. The results, however, still indicate rapid loss at temperatures above 80 °F.

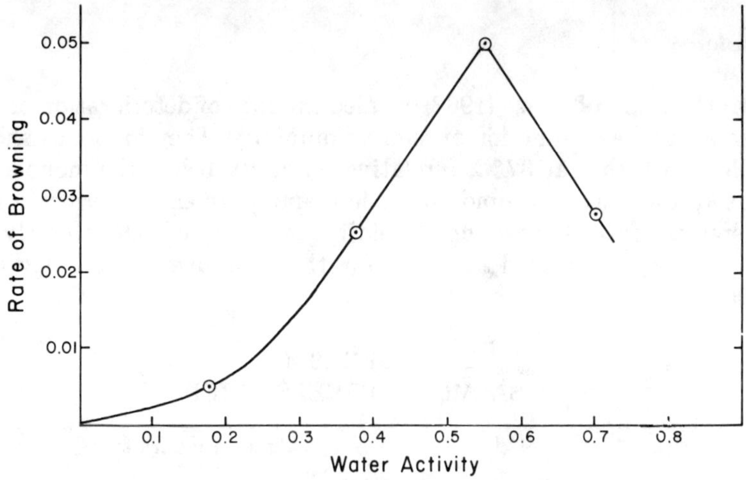

FIG. 18.14. FREEZE-DRIED PORK AT 37 °C (From Sharp 1963).

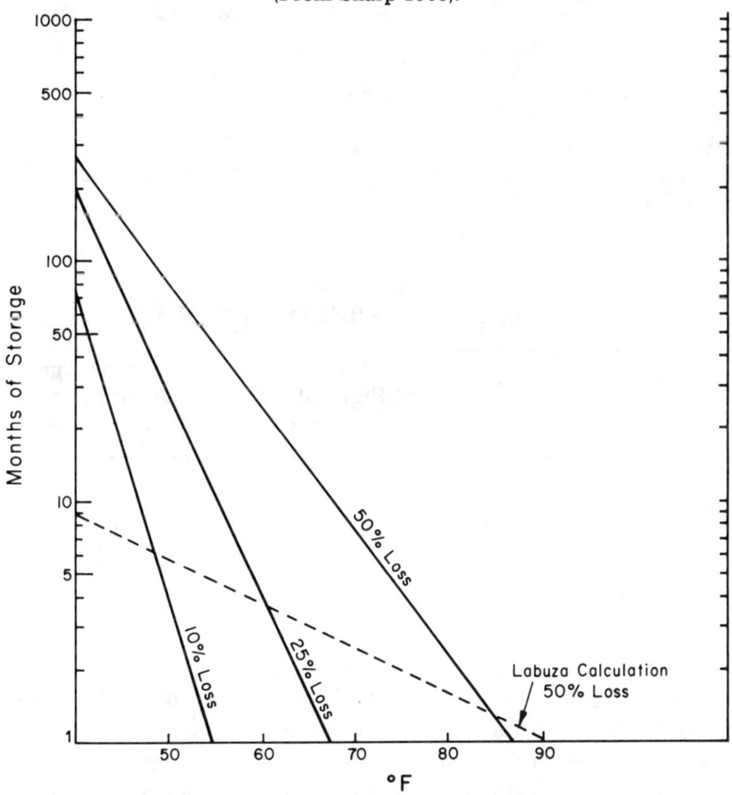

FIG. 18.15. MONTHS OF STORAGE VERSUS TEMPERATURE (°F) TO 10, 25, AND 50% LOSS OF THIAMIN IN DEHYDRATED PORK

(From Rice and Robinson 1944 as cited in Kramer 1974).

Seafood

Martinez and Labuza (1968) studied the rate of deterioration of freeze-dried salmon as a function of relative humidity. They found, as shown in Table 18.10, that at 37 °C, a relative humidity below the monolayer increased the rates of lipid oxidation and pigment deterioration, but lowered the rate of browning. A relative humidity of 32%, slightly above the monolayer, seemed to allow for the best overall stability during storage.

TABLE 18.10
SALMON — FREEZE-DRIED

% RH	Time in Hours to: 2,000 μl O_2/g lipid (oxidation)	300 optical density (browning)	1.6 OD (475/390nm) (pigment deterioration)
0.1 (dry)	240	160	90
11.0 (below monolayer)	340	—	110
32.0 (above monolayer)	640	100	200
41.0 (above monolayer)	—	60	—

Martinez and Labuza (1968).

TABLE 18.11
SHRIMP — FREEZE-DRIED

% O_2	Rate of Pigment Loss dA_s/dt (amount/day)	Rate of Oxygen Absorption dO_2/dt (μl/g/day)
21.0	.073	8.6
7.8	.044	5.2
7.0	.037	4.3
2.5	.017	2.0

Simon *et al.* (1971).

Simon *et al.* (1971) studied the effect of oxygen partial pressure on oxidation and pigment loss of freeze-dried shrimp at 37 °C. Their data, shown in Table 18.11, demonstrate the importance of vacuum packing at high temperatures. If data were available for the temperature sensitivity of the reaction, the temperature necessary to give protection equal to that of vacuum packing could be found. Figure 18.16 demonstrates the effect of this oxidation on the flavor score. A value of 5 is borderline acceptability. As can be seen, the air packed shrimp is unacceptable right at the start, and even 3.5% oxygen gives a shelf-life of only 45 days.

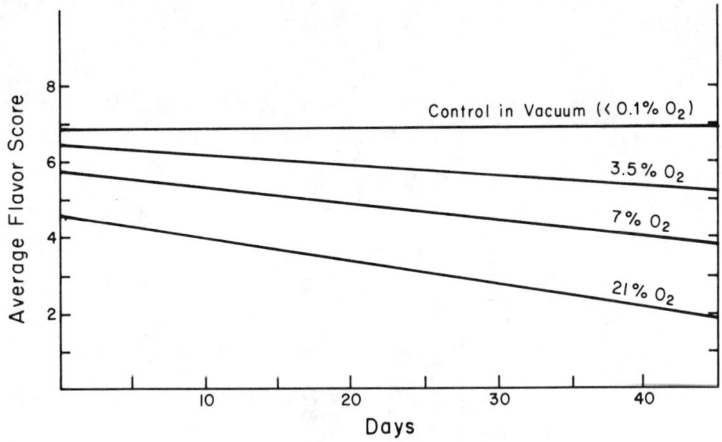

FIGURE 18.16. FREEZE-DRIED SHRIMP (37 °C)
(From Simon *et al.* 1971).

DRIED FRUITS

Enzymatic, and in some cases nonenzymatic browning reactions leading to color darkening and flavor change are the major modes of deterioration of dried fruits. Enzymatic reactions predominate since the fruits are not blanched and are usually not dried below 0.5 to 0.6 a_w. Powdered fruits, however, have lower a_w and nonenzymatic reactions would predominate. This is most often measured by the optical density of alcohol-extracted pigments. Sulfur dioxide is added to inhibit the color change, but it is used up in the reaction. Thus, loss of sulfur dioxide with storage time and temperature is often a deciding factor in shelf-life. Since nonenzymatic browning is a reaction between amino acids and reducing sugars, with loss of both occurring, the extent of the reaction is sometimes measured by following the change in sugar and amino acid content. Flavor change is another criterion which is measured by taste panels.

Apricots, Figs and Raisins

In 1946 Stadtman *et al.* (as cited in Copley and Van Arsdel, 1964) concluded that the activation energy of darkening due to enzymatic browning in dried apricots is about 26 Kcal/mole (Q_{10} of 3.9). It should be noted that enzymatic browning predominates because the fruit is not blanched. It was found that the rate was sufficiently independent of

TABLE 18.12
DARKENING OF DRIED FRUITS

Fruit	Q_{10}	End-point Optical Density	k = Rate of Darkening (0.D./day) × 10^{-1}					
			Days to End-point 50°F	k 50°F	Days to End-point 70°F	k 70°F	Days to End-point 90°F	k 90°F
Calimyrna Figs	2.2	0.75	1,300	5.8	403	18.6	100	74.7
Apricots*	5.8	0.3	2,140	1.4	190	15.8	29	103.1
Raisins	3.6	1.0	4,200	2.5	855	11.7	137	73.0
Golden raisins	2.8	0.3	2,500	1.2	732	4.1	120	25.1

Nury *et al.* 1960, cited in Copley and Van Arsdel, 1964.
*Rate measured after initial induction time: 176 days at 50°F, 141 days at 70°F and 63 days at 90°F.

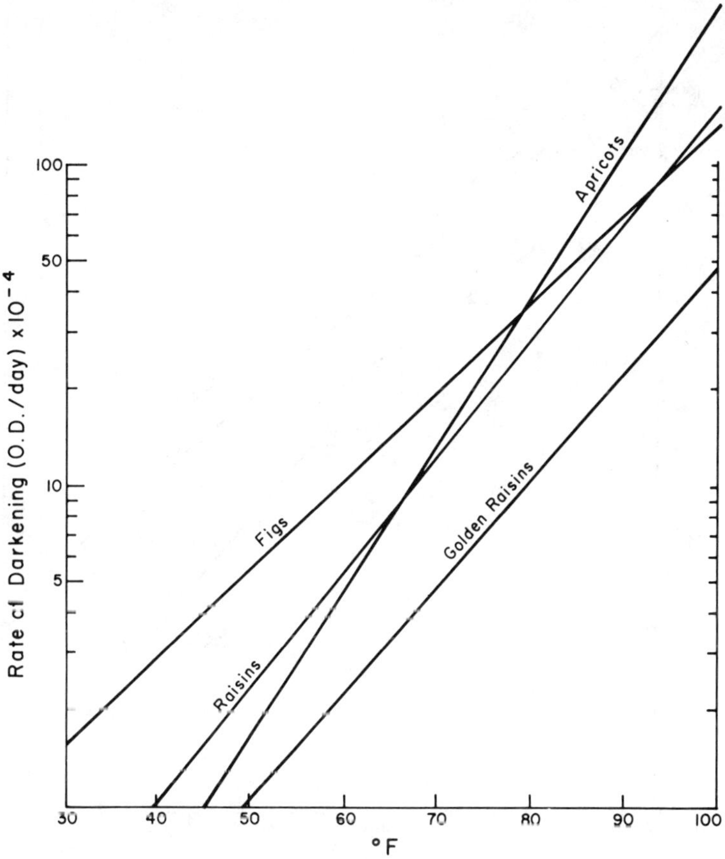

FIG. 18.17. DRIED FRUITS — RATE OF DARKENING VERSUS TEMPERATURE °F

(From Nury *et al.* 1960 as cited in Copley and Van Arsdel 1964).

sulfur dioxide loss, moisture content, oxygen concentration and storage time, so that the shelf-life can be determined in terms of temperature. However, this leaves out the fact that the fruit can dry out and become too hard to eat.

In 1960, Nury *et al.* (as cited in Copley and Van Arsdel 1964) at the USDA Western Regional Laboratory used Stadtman's method for measuring color darkening and determined the Q_{10}s for enzymatic darkening of apricots, figs and raisins. They also determined a color cutoff point based on a specified value of optical density. The results are

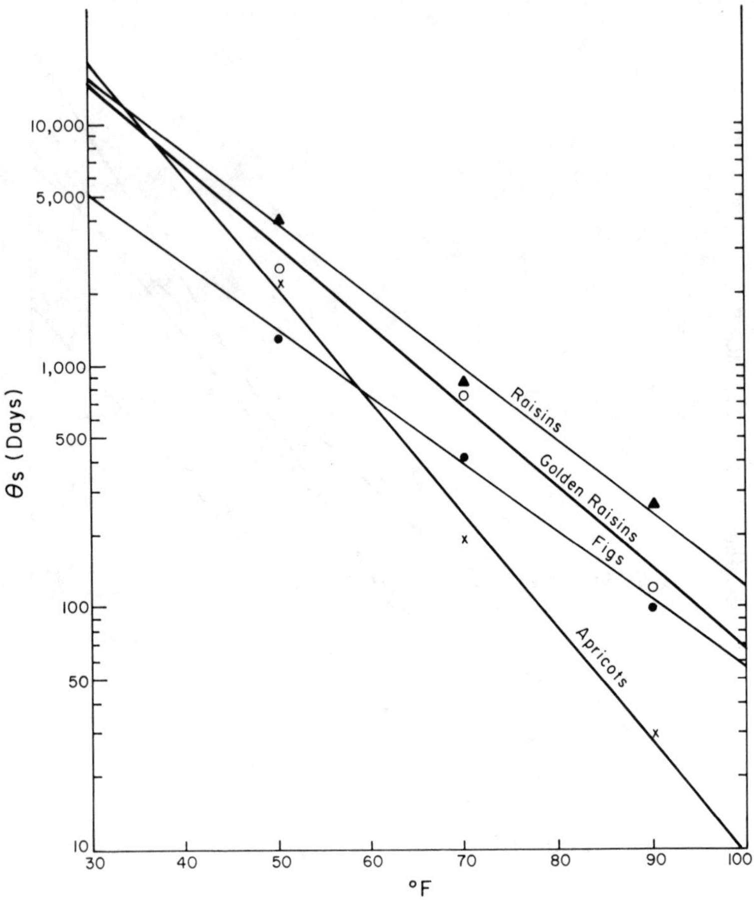

FIG. 18.18. DRIED FRUITS — DAYS TO UNACCEPTABLE DARKNESS VERSUS TEMPERATURE °F

(From Nury *et al.* 1960 as cited in Copley and Van Arsdel 1964).

TABLE 18.13
STORAGE STABILITY OF RAISINS

Drying Method	Weeks to Noticeable Difference 70 °F	90 °F	Q_{10}	Weeks to 0.1 Unit Increase in Optical Density 70 °F	90 °F	Q_{10}
Tunnel dried	34	8.8	3.7	24	5	4.0
On-the-vine dried	41	14.0	2.8	50	10	4.5
Sun dried	31	11.0	2.6	19	3	5.4

From Stafford and Guadagni (1977).

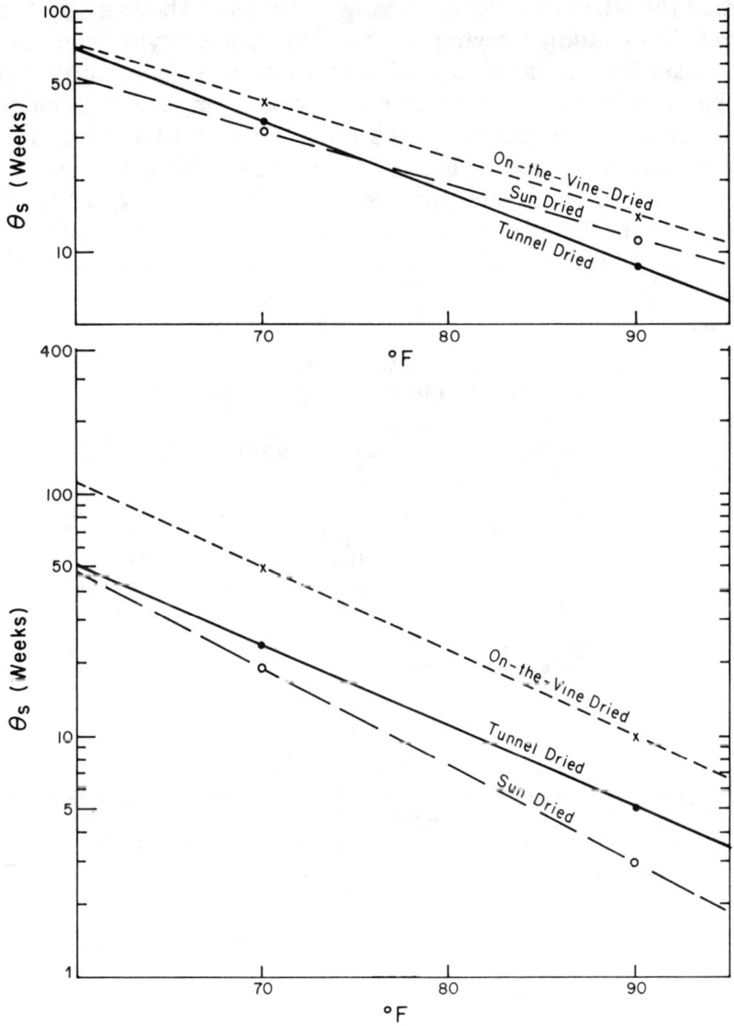

FIG. 18.19.(TOP) RAISINS — WEEKS TO NOTICEABLE FLAVOR CHANGE VERSUS TEMPERATURE °F
(BOTTOM) RAISINS — WEEKS TO 0.1 UNIT INCREASE IN OPTICAL DENSITY VERSUS TEMPERATURE (°F)
(From Stafford *et al.* 1977).

shown in Table 18.12 and Fig. 18.17. The shelf-life plot, Fig. 18.18, shows the shelf-life to be very long below 65 °F. In 1977, Stafford and Guadagni studied the effect of different drying methods on the storage stability of raisins. They studied drying on the vine, tunnel drying and sun drying and measured the flavor stability and rate of enzymatic darkening at 70 °F and 90 °F. They found that on-the-vine drying yielded a longer shelf-life based on flavor and color, as seen in Table 18.13 and Fig. 18.19. The longer shelf-life is due to better initial quality since the Q_{10}s are comparable for each product. However, as is shown in Fig. 18.19 the color change occurs faster than the flavor change. This would only be important in light products initially, but could lead to severe loss of shelf-life.

Apples

TABLE 18.14
DRIED APPLESAUCE STORAGE

% RH at 37 °C	Loss of Flavor Score/Day	Shelf-Life Days
1	0.02	225
11	0.035	110
33	0.11	41
50	0.19	24

From Karel and Labuza (1967).

TABLE 18.15
APPLE FLAKES

Temperature	Rate of SO_2 Loss (ppm/day)	Months to Brown Color
50 °F	3.8	over 15
70 °F	7.3	11
90 °F	20.0	3

Bolin and Boyle (1971).

Karel and Labuza (1967) studied the effect of moisture content on dried applesauce. They found the rate of flavor loss at 37 °C to change with percent relative humidity as shown in Table 18.14. When stored at 37 °C and two different relative humidities in package films of varying moisture permeability, dried applesauce with an initial relative humidity of less than 1% took from 24 to 225 days to reach unacceptable flavor. The prediction of loss following the methods described in Chapter 3 were very close to actual changes.

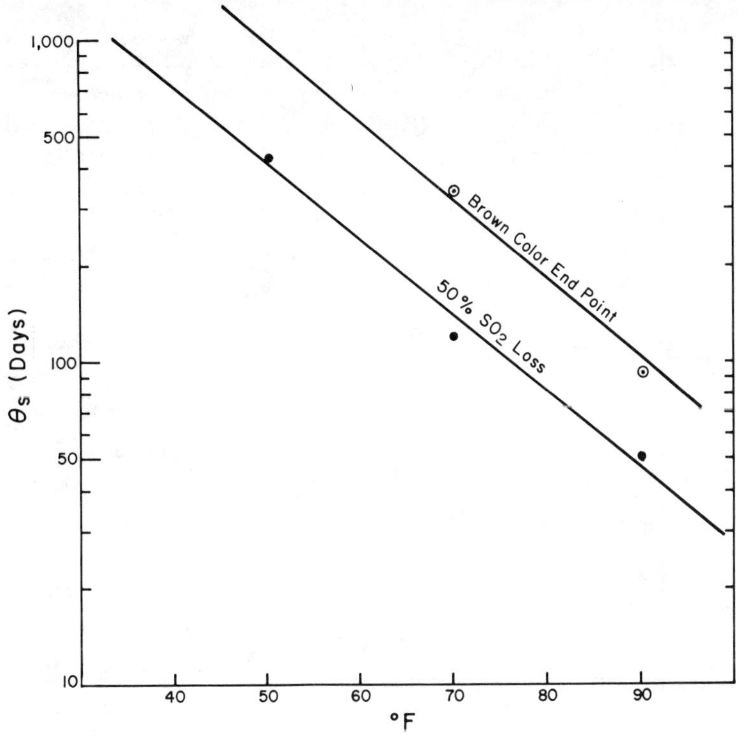

FIG. 18.20. TIME TO 50% SO_2 LOSS IN DRIED APPLES (From Bolin and Boyle 1972).

Bolin and Boyle (1972) at the Western Regional Research Laboratories studied the effect of storage and processing on sulfur dioxide in commercial dried apples. They found, as seen in Table 18.15, that the rate of SO_2 loss per day increased, and the shelf-life decreased, with higher temperatures. Figure 18.20 shows the number of days to 50% loss of SO_2. The Q_{10} of sulfur dioxide loss is 2.7. Loss of acceptability based on color has the same Q_{10} as SO_2 loss. More than 50% SO_2 is lost before the color becomes unacceptable.

Peaches

Bolin and Stafford (1976) have also studied the color stability of dried peaches. Time found to unacceptable darkness of color vs temperature is shown in Fig. 18.21 and the Q_{10}s are listed. The difference in shelf-life

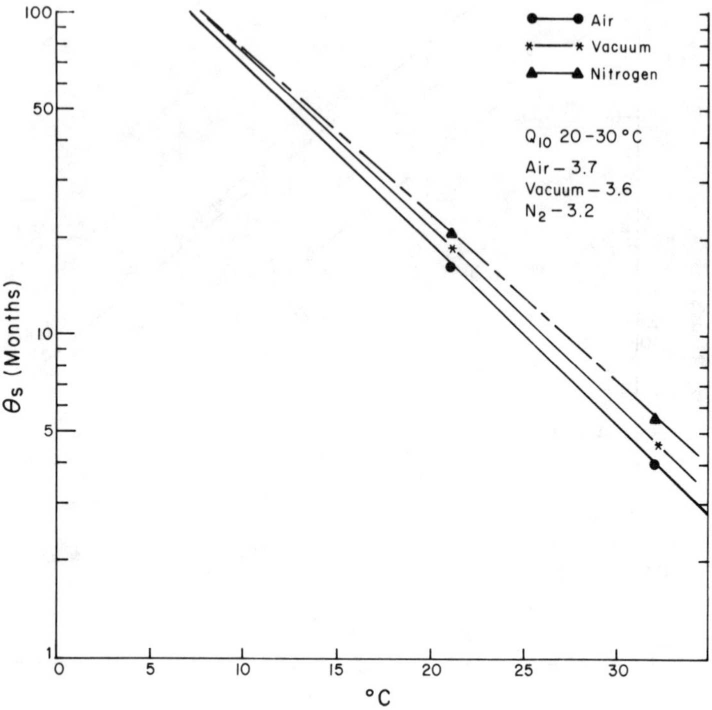

FIG. 18.21. SHELF-LIFE OF DRIED PEACHES
(From Bolin and Stafford 1976).

with storage in air, vacuum and nitrogen means that the packaging film used is also important. Packages with greater resistance to oxygen permeation would give a longer shelf-life since lower oxygen levels slow the reaction significantly.

Dried Orange Powder

In 1969, studies by Gee *et al.* (1969) showed that the principal mode of deterioration of dried orange powder was nonenzymatic browning (NEB) reactions between sugars and amino acids. In this case the a_w is low so enzymatic reactions are slow. They stored samples at 0, 70, and 90 °F (above 90 °F NEB is accelerated out of proportion to any other possible degradation reaction) and measured the sugar and amino acid content after 1, 3, 7, and 10 months of storage. Their results are shown in Table 18.16 and Fig. 18.22. The Q_{10} for 10% amino acid loss is 1.3, which is quite low for NEB. This means that the amino acids possibly were lost by some other degradation mechanism.

TABLE 18.16.
DRIED ORANGE POWDER

Total Amino Acid Content			
Initial (μ mole Amino Acid/g Solids)	% of Initial After 10 Months Storage		
	0°F	70°F	90°F
202.6	94%	86%	76.5%

Gee *et al.* (1969).

Sour Cherries

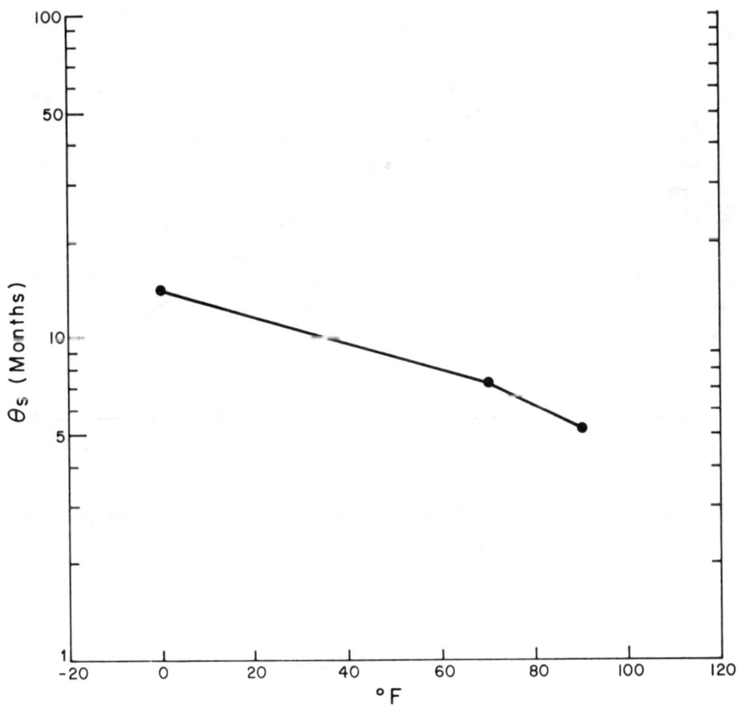

FIG. 18.22. DRIED ORANGE POWDER — MONTHS TO 10% LOSS OF AMINO ACIDS VERSUS TEMPERATURE °F
(From Gee *et al.* 1969).

The decrease of the anthocyanin pigment content of freeze-dried sour cherries has been studied by Do *et al.* (1976). The pigment loss and time to 54% loss is shown in Table 18.17 and Fig. 18.23.

TABLE 18.17
FREEZE-DRIED SOUR CHERRIES

Storage Time (months)	Pigment Content Anthocyanin — mg/100 g (Initial 13.2 mg/100 g) 21 °C	38 °C
0	9.28	9.28
2	~6.90	~4.40
4	~5.80	~2.20
6	5.04	1.10

Do *et al.* (1976). Q_{10} = 2.2

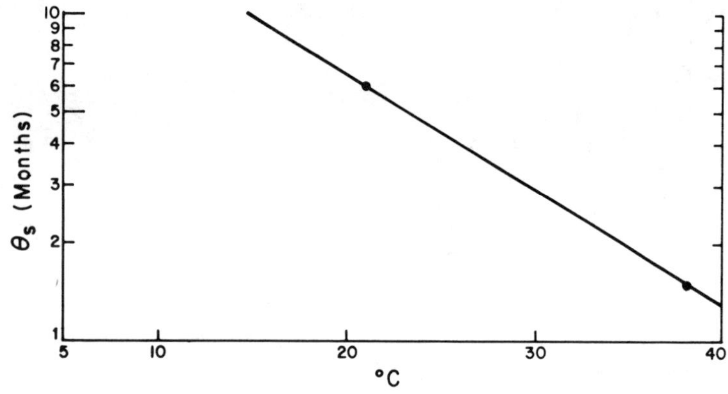

FIG. 18.23. SOUR CHERRIES — MONTHS TO 54% LOSS OF PIGMENT
(From Do *et al.* 1976).

CANDIES

The changes in moisture, texture and flavor of five different types of candies stored for two years at −23 °C, 21 °C and 37 °C were studied by Cecil and Woodroof (1962). A summary of rate constants, activation energy and temperature coefficients (Q_{10}s) is shown in Table 18.18. Only the change in texture and flavor of the starch jelly when fruit is added showed much sensitivity to temperature.

TABLE 18.18.
CHANGES IN MOISTURE, TEXTURE AND FLAVOR OF CANDY STORED TWO YEARS AT −23 °C, 21 °C AND 37 °C, (ASSUMING FIRST ORDER)

	k at 21 °C (months^{-1})	E_a (Kcal/mole)	Q_{10}
Caramel Nougat (stnd)			
Texture	.1993	4.85	1.34
Moisture	.1355	0.3	1.02
Flavor	.2164	4.85	1.34
Caramel Nougat (coated)			
Texture	.1018	3.03	1.20
Moisture	.0916	1.99	1.13
Flavor	.1481	3.67	1.25
Coconut Cream (coated)			
Texture	.1351	3.62	1.25
Moisture	.1403	2.42	1.16
Flavor	.2965	4.02	1.28
Starch Jelly and Fruit			
Texture	.0955	21.34	3.66
Moisture	.1438	2.36	1.15
Flavor	.0771	21.50	3.69
Starch Jelly Plain			
Texture	.1212	2.37	1.15
Moisture	.1182	2.56	1.17
Flavor	.0938	3.72	1.25

OPEN DATING

With respect to dehydrated foods, this chapter shows that a myriad of reactions can occur in dehydrated foods which are a function of initial quality and processing conditions, and are influenced by temperature, moisture change, oxygen level, light and the package permeability. Since consumers are unaware of these factors, a "pack date" would seem to be useful only from the standpoint of stock rotation.

The most logical method of open dating would be to either have a "sell by date" with instructions as to how the product should be stored in the home or have a "best if used by date" with similar instructions. For example, the instructions to keep in a cool, dry, dark place (not in a cabinet next to the stove or sink) could be placed on the package along with the estimated shelf-life for various environments such as: (1) a cool dry area, e.g. 60 °F and 40% RH; (2) a warm moist area, 70 °F and 60% RH; (3) a hot dry area, 85 °F and 30% RH; (4) a cool moist area, 60 °F and 60% RH.

In fact, these standards might be set up similar to the British Three Star System, for frozen storage, assigning a letter to each of them. To implement this, of course, the manufacturer must assess the mode of deterioration of each product and gather information on the distribution system. From this, an average sale date could be instituted which could be used in all areas. If a product were sold beyond this date but still within the shelf-life (which could be quite long), it could be offered at a reduced price. This would force the marketing segment to turn over the product sooner. On the other hand a "best if used by date" might be difficult to implement since it has not known to which region the food is going when it is manufactured.

REFEERENCES

BOLIN, H.R. and BOYLE, F.P. 1972. Effect of storage and processing on sulfur dioxide in preserved fruit. Food Prod. Dev. Nov. 82-86.

BOLIN, H.R. and STAFFORD, A.E. 1976. Color stability of dried peaches. Food Prod. Dev. Oct., 74-76.

BROCKMAN, M.C. 1966. Storage stability of freeze-dried foods. ASHRAE J. August, 54-58.

Burton, W.G. 1949. Mashed potato powder. IV. Deterioration due to oxidative changes. J. Soc. Chem. Ind. *68,* 149-151.

BURTON, W.G. 1945. Mashed potato powder. III. The high temperature browning of mashed potato powder. Soc. Chem. Ind. *641,* 215-218.

CECIL, S.R. and WOODROOF, J.G. 1962. Long term storage of military rations. G. Agric. Exp. Stn. Tech. Bull. 25.

COPLEY, M.J. and VAN ARASDEL, W.B., 1964. Food Dehydration. AVI Publishing Co. Westport, Conn.

DAOUD, H.N. and LUH, B.S. 1967. Packaging of food in laminate and aluminum film combination pouches. IV. Freeze-dried red bell peppers. Food Technol. *21,*(3), 21.

DO, J.Y., POTEWIRATANANOND, G., SALUNKHE, D.K. and RAHMAN, A.R. 1976. Freeze-dehydrated compressed sour cherries. II. Stability of anthocyanins during storage. J. Food Technol. *11,* 265-272.

GEE, M., GRAHAM, R.P. and MORGAN, A.I. Jr. 1969. Stability of foam-mat dried orange powder. Food Technol. *23*(5), 83-84.

HENDEL, C.E. 1959. Dehydrated mashed potatoes. *In* Potato Processing. W.F. Talburt and O. Smith (Editors). AVI Publishing Co., Westport, Conn.

KAPSALIS, J.G., WOLF, M., DRIVER, M. and WALKER, J. 1967. The effect of moisture content on flavor and texture stability of dehydrated foods. No. TP-330. U.S. Army Natick (Mass.) Laboratories.

KAREL, M. and LABUZA, T.P. 1967. Mechanisms of deterioration and formulation of space diets. AFSC Aerospace Medical Division, Brooks Air Force Base, Texas. Project No. 41-609-66-46.

KAREL, M. and LABUZA, T.P. 1969. Optimization of protective packaging of space foods. AFSC Aerospace Medical Division, Brooks Air Force Base, Texas. Project No. 41-609-66-46.

KAPSALIS, J.G. 1973. Moisture and food characteristics. U.S. Army Natick Activities R&D Report. Assoc. Military Food and Packaging Systems, *25*(1) 60.

KAREL, M. and LABUZA, T.P. 1969. Optimization of protective packaging of space foods. AFSC Aerospace Medical Division, Brooks Air Force Base, Texas, Contract No. F41-609-68-C-0015.

KRAMER, A. 1974. Storage retention of nutrients. Food Technol. *28*(1), 65-72.

LABUZA, T.P. 1972. Nutrient losses during drying and storage of dry foods. Crit. Rev. Food Technol. *3*, 217.

LAJOLLA, F., TANNENBAUM, S.R. and LABUZA, T.P. 1971. Reaction at limited water concentration. 2. Chloropohyll degradation. J. Food Sci. *36*, 850-853.

LEGAULT, R.R., HENDEL, C.E., TALBURT, W.F. and POOLE, M.F. 1951. Browning of dehydrated sulfited vegetables during storage. Food Technol. *5*, 417-423.

MARTINEZ, F. and LABUZA, T.P. 1968. Rate of deterioration of freeze-dried salmon as a function of relative humidity. J. Food Sci. *33*, 241-247.

MASURE, M.P., BOHART, G.S., EASTMOND, E.J. and BOGGS, M.M. 1950. Value of starch coating in the preservation of quality of dehydrated carrots. Food Technol. *4*, 94-97.

NURY, F.S., TAYLOR, D.H. and BREKKE, J.E. 1960. Research for better quality in dried fruits: Figs — USDA ARS-74-16; Raisins — USDA ARS-74-17; Apricots — USDA ARS-74-19. Albany, CA.

RICE, E.E. and ROBINSIN, H.E. 1944. Nutritive value of canned and dehydrated meat and meat products. Am. J. Public Health. *34*, 587.

ROSS, A.F. 1948. Deterioration of processed potatoes. *In* Advances in Food Research, *1*, 257-290. Academic Press, New York.

SAPERS, G.M. 1975. Flavor and stability of dehydrated potato products. Agric. Food Chem. *23*, 1027.

SAPERS, G.M., PANASIUK, O., TALLEY, F.B. and SHAW, R.L. 1973. Flavor, quality and stability of potato flakes — effects of raw material and processing. J. Food Sci. *38*, 586-589.

SAPERS, G.M., PANASIUK, O., TALLEY, F.B. and SHAW, R.L. 1974. Flavor, quality and stability of potato flakes: Effects of drying conditions, moisture content and packaging. J. Food Sci. *39*, 555-558.

SHARP, J.G. 1962. Non-enzymatic browning deterioration in dehydrated meat. Recent Adv. Food Sci. *2*, 65-73.

SHARP, J.G. and ROLFE, E.J. 1958. Deterioration of dehydrated meat during storage. *In* Fundamental Aspects of Dehydration of Foodstuffs. Soc. Chem. Ind. 197-210.

SIMON, I.B., LABUZA, T.P. and KAREL, M. 1971. Computer-aided predictions of food storage stability: Oxidative deterioration of a shrimp product. J. Food Sci. *36*, 280-286.

STADTMAN, E.T., BARKER, H.A., HAAS, V., MRAK, E.M. and MACKINNEY, G. 1946. Storage of dried fruit. Ind. Eng. Chem. *38*, 99-104, 324-329.

STAFFORD, A.E. and GUADAGNI, D.G. 1977. Storage stability of raisins dried by different procedures. J. Food Sci. *42*(2), 547-548.

SULLIVAN, J.F., KONSTANCE, R.P., CALHOUN, M.J., TALLEY, F.G., CORDING, J. and PANASIUK, O. 1974. Flavor and storage stability of explosion puffed potatoes. J. Food Sci. *39*, 58.

TALLEY, F.B., KOMANOWSKY, M., CORDING, J., Jr. and ESKEW, R.K. 1966. Flavor and storage stability of dehydrated pumpkin. Food Technol. *20*, 1369-1370.

THOMPSON, J.S., FOX, J.B. Jr. and LANDMAN, W.A. 1962. Effect of water and temperature on freeze-dried beef during storage. Food Technol. *16*, 131.

TRESSLER, D.K. 1956. New developments in the dehydration of fruits and vegetables. Food Technol. *10*, 119-124.

TOUMY, J.M. and HINNERGARDT, L.C. 1968. Effect of headspace oxygen on the quality of freeze-dried raw beef patties. U.S. Army Natick (Mass.) Laboratories Technical Report 69-54-FL.

WATTS, B.M. 1962. Meat products. *In* Symposium on Foods: Lipids and Their Oxidation. H.W. Schultz (Editor). AVI Publishing Co., Westport, Conn.

CHAPTER 19

SHELF-LIFE OF FROZEN CONVENIENCE FOODS

INTRODUCTION

The group of foods discussed here is best described collectively as frozen convenience foods. The major group of products included are precooked foods, predominantly TV dinners and entrees. Definitions of these products may be found in military meals specifications (Anon. 1956). A dinner generally is considered to consist of a main course dish, usually meat, with at least two other vegetables. An entree is a main course dish served with one, or no vegetable courses. The distinguishing key word here is "precooked", for the convenience of these items lies in the fact that heating is all that is necessary before consumption.

PROCESSING

Individual meal components (e.g., meat, gravy, vegetables, etc.) are prepared and processed to varying degrees using the methods described in other sections, and then are held in various forms, before final meal assembly and packaging. The components are put together on manual and/or automated filling lines. The products may then be frozen by a variety of methods (Fennema 1975). Two types of containers are basically used today; the rigid aluminum tray (with or without packets) covered with a foil sheet overlay, and the "boil-in-bag" (Tressler 1968a). Oven-proof laminated paperboard has begun to appear as a replacement for aluminum trays (Anon. 1977).

DISTRIBUTION

The time-temperature exposure of products in the frozen distribution chain remains the largest question mark facing decision makers in the food industry. Any reliable prediction of the performance of any given product must reasonably account for the entire temperature history of the product, from the initial freezing process all the way through storage in the consumer's freezer. In fact, if home freezers in the U.S. were rated by a system similar to the English Three Star System, then good recommendations for home storage periods could be made.

The association of Food and Drug Officials of the United States (Association of Food and Drug Officials of the United States 1961) recommended a series of operating standards for the frozen food industry. Significant among these was the recommendation of 0 °F as the maximum storage temperature for a food product in the distribution chain. The energy crunch has encouraged the replacement of the old style open freezer cases with newer types with doors. This saves energy, but also produces lower, more uniform temperatures in the display case and thus gives better control over frozen food quality.

Space in the supermarket freezer case is, as always, expensive (due to energy costs) and highly competitive. A product which does not sell in the freezer case has an added drawback in that it takes up expensive space. Brand identification and loyalty are important in frozen food marketing. In addition, frozen foods have come to be associated with high quality at premium prices (Martin 1968). A product which does not satisfy the customer has the added disadvantage of lowering the consumer's opinion of the entire product line.

The requirements of S-641, "The Consumer Food Act of 1976" (Federal Register 3-22-76), seek to "protect consumers from adulterated food" and "to promote honesty and fair dealing in the interest of the consumers" by classification and standardization of the labeling, including code dating, regulations for various groups of food products "to which the Secretary (of Health, Education and Welfare) has made a finding that date information is necessary."

The major problem with this proposed regulation can be found in its vagueness. What type of date information is necessary to "promote honesty and fair dealing" with consumers? First, we must ascertain what constitutes fair dealing with the consumer. This seems best defined simply as satisfying the expectation of the consumer. While also vague, this definition is broad enough to permit changes in expectations as consumers become more knowledgeable about foods and nutrition. Even now, different segments of the consumer market buy different products for different reasons and with different intentions. Quick Frozen Foods magazine (Anon. 1974) equated overall satisfaction with value received and generally noted that "customers with smaller incomes rated the value they received from frozen foods lower than customers with larger incomes". This same source noted the following market segmentation: frozen TV dinners showed the greatest sales strength in the "low income" (< $5,000) group while the higher priced entrees and specialty items were brought predominantly by the high income (> $15,000) groups.

MODES OF DETERIORATION

The major difficulties encountered in discussing the deterioration of precooked frozen TV dinners and entrees stem from their heterogeneity. This group covers the spectrum of foods from the plain chicken pot pie, to elegant prepared entrees such as lobster Newburgh and chicken Kiev. The serving cost range reflected here was from about 39 cents to over $3.00 per serving (Personal Market Survey 1977). The variables encountered in the production of these foods covers a broad range of raw ingredients, processing methods and packaging materials. These factors are commonly termed the "PPP" factors representing the specific product, processing and packaging of the frozen food. The influence of these factors on initial frozen quality, and subsequent deterioration rates is discussed in a number of general references (Tressler *et al.* 1968; Van Arsdel *et al.* 1969).

Before listing modes of deterioration expected by prepared frozen foods, two qualifications are necessary. First, high temperature abuse in the distribution chain cannot be tolerated if meaningful dating provisions are to be enacted. While certain specific product groups require very low storage temperatures and others are more tolerant of higher temperatures, the AFDOUS code recommendation of 0 °F at all points in distribution seems to occupy a satisfactory middle ground. Unfortunately, in 1969, Maryland was the only state to actively enforce a regulation maintaining retail freezer cases below this temperature (Rutgers University 1971). If 0 °F could be maintained throughout the distribution of frozen foods, then the single largest source of uncertainty in the storage quality of frozen foods would be removed. The significance of this is not to be missed. Among the food industry comments following the frozen foods section of the Rutgers Survey, we find numerous industrial sources specifying temperatures of 0 °F or below in their own distribution systems, but indicating that this condition was not being met in many retail display cases. The second qualification is that the deterioration discussed here refers to loss of organoleptic attributes, the importance of which is determined in terms of consumer satisfaction. The danger of microbial spoilage becomes a factor only if high temperature abuse occurs; at temperatures in the neighborhood of 0 °F microbial growth is not a problem (Jul 1969; Van Arsdel *et al.* 1969). Nutrient loss in frozen storage is not covered in this section because of the great variety of ingredient histories and processing combinations which ultimately appear in the freezer case.

The predominant (by frequency of reference) mode of deterioration of precooked frozen foods is lipid oxidation, causing rancidity in the meat portion of the product. However, the susceptibility of the product to lipid oxidation is, as noted earlier, strongly influenced by the ingredients, processing and packaging which go into the product. Changes in gravies and sauces (weeping and curdling) is the other deteriorative mechanism reported in the literature concerning the storage stability of precooked frozen foods. Protein denaturation, which has been found to cause toughening and loss of solubility of proteins in frozen uncooked meats is not discussed with reference to precooked frozen foods.

SHELF-LIFE

The actual shelf-life data on precooked frozen foods in the literature is quite sparse and, without exception, quite dated (over 10 years old). Newer techniques of quality determination (e.g., taste panel and statistical design of experiments) and data treatment (e.g., shelf-life plot, use of Q_{10}, E_a) in use today, can provide a great deal of information regarding the storage stability and mode of deterioration of a product. However, much of the data presented in the literature are not in a form which allows adaptation of the data to this form without the introduction of additional error.

A number of reviews of the frozen food shelf-life data available have been presented in various forms (Tressler *et al.* 1968; Van Arsdel *et al.* 1969), but no summary of Q_{10} values and shelf-lives has been presented. Frozen fried chicken dinners and entrees occupy a dominant place in the freezer case. As in the rest of the frozen dinner market, a few national brands take up most of the space. They are selling quality by brand loyalty.

The original time-temperature tolerance (TTT) study on frozen fried chicken (Hanson *et al.* 1959) showed three degrees of flavor deterioration; loss of "fresh" flavor, which might correspond to the Just Noticeable Difference (JND), "stale" comments by 20% of the panelists, and "rancid" comments by 20% of the panelists. The data in Fig. 19.1 give Q_{10} values (all Q_{10} values given are for the range $-10\,°C$ to $-20\,°C$) of 2.55 (JND endpoint), 1.94 (stale), and 2.67 (rancid). Apparent activation energy (E_a) values ranging from 11.8 to 17.8 Kcal/mole support lipid oxidation as the predominant mode of failure. As seen in Fig. 19.1, the JND occurs earliest with "rancid" comments last. Shepard (1960) reviewded these same data (Fig. 19.2) and came up with a $Q_{10} = 3.5$ and $E_a = 18.4$ Kcal/mole, using an incorrect equation. The importance of the PPP factors mentioned earlier cannot be stressed too much since they are all important.

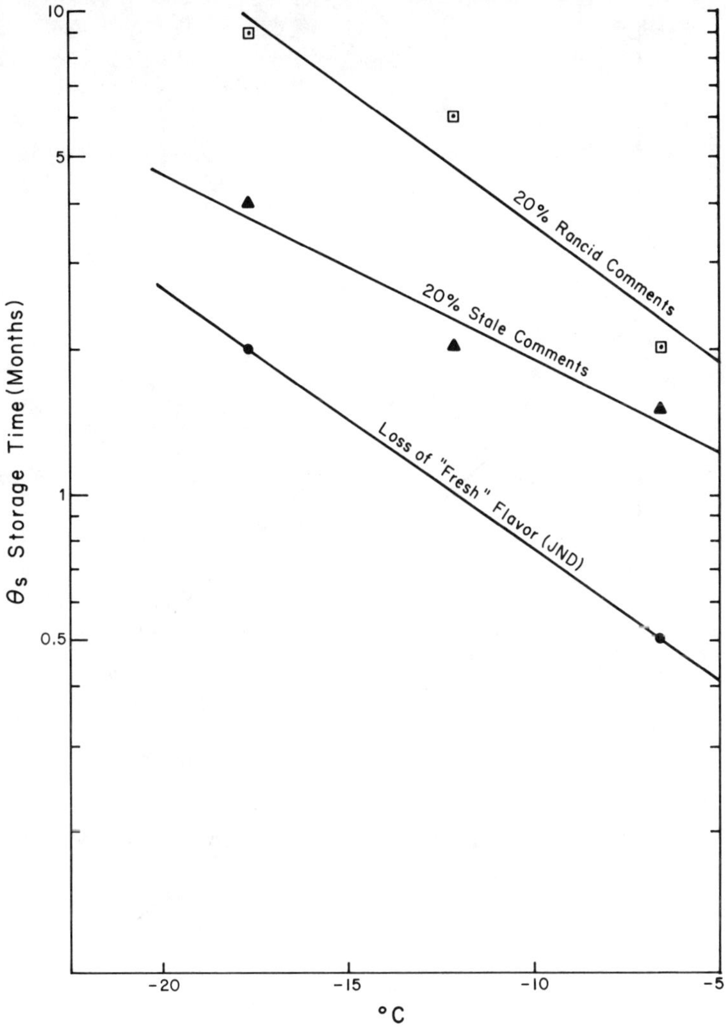

FIG. 19.1. SHELF-LIFE PLOTS FOR FROZEN FRIED CHICKEN IN RETAIL PACKAGES
(From Hanson *et al.* 1959).

The effect of packaging on shelf stability is seen in the data of Hanson *et al.* (1957a), and Klose *et al.* (1959). In this study cut-up chicken was wrapped in one of two packages considered either "good" or "inferior". The fried chicken was also included, packaged in the "good" package.

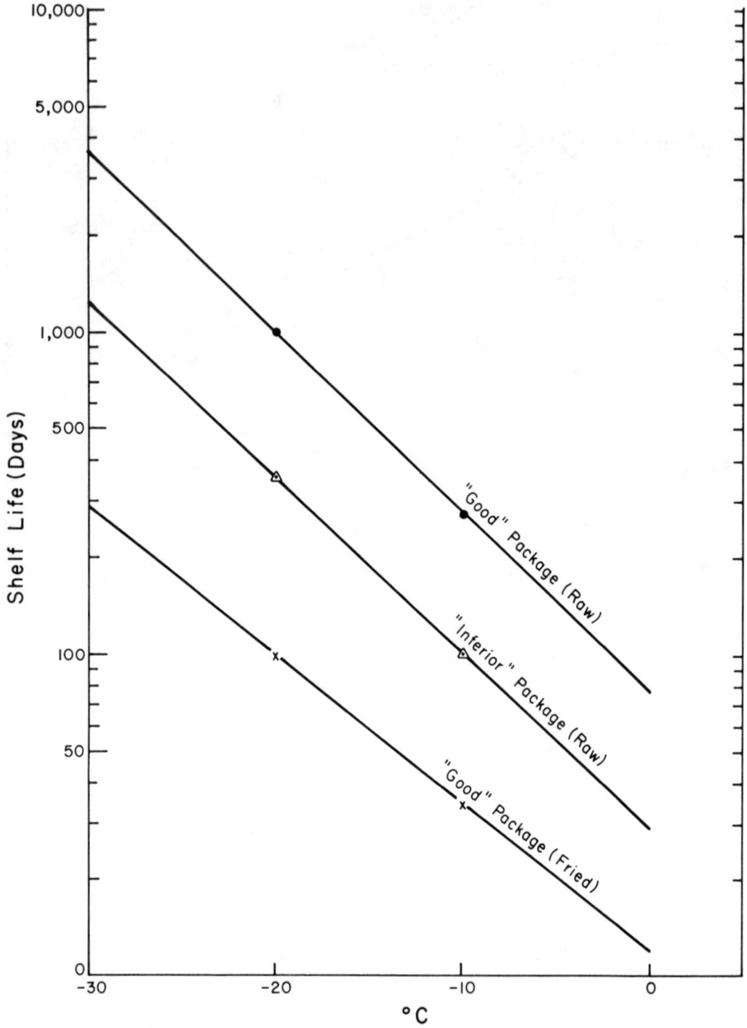

FIG. 19.2. SHELF-LIFE PLOTS FOR CUT-UP CHICKEN PRODUCTS (From Hanson *et al.* 1957; Klose *et al.* 1958).

Figure 19.2 indicates that the inferior package allowed deterioration more rapidly than the good package, while the fried chicken deteriorated faster. E_a values ranged from 14.1 to 17.3 Kcal/mole again suggesting rancidity as the mode of failure. The Q_{10}s were about 3 to 3.5.

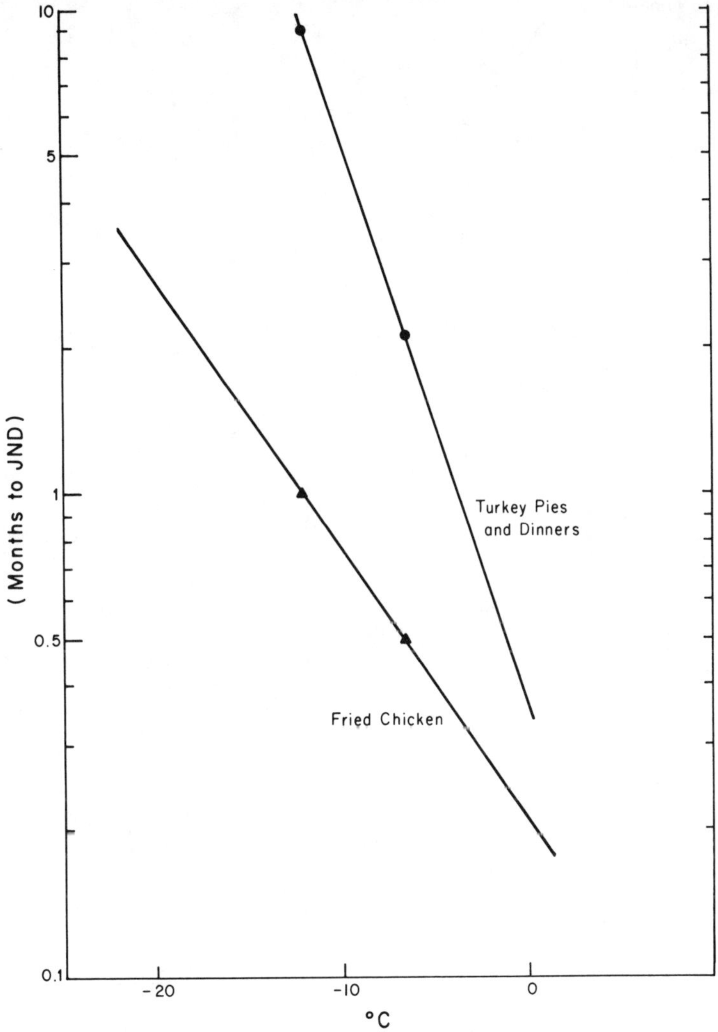

FIG. 19.3. SHELF-LIFE PLOTS FROM USDA TEST DATA
(From Hanson and Fletcher 1958).

The USDA also performed the only TTT study on turkey pies and dinners (Hanson and Fletcher 1958), shown in Fig. 19.3. One problem with these data is that good shelf-life data are only obtained at 10 °F (—12 °C) and 20 °F (—7 °C). The E_a of 37.5 Kcal/mole as calculated from these data, is much higher than might be expected from a rancidity end-point. The

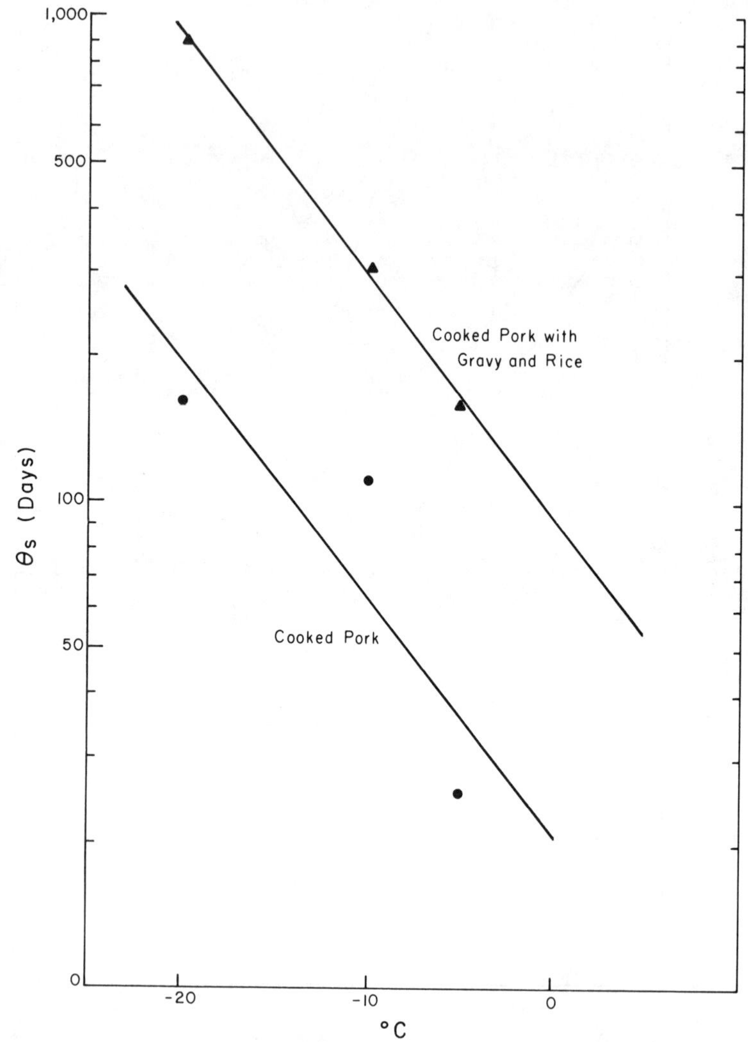

FIG. 19.4. SHELF-LIFE PLOTS OF COOKED PORK FROZEN WITH AND WITHOUT GRAVY

(From Dalhoff and Jul 1965).

effect of antioxidants and of fluctuating temperatures were investigated in this study but neither were noted to have a significant effect on shelf-life. Interestingly enough, a recent trip to the supermarket revealed that few products containing antioxidants were in the frozen food section; no antioxidants were found on any TV dinner of frozen entree ingredient statement.

All published shelf-life work on cooked pork and beef has been done by European workers. Mogens Jul has compiled just about all the data that exist outside food company files and produced a number of reviews of frozen meat processing and the effect of the PPP factors on storage quality (Jul 1968; 1969). The effective use of gravy cover as a physical antioxidant by acting as a barrier to oxygen uptakes was discussed. Figure 19.4 illustrates the effect of adding gravy to cooked pork (Dalhoff and Jul 1965). While the slopes of the two lines are similar (a Q_{10} of about 3) the time to JND, days of high quality life (HQL) at 0 °F, is 150 days without gravy and about 700 days with gravy; an increase of over 400%. The effect of form of the products on HQL is shown in Fig. 19.5 (Jul 1969). Goulash, cooked beef with gravy, onions and carrots has an HQL of about 52 months at 0 °F, while cooked chopped beef with gravy and onions had an HQL of approximately 29 months. These periods seem rather long, but here again, we see the problem with data collected at relatively high (around 20 °F) freezer temperatures. The indicated mode of failure was rancidity; however, the apparent E_a values were 30.9 and 35.7 Kcal/mole for the goulash and chopped beef, respectively. These values are somewhat higher than the range expected for lipid oxidation (10—25 Kcal/mole). Then again, these data may actually reflect some enhanced resistance to rancidity due to the effect of gravy, spices or any one of many related factors.

Some data are also available on the stability of white sauces in frozen storage. Hanson *et al.* (1957b) performed a TTT study on thickened precooked frozen foods. Weeping and curdling of the sauces and puddings were noted, respectively attributable to starch retrogradation and protein denaturation. The only data which could be used for the shelf-life plot format was a study on the frozen stability of white sauce thickened with waxy rice flour, as shown in Fig. 19.6. The time to 3% weep (maximum) after storage at three temperatures was determined. The calculated Q_{10} was 31 and the E_a was 45 Kcal/mole for these data, while the shelf-life at 0 °F was about 12 months (from reported data) and is actually only about 6.8 months (from the linear regression of data).

In his discussion of the importance of low storage temperature, Tressler (1968a) presents a series of "roughly equivalent storage periods" (Fig. 19.7). The data gives a shelf-life of 11 months at 0 °F with Q_{10} = 3.45. This is close to some of the values reported above.

The Refrigeration Research Foundation (1973) published the results of an extensive review of previous studies on the time-temperature tolerance of frozen foods compiled by Olsson and Nilsson in 1972. In this review, the range of values are noted for HQL and Practical Storage Life (PSL) for some general classifications of frozen foods. Groups of interest

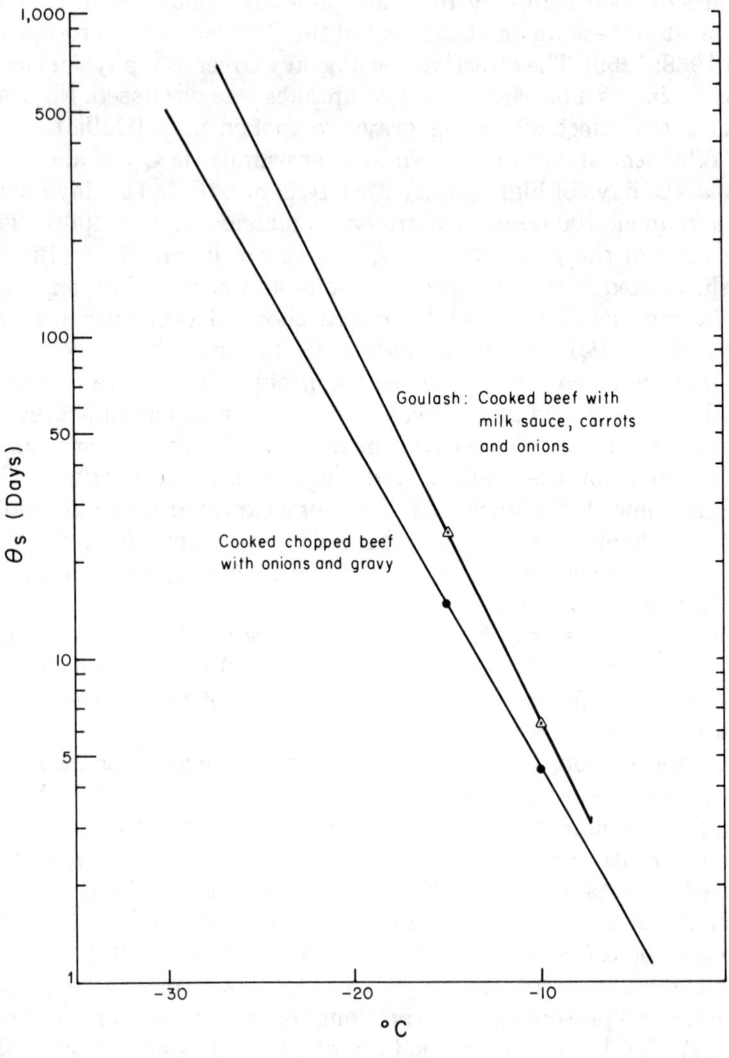

FIG. 19.5. SHELF-LIFE PLOTS OF COOKED PREPARED DISHES
(From Jul 1969).

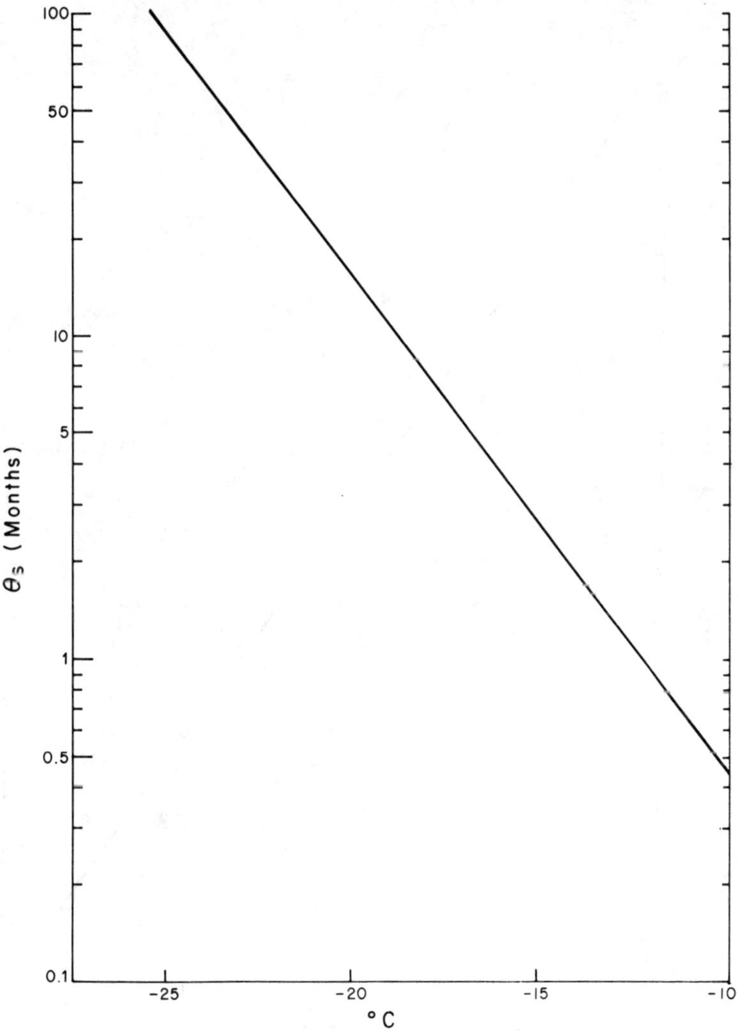

FIG. 19.6. SHELF-LIFE PLOT FOR WHITE SAUCE STABILITY
(From Hanson *et al.* 1957b).

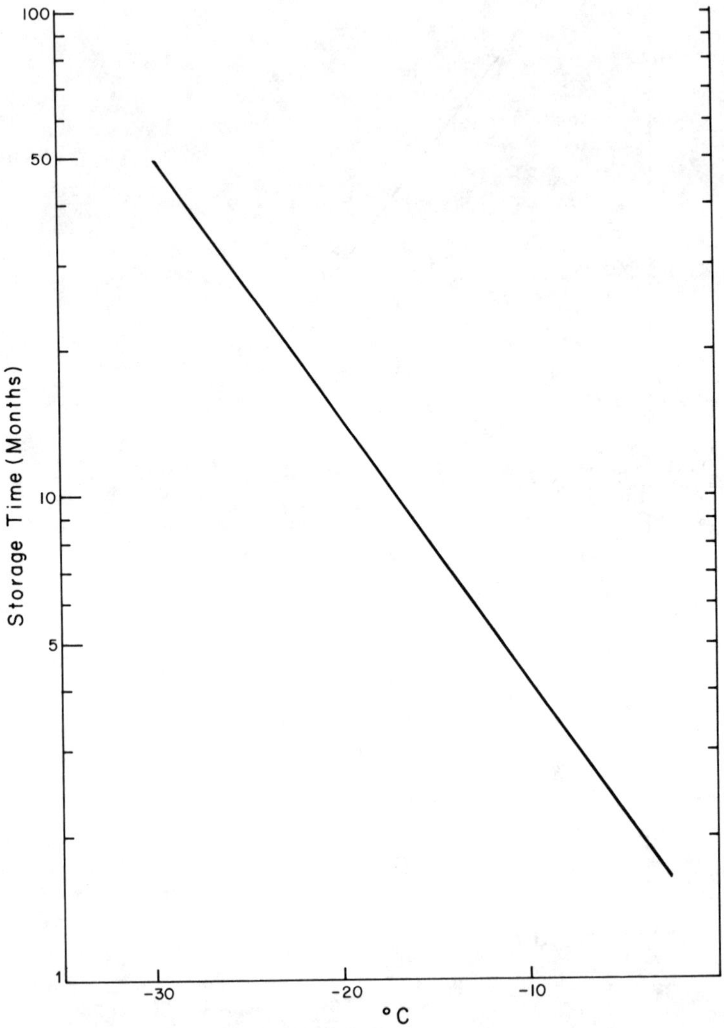

FIG. 19.7. SHELF-LIFE PLOT OF ROUGHLY EQUIVALENT STORAGE PERIODS FOR FROZEN PRECOOKED FOODS
(From Tressler 1968b).

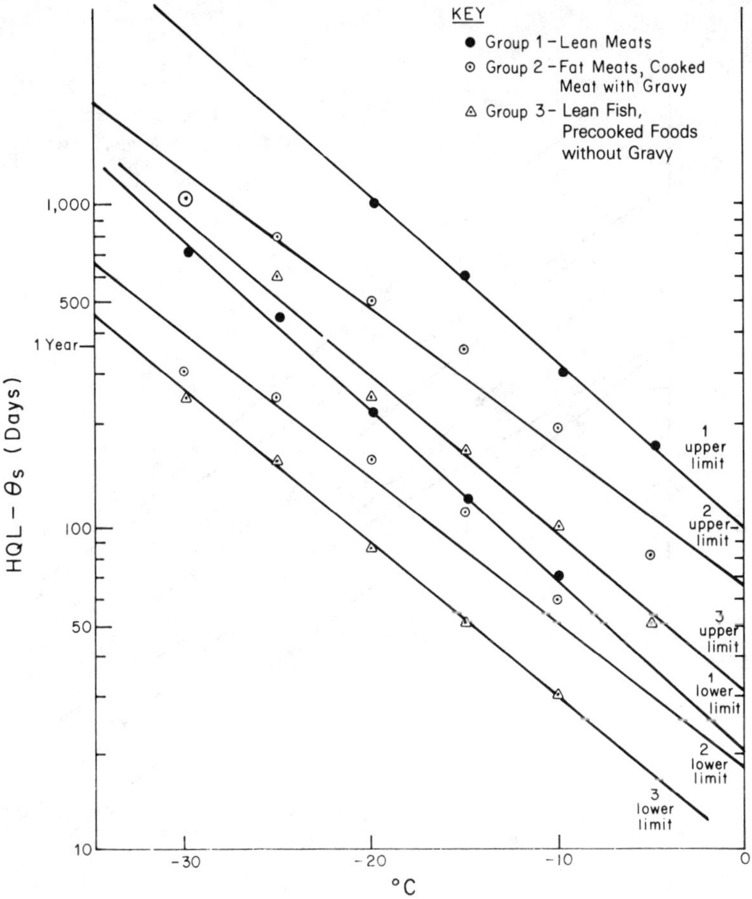

FIG. 19.8. SHELF-LIFE PLOTS FOR RANGES OF HIGH QUALITY LIFE (DAYS) FOR SOME FOOD GROUPS OF REFRIGERATION RESEARCH FOUNDATION

(From Refrigeration Research Foundation 1973).

here are: Group 1 — raw and precooked raw meat; Group 2 — raw and precooked fat meat and all cooked meat with gravy; and Group 3b — precooked foods without gravy. The ranges of values found are shown in Fig. 19.8 (HQL) and 19.9 (PSL). The data of all the studies are summarized in Table 19.1.

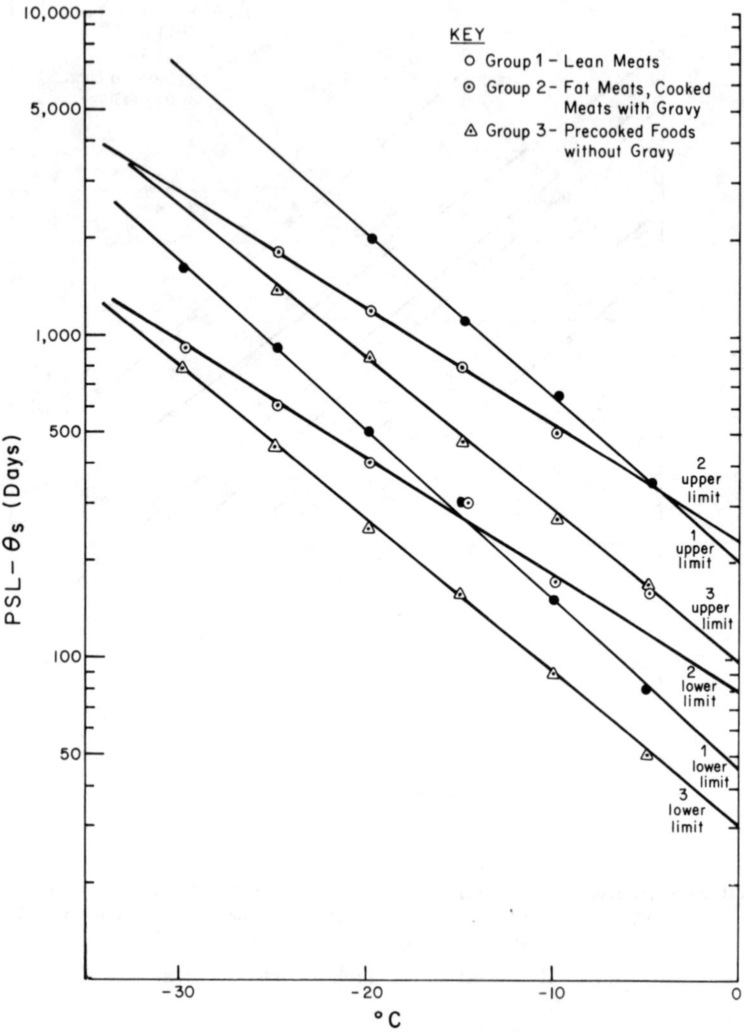

FIG. 19.9. SHELF-LIFE PLOTS: RANGES OF PRACTICAL STORAGE LIFE FOR SOME FOOD GROUPS OF THE REFRIGERATION RESEARCH FOUNDATION

(From Refrigeration Research Foundation 1973).

TABLE 19.1.
SUMMARY OF SHELF-LIFE DATA

Product	Shelf-Life at 0°F	Q_{10} (−10 to −20°C)	Apparent Activation Energy	Reference
Fried chicken				
"Fresh flavor"	60 days	2.55	16.9 Kcal/mole	Hanson *et al.*
"Stale"	110 days	1.94	11.8	(1959)
"Rancid"	285 days	2.67	17.8	(Fig. 19.1)
Cut-up chicken				
"Good" package	750 days	3.70	17.3	Klose *et al.*
"Inferior" package	265 days	3.50	16.7	(Fig. 19.2)
"Fried"	80 days	2.94	14.1	
USDA data				
Fried chicken	61 days	3.55	18.4	Shepard
Turkey pies and				(1960)
dinners	~1200+	13.73	37.5	(Figure 19.3)
Cooked pork				
Without gravy	155 days	3.14	14.7	Dalhoff and Jul
With gravy	710 days	3.04	15.2	(1965)(Fig. 19.4)
Cooked beef				
Chopped beef	840 days	10.4	35.7	Jul (1968)
Goulash	~1560 days	14.7	30.9	(Fig. 19.5)
White sauce	205 days	30.8	45.0	Hanson *et al.* (1957)(Fig. 19.6)
"Roughly Equivalent Storage periods"	330 days	3.45	16.5	Tressler (1968a) (Fig. 19.7)
HQL Range				
Group 1	175—800 days	3.21—3.34	15.9—17.4	Refr. Res. Fdn.
Group 2	115—380 days	2.66—2.83	13.1—13.6	(1973)
Group 3	70—260 days	3.01—3.07	14.6—14.9	(Fig. 19.8)
PSL Range				
Group 1	380—1550 days	3.16—3.30	15.2—15.7	Refr. Res. Fdn.
Group 2	340—980 days	2.24—2.34	10.7—11.2	(1973)
Group 3	210—660 days	2.92—2.98	14.2—14.5	(Fig. 19.9)

OPEN DATING

An open "pack date" would be of little use in any frozen food, including frozen convenience foods, since exposure to high temperatures for relatively short times can be more detrimental to quality than long storage at low temperature. However, this does not mean an open date system should not be used. It says that control of abuse should be exercised. An open date is also not insurance of food safety, since if abused, pathogens can grow, but normal deterioration will not harm the consumer. An important selling point is that the quality of frozen convenience products, and the competitive nature of the frozen food market will not permit a product that does not sell to remain in the freezer case for long. This forces frozen food packers to meet or exceed the consumers' expectations of quality or suffer the possibility of financial loss. The food companies must rely on their sales force in the field to see that out-of-date or problem merchandise does not remain in the market. If the uncertainty of the frozen distribution system could be removed by assuring that some maximum time-temperature exposure would not be exceeded, then an open code of the "best if used by" date would seem to be most appropriate as for the other frozen foods, while a "pack date" would be the least desirable.

As can be seen, a "sell by date" is less appropriate than a "best if used by date". However, if it is reasonable to expect that many industry sources have some idea as to the shelf-life data most applicable to the specific products they market, and the performance of the product in the distribution channels, either type of date could be used. It may be unreasonable however, to require that a food company make public this information, which is likely to be considered proprietary information, and relates only to a specific product. Given the current stance of the regulatory agencies, and the good quality record of the frozen food industry, it becomes apparent that these companies do have some idea of the treatment their products receive in distribution, and the length of time they can be expected to maintain quality in the marketplace (practical storage life). This being the case, it seems that an open "sell by" or "best if used by date" accompanied by a consumer education program, to assure that the significance of the dates is apparent to the consumer, makes most sense. The ultimate result of an effective open coding system working to the benefit of producer and consumer would be to improve quality in the marketplace and to earn greater confidence in our processed food supply.

REFERENCES

ANON. 1956. Meal, precooked, frozen. Military Specification Military. 13966 A, May 7.

ANON. 1974. Frozen foods acclaimed by rich, poor alike. Quick Frozen Foods *36*(7), 24-26.

ANON. 1977. Ovenable paperboard is hot. Packaging Digest *14*(11), 42.

ASSOCIATION OF FOOD AND DRUG OFFICIALS OF THE UNITED STATES. 1961. Frozen Food Code. Assoc. Food Drug Off. U.S., Washington, DC. (Adopted June 22nd).

DALHOFF, E. and JUL, M. 1965. Factors affecting the keeping quality of frozen foods. *In* Progress in Refrigeration Science and Technology, Vol. 1. W.T. Penzer (Editor). AVI Publishing Co., Westport, Conn.

FEDERAL REGISTER. 1976. The Consumer Food Act of 1976. S-641, March 22.

FENNEMA, O.R. 1975. Freezing preservation. *In* Principles of Food Science, Part 2. Owen R. Fennema (Editor). Marcel Dekker, New York.

FENNEMA, O.W., POWRIE, W.D. and MARTH, E.H. 1973. The Low Temperature Biology of Foods and Living Matter. Marcel Dekker, New York.

HANSON, H.L., FLETCHER, L.R. and CAMPBELL, A.A. 1957. Time-temperature tolerance of frozen foods. V. Texture stability of thickened, precooked frozen foods as influenced by composition and storage conditions. Food Technol. *11*, 339-342.

HANSON, H.L. and FLETCHER, L.R. 1958. Time-temperature tolerance of frozen foods. XII. Turkey dinners and turkey pies. Food Technol. *12*, 40-43.

HANSON, H.L., FLETCHER, L.R. and LINEWEAVER, H. 1959. Time-temperature tolerance of frozen foods. IVII. Frozen fried chicken. Food Technol. *13*, 221-224.

JUL, M. 1968. Frozen meats. *In* Recent Advances in Food Science, Vol. 4. The Low Temperature Biology of Foodstuffs. J. Hawthorne and E.J. Rolfe (Editors). Pergamon Press, New York.

JUL, M. 1969. Quality and stability of frozen meats. *In* Quality and Stability of Frozen Foods. W.B. Van Arsdel, M.J. Copley and R.L. Olson (Editors). John Wiley & Sons, New York.

KLOSE, A.A., POOL, M.F., CAMPBELL, A.A. and HANSON, H.L. 1959. Food Technol. *13*, 477.

MARTIN, S. 1968. The rise of prepared and precooked frozen foods. *In* Freezing Preservation of Food, Vol. 4, 4th ed., D.K. Tressler, W.B. Van Arsdel, M.J. Copley (editors). AVI Publishing Co., Westport, Conn.

PERSONAL MARKET SURVEY, December, 1977.

REFRIGERATION RESEARCH FOUNDATION. 1973. TTT and PPP. Information Bulletin No. 73-1, January.

RUTGERS UNIVERSITY. 1971. Food Stability Survey. Rutgers University Department of Food Science, for the State of New Jersey Department of Health. In cooperation with the U.S. Department of Agriculture/Economic Research Service.

SHEPARD, A.D. 1960. *In* Conference on Frozen Foods Quality. USDA Western Regional Research Laboratory, Albany, CA. November 4th. ARS 74-21.

TRESSLER, D.K., VAN ARSDEL, W.B. and COPLEY, M.J. 1968a. The Freezing Preservation of Foods, Vol. 4. Freezing of precooked and prepared foods. AVI Publishing Company, Westport, Conn.

TRESSLER, D.K. 1968a. The packaging of precooked and prepared frozen foods. *In* The Freezing Preservation of Foods, Vol. 4, 4th Ed. D.K. Tressler, W.B. Van Arsdel, M.J. Copley (Editors). AVI Publishing Co., Westport, Conn.

TRESSLER, D.K. 1968b. Special problems encountered in preparing, freezing, storing, transporting and marketing frozen precooked and prepared foods. *In* The Freezing Preservation of Foods, Vol. 4, D.K. Tressler, W.R. Van Arsdel and M.J. Copley (Editors). AVI Publishing Co., Westport, Conn.

VAN ARSDEL, W.B., COPLEY, M.J. and OLSON, R.L. 1969. Quality and Stability of Frozen Foods — Time-Temperature Tolerance and its Significance. John Wiley and Sons, New York.

CHAPTER 20

SHELF-LIFE OF FROZEN MEAT AND SEAFOOD

PRESERVATION

Seafoods

Glazing. — Glazing of whole and dressed frozen fish with water protects against excessive dehydration and weight loss (Harris and Von Loesecke 1960; Lane 1964; U.S. Department of the Interior). It has also been shown to retard oxidative rancidity (Harris and Von Loesecke 1960). Various glazing solutions are prepared with phosphates, sugars, benzoic acid and polyhydric and other alcohols (Harris and Von Loesecke 1960). Glazing with monosodium glutamate (MSG) is an effective preservation method for salmon, haddock, mackerel and rosefish (Borgstrom 1968). When glazing is used, wrapping of the fish is not done. Due to possible cracking of the glazes, suitable wrapping material tightly applied is preferable but more expensive (Harris and Von Loesecke 1960).

Antioxidants. — Ascorbic acid, gallate esters, cysteine and glutamate have been used for retardation of fat oxidation with little to no improvements (Van Arsdel *et al.* 1969; Borgstrom 1968; Lane 1964). Some off-flavors may develop and antioxidants are, therefore, not a feasible method for preservation (Lane 1964).

Additives. — Salt brine dips and polyphosphates modify thaw drip of frozen seafood, but may contribute to fat and protein denaturation (U.S. Department of the Interior).

Protective coatings. — Alginate and carrageenan gels have been successfully applied to frozen fish. Further investigation is needed (Borgstrom 1968).

Freezing. — Most fish fillets sold commercially are placed in retail-shaped block compartments and frozen on plates in indirect contact freezers (Rutgers University 1971; U.S. Department of the Interior 1956a). Whole fish are frozen in blast freezers or in contact freezers (U.S. Department of the Interior). Whole fish frozen on contact freezers have longer storage lives than fillets frozen in blast freezers (Nikkila and Linko 1956).

Freezing whole fish at sea for later thawing, filleting and refreezing is a growing practice which significantly decreases shelf-life after refreezing

(Van Arsdel *et al.* 1969). The quality decrease is similar to that found to occur when frozen cod stored at −18 °F is exposed to higher temperatures (−10 °C) for short periods of time (Dyer *et al.* 1957a,b; Van Arsdel *et al.* 1969). Some species of fish like ocean perch (rosefish) and flounder suffer no damage by double freezing, but other species like cod are more sensitive (Van Arsdel *et al.* 1969).

Within established commercial techniques, the rate of freezing has little to no effect on product shelf-life in comparison to the length of frozen storage (Lane 1964; U.S. Department of the Interior; Van Arsdel *et al.* 1969).

Meats

Antioxidants. — No antioxidants are effectively used commercially for frozen meats. The problems of getting the antioxidants into the fat have not been solved (Borgstrom 1968).

Glazing. — Glazing with water retards off-flavor production and discoloration of frozen lean meat upon storage. However, wrapping of meat is used commercially (Lawrie 1966).

Freezing. — Fresh meat may be cut into retail cuts, packaged and then frozen in tunnel blast freezers (−40 °F) or may be frozen whole, unpackaged (Chain Store Age 1977; Hawthorne and Rolfe 1968). Freezing rates used commercially do not appreciably affect the product shelf-life (Hawthorne and Rolfe 1968). For retail market distribution the prepackaged retail cuts are used.

PACKAGING

The importance of effective packaging of frozen meat and seafood is often overlooked. Effective packaging increases shelf-life and overall product quality by protecting the product from excessive dehydration, denaturation, oxidative rancidity and microbial recontamination (Rutgers University 1971; Lane 1964; Van Arsdel *et al.* 1969). Adequate packaging materials for frozen seafood and meats should have the following properties: (a) Impermeable to oxygen and moisture transmission; (b) resistant to tearing and puncturing; (c) pliable, to form tight wraps; (d) easily sealable; (e) greaseproof; (f) durable at low temperatures; and (g) free from imparting odors or off-flavors (Commonwealth Scientific Industrial Research Organization 1977; Rutgers University 1971; Hiner *et al.* 1951; Lane 1964, 1966; Harris and Von Loesecke 1960; Palmer *et al.* 1953; U.S. Department of the Interior; Van Arsdel *et al.* 1969).

Films and wraps commercially used which meet these requirements are cellophane, aluminum foil, polyvinylidene chloride (Saran, Cryovac), and rubber hydrochloride film (Pliofilm) (Chain Store Age 1977; Lawrie 1966; Nikkila and Linko 1956; U.S. Department of the Interior 1956). Polyethylene is also used for meat, but is not as suitable for fish due to its higher permeability to oxygen and solvent vapors (Lawrie 1966; U.S. Department of the Interior 1956).

Coated papers are also effective packaging materials used for frozen fish. These include waxed paper, vinyl and Saran-coated papers and polyethylene-coated cellophane (U.S. Department of the Interior 1956a).

Packaging cartons, which are often used for frozen fish are usually wax or otherwise coated cardboard or paper (U.S. Department of the Interior 1956b). Polystyrene trays surrounded by films and wraps are used often for fish and meats. These provide easy handling of the package and prevent piercing of the film or wrap by hard frozen meat (Lawrie 1966). When films or coated papers are not used around frozen fish, inside the cartons, carton overwraps provide the primary protection.

The palatability losses of frozen retail meat cuts, resulting from desiccation, are minimized when they are packed in nitrogen or vacuum, although this is a more expensive method (CAS 1977; Hiner *et al.* 1951; Lawrie 1966). Fatty fish benefit from vacuum packing more than leaner fish (Van Arsdel *et al.* 1969).

DISTRIBUTION

Correct handling practices and stock rotation throughout transportation, warehoushing and retailing of frozen meat and seafood are very important to the product quality (Rutgers University 1971). Time-temperature tolerance for frozen fish products during commercial distribution is summrized in Table 20.1.

Ships and mechanically refrigerated railroad cars are also used for distribution to freezer warehouses. The railroad cars are capable of maintaining temperatures below −18 °C and constant relative humidity. The ships contain freezers similar to warehouses (Lane 1966).

All stages of distribution should maintain temperatures of −18 °C or lower to prevent deterioration of frozen meats and seafoods (Awad *et al.* 1969; Commonwealth Scientific Industrial Research Organization 1977; Connell 1964; Rutgers University 1971; Hawthorne and Rolfe 1968; Desrosier and Desrosier 1977). Small fluctuations in temperature (1—2 °C) during distribution and storage do not appreciably affect the shelf-life of these products (Van Arsdel *et al.* 1969). However, larger

TABLE 20.1
TIME-TEMPERATURE TOLERANCE FOR FROZEN FISH PRODUCTS DURING DISTRIBUTION[1]

Phase of Distribution	Temperature Mean	Temperature Range	Mean Time Held
Refrigerated trucks from processor	−13 °C	−15° to 0 °C	3 days, 14 hr
Freezer warehouses	−22 °C	−23° to −20 °C	—
Retail distribution trucks	−4 °C	−20° to −7 °C	3.5 hr
Retail freezer cases	−15 °C	—	—

[1]From Lane (1966).

fluctuations in the higher temperature ranges significantly affect the shelf-life (Connell 1964; Lane 1964; Van Arsdel *et al.* 1969). Frozen cod fillets normally held at −18 °C for short periods — 3 days to 2 weeks — to −10 °C were shown to undergo significantly increased deterioration. The longer the exposure to −10 °C, the greater the deterioration (Dyer *et al.* 1957a,b).

Fresh frozen retail-cut meats are usually held in the processors' freezer (−20 °F) for about one week. Mechanically refrigerated trucks transport the meat to retail stores. The trucks are equipped with frozen food compartments capable of maintaining −22 °C temperatures. Retail stores keep their frozen meats in storage cases at about −18 °C (Chain Store Age 1977).

MODES OF DETERIORATION

The major deterioration in freezer storage in fish occurs in the protein and lipid components. The stability of seafood varies greatly with species and especially with differences in fat content (Hawthorne and Rolfe 1968; Van Arsdel *et al.* 1969). Off-flavors develop with increased storage time due to oxidative changes of the fat. This is more quickly developed in fatty fish than lean fish, and can be measured by taste panel evaluations (Dyer and Morton 1959; Rutgers University 1971; Lane 1964; Hawthorne and Rolfe 1968; Van Arsdel *et al.* 1969).

Deterioration of seafoods with freezer storage causes increased toughness and increased tendency to dry when cooked (Connell 1964; Hawthorne and Rolfe 1968; Van Arsdel *et al.* 1969). The toughening with storage is due to gradual denaturation of the proteins (Connell 1964; Rutgers University 1971; Hawthorne and Rolfe 1968; Harris and Von Loesecke 1960). The effect of frozen storage times and temperatures seems to be effectively measured by protein extractability and can be fairly well paralleled with sensory evaluations of toughness (Dyer and Morton 1956, 1959; Dyer *et al.* 1957b; Hawthorne and Rolfe 1968; Van Arsdel *et al.* 1969). However, sensory evaluations of toughness are due primarily to pH changes in the tissue and, therefore, may not satisfactorily measure deterioration due to storage, especially at very low (−29 °C) temperatures (Cowie and Little 1966). The higher the temperature of frozen storage (below about −5 °C, the freezing point of the muscle), the faster the rate of protein denaturation (Connell 1964; Cowie and Little 1967; Love and Elerian 1964; Lovern 1962). Below about −30 °C alterations may take a year to develop (Connell 1964; Love 1962).

Extensive research has been done on the measurement of protein denaturation in cod muscle during frozen storage (Hawthorne and Rolfe 1968). Very good correlation was seen between toughness measured by cell fragility and protein denaturation (Love 1962). However, in fatty fish, the correlation was not satisfactory (Love and Muslemuddin 1975).

A parallel effect of temperature on the rate of protein denaturation (loss of solubility) and the rate of lipid deterioration and its off-flavor production was seen in cod, rosefish, halibut, plaice and whitefish (Dyer *et al.* 1956; Lovern 1962; Olley and Lovern 1960).

The myofibrillar proteins (actomyosin) but not the sarcoplasmic proteins become insoluble with frozen storage (Awad *et al.* 1969; Connell 1964; Hawthorne and Rolfe 1968; Van Arsdel *et al.* 1969). A mechanism postulated for the protein insolubilization in frozen fish may be the destruction of a stabilizing lipid (phospholipid) or actomyosin and/or the interaction of free fatty acids with actomyosin producing hydrophobic areas on the protein surface (Awad *et al.* 1969; Connell 1964). The measurement of free fatty acid production (lipolysis) as opposed to peroxide values (oxidation) in rosefish correlated with the protein denaturation (Dyer *et al.* 1956). Free fatty acid accumulation in cod and rosefish due to enzymatic action paralleled the hydrolysis of phospholipids (Dyer *et al.* 1956; Lovern 1962; Olley and Lovern 1960). The lipolysis of the phospholipids is unaffected by bacterial enzymes on the fish surface, accumulated prior to freezing (Lovern 1962). Therefore, phospholipid hydrolysis is promoted entirely by tissue enzymes and is a measure of deterioration (Lovern 1962; Olley and Lovern 1960). Freezing activates this system (Olley and Lovern 1960).

Deterioration of meat due to frozen storage is very similar to that of fish, except that in meat it occurs more slowly (Lawrie 1968; Van Arsdel *et al.* 1969). Protein denaturation, fat off-flavor production, desiccation of the tissue and myoglobin color changes all occur with extended frozen storage (Hiner *et al.* 1951; Lawrie 1968). Flavor deterioration due to oxidation of fats is usually the primary limiting factor in shelf-life of frozen meats (Commonwealth Scientific Industrial Research Organization 1977; Hiner *et al.* 1951). Frozen pork deteriorates more rapidly than beef or lamb (Commonwealth Scientific Industrial Research Organization 1977; Lawrie 1966, 1968; Palmer *et al.* 1953). This is primarily due to greater unsaturation of the pork fat and therefore a higher susceptibility to oxidation. Also, most pork cuts contain higher percentages of fat than beef or lamb (Palmer *et al.* 1953).

Microbial deterioration of frozen meats and seafoods is not a major mode of deterioration since temperatures of freezing inhibit activity of most microbes (Desrosier and Desrosier 1977).

Nutrients in frozen meats are generally well preserved (Rutgers University 1971). Thiamin, riboflavin and niacin have shown changes upon freezer storage but no relationship between these changes and storage time and temperature have been seen (Harris and Von Loesecke 1960). The nutrient changes are nutritionally insignificant and are not a good measure of shelf-life in frozen meats (Lehner *et al.* 1951, 1952; Meyer *et al.* 1963; Harris and Von Loesecke 1960; Van Arsdel *et al.* 1969).

SHELF-LIFE DATA

Figures 20.1 through 20.6 show the shelf-life data for various species of fish measured organoleptically for either flavor or texture changes. As seen, the Q_{10} is dependent on species and increases for fatty fish. The values also vary based on the source, with Q_{10}s ranging from about 1.3 to 4.5. It is interesting that no data are available for frozen fresh water fish such as trout.

Figure 20.7 shows data for the rate of protein insolubility (first order reaction assumed) in cold fillets as compared to a laboratory texture measurement. Both give much higher Q_{10}s (>10) than those based on the organoleptiic shelf-life of lean ocean fish (Q_{10} of 2.5). Data for phospholipid hydrolysis which might lead to the toughness also show a high Q_{10} of about 12 (Lovern 1962), whereas free fatty acid production which may affect flavor (assuming a first order reaction) has a Q_{10} of 4.6 (Olley and Lovern 1960). Other protein solubility data (Cowie and Little 1966, 1967), give a Q_{10} of around 4.7 which is closer to the shelf-life Q_{10}. These results make it difficult to decide what mode of reaction causes the end of shelf-life.

Figures 20.8 to 20.14 give the data reported on shelf-life of frozen meats. In most cases the Q_{10} is about 2 to 3. Thus, frozen meat is much less sensitive to storage temperature changes than poultry or fish. More

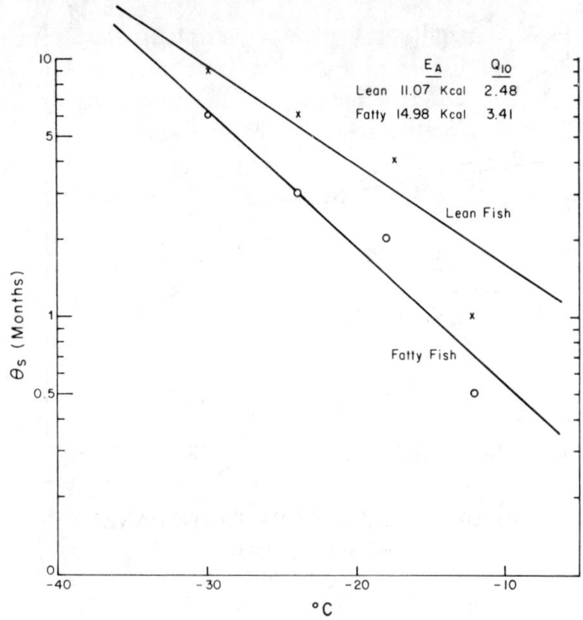

FIGURE 20.1. SHELF-LIFE OF COMMERCIAL FISH (From Lawrie 1966).

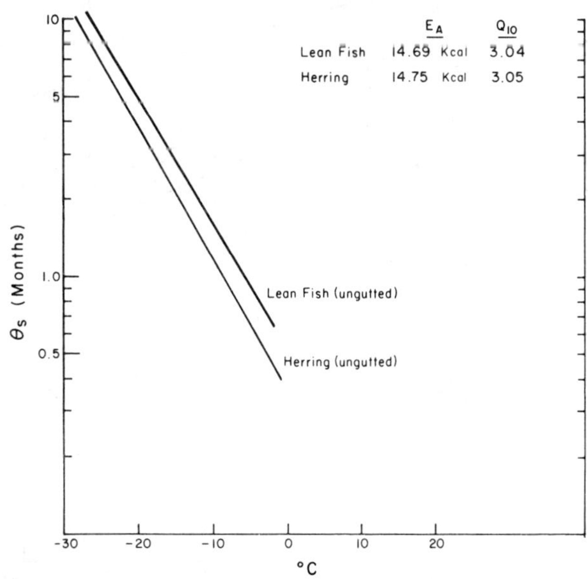

FIG. 20.2. SHELF-LIFE OF LEAN FISH AND HERRING (From Borgstrom 1968).

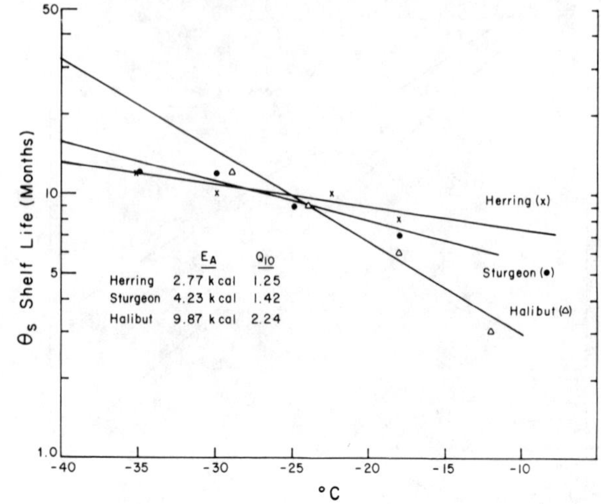

FIG. 20.3. SHELF-LIFE BY TASTE PANEL (From Lane 1964).

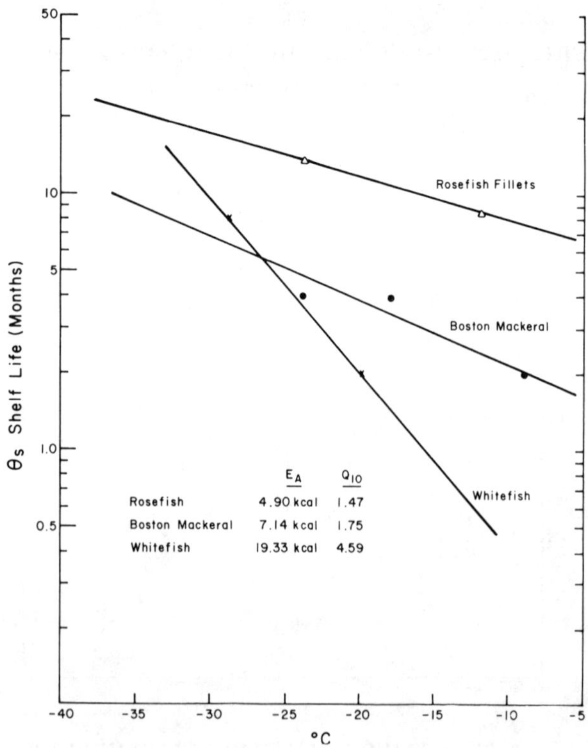

FIG. 20.4. SHELF-LIFE PLOTS OF VARIOUS FISH SPECIES (From Lane 1964).

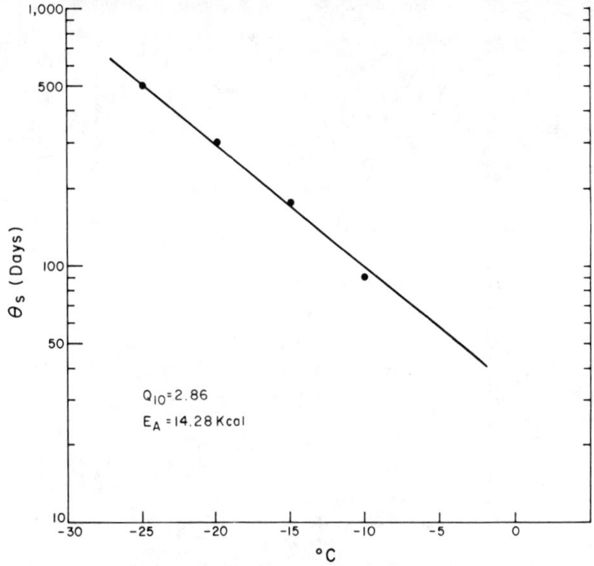

FIG. 20.5. SHELF-LIFE PLOT OF AMERICAN POLLACK (From Van Arsdel *et al.* 1969).

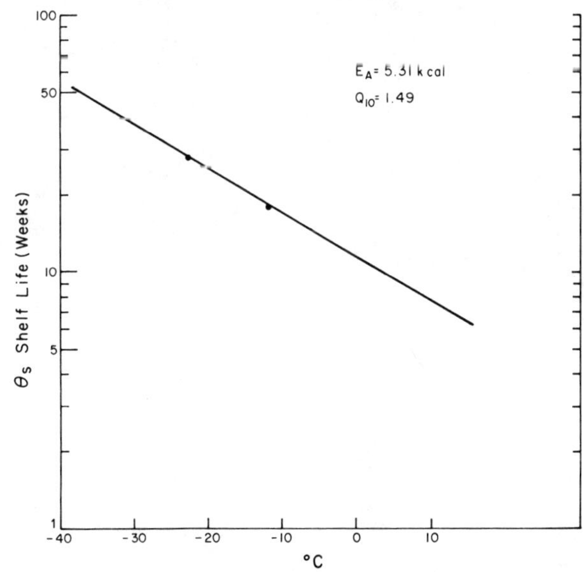

FIG. 20.6. ROSEFISH FILLETS — SHELF-LIFE PLOT — TASTE PANEL RESULTS

(From Dyer *et al.* 1956).

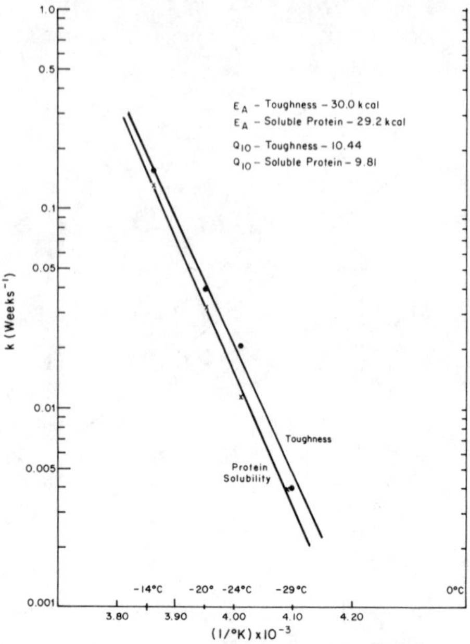

FIG. 20.7. COD FILLETS — PROTEIN SOLUBILITY (% OF TOTAL N) — ARRHENIUS PLOT — TOUGHNESS BY CELL FRAGILITY METHOD

(From Lane 1962).

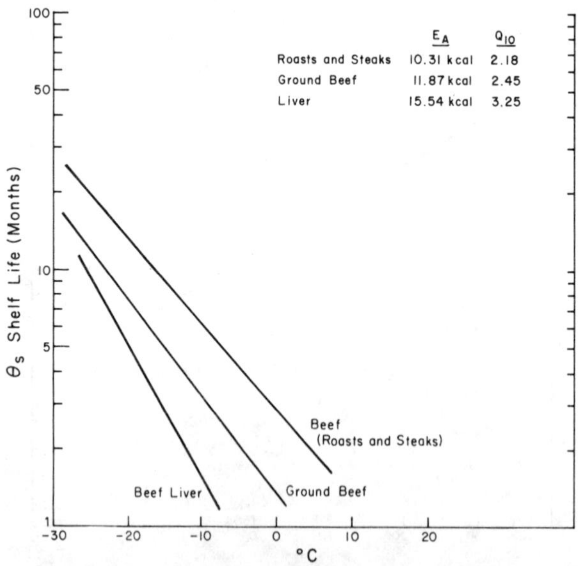

FIG. 20.8. SHELF-LIFE PLOTS OF BEEF COMMERCIALLY PACKAGED

(From Commonwealth Scientific Industrial Research Organization (Australia)).

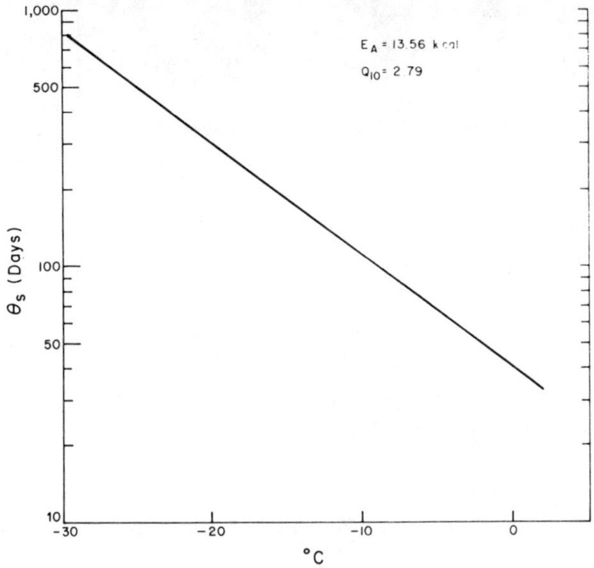

FIG. 20.9. HIGH QUALITY LIFE — CHOPPED BEEF
Normal commercial quality; good commercial package.
(From Hawthorne and Rolfe 1968).

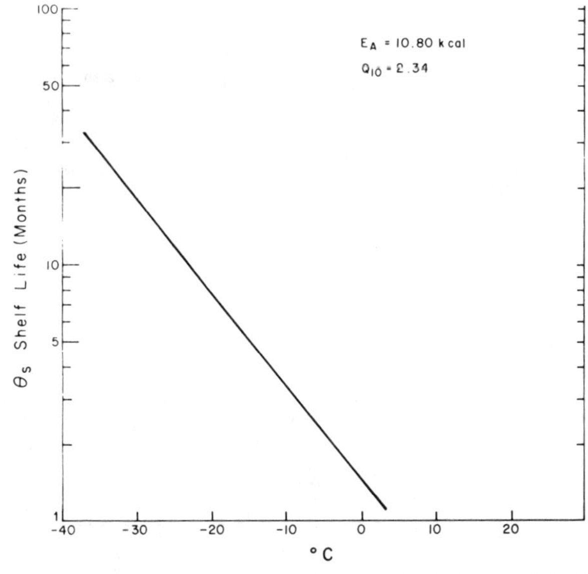

FIG. 20.10. FROZEN PORK SHELF-LIFE PLOTS (ROASTS AND CHOPS)

(From Commonwealth Scientific Industrial Research Organization 1977).

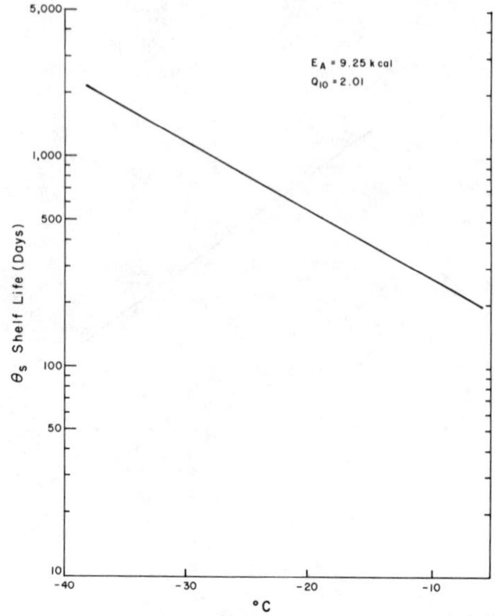

FIG. 20.11. TASTE PANEL DETERMINATION OF SHELF-LIFE OF PORK CHOPS (PACKAGED IN POLYETHYLENE IN A FREEZER CARTON)
(From Van Arsdel *et al.* 1969).

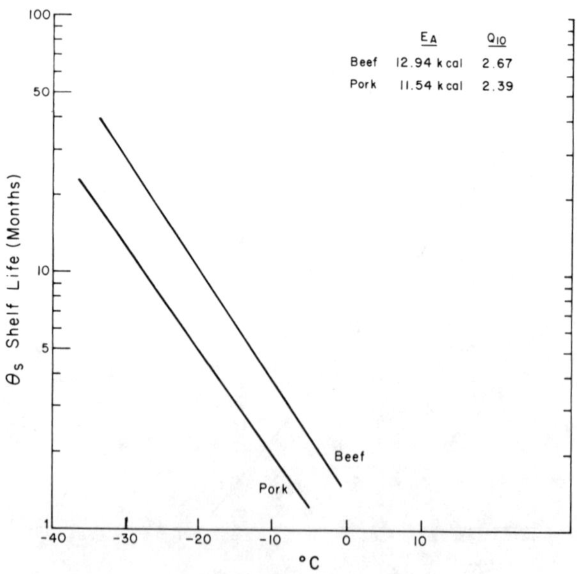

FIG. 20.12. BEEF AND PORK — TIME FOR APPEARANCE OF FATTY OFF-FLAVORS
(From Lawrie *et al.* 1966, 1968).

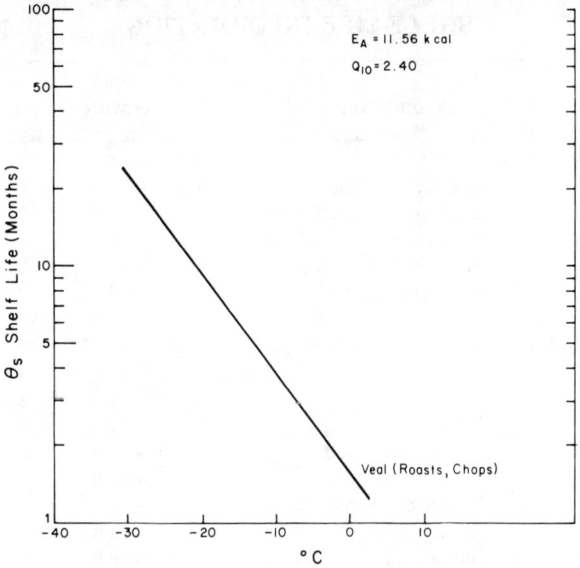

FIG. 20.13. FROZEN VEAL SHELF-LIFE PLOTS (COMMERCIALLY PACKAGED)

(From Commonwealth Scientific Industrial Research Organization 1977).

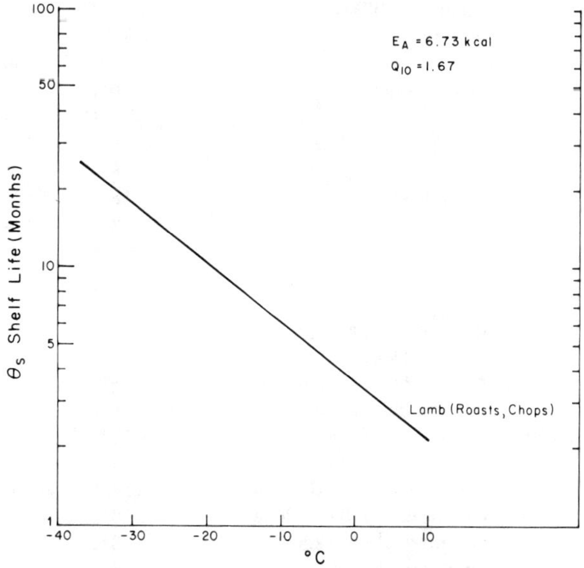

FIG. 20.14. FROZEN LAMB SHELF-LIFE PLOTS (COMMERCIALLY PACKAGE)

(From Commonwealth Scientific Industrial Research Organization 1977).

TABLE 20.2
SHELF-LIFE INFORMATION

Product	Packaging/Notes	Temp-erature	(mos)	Refer-ences
Seafood				
Lean fish (L)	ungutted or glazed, packaged	−18 °C	3—4	1
Fatty fish (F)	packaged or glazed whole	−18 °C	2—3	2
sprat (F)	packaged or glazed whole	−18 °C	2—3	
smelt (F)	packaged or glazed whole	−18 °C	2—3	
sole (L)	packaged fillet	−18 °C	3—4	
halibut (F)	fillets	−18 °C	6	6
Boston mackerel (F)	packaged or whole glazed	−18 °C	2—4	7
Herring (F)		−18 °C	8	8
Whitefish (L)		−20 °C	2—4	9
Rosefish (L)	fillets	−12 °C	4—8	10
Striped bass (L)	fillets or dressed	−18 °C	3—4	11
Sturgeon (F)		−18 °C	7	12
Plaice (L)	fillets, packaged	−18 °C	3—4	13
Cod (L)	fillets	−18 °C	3—4	14
American pollack (L)	fillets	−18 °C	6—8	15
Flounder (L)	fillets	−18 °C	(3—4),6	16
Whiting (L)	drawn	−18 °C	4	17
Haddock (L)	fillets	−18 °C	(3—4),6	18
Sea trout (L)	fillets	−18 °C	6	19
Mullet (L)	fillets	−18 °C	6	20
Pacific Ocean perch (L)	packaged fillets	−18 °C	2—4	21
Salmon (F)	steaks	−18 °C	2	22
Trout (F)	vacuum packed	−20 °C	8	23
Trout (F)	cellophane wrap and carton	−20 °C	2	24
Scallops		−18 °C	3—4	25
Clams	shucked	−18 °C	3	26
Crab	King	−18 °C	3	27
Crab	Dungeness	−18 °C	10	28
Oysters	shucked	−18 °C	2—4	29
Shrimp		−18 °C	3—4,(12)	30
Meat				
Beef	commercial package	−18 °C	6—12	31
chopped	commercial package	−18 °C	2—3	32
ground	commercial package	−18 °C	6—7	33
liver	commercial package	−18 °C	4	34
roasts and steaks	commercial package	−18 °C	10—12	35
Pork	carton and polyethylene	−18 °C	4—12	36
chops	carton and polyethylene	−18 °C	4-5,(6—7)	37
roasts	carton and polyethylene	−18 °C	6—7,(8)	38
Veal	commercial package	−18 °C	4—14	39
roasts and chops	commercial package	−18 °C	7—8	40
cutlets, cubes	commercial package	−18 °C	6—8,(4)	41

continued . . .

TABLE 20.2 (continued)

Product	Packaging/Notes	Temperature	(mos)	References
Lamb	commercial package	−18 °C	6–16	42
roasts	commercial package	−18 °C	9-10,(12)	43
chops	commercial package	−18 °C	9–10	44
ground	commercial package	−18 °C	12	45

[1]Hawthorne and Rolfe (1968); Van Arsdel *et al.* 1969); Borgstrom (1968
[2]Hawthorne and Rolfe (1968); Van Arsdel *et al.* (1969)
[3]Van Arsdel *et al.* (1969)
[4]Van Arsdel *et al.* (1969)
[5]Van Arsdel *et al.* (1969)
[6]U.S. Department of the Interior, Fish and Wildlife Service (1956b); Lane (1964)
[7]Lane (1964); Van Arsdel *et al.* (1969)
[8]Lane (1964)
[9]Lane (1964); U.S. Department of the Interior, Fish and Wildlife Service (1956b); Dyer *et al.* (1956)
[10]Lane (1964); U.S. Department of the Interior, Fish and Wildlife Service (1956b)
[11]Lane (1964); U.S. Department of the Interior, Fish and Wildlife Service (1956b)
[12]Lane (1964)
[13]Van Arsdel *et al.* (1969)
[14]Van Arsdel *et al.* (1969)
[15]Van Arsdel *et al.* (1969); U.S. Department of the Interior, Fish and Wildlife Service (1956b); Hawthorne and Rolfe (1968)
[16]Van Arsdel *et al.* (1969); U.S. Department of the Interior, Fish and Wildlife Service (1956b)
[17]U.S. Department of the Interior, Fish and Wildlife Service (1956b)
[18]Van Arsdel *et al.* (1969); U.S. Department of the Interior, Fish and Wildlife Service (1956b)
[19]U.S. Department of the Interior, Fish and Wildlife Service (1956b)
[20]U.S. Department of the Interior, Fish and Wildlife Service (1956b)
[21]U.S. Department of the Interior, Fish and Wildlife Service (1956b); Van Arsdel *et al.* (1969)
[22]U.S. Department of the Interior, Fish and Wildlife Service (1956b); Van Arsdel *et al.* (1969)
[23]Van Arsdel *et al.* (1969)
[24]Van Arsdel *et al.* (1969)
[25]Van Arsdel *et al.* (1969)
[26]Van Arsdel *et al.* (1969); U.S. Department of the Interior, Fish and Wildlife SErvice (1956b)
[27]U.S. Department of the Interior, Fish and Wildlife Service (1956b)
[28]U.S. Department of the Interior, Fish and Wildlife Service (1956b)
[29]U.S. Department of the Interior, Fish and Wildlife Service (1956b); Van Arsdel *et al.* (1969)
[30]U.S. Department of the Interior, Fish and Wildlife Service (1956b); Van Arsdel *et al.* (1969)
[31]U.S. Department of the Interior, Fish and Wildlife Service (1956a); U.S. Department of the Interior, Fish and Wildlife Service (1956b); Research Organization (1977)
[32]U.S. Department of the Interior, Fish and Wildlife Service (1956a)
[33]Commonwealth Scientific Industrial Research Organization (1977); U.S. Department of the Interior, Fish and Wildlife Service (1956b)
[34]Commonwealth Scientific Industrial Research Organization (1977)
[35]Commonwealth Scientific Industrial Research Organization (1977); U.S. Department of the Interior, Fish and Wildlife Service (1956b); Lawrie (1966)
[36]Commonwealth Scientific Industrial Research Organization (1977); Lawrie (1966); Lawrie (1968); Hiner *et al.* (1951)
[37]Van Arsdel *et al.* (1969); Commonwealth Scientific Industrial Research Organization (1977); U.S. Department of the Interior, Fish and Wildlife Service (1956b)
[38]Commonwealth Scientific Industrial Research Organization (1977); U.S. Department of the Interior, Fish and Wildlife Service (1956b)
[39]Commonwealth Scientific Industrial Research Organization (1977)
[40]Commonwealth Scientific Industrial Research Organization (1977); U.S. Department of the Interior, Fish and Wildlife Service (1956b)

[41]Commonwealth Scientific Industrial Research Organization (1977); U.S. Department of the Interior, Fish and Wildlife Service (1956b)
[42]Commonwealth Scientific Industrial Research Organization (1977); U.S. Department of the Interior, Fish and Wildlife Service (1956b); Hiner *et al.* (1951)
[43]Commonwealth Scientific Industrial Research Organization (1977); U.S. Department of the Interior, Fish and Wildlife Service (1956b)
[44]Commonwealth Scientific Industrial Research Organization (1977)
[45]U.S. Department of the Interior, Fish and Wildlife Service (1956b)

importantly, it is much less sensitive than frozen vegetables, so meat is not the major problem in the storage of mixed meals, such as TV dinners or frozen pizza.

Shelf-life data for which no Q_{10} could be calculated are listed in Table 20.2.

OPEN DATING

Frozen meats and seafoods vary greatly with species in their expected shelf-life. Pack dates may therefore mislead the consumer to believe "all" fish and meat are equivalent in shelf-life quality. Expiration dates are too restrictive in their date of quality life termination. The consumer of frozen meats and seafoods would most probably freeze these items in the home freezer. Home freezer temperatures vary greatly and many are above −18 °C (0 °F). Predetermination of this home freezer storage is unreasonable.

A "sell by date" or "best if used by date" seems most feasible for frozen meats and seafoods. Both the product varieties and distribution system can be incorporated into determining the "sell by date" and home storage to give a "best if used by date". The frozen foods distribution system within and to the U.S. seems fairly consistent although improvements, especially in refrigerated truck temperatures, should be made. No Federal regulation exists as to the maximum temperatures of frozen food storage cases in retail stores. This regulation would be an advancement in the system. The "best if used by date" puts more responsibility on consumers and their handling of their purchases, if storage informaiton is given. Cooperation and education in all cases would promote the feasibility of these systems.

REFERENCES

AWAD, A., POWRIE, W.D. and FENNEMA, O. 1969. Deterioration of freshwater whitefish muscle during storage at −10 °C. J. Food Sci. *34*, 1

CHAIN STORE AGE/SUPERMARKETS. 1977. CSA Meat Manual Distribution. (Nov.) p 56.

COMMONWEALTH SCIENTIFIC INDUSTRIAL RESEARCH ORGANIZATION (Australia). 1977. Storage temperature for frozen meats. Na. Provis. 12. (March 12).

CONNELL, J.J. 1964. Fish muscle proteins and some effects on them of processing. Symposium on Foods: Proteins and Their Reactions. AVI Publishing Co., Westport, Conn.

CONNELL, J.J. and HOWGATE, P.F. 1968. Sensory and objective measurements of the quality of frozen stored cod of different initial freshness. J. Sci. Food Agric. *19* (June).

COWIE, W.P. and LITTLE, W.T. 1966. The relationship between toughness of cod stored at −29 °C and its muscle protein solubility and pH. J. Food Technol. 1, 335.

COWIE, W.P. and LITTLE, W.T. 1967. The relationship between the toughness of cod stored at −7 °C and −14 °C. Its muscle protein solubility and muscle pH. J. Food Technol. *2,* 217.

DESROSIER, N.W. and DESROSIER, J.N. 1977. The Technology of Food Preservation. AVI Publishing Co., Westport, Conn.

DYER, W.J. and MORTON, M.L. 1959. Storage of frozen rosefish fillets. J. Food Res. Board of Canada. *16*, 43.

DYER, W.J. and MORTON, M.L. 1956. Storage of frozen plaice fillets. J. Food Res. Board of Canada. *13*, 129.

DYER, W.J., FRASER, D.I., ELLIS, D.S. and MacCALLUM, W.A. 1957. Influence of intermittent short storage periods at 15 °F, as encountered during refrigerator car transportation, on the quality of frozen cod stored at 0 °F. J. Fish Research Board of Canada. *14*, 627.

DYER, W.J., FRASER, D.I. and MacCALLUM, W.A. 1957. Further study of Canada. *13*, 569.

DYER, W.J., FRASER, D.I. and MacCALLUM, W.A. 1957. Further study of the influence of short storage periods, 3 days to 2 weeks at 15 °F, on the quality of frozen cod stored at 0 °F. J. Fish Res. Board of Canada. *14*, 925.

ELERIAN, M.K. 1965. The refractive index of the muscle of fish and shellfish. I. A possible method for measuring protein deterioration in fresh and frozen cod. J. Sci. Food Agric. *16*(4) 228.

HAWTHORNE, J. and ROLFE, E.J. 1968. Recent Advances in Food Science, Vol. 4. Pergamon Press, Oxford, England.

HARRIS, R.S. and Von LOESECKE, H. 1960. Nutritional Evaluation of Food Processing. AVI Publishing Co., Westport, Conn.

HINER, R.L., GADDIS, A.M. and HARKINS, O.G. 1951. Effects of methods of protection on palatability of freezer stored meat. Food Technol. *5*(6), 223.

LANE, J.P. 1964. TTT of Frozen Seafoods. I. Review of some of the recent literature on the storage life of frozen fishery products. Food Technol. *18*, 1100.

LANE, J.P. 1966. Time-temperature tolerance of frozen seafoods. II. Temperature constants during commercial distribution of frozen fishery products. Food Technol. *20,* 549.

LAWRIE, R.A. 1966. The storage and preservation of meat. *In* Meat Science. Pergamon Press, Oxford, England.

LAWRIE, R.A. 1968. Chemical changes in meat due to processing — a review. J. Sci. Food Agric. *19*(5), 233.

LEHNER, W.P. Jr. *et al.* 1951. Effect of frozen storage and subsequent cooking on the thiamin, riboflavin and niacin content of pork chops. Food Res. *16*, 485.

LEHNER, W.P. Jr. *et al.* 1952. Stability of thiamin, riboflavin, and nicotinic acid of lamb chops during frozen storage and subsequent cooking. Food Res. *17*, 24.

LOVE, R.M. 1962. Protein denaturation in frozen fish. VI. Cold storage studies on cod using the cell fragility method. J. Sci. Food Agric. *13*, 269.

LOVE, R.M. and ELERIAN, M.K. 1964. Protein denaturation in frozen fish. VIII. The temperature of maximum denaturation in cod. J. Sci. Food Agric. *11*, 805.

LOVE, R.M. and MUSLEMUDDIN, M. 1975. Protein denaturation in frozen fish. XIII. A modified cell fragility method insensitive to the pH of the fish. J. Sci. Fd. Agric. *23*, 1239.

LOVERN, J.A. 1962. The lipids of fish and changes occurring in tem during processing and storage. *In* Fish in Nutrition. E. Heen and R. Kreuzer (Editors). Fishing News, London.

MEYER, B., MYSINGER, M. and BUCKLEY, R. 1963. The effect of 3 years of freezer storage on the thiamin, riboflavin and niacin content of ripened and unripened beef. J. Agric. Food Chem. *11*, 525.

NIKKILA, O.E. and LINKO, R.R. 1956. Freezing, packaging and frozen storage of fish. Food Res. *21*, 42.

OLLEY, J. and LOVERN, J.A. 1960. Phospholipid hydrolysis in cod flesh stored at various temperatures. J. Sci. Food Agric. *11*, 644.

PALMER, A.Z. *et al.* 1953. Deterioration of frozen pork as related to fat composition and storage treatment. Food Technol. *7*, 90.

RUTGERS UNIVERSITY. 1971. Food Stability Survey. Rutgers University Department of Food Science, for the State of New Jersey Department of Health. In cooperation with the U.S. Department of Agriculture/Economic Research Service.

U.S. DEPARTMENT OF THE INTERIOR, FISH AND WILDLIFE SERVICE. 1956a. Factors to be considered in the freezing and cold storage of fishery products. Fishery Leaflet No. 429.

U.S. DEPARTMENT OF THE INTERIOR, FISH AND WILDLIFE SERVICE. 1956b. Preparation, freezing and cold storage of fish, shellfish and precooked fishery products. Fishery Leaflet No. 430.

U.S. DEPARTMENT OF THE INTERIOR, FISH AND WILDLIFE SERVICE. 1956c. Distribution and marketing of frozen fishery products. Fishery Leaflet No. 431.

VAN ARSDEL, W.B., COPLEY, M.J. and OLSON, R.D. 1969. Quality and Stability of Frozen Foods. John Wiley & Sons, New York.

CHAPTER 21

SHELF-LIFE OF FRESH FRUITS AND VEGETABLES

INTRODUCTION

In the regulations on open dating proposed for Massachusetts (Massachusetts Department of Public Health 1973), Minnesota (1973), and by the United States Congress (1976) there is a specific exclusion of fresh fruits and vegetables from open dating requirements. This is perhaps an indication of the difficulty in enforcing such a law as well as an indication that there may not be a great need for regulation of these foodstuffs. The consumer can generally view the product at least partially and judge it by appearance and touch. Perhaps this is adequate control for consumer protection since such physical measurements are indeed indicative of quality to some extent.

PREHARVEST FACTORS

One complication with biological materials is that the products do not consistently contain the same amounts of various constituents, nor do these constituents change at consistent rates. There are many preharvest factors which will influence the post-harvest life of the product. For instance, seasonal variations can have some effect. Higher temperatures during the growing season can cause an increase in the sugar content of oranges. The temperature just prior to harvest can also affect postharvest life. With higher harvesting temperatures the product will degrade quicker. Stone fruits will get brown around the pits, and watery breakdown will occur in onions during storage, after high temperature harvest. Lettuce is more susceptible to russet spotting if the temperature exceeds a 30 °C for two or more days before harvest.

Extremes in soil moisture also cause changes in postharvest life. Low soil moisture inhibits calcium uptake, which makes the product more susceptible to breakdown. A high relative humidity prior to harvest can increase the extent of fungus infection.

Chemicals applied either as pesticides or as agents to prevent the commodity dropping from the tree can either inhibit or enhance ripening, color production and chlorophyll breakdown.

Too much or not enough fertilizer applied to provide nitrogen and trace metals can cause problems with the quality of the commodity.

With too much nitrogen, maturation is delayed and when the product does mature it is larger and softer, making it more susceptible to physical injury. High potassium can increase the chance of certain physical disorders occurring, such as bitter pit, cork spot, and internal breakdown. A calcium deficiency can lead to early maturity and faster senescence due to a higher rate of respiration.

STAGES OF GROWTH

Since fresh fruits and vegetables are dynamic living systems, some consideration should be given to the stages that they go through in their life span. Gortner *et al.* (1967) outlined the growth patterns as follows.

Development starts with the formation of the edible part: the setting of fruit, the emergence of a seedling, the swelling of a root, tuber or bulb, or the elongation of a stalk or petiole. Development ceases with the termination of the desirable or natural enlargement or when the growth pattern of the edible part changes. This occurs mainly before harvest and includes prematuration and some of maturation.

Prematuration starts with development and lasts until the beginning of edible use. Maturation is further development of the edible part, up to where senescence begins. This includes ripening, which is a set of physical and biochemical changes by which the plant material reaches an edible state.

Senescence begins at the end of ripening. In this stage, the plant material goes through natural physiological changes which cause a loss of disease resistance and quality and lead to the death of the organelle. Deterioration refers to senescence as well as changes caused by wilting, freezing or mechanical injury and can occur any time during the life span of a product.

CHANGES DURING POST-HARVEST LIFE

The major, but by no means only, contribution of fresh fruits and vegetables to our diet is their supply of L-ascorbic acid or vitamin C. Nelson (1972) stated that other nutrients are more stable than vitamin C. Consequently, vitamin C retention is often used as an index of nutrient retention (Tressler and Evers 1957). However, vitamin C is usually not used in economic studies of fruit and vegetable breakdown. Instead, aesthetic factors such as sight, touch, smell and taste are often used. Use of these factors is justifiable since there is a direct relationship between market quality and nutrient retention. To better understand the changes taking place, the generalized sequence of steps which are often used before a product reaches market will be described, along with a discussion of the factors which affect deterioration.

Harvest

During the growth and maturation of fruits and vegetables, they are dependent on the parent plant for photosynthesis, minerals and maintenance of water balance. Once they are detached, fruits and vegetables become independent units and their own respiration and transpiration play a dominant role in their ultimate fate (Eskin *et al.* 1971). After harvest the quality tends to decline due to the aforementioned processes, as well as by other biochemical and physical mechanisms. Eventually the product will become unusable due to enzyme activity and/or microbial spoilage. One consideration for proper development and subsequent storage stability is the stage of development at which the commodity is harvested.

In fruits, time of harvest is determined by maturity. If a fruit is picked very early the development of flavor and nutrients may be interrupted, leading to abnormal ripening. If a fruit is overmature when picked, some food value has already been lost and the storage life is shortened. Wilkinson (1970) discusses the relationship between the stage of growth at which a fruit is picked and the possible storage disorders. The factor determining the best time for harvest is the type of fruit being considered.

There are two types of fruit. Each type is harvested at a different stage of maturity. A climacteric fruit is one which exhibits a sharp rise in respiration, triggered by the accumulation of ethylene gas. This sharp rise, or climacteric, signals the beginning of ripening in these fruits. Once the climacteric has started it is difficult to stop without imposing extreme conditions even if all the ethylene is removed from the fruit tissues. The maximum respiration rate at the top of the climacteric rise is the climacteric peak. It is at this peak that climacteric fruits are of most acceptable eating quality. Following the climacteric peak the respiration rate drops and senescence begins. Fruits which do not exhibit a climacteric are known as nonclimacteric fruits. A list of some climacteric and nonclimacteric fruits can be seen in Table 21.1.

Most climacteric fruits, except the avocado, can ripen on the tree. Although the maximum eating quality in apples and many other climacteric fruits is obtained when they are tree ripened, they are generally now allowed to do so since this can greatly reduce the storage life

TABLE 21.1
CLIMACTERIC AND NONCLIMACTERIC FRUITS

Climacteric Fruits		
Apple	Fig	Peach
Apricot	Mango	Pear
Avacado	Melon	Persimmon
Banana	Papaya	Plum
Blueberry	Passion fruit	Tomato
Nonclimacteric Fruits		
Cherry	Grapefruit	Orange
Cucumber	Guava	Pineapple
Grapes	Lemon	Strawberry

(Hulme and Rhodes, 1971). There are a few exceptions to maximum quality being obtained by tree ripening, like the pear which will become mealy due to the formation of stone cells. Ethylene gas can be used to trigger the climacteric in these fruits for uniform ripening just before marketing. This is often done in bananas. Nonclimacteric fruits are sometimes exposed to ethylene to degreen them.

Nonclimacteric fruits, such as citrus, are generally allowed to ripen on the tree. In this way the proper water balance in the fruit is maintained by the tree except when there is extended severe weather. Nonclimacteric fruit is generally sent to market without prolonged storage. This is especially true of citrus fruits (Ting and Attaway 1971).

Immature lettuce (McKenzie 1931) and potatoes (Smith 1967) respire more rapidly than mature produce directly after harvest. Eventually the respiration rate equilibrates to the levels of those harvested at a mature stage.

Mechanical injury is another factor which can shorten the postharvest life of a commodity. This is becoming increasingly important as the amount of machine harvesting continues to rise, and is important in such fruits as Golden Delicious and McIntosh apples, as well as peaches and nectarines.

Injury

Mechanical injury causes bruises or cuts which disrupt the cells and allow undesirable reactions to occur. Vitamin C is highly oxidizable when exposed to air or when the cells are disrupted, allowing certain enzymes to come into contact with it. Damage or leafy tissue can lead to mixing of enzyme and substrate which results in loss of carotenoids. At the site of the injury either Maillard, enzymatic or phenolic browning takes place. Mechanical injuries also disrupt the protective outer layers, or cuticle, allowing for further moisture loss and for microbial infection and growth.

Quickly cooling fruit after mechanical harvesting can delay the symptoms of mechanical injury in some cases. For instance, it allows tomatoes to be processed before appreciable loss of vitamin C occurs (National Canners Association 1973). Quickly cooling a commodity after harvest is generally advantageous, as it slows the rate of respiration and of moisture loss (which can lead to quality degradation). It is essential that highly perishable products be cooled quickly in order to maintain a reasonable storage life.

TRANSPORTATION

For many years the standard box for transportation of fruits and vegetables was the lug box with 50 to 110 lb capacity. It is still used today in small operations but it is bulky and hard to handle, involves much labor, and can damage the commodity when the boxes are overfilled and stacked. Today pallet boxes with capacities of 20 to 30 bu (800—1000 lb) are used for many soft fruits such as apples, peaches, pears, and plums as well as for vegetables such as potatoes. These boxes greatly reduce the labor involved by facilitating mechanical handling. Bulk trucks are used for citrus fruits and many vegetable crops. Most berries which need no washing or sorting are packed into small shipping containers to protect them from damage. Berries, such as blueberries and cranberries that are mechanically harvested, are exceptions.

Damage can and does occur in the commodities due to packing in these containers as well as due to shipment in them. Pressure bruises caused by overfilling pallet boxes are often deeper and more decay-prone than impact bruises. Vibrations during shipment can cause friction bruises which lead to browning in pears. O'Brien and Kasmire (1972) found that leaf suspension caused much more damage to peaches than did air-ride suspension after similar 100 mile journeys. The railroads still pay high claim losses because of inadequacies in their systems such as heavy impacts and delays in service (Ryall and Lipton 1972).

When commodities are being transported long distances to market they are generally kept cool by mechanical refrigeration in the trailer truck or railroad car. Some railroad cars use ice but Ryall and Pentzer (1974) claim that this will soon be a thing of the past. Refrigeration is especially important in transporting fruits and vegetables because not only can the ambient air raise the temperature of the commodity but the respiration of the commodity itself also produces heat proportional to the rate of respiration. In this way, the center of the produce can become much warmer than the ambient temperature and great quality losses can occur.

PRECOOKING AND WASHING

Before going to market fresh fruits and vegetables are generally precooled and/or washed and/or fumigated or disinfected. Care has to be taken in unloading the produce to minimize the damage. Slow tilting mechanisms are used as well as dumping produce into water, and submerging the boxes in water to let the commodity float out.

Washing can be accomplished by soaking in a cleaning solution followed by a rinsing, a spraying (which can also be used to cool the product), or brushing with either dry or wet brushes. The residual insecticides are easily removed, as the ones used today are more effective and less stable than ones used in the past. Often disinfectants are added to washing solutions although these will not stop infections which have already penetrated the surface. Waxes are also applied in some cases to slow water loss.

Besides spraying, precooling can be accomplished by either forced air or vacuum cooling. The method used depends on the commodity's rate of deterioration, configuration and ability to be exposed to water without further complications. Grapes are generally fumigated with sulfur dioxide to prevent mold growth and slow down respiration. It should be noted that sulfur dioxide treatment contributes to thiamin destruction in grapes.

SHELF-LIFE DATA

Not all fruits and vegetables are stored for extensive periods before going to market but there is always some delay between harvest and consumption during which the changes described below can take place. The length of postharvest life depends on the kind of produce and the environment in which it is kept. Very soft fruits, such as berries, will keep reasonable quality for only about 72 hr after harvest if they are not treated in some way. The most widely used method for lengthening the postharvest life of these and other commodities is temperature control. Most fruits and vegetables maintain their best quality at temperatures just above their freezing point, as shown in Tables 21.2 and 21.3.

TABLE 21.2

RECOMMENDED TEMPERATURE AND RELATIVE HUMIDITY, APPROXIMATE STORAGE LIFE AND HIGHEST FREEZING POINT OF FRESH VEGETABLES IN COMMERCIAL STORAGE[1]

Commodity	Recommended Temp. (°F)	Recommended Relative Humidity	Approx. Length of Storage Period	Highest Freezing Point (°F)
Artichokes (Jerusalem)	31—32	90—95	2—5 months	—
Asparagus	32—36	95	2—3 weeks	30.9
Beans, green or snap	40—45	90—95	7—10 days	30.7
Beans, lima	32—40	90	1—2 weeks	31.0
Broccoli	32	90—95	10—14 days	30.9
Cabbage (late)	32	90—95	3—4 months	30.9
Carrots, mature (topped)	32	90—95	4—5 months	29.5
Cauliflower	32	90—95	2—4 weeks	30.6
Corn, sweet	32	90—95	4—8 days	30.9
Cucumbers	45—50	90—95	10—14 days	31.1
Eggplants	45—50	90	1 week	30.6
Lettuce	32	95	2—3 weeks	31.7
Melon, honeydew	45—50	85—90	3—4 weeks	30.3
Mushrooms	40—50	80—85	2—3 weeks	31.3
Onions (dry) and onion sets	32	65—70	1—8 months	30.6
Peas, green	32	90—95	1—3 weeks	30.9
Peppers, sweet	45—50	90—95	2—3 weeks	30.7
Spinach	32	90—95	10—14 days	31.5
Squashes, summer	32—50	90	5—14 days	31.1
Sweetpotatoes	55—60	85—90	4—6 months	29.7
Tomatoes, mature green	55—70	85—90	1—3 weeks	31.0
Tomatoes, firm-ripe	45—50	85—90	4—7 days	31.1

[1]From USDA (1968).

As temperature is decreased, the rate of most changes in fruits and vegetable produce will also decrease. It can be seen from Table 21.4 that as the temperature approaches the freezing point an increasing proportion of benefit is gained; that is, the amount of decrease occurring for each 1 °C drop in temperature is greater at lower temperatures than at the higher temperatures. This is why it is most beneficial to cool highly perishable commodities quickly and maintain a low temperature to maintain good quality.

Other environmental factors which can be controlled to extend the postharvest life of produce are the gaseous content of the atmosphere and the humidity. Modifying the atmosphere by either lowering the oxygen content (usually to 10% or less) or raising the carbon dioxide content, can decrease the respiration rate. Lowered oxygen content also

TABLE 21.3

RECOMMENDED TEMPERATURE AND RELATIVE HUMIDITY, APPROXIMATE STORAGE LIFE AND HIGHEST FREEZING POINT OF FRESH FRUITS IN COMMERCIAL STORAGE[1]

Commodity	Recommended Temp. (°F)	Recommended Humidity	Approximate Length of Storage Period	Highest Freezing Point (°F)
Apples	30—40	90	3—8 months	27.6
Avocados	40—55	85—90	2—4 weeks	31.5
Bananas	56—58	90—85	1—2 weeks	30.6
Berries				
Blueberries	31—32	90—95	2 weeks	29.7
Cranberries	36—40	90—95	2—4 months	30.4
Strawberries	32	90—95	5—7 days	30.6
Cherries, sweet	30—31	90—95	2—3 weeks	30.6
Grapefruit, Florida and Texas	50	85—90	4—6 weeks	30.0
Grapes, American	31—32	85	2—8 weeks	29.7
Lemons	—	85—90	1—6 months	29.4
Limes	48—50	85—90	6—8 weeks	29.1
Oranges, California and Arizona	38—48	85—90	3—8 weeks	29.7
Peaches	32—32	90	2—4 weeks	30.3
Pears	29—31	90—95	2—7 months	29.2
Tangerines, Temple oranges and related citrus fruits	32—38	85—90	2—4 weeks	30.1

[1]From USDA (1968).

TABLE 21.4

Q_{10} FOR LOSS OF SALEABILITY[1]

Temp. (°C)	Asparagus	Peas	Brussels Sprouts	Celery	Head Lettuce	Sweet Corn
0—10	2.7	3.3	3.8	4.1	2.5	3.9
10—20	2.4	2.8	2.7	2.3	2.2	3.6
20—30	1.8	2.0	1.9	1.9	1.9	1.5

[1]From Ryall and Lipton (1972).

suppresses the production of ethylene, therefore delaying the onset of ripening. By using these techniques along with low temperatures, the storage life of some commodities can be greatly extended. Controlled atmosphere storage is used mainly for apples and somewhat for pears.

For each commodity as well as for each variety of each commodity there is a unique combination of oxygen, carbon dioxide level and temperature which will work best. This is a result of the fact that each commodity has a unique threshold level of low oxygen and high carbon dioxide tolerance before injury is induced. The tolerance level is also temperature dependent.

Even when care is taken to employ the storage methods above, unless one pays particular attention to relative humidity, excessive moisture loss will occur and make the product unsaleable. Starting right after harvest, plant materials begin to lose water due to evaporation since the parent plant is no longer available to replenish what is lost. The extent to which water is lost is dependent on both the product's environment and configuration. Two of the environmental factors that determine the rate of water loss are temperature and relative humidity. These parameters are related by a parameter known as the vapor pressure deficit (VPD). With a higher VDP there is a greater potential for water loss. VPD will decrease with increasing relative humidity and with decreasing temperature. High air velocities past products will also increase the rate of moisture loss. The effects of humidity, temperature, and air movement on weight losses can be seen in Table 21.5. A product with a high surface to volume ratio and/or a highly permeable surface will lose water more rapidly than products without these attributes. The storage life of carrots can be doubled by the removal of the leafy tops which are very permeable and have a high surface to volume ratio (USDA 1966).

Moisture loss can cause both an economic and nutritive loss of the produce. Shrivel due to water loss is unsightly and makes the products unsaleable. Shrivel is noticeable when grapes lose 5 to 6% or their original weight (Allen and Pentzer 1934) or when apples lose 5 to 8% of their weight (Smock and Neubert 1950). During storage potatoes lose weight and therefore market value, mainly due to water evaporation (Talburt and Smith 1975).

In kale, Ezell and Wilcox (1959) found that slight to moderate wilting caused 90% of the original vitamin C to be lost in three weeks at 0 °C, four days at 10 °C and in two days at 21 °C. With rapid wilting the same losses took place in 9 days, 2 days and 1 day, respectively. Wilting may also enhance carotene oxidation and high carotene vegetables causing them to lose some of their vitamin A activity.

The package in which the commodity is kept can raise the relative humidity and modify the internal atmosphere by offering resistance to water and gas exchange, respectively. The USDA (1966) points out benefits to carrots, pears, sweet cherries and Golden Delicious apples by using various plastic films. Care must be taken to prevent the build-up

TABLE 21.5
WEIGHT LOSSES IN VARIOUS FRUITS DURING STORAGE AS AFFECTED BY HUMIDITY, TEMPERATURE AND AIR MOVEMENT[1]

Fruit	Temperature (°)	Air Movement Changes/hr	RH %	Weight Loss, Percent of Original Weight 30 days	60 days	90 days	120 days
Pears	32	3—4	65	2.9	5.8	7.7	10.7
Pears	32	3—4	80	2.5	4.8	6.5	8.3
Pears	32	3—4	98	2.0	3.5	4.6	5.5
Pears	41	4	65	5.6	9.9	14.0	19.7
Pears	41	4	80	3.5	6.2	8.5	11.3
Pears	41	4	98	2.6	4.2	5.0	6.4
Pears	41	8—9	65	8.4	15.5	22.5	29.3
Pears	41	8—9	80	5.2	9.5	13.8	18.3
Pears	41	8—9	98	3.0	4.5	6.0	7.8
Apples	39	4	65	2.5	4.7	6.9	9.3
Apples	39	4	75	2.1	4.0	6.0	8.3
Apples	39	4	100	1.2	1.8	2.7	—
				2 days	**4 days**	**8 days**	**10 days**
Strawberries	32	4	65	4.7	7.3	12.4	15.0
Strawberries	32	4	80	4.4	7.0	11.6	13.3
Strawberries	32	4	98	4.4	6.8	11.8	14.0
Strawberries	32	9	65	4.7	8.4	15.7	20.4
Strawberries	32	9	80	4.4	6.3	11.1	13.8
Strawberries	32	9	98	4.2	6.6	11.2	13.9

[1]From Ryall and Penter (1974).

of too much carbon dioxide, the depletion of the oxygen, or the relative humidity from reaching 100% at which point moisture may condense and the potential for microbial growth increased.

The storage conditions mentioned above are meant to slow down, but not stop, the metabolic activities of the commodities so that they may be maintained for longer periods. The maturation processes continue to some extent. An overview of the chemical changes during maturation in fruits and vegetables can be summarized as follows.

In fruits there is an increase in sugars due to the breakdown of starch. Acidity also decreases. Oil in nuts and avocados increases. There is a loss of tannins and astringency which is important in persimmons and bananas. For produce in general there will be a softening resulting from changes in the pectic substances, a development of volatiles which contribute to flavor and aroma, the formation of pigments in the skin, a loss of chlorophyll, an initial increase in vitamin C followed by a decrease, and an increase in provitamin A (Ryall and Pentzer 1974). Some of these changes and others will now be considered in relation to storage effects on them.

Respiration rates vary from commodity to commodity, depending mainly on the type of tissue. Active tissue will respire much faster than storage tissue as shown by Platenius (1942) who found that asparagus respires 59 times faster than potatoes at 24 °C. A commodity which is respiring more rapidly will degrade faster. Respiration not only leads to senescence but can also cause weight loss as the product consumes its food supply. Sistrunk (1965) found that snap beans stored at 21 °C for 10 days lose 30% of their weight due to respiration.

Controlled atmospheres and low temperatures can be used to slow the respiration process. The Q_{10}s of respiration for some products can be seen in Table 21.6. Once again it can be noted that at lower temperatures the rate of decrease is greater than at higher temperatures. The Q_{10} between 0 and 30 °C is usually around 2.5. Temperatures of 30 °C or above generally inhibit respiration as shown in Fig. 21.1. It was noticed in this experiment that the climacteric pattern at 30 °C was drastically altered from the norm (Biale and Young 1971).

As produce matures it usually softens, which makes it more desirable to eat but also more susceptible to mechanical damage. Softening is due to changes in the cell wall materials and in climacteric fruits it precedes the climacteric, so softening is often used as an index of when to harvest. The effect of storage temperature on softening rate can be seen in Fig. 21.2.

TABLE 21.6
Q_{10}s FOR RESPIRATION OF SOME VEGETABLES[1]

Vegetable	Temperature Range 5—10 °C	10—24 °C
Asparagus	3.7	2.5
Peas	3.9	2.0
Carrots	3.3	1.9
Tomatoes	2.0	2.3
Potatoes	2.1	2.2

[1]From Platenius (1942).

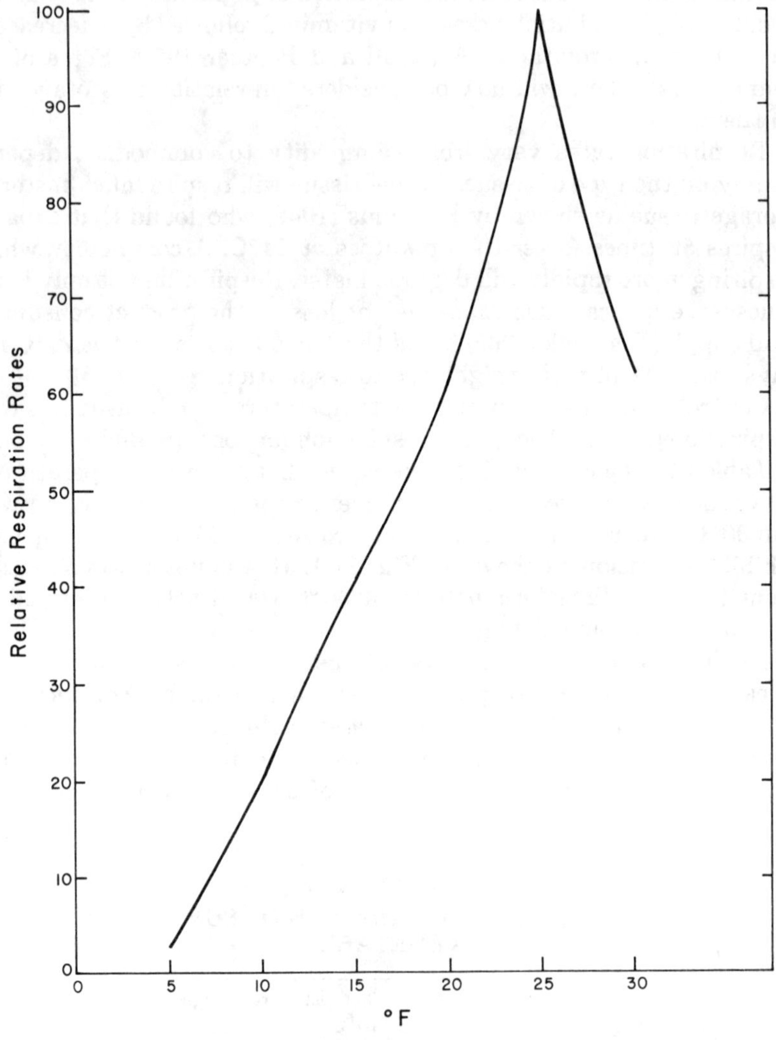

FIG. 21.1. EFFECT OF TEMPERATURE ON RESPIRATION RATES OF FUERTE AVOCADO
(From Biale and Young 1971).

Lignification is a process by which produce can toughen, as in the case of asparagus and broccoli. Achieving low temperatures immediately after harvest is important in slowing this process especially where asparagus is concerned. Lignification is also responsible for mealiness in tree ripened pears.

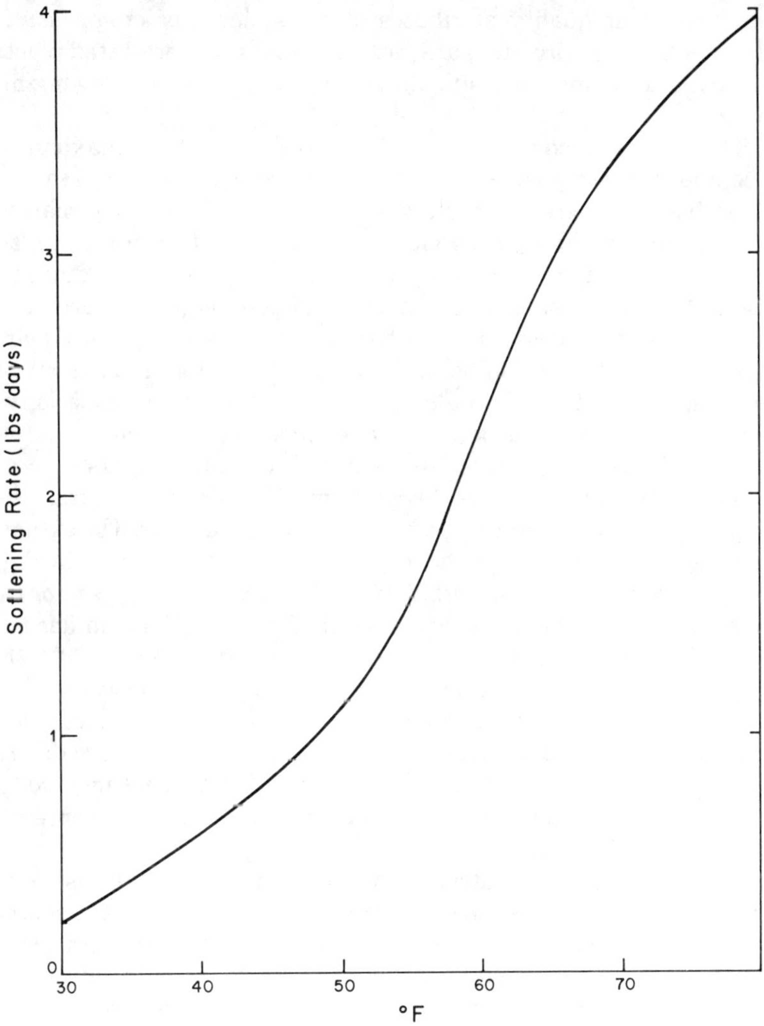

FIG. 21.2. EFFECT OF TEMPERATURE ON SOFTENING RATES OF PEACHES

(From Haller and Harding 1939).

The firmness in fruits and vegetables is to some extent maintained by the pressure inside the cells exerted by water. This is known as turgor. Turgor is lost by the plant material due to transpiration and respiration water losses. This can be tolerated to a greater extent in some products than in others. Products such as celery and lettuce depend upon turgor to maintain their quality attributes of crunchiness or crispness. This explains why these products are generally found in perforated plastic bags or loose plastic overwraps to allow gas exchange while slowing moisture loss.

The total acid content of a fruit generally reaches a maximum on the tree and declines postharvest. This, coupled with an increase in sugars, gives fruits a more desirable sugar-to-acid ratio as they mature. Conversely, in maturing seeds (such as peas, sweet corn and lima beans) sugar content decreases and starch synthesis increases during maturation. After harvest, the rate of conversion of sugar to starch increases. For this reason these commodities should be cooled quickly and soon after harvest. Tubers, bulbs, and roots contain a lot of starch which, as in the case of potatoes, degrades to sugar after harvest, especially at low temperatures. When a potato is re-exposed to warmer temperatures it has the ability to resynthesize the starch from the sugars.

All fruits and vegetables lose vitamin C after harvest, but usually to not too great an extent except in the case of asparagus. The extent of loss and the temperature dependence in asparagus can be seen in Fig. 2.3.

Tomatoes that are harvested when they are mature green for the fresh market generally have a lower vitamin C content than similar tomatoes ripened on the vine (18—19 mg/100 g compared to 25 mg/100 g) (Krochta and Feinberg 1975). Ripening on the plant does not always lead to an increase in vitamin content. Singleton (1959) found that pineapples which are harvested and then stored at 24 °C during the normal ten day ripening period have an increase in vitamin C to 12.4 to 13.0 mg/100 g, while similar fruit ripened in the field decreases in vitamin C content to between 9.1 to 12.4 mg/100 g.

Another important nutrient from fruits and vegetables is supplied by the carotenes, which possess provitamin A activity. Fruits generally contain a fair amount of carotene as exemplified by the 40 to 100 IU/100 g in apples and the 190 to 400 IU/100 g in orange juice (Holme and Rhodes 1971). Fruit carotenes tend to accumulate during harvest as shown for "Shamouti" oranges by Eilati *et al.* (1969). Root crops such as carrots and sweet potatoes also contain relatively large amounts of carotenes. Carotenes usually degrade during senescence, especially in leafy vegetables. The degradation reactions are catalyzed by light and enzymes.

Carotenes are colored derivatives of carotenoids. Carotenoids cause the yellow colors which are often unmasked as chlorophyll degrades. This occurs in some fruits as well as in vegetables. In bananas, the levels of carotenoids after harvest remain constant, in apples the levels increase,

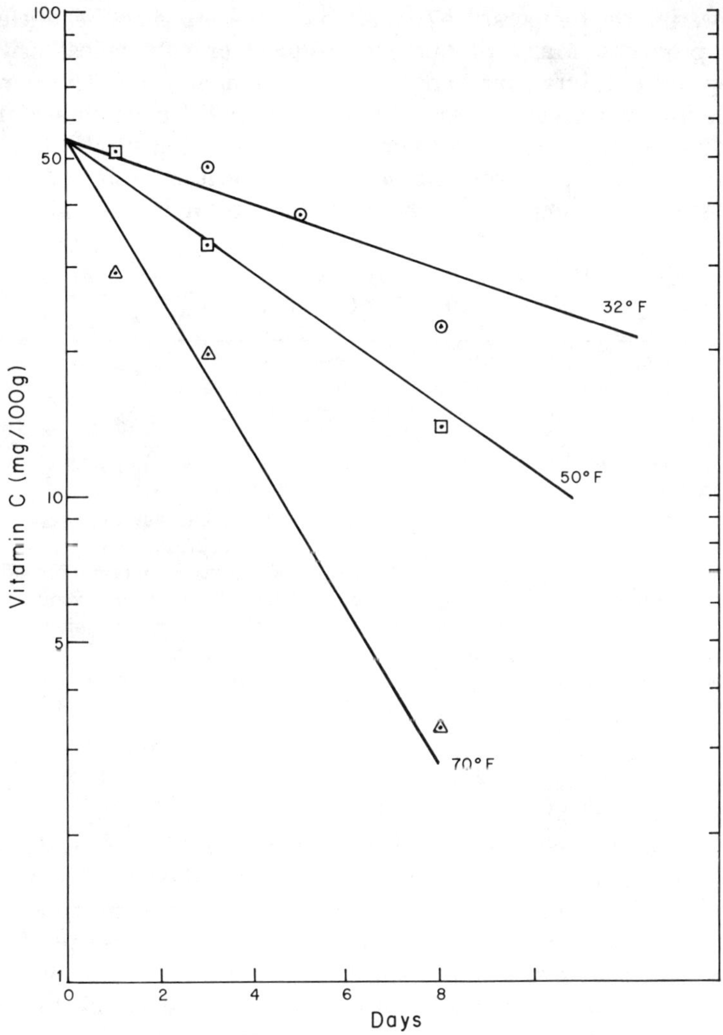

FIG. 21.3. EFFECT OF TEMPERATURE ON VITAMIN C LOSS IN ASPARAGUS

(From Scott and Kramer 1944).

and in pears carotenoids decrease with time. In vegetables, yellowing is usually undesirable and it is best inherited by diligent temperature control. It has been noted that controlled atmosphere storage delays yellowing in several vegetables. This does not always produce an acceptable product but some controlled atmospheres are being used successfully, especially during transit.

Lowering the temperature to just above freezing is not beneficial to all plant products. Many products of tropical or subtropical origin are susceptible to injury from exposure to cool temperatures. The symptoms of this injury are very diverse, but all commodities which are afflicted lose disease resistance. The temperature range of susceptibility is also varied and depends on the commodity, as shown in Table 21.7. Another variation is the exposure time necessary to induce chilling injury.

TABLE 21.7
CHILLING INJURY

Commodity	Lowest Safe Temp. (°F)	Characteristics of Chilling Injury
Apples (McIntosh)	36	brown core (core flush)
Bananas	56	dull to black color, skin
Beans, snap	45—50	pitting and russeting
Cranberries	34	internal breakdown
Grapefruit	45	scald, pitting, internal breakdown
Oranges, California	50	rind pitting and browning
Peppers, sweet	45	pitting, surface browning
Potatoes (Chippewa and Sabago)	40	surface browning
Tomatoes, green	55	improper ripening, decay
Tomatoes, ripe	50	decay

[1]From USDA (1968).

For bananas it is only a matter of hours before the damage is done, while for beans, tomatoes, and peppers it can take ten days to two weeks, and for apples, citrus fruits, winter squash, and cranberries the time is on the order of weeks or months. Immature fruits are more susceptible to this injury than mature ones. Often the damage that is done does not show up while the commodity is in cold storage, but will only manifest itself after exposure to higher temperatures for some specific time. Even then internal damage to some items is not visible unless they are cut open and examined. Chilling can also reduce the nutritive value of some crops. In some vegetables, chilling reduces the vitamin C content, while in most the opposite is true. Ezell *et al.* (1952) reported that carotene in sweet potatoes is reduced in the chilling range around 10°C. Chilling also affects respiration as the rate increases with the onset of injury.

OPEN DATING

Because fresh fruits and vegetables are living systems of many different kinds, it is difficult to predict their postharvest lives. It is essentially impossible to make predictions if the conditions of handling the product are not known, therefore a "pack date" is essentially useless. It would be very beneficial to the survival of the commodity and to assurance of a minimal postharvest life if proper handling conditions could be ensured.

The consumer is often able to judge quality based on physical characteristics, which are generally related to other aspects of quality such as nutritional quality. However, a consumer may not be able to scrutinize all of the produce to be purchased, especially since prepackaging is becoming more prevalent. Perhaps a "sell by date" on these packages that indicates the date up to which all the produce is guaranteed to be of good quality, based on a reasonable life at proper conditions, would help ensure good practices by produce marketers. Higher quality specifications would be demanded and proper care would have to be followed for maximal economic return. To assist in maintaining high quality, a set of guidelines would probably be helpful to all those involved with the fresh market sale of fruits and vegetables. An expiration date of "best if used by date" would not be useful because handling and storage conditions after purchase are extremely variable and unpredictable.

REFERENCES

ALLEN, F.W. and PENTZER, W.T. 1934. Studies on the effect of humidity in the cold storage of fruits. Proc. Am. Soc. Hortic. Sci. *3*, 215-233.

BIALE, J.B. and YOUNG, R.E. 1971. The avacado pear. *In* The Biochemistry of Fruits and Their Products, Vol. 2. A.C. Hulme (Editor). Academic Press, New York.

EILATI, S.K., MONSELIZE, S.P. and BUDOWSKI, P. 1969. Seasonal development of external color and carotenoid content in the peel of ripening 'Shamouti' oranges. J. Amer. Soc. Hortic. Sci. *94*(4), 346-348.

ESKIN, N.A.M., HENDERSON, H.N., and TOWNSEND, R.J. (1971). Biochemistry of Foods. Academic Press, New York.

EZELL, B.D. and WILCOX, M.S. 1959. Loss of vitamin C in fresh vegetables as related to wilting and temperature. J. Agric. Food Chem. *10*, 124-126.

EZELL, B.D., WILCOX, M.S., and CROWDER, J.N. 1952. Pre- and post-harvest changes in carotene, total carotenoids, and ascorbic acid of sweet potatoes. Plant Physiol. *27*, 355-369.

GORTNER, W.A., DULL, C.G., and KRAUSE, B.H. 1967. Fruit development, maturation, ripening and senescence: a biochemical basis for horticultural terminology. Hortic. Sci. *2*, 141-144.

HALLER, M.H. and HARDING, P.L. 1939. Effect of Storage Temperature on Peaches. USDA Tech. Bull. No. 680.

HULME, A.C. and RHODES, M.J.C. 1971. Pome fruits. *In* The Biochemistry of Fruits and Their Products, Vol. 2 A.C. Hulme (Editor). Academic Press, New York.

KROCHTA, J.M. and FEINBERG, B. 1975. *In* Nutritional Evaluation of Food Processing. R.S. Harris and E. Karmas (Editors). AVI Publishing Co., Westport, Conn.

McKENZIE, K.A. 1931. Respiration studies with lettuce. Proc. Am. Soc. Hortic. Sci. *28*, 244.

MASSACHUSETTS DEPARTMENT OF PUBLIC HEALTH. 1973. Labeling Resolutions. Massachusetts Department of Public Health, Division of Food and Drugs.

MINNESOTA 1973. S.F. No. 160. Sixty-Eighth Legislature.

NATIONAL CANNERS ASSOCIATION. 1973. Report of technical data on cans examined from the 1972 fruit and vegetable pack. Canners Leagues of California, Berkeley.

NELSON, P.E. 1972. Processing effects on the nutritional components of horticulture crops. Hortic. Sci. *7*, 151-153.

O'BRIEN, M. and KASMIRE, R.F. 1972. Engineering developments and problems at production source of fresh product. Trans. ASAE *15*, 566-568.

PLATENIUS, H. 1942. Effect of temperature on the respiration rate and the respiratory quotient of some vegetables. Plant Physiol. *17*, 179.

RYALL, A.L. and LIPTON, W.J. 1972. Handling, Transportation and Storage of Fruits and Vegetables. Vol. 1, Vegetables and Melons. AVI Publishing Co., Westport, Conn.

RYALL, A.L. and PENTZER, W.T. 1974. Handling, Transportation and Storage of Fruits and Vegetables. Vol. 2, Fruits and Tree Nuts. AVI Publishing Co., Westport, Conn.

SCOTT, L.E. and KRAMER, A. 1949. Physiological changes in asparagus after harvest. Proc. Am. Soc. Hortic. Sci. *54*, 357-366.

SINGLETON, V.L. 1959. Pineapple Research Institute of Hawaii, Research Report No. 69.

SISTRUNK, W.A. 1965. Influence of post-harvest storage of snap beans on chemical and physical changes during canning. J. Food Sci. *30*, 240.

SMITH, O. 1967. *In* Potato Processing, 2nd Edition. W.F. Talburt and O. Smith (Editors). AVI Publishing Co., Westport, Conn.

SMOCK, U.J. and NEUBERT, A.M. 1950. Apples and Apple Products. John Wiley and Sons, New York.

TALBURT, W.F. and SMITH, O. 1975. Potato Processing, 2nd Ed. AVI Publishing Co., Westport, Conn.

TING, S.B. and ATTAWAY, J.A. 1971. *In* The Biochemistry of Fruits and Their Products, Vol. 2 A.C. Hulme (Editor). Academic Press, New York.

TRESSLER, D.K. and EVERS, C.F. 1957. The Freezing Preservation of Foods, Vol. 1. AVI Publishing Co., Westport, Conn.

USDA. 1966. Protecting our Food — The Yearbook of Agriculture. 89th Congress, 2nd Session, House Document #349.

USDA. 1968. The Commercial Storage of Fruits, Vegetables and Florist and Nursery Stock. USDA Agric. Handbook 66.

UNITED STATES SENATE (1976). S. 641, 94th Congress, 2nd Session.

WILKINSON, B.G. 1970. Physiological disorders of fruit after harvesting. *In* The Biochemistry of Fruits and their Products, Vol. 1. A.C. Hulme (Editor) Academic Press, New York.

CHAPTER 22

BASIC INFORMATION NEEDED TO IMPLEMENT OPEN DATING

INDUSTRY

The previous chapters described literature data available on the shelf-life of foods. Each food item must be considered by itself, and large variations in shelf-life can exist based on preharvest/slaughter conditions, genetic variety and process/package system utilized. Additionally, knowledge must be obtained as to the marketing scheme for each food product before predictions of shelf-life can be made. To do this the industry must develop scientifically based, accelerated shelf-life data. Government cannot mandate a particular shelf-life for a particular product as there are too many variables.

A survey of testing procedures currently used by the major food industries was made using the attached questionnaire. The results are as follows.

Cereal Grain Products

One leading manufacturer of breakfast cereals uses three different types of time-temperature testing procedures for its cereals. (1) The first type approximates severe distribution conditions with a 24 hr fluctuating temperature cycle at 65% RH. The cereal is held (in its normal package) for 5 hr at 70 °F, equilibrated to 90 °F over a 2 hr period, held at 90 °F for 11 hr and then equilibrated back to 70 °F over 6 hr. The cereal must still be of high quality after 12—16 weeks to be acceptable. (2) The second procedure uses a constant temperature of 100 °F at ambient humidity. Again, the cereal in its package must survive 12—16 weeks of storage with high quality. This gives a Q_{10} of about 2.6. In both of these procedures the cereal is tested by an expert taste panel for loss of the toasted, highly fresh flavor and for loss of crispness. (3) The third procedure is used to test for lipid oxidation reactions. The cereals are held in sealed glass containers at 115 °F and 140 °F and are assayed for intermediates in the oxidation reaction. They should survive 3—4 weeks at 115 °F and 102 weeks at 140 °F (a Q_{10} of 1.5).

A second manufacturer of breakfast cereals uses 73 °F or 77 °F constant temperature storage at 50% RH as being most typical of real conditions. Storage of the cereals in their packages at 20, 50 and 80% RH is used but rarely to accelerate lipid oxidation. (Nonenzymatic browning occurs so quickly at this temperature that it tends to dominate.) Moisture absorption is the major mode of deterioration of these cereals although staling and rancidity are also important. During and after storage the cereals are tasted by an expert panel and/or a 36-member taste panel. The expert panel does "profile curves" over a period of months. They do a description of the flavor, appearance, aroma and texture of the cereal at each tasting and plot the changes with storage. The 36-member panel tastes stored cereal along with a control cereal and looks for a "just noticeable difference." As a general rule of thumb, this company considers one week survival at 100 °F to equal 6 weeks survival at 73 °F (which is a Q_{10} of 3.33). This ratio, however, varies considerably with each type of cereal.

A third cereal company replied that they use 98 °F constant temperature to "check organoleptic stability" and estimate that 3 months' stability at 98 °F is equal to 2 years of high quality life at 70 °F. This is a Q_{10} of 3.75. It can be seen, therefore, that the industry experts do not agree on the sensitivity of cereals to temperature in predicting shelf-life. This is probably because of the large variety in the types of products.

One company that produces cake mixes states that they should survive 12—16 weeks at 100 °F at ambient % RH and also in a room at 56% RH cycling from 70 °F to 90 °F each 24 hr period. Survival for 12—16 weeks under these conditions indicates a survival with high quality life for about 48 weeks under distribution conditions, giving a Q_{10} of 2. Loss of leavening power is the first failure to occur in cake mixes and is the major emphasis of testing. Some flavor loss will occur secondarily. Little or no rancidity occurs.

The Q_{10}s derived from these data are consistant with the shelf-life data presented in the preceding chapters.

Frozen Foods

A number of different tests that accelerate deterioration are used for frozen foods.

One company holds samples of their frozen foods (mostly foods with low moisture content) at 0 °F for 72 weeks, 10 °F for 30 weeks, and 20 °F for 20 weeks. The food must survive at least 52 weeks at 0 °F with high quality, and at least 10—12 weeks at 20 °F. This is a Q_{10} of only 4, which is quite low for most frozen foods and might underestimate quality losses.

Moisture migration from the food into the surrounding air with resulting dessication of the food and ice crystal formation in the package is a major mode of deterioration of frozen foods under fluctuating temperature conditions. Cycling temperature storage is used to test for this; i.e., from 0 °F or 10 °F up to 20 °F with one day at each temperature and then repeated several times.

Oxidative rancidity is the principal mode of deterioration for frozen processed meat products. Samples are held frozen at 0 °F, then defrosted at refrigeration temperatures and evaluated for flavor change. Since 0 °F is the normal distribution temperature, no accelerated testing was reported. In one "freeze-thaw" test, five packages of the food tested are put in a 0 °F room on Day 0. On Day 1 four of the packages are put into a 70 °F room for 4 hr and then back to the 0 °F room. On Day 2, three packages are thawed; on Day 3, two packages, and on the fourth day only one package is thawed. All five of the packages should survive this treatment with little texture change and flavor loss.

Microbial growth is also a problem under cycling temperatures. The extent to which this is a problem for each type of frozen food can be determined by a storge procedure similar to the above freeze-thaw test except that 100 °F is used for the 4-hr thawing periods instead of 70 °F.

Representatives of the Birdseye Company presented a paper at the 1965 Institute of Food Technologists Meeting entitled "Times and temperature encountered in distribution of frozen foods" (C.H. Byrne, F. Zobel and C.J. Harrigan, General Foods, White Plains, NY 10625). These times and temperatures are used by some companies to test the reactions of their products under actual conditions.

Canned Fruits and Vegetables

One major manufacturer of canned foods uses constant temperature storage at four different temperatures: 100 °F (accelerated deterioration), 85 °F (high ambient), 65 °F (ideal storage) and 37 °F for relatively stable reference control samples. In canned foods organoleptic qualities fail before nutrient losses occur, therefore the samples are tested periodically for color, flavor and texture. The condition of the containers is also monitored. No data were reported to estimate a Q_{10} value.

Bakery Products

Fresh, moist bakery products such as breads and cakes are stored at ambient temperatures and humidities and tested for staling, mold growth and "firming." Drier products such as crackers and cookies are stored at high temperatures with low humidities to test the stability of the fats and oils used, and at high temperatures with high humidities to test for staling and textural changes due to moisture pickup. Dry storage temperatures used are: 126 °F, 108 °F, 90 °F, 72 °F, 32 °F and −10 °F.

Temperatures and % RHs used to test for moisture pickup are as follows: 100 °F with 90% RH, 75 °F with 70% RH, 75 °F with 50% RH and −10 °F with ambient RH.

Salad Dressing

One company listed the major mode of deterioration of salad dressing as the breakdown of the emulsion into its separate components. This is hastened by fluctuating temperatures, so cycling temperatures are used in accelerated shelf-life testing. Color change and significant flavor change are also modes of deterioration. 100 °F with 90% RH is used to accelerate deterioration and 70 °F with 50% RH is used to simulate ambient conditions.

A second company listed oxidation leading to off-flavors or off-odors as a mode of deterioration in addition to emulsion breakdown. They use elevated temperature and high humidity to accelerate deterioration and consider the Q_{10} to be 2 for these reactions. They use a "best if purchased by" open dating and allow one year beyond this for consumer storage and use.

Dry Mixes

In dry mixes the differing equilibrium relative humidities of the various components can cause accelerated deterioration due to caking, oxidation, nonenzymatic browning, etc., of one or two of the components if they are allowed to freely equilibrate with each other. For this reason one company stated that "all storage studies include product/package system evaluations involving evaluation of different protective packaging modes to optimize shelf-life. Equilibrium relative humidity studies are carried out on all mixes to establish protective packaging parameters." Accelerated tests are conducted at 100 °F with 90% RH and ambient tests use 70 °F with 50% RH. No Q_{10}s were reported.

Dehydrated Vegetables

Lipid and hydrolytic oxidation, nonenzymatic browning and chlorophyll breakdown are the major modes of deterioration reported for dehydrated vegetables. Elevated temperatures of 100 °F to 120 °F at constant low % RH are used to accelerate deterioration. Exposure to light aids oxidation and is also used in accelerated shelf-life testing.

Margarine and Vegetable Shortening

Margarine and vegetable shortenings oxidize slowly due to relatively high natural lavels of tocopherols (Vitamin E). Other modes of failure which occur more quickly are monitored in accelerated shelf-life tests.

Margarine develops a slow, pasty melt and loses flavor with age. Exposure to elevated temperatures of 70 °F and 80 °F are used to accelerate these changes.

Shortenings lose gas and color and develop poor texture with storage. Storage at a constant temperature of 105 °F is used in accelerated tests.

Aerosol Toppings

Fluctuating temperatures accelerate the development of curdled or fluid texture in aerosol toppings. Cycling temperature storage of 45 °F, up to room temperature, back to 45 °F, and then down to −10 °F are used in tests by one major manufacturer.

Refrigerated Processed Meats

One company listed the following modes of deterioration for processed refrigerated meats: (1) Bacteriological milkiness of accompanying or adjacent fluid; (2) bacteriological slime formation; (3) Oxidative rancidity; (4) Fading or noticeable color change; and (5) Mold or yeast formation in non-vacuum packages. Canned ham degradation occurs at refrigeration temperatures via (1) deterioration of the can, (2) flavor change and (3) swelling due to gas formation (chemical reaction).

This company stated that "no accelerated testing is done except for slight evaluation of temperature." Normal distribution temperatures of refrigeration meats are 25—40 °F. "Random boxes of packaged product are picked from production lines and placed into a holding cooler at 43 °F ± 1°. At weekly intervals these samples are visually inspected and organoleptically evaluated for signs of spoilage of flavor change."

A second company listed similar modes of deterioration for their refrigerated processed meat products. They also do not run accelerated shelf-life tests, but hold samples at 40—42 °F (normal distribution temperatures) until signs of deterioration are present.

Canned Meat

One producer of a canned meat product listed production of hydrgen gas resulting from can deterioration as the major mode of degradation.

They store samples at 100 °F to accelerate this deterioration and consider the shelf-life at 100 °F to be about 40% of the shelf-life at 40 °F, but feel that the ratio is very variable. This is a Q_{10} of 1.3.

Soft Drinks and Fountain Syrups

Acid hydrolysis and/or oxidation of the essential flavor oils leading to loss of flavor is the major mode of deterioration of soft drinks and fountain syrups. Fountain syrups are more acid (pH = 1.5 to 3.0) than canned or bottled soft drinks (pH 2.5 to 4.0) so the degradation of the flavor oils occur at a faster rate in the syrups.

One major soft drink company reported storage at 40 °C as a method of accelerating deterioration but said that the accelerating factor in comparison to normal conditions (Q_{10}) had not yet been determined. The "accelerated testing is used only as an indicator and not a substitute for long-term testing at ambient conditions."

Distribution Conditions

Cereals, dry mixes, bakery products, snack foods, soft drinks, fountain syrups, and canned goods are generally shipped under ambient temperatures and relative humidities. For nationwide distribution systems this includes hot and humid conditions in the southeast, hot and dry in the southwest, moderate temperatures and humidity in coastal areas and much seasonal variation in the midwest. One nationwide company stated that "Based on more than 40-year records compiled by the U.S. Weather Bureau, *et al.*, our products are generally exposed to 40—60% RH and 60—80 °F. For brief periods, while in transit there may be exposure to higher or lower conditions which do not influence total shelf-life measurably." Most warehouses in the north are heated in the winter to above freezing and many in the south are cooled in the summer to about 70 ° or 80 °F.

AFDOUS has recommended a maximum temperature of 0 °F for distribution of frozen foods. Of the companies responding to the questionnaire, two cited 0 °F as the general distribution temperature, another said that their distribution temperature was never higher than —5 °F, and a fourth stated that "frozen products are shipped at —20 °F."

Processed meats are generally refrigerated at 25—40 °F. One company listed holding temperatures of 32—40 °F after packaging, shipping temperatures of 28—32 °F and holding temperatures of 33—38 °F in distribution centers.

Table 22.1 lists the distribution times, shelf-life and percentage of food over age reported in this survey. It must be assumed that these are fairly good guesses but the survey pointed out that the scientific approach

TABLE 22.1
DISTRIBUTION TIMES AND SHELF-LIVES CITED BY COMPANIES

Item	Distribution Times Average	Minimum	Maximum	Shelf-life	Average % of food held longer than shelf-life
Dry mixes	3 months	1 months	6 months	12—18 months	*
Tea	3 months	1 month	6 months	6—9 months	*
Salad dressing	3 months	1 month	6 months	12—18 months	*
Ice cream	1 month	1 day	2 months	3—6 months	*
Instant tea	3 months	1 month	6 months	3 years	*
Canned meats	3 months	1 month	6 months	3 years	*
Pet foods	3 months	1 month	6 months	3 years	*
Margarines	3 months	2 weeks	6—9 months	1 year	1
Buttered syrups	3 months	2 weeks	1 year	2 years	1
Shortenings	2 months	2 weeks	1 year	2½ years	2
Aerosol toppings	2 months	2 weeks	4 months	1 year	2
Fresh bakery products	48 hours	8 hours	240 hours	10 days	<5
Frozen foods	60 days	20 days	2 years	2 years	<5
Fresh pork	3 days	1 day	—	—	<5
Candy	60 days	20 days	1 year	1 year	<5
Potato chips, etc.	10 days	3 days	3 months	3 months	<5
Ham	3 days	—	1 year	1 year	5
Dry baked goods	1 month	1 month	1 month	6 months	*
Dry vegetables	6 months	1 month	3 years	1—2 years	—
Canned purees	10 months	1 month	36 months	3—5 years	2—3
Cereals	6 months	1 month	24 months	3—5 years	2—3
Canned fruits and vegetables	9 months	—	3 years	3 years	0
Ready-to-eat dry cereals	1 month	—	—	6—9 months	<5
Cereal, to be cooked	1 month	—	—	9 months	<5
Dry cereals	2 months	6 weeks	—	1 year	2
Cake mixes	3½ months	—	—	1—2 years	<2
Refrigerated processed meats	50 days	7 days	90 days	(vacuum packed) 35—120 days (non-vacuum packed) 15—25 days	<1
Canned hams	3 months	1 month	1 year	1½ years	<1
Frozen meats	2 months	20 days	6 months	3—9 months	<1
Refrigerated canned pickles	50 days	7 days	90 days	4 months	<1

continued . . .

TABLE 22.1 (continued)

	Distribution Times				Average % of food held longer than
Item	Average	Minimum	Maximum	Shelf-life	shelf-life
Frankfurters	5 days	3 days	15 days	38—50 days**	0
Bacon	5 days	2 days	15 days	55—60 days***	0
Soft drinks	1 month	††		12 months	negligible
Fountain syrups	1 month	††		6 months	negligible
Pourable salad dressing	3 weeks	2 weeks	6 weeks	18 months	5

*Company uses a salesman pickup plan whereby "all products are picked up at termination of established shelf-life limits."
**Varies with plant — Plant A = 55—55 days; Plant B = 48—53 days; Plant C = 35—43 days; Plant D = 50—55 days.
***Varies with plant — Plant A = 55 days; Plant B = 60 days.
††Varies with the season: Summer — 87.9% <1 month old, 97.2% <3 months old, 0% >1 year old. Winter — 61.6% <1 month old, 82.9% <3 months old, 0% >1 year old.

described in Chapter 3 is generally not utilized, probably because of lack of knowledge, cost involved and more importantly, the amount of time necessary to do it for already established foods. Mandating open dating would certainly force the issue but whether it would reduce the percentage of foods beyond acceptable shelf-life as reported in Table 22.1 is not known.

MARKETING PRACTICES

Perhaps the key to setting "open dates" on food packages is a knowledge of the marketing practices used to handle foods. Many manufacturers lose control once the food is processed. Much more information must be gained on how long products are held in distribution centers, broker warehouses, and market warehouses. For products with large seasonal/yearly variations in quality and quantity, dating by pack date would seem to be unreasonable if the product is held at low enough temperatures for long times. Industry, however, must monitor these situations to insure the consumer is getting good quality, especially in years of increased harvest yields. Supermarkets must also be made aware of the problems involved.

GOVERNMENT

The government has several alternatives: (1) Do nothing — this is the worst alternative, since increased state legislation with wide variations in open dating practices would tend to reduce food availability and competition. (2) Mandate required open dating — This is also a poor choice, since not enough data are available for each type of food and most processors would not know how to go about setting a legitimate endpoint. The consumer would not be served by this unless the government took on the job of doing all the shelf-life testing under contract or setting up courses such as done in the Better Process Control schools for thermal processing. (3) Set regulations as to what should be on the label if open dating is used (i.e., voluntary industry practice with mandated label requirement).

This latter alternative would be the most logical government action, as was done with nutritional labeling. Based on data discussed previously, the FDA or Congress could decide for each food type which system of dating is best, if any. This decision should be based on two aspects: (1) increased quality for the consumer and (2) a shoring up of the distribution system. It could be required that the industry make known the method used to assess the shelf-life, with the tests used to insure acceptability. Only in this way can the regulatory agency determine whether indeed a food is out of compliance. This document could be on public file but other companies producing similar products should not be allowed to just follow example; they should do their own testing since product variability can be great. Some sort of reliability testing program should also be instituted such as through the use of time-temperature indicators.

Currently, in states where open dating is used, compliance monitoring has not been carried out. Thus, little information is known as to how truthful the shelf-life dates are. The regulatory agency should keep records of compliance so that logical changes can be done in the future.

CONSUMERS

Consumers have the last say on product quality, as is reflected in their complaints and their buying habits. Open dating should assure them of better quality products but, it also has an educational goal of teaching them how to store foods properly for maximum quality and shelf-life. This type of education should lead to better buying practices and elimination of searching for freshest product — the consumer could learn to trust the system.

Shelf Life Information

Company ______________________________

Respondent ______________________________

1. Types of Foods produced

   a. Packaging used.

   b. General process used.

   c. General distribution conditions (% RH and temperature)

   d. Average, minimum and maximum distribution times.

   e. Average % of food held longer than predicted shelf-life.

2. Accelerated Shelf-Life Testing

   a. Type of methods used to accelerate deterioration.

   b. Deterioration mode for type of food.

   c. Is the product/package system studied together.

   d. Accelerating factor in comparison to normal conditions.

   e. Actual shelf-life of product.

3. Open Dating Practices

a. For each product above should the date used be manufactured date, sell by date (with some given life left) or use before date.

b. Risks and benefits of open dating.

INDEX